CEREBRAL PALSY

A JOHNS HOPKINS PRESS HEALTH BOOK

FREEMAN MILLER, MD, is Co-Director of the Cerebral Palsy Program at the Nemours / Alfred I. duPont Hospital for Children, Wilmington, Delaware; Assistant Professor of Orthopaedic Surgery at Sidney Kimmel School of Medicine of Thomas Jefferson University, Philadelphia, Pennsylvania; and Affiliated Associate Professor of Kinesiology and Mechanical Engineering at the University of Delaware, Newark.

STEVEN J. BACHRACH, MD, is Co-Director of the Cerebral Palsy Program and former Chief of the Division of General Pediatrics at the Nemours / Alfred I. duPont Hospital for Children, Wilmington, Delaware, and Professor of Pediatrics at Sidney Kimmel School of Medicine of Thomas Jefferson University, Philadelphia, Pennsylvania. He is also Medical Director at the HMS School for Children with Cerebral Palsy, in Philadelphia.

❧ *Cerebral Palsy*

A Complete Guide for Caregiving

THIRD EDITION

Freeman Miller, MD
Steven J. Bachrach, MD

and The Cerebral Palsy Center
at Nemours / Alfred I. duPont
Hospital for Children

JOHNS HOPKINS UNIVERSITY PRESS   BALTIMORE

Note to the Reader: This book is not meant to substitute for medical care of people with cerebral palsy, and treatment should not be based solely on its contents. Instead, treatment must be developed in a dialogue between the individual or the individual's parent and his or her physician. Our book has been written to help with that dialogue.

Drug dosage: The author and publisher have made reasonable efforts to determine that the drugs discussed in this text conform to the practices of the general medical community. The medications described do not necessarily have specific approval by the US Food and Drug Administration for use in treatment of the diseases for which they are recommended. In view of ongoing research, changes in governmental regulation, and the constant flow of information relating to drug therapy and drug reactions, the reader is urged to check the package insert of each drug for any change in indications and dosage and for warnings and precautions. This is particularly important when the recommended agent is a new and/or infrequently used drug.

© 1995, 2006, 2017 Johns Hopkins University Press
All rights reserved. Published 2017
Printed in the United States of America on acid-free paper
9 8 7 6 5 4 3 2 1

Johns Hopkins University Press
2715 North Charles Street
Baltimore, Maryland 21218-4363
www.press.jhu.edu

Library of Congress Cataloging-in-Publication Data

Names: Miller, Freeman, author. | Bachrach, Steven J., author.
Title: Cerebral palsy : a complete guide for caregiving / Freeman Miller, MD, Steven J. Bachrach,
    MD, and the Cerebral Palsy Center at Nemours / Alfred I. duPont Hospital for Children.
Description: Third edition. | Baltimore : Johns Hopkins University Press, 2016. | Series: A Johns
    Hopkins Press health book | Includes bibliographical references and index.
Identifiers: LCCN 2016028464| ISBN 9781421422152 (hardcover : alk. paper) | ISBN 1421422158 (hard-
    cover : alk. paper) | ISBN 9781421422169 (pbk. : alk. paper) | ISBN 1421422166 (pbk. : alk. paper) |
    ISBN 9781421422176 (electronic) | ISBN 1421422174 (electronic)
Subjects: LCSH: Cerebral palsied children. | Cerebral palsy—Popular works.
Classification: LCC RJ496.C4 M53 2016 | DDC 618.92/836—dc23
LC record available at https://lccn.loc.gov/2016028464

A catalog record for this book is available from the British Library.

The preparation of illustrations for this book was supported in part by funding from the Nemours Research Programs of the Nemours Foundation. Unless otherwise noted, illustrations are by Jacqueline Schaffer.

Special discounts are available for bulk purchases of this book. For more information, please contact Special Sales at 410-516-6936 or specialsales@press.jhu.edu.

Johns Hopkins University Press uses environmentally friendly book materials, including recycled text paper that is composed of at least 30 percent post-consumer waste, whenever possible.

❧ CONTENTS

PART THREE: CEREBRAL PALSY ENCYCLOPEDIA

PROBABLY EVERY PARENT of every child who has a health problem remembers the first time someone gave that problem a name. It may have been
in the hospital, soon after the baby was born, or it may have been months, or
even years, later. Hearing those words about your child, and wanting so much
for them not to be true, is something that stays forever in your mind.

For my husband and me, that moment occurred more than twenty-five
years ago. It was when our son Joshua was six months old. We suspected something was wrong with Josh, and our pediatrician had recommended that we
consult with a specialist. But we were not prepared to have the doctor tell us
that Josh had cerebral palsy and that his development was going to be delayed.

Cerebral palsy. We had heard the words, of course, but they had never
before had any relation to us. What did these words mean for the future of our
precious son? As time went on, we found out that it's difficult to know in the
early years of childhood just what cerebral palsy does mean for an individual
child. With cerebral palsy, as with many things in life, only time will tell. But
waiting, and not knowing, is a very difficult thing when it involves your child.

While we were searching for answers, my husband and I met Dr. Freeman
Miller and Dr. Steven Bachrach. We were so impressed with the concern and
sensitivity they showed toward Josh and toward us that we knew we'd found
the doctors who would not only help our family through the difficult times
but cheer along with us when times were good. Their medical advice proved
to be among the most valuable we'd ever received, and their open, caring, and
honest approach let us know that they would be there for us when we needed
them. Drs. Bachrach and Miller have been there all through the years, even after Josh was no longer eligible for treatment at the Nemours / Alfred I. duPont
Hospital for Children because of age restrictions. Both my husband and I will
be ever appreciative and grateful.

Sound professional advice and a caring commitment to do what's best for
your child. That's what anyone who is the parent of a child with cerebral palsy
wants. And that's what Drs. Miller and Bachrach and their colleagues offer
in this book. They will help you understand cerebral palsy and how it affects
your child. They will answer your questions. They will help you cope. They
will show you on every page that they understand, at least a little bit, what it's
like to be the parent of a child with cerebral palsy. Perhaps most importantly,
they will do all this because they care so much about the children.

Whether you've just learned that your own precious child has cerebral palsy
or you and your family have been living with this condition for several years,

you will find that this book is a wonderful resource, as valuable to someone with an infant as to someone with a young adult. I still open the book and glance through it from time to time. I still learn from its masters, and it's still a timely fit. I urge you not to put it on your bookshelf, but to keep it handy and turn to it often. The information it provides will give strength and hope and courage to both you and your child.

I wish you luck and success in your journey.

JOAN LENETT WHINSTON

❧ PREFACE

THE INFORMATION in these pages represents the current thinking of professionals who specialize in the medical, psychological, educational, and legal aspects of caring for children who have cerebral palsy. The book was written for everyone who provides the daily care of a child with cerebral palsy, whether parent, grandparent, great-grandparent, brother, sister, aunt, or uncle. We hope that teachers, physicians, and anyone else who cares about the well-being of such a child will also benefit from it. Our goal in writing this book is to help those who care for a child with cerebral palsy understand the child's needs and how these needs can best be met. In helping the caregivers, of course, our ultimate goal is to help the child.

By learning about CP and the many options for treatment, parents and others will be better prepared to ask direct questions of the professional, who will probably respond by providing additional information or clarification. Thus, one of our purposes in writing this book is to improve communication between the professional and the caregiver—again, resulting in better treatment for and care of the child.

Cerebral Palsy: A Complete Guide for Caregiving is arranged in three parts. The first part is composed of chapters that address a range of issues, usually progressing in sections by the chronological age of the child. You may want to read this part of the book from beginning to end, or you may prefer to turn to the specific section of this part of the book that addresses the issues that are relevant for your child right now. For example, if your child is 5 years old and has a hemiplegic pattern of involvement, you may want to begin by reading the introduction to Chapter 5, plus the section of that chapter that focuses on children with hemiplegia from age 4 to age 6.

The twelve chapters in Part 1 are arranged as follows: Chapter 1 provides an overview of cerebral palsy, and Chapter 2 presents normal developmental milestones from a pediatric perspective, including a discussion of normal and abnormal behavior. Chapters 3 and 4 describe medical problems and intellectual and psychosocial issues associated with CP. Specific patterns of involvement and their orthopedic treatment are discussed in Chapters 5, 6, and 7. Although problems encountered in childhood provide the primary focus of this book, one chapter—Chapter 8—looks at issues confronted by the adult with CP. Chapter 9 describes the medical system and introduces the various kinds of professional caregivers you and your child may meet. In Chapter 10, health insurance and other financial aspects of care are addressed. Finally,

Chapters 11 and 12 explain how the educational and legal systems can benefit your child—and how you can make sure that they do.

Part 2 provides practical information for the caregiver. Subjects covered range from wheelchair maintenance to daily hygiene tips such as toothbrushing, and entries are intended to help caregivers provide exceptional care for children with cerebral palsy. We must add a word of caution here, and that is that caregivers need to learn the techniques described in this section *from an experienced professional.* The instructions in Part 2 are *memory refreshers* for those who have already been taught these caregiving techniques by professionals.

Part 3 is an encyclopedia, arranged in alphabetical order. Listed, defined, and described in this section are the medical terms and diagnoses and the medical and surgical procedures that are encountered by families and others who provide care to children with cerebral palsy. Parents can use this reference as a guide and consult it when new problems arise or new treatments are being considered. Those caring for a child whose doctor recommends that a *pelvic osteotomy* be performed, for example, can find out what this procedure involves, why and when it is recommended, and what the preoperative and postoperative course will be like for the child.

The Resources section, at the back of the book, lists the names, addresses, phone numbers, and web pages of organizations that provide professional support for children with CP and their caregivers.

A final thought before we begin: Each child is an individual, and no book can provide information that applies specifically to an individual child at any given time. We have written this book to provide information that applies generally to all children with CP, but specific information about *your child* can only be obtained directly from a medical professional who knows the child.

❧ ACKNOWLEDGMENTS

A WORK OF this scope depends on the efforts and contributions of many people, and we truly thank them all. The following colleagues and health care professionals, most of whom have worked with us at the Nemours / Alfred I. duPont Hospital for Children, contributed to the first and/or second edition of this book:

Michael Alexander, MD
Benjamin Alouf, MD
Ellen Arch, MD
Joan Blair, MSN, RN, APRN-BC
Millie Boettcher, MSN, CPNP, CNSN
Mary Bolton, PT
Marilyn L. Boos, RNC, MS
Winslow Borkowski, MD
Aaron Chidekel, MD
Steven Cook, MD
Kirk Dabney, MD
Linda Duffy, BS, PA-C
Maureen Edelson, MD
Stephen Falchek, MD
T. Ernesto Figueroa, MD
Diane Gallagher, EdD
Rochelle Glidden, PsyD
H. Theodore Harcke, MD
Brian J Hartman, Esq.
Douglas Huisenga, PT, ATC

Heidi Kecskemethy, RD, CSP
Maura McManus, MD
Robin C. Meyers, MPH, RD
Ralph Milner, MD
Robert O'Reilly, MD
Douglas T. Pearson, PhD
Denise Peischl, BSBME
Joseph Queenan, MD
Rochelle Sassler
Mena Scavina, DO
Ellen Scharff, MSW
David Sheslow, PhD
Bart Stevens, ChLAP
Susan Stine, MD
Kathleen Trzcinski, RN, MSN, CRNP
Rhonda S. Walter, MD
Joan Lenett Whinston
Joshua Whinston
Philip Wolfson, MD

The following colleagues from Nemours / AI DuPont Hospital for Children contributed to this new, third edition of the book. We appreciate the thought and work that went into their contributions:

Judith Adelizzi-DeLany, MSN, APRN, PPCNP-BC
Joan L. Blair, MSN, RN, PNP-BC
Aaron Chidekel, MD
Stephanie Chopko, PhD

Justin Connor, MD
Jaclyn M. Costantino, RD, LDN
Allan R. De Jong, MD
Linda Duffy, BS, PA-C
Maureen L. Egan, MSN, APRN

T. Ernesto Figueroa, MD

Mark S. Finkelstein, DO

Sharon W. Gould, MD

Samantha V. Hill, MD

Tracy Hills, DO

Denise A. Hughes, MS

Heidi H. Kecskemethy, MS Ed,
    RDN, CSP, LDN, CBDT

Lance E. Kisby, DMD

Erika M. Kutsch, DO

Jennifer M. LeComte, DO

Sharon S. Lehman, MD

Richard Lytton, MA, CCC-SLP

Katherine M. McKee-Cole, MD

Maura McManus, MD

Anne Meduri, MD

Betsy Mullan, PT, PCS

Cory Ellen Nourie, MSS, MLSP

Robert O'Reilly, MD

Laura L. Owens, MD

Vandna Passi, MD

Denise Peischl, BSBME

Joseph H. Piatt Jr., MD

David Pressel, MD, PhD

Julieanne P. Sees, DO

Dawn M. Selhorst, BS, RRT-NPS

Sara Slovin, MD, MSPH

Abigail Strang, MD

Rhonda S. Walter, MD

Krishna White, MD, MPH

We had special contributions from colleagues with expertise in fields outside medicine who also work with children with cerebral palsy. These include Diane Gallagher, EdD, and Christina R. Coia, MEd, of the HMS School for Children with Cerebral Palsy in Philadelphia, who wrote the educational chapter, and Brian J. Hartman, Esq., of the Community Legal Aid Society of Delaware, who wrote the chapter on legal issues. Special thanks to Joshua Whinston, a young man with CP, his mother, Joan Lenett Whinston, and two other parents of children with CP, Michele Shusterman and Nancy Lemus. Thanks also to many of the staff and students of the HMS School, whose pictures appear in this book.

We also acknowledge the support of our editors at Johns Hopkins University Press, especially Jacqueline Wehmueller, who has been with this project for more than 20 years, from the first through this third edition.

We especially acknowledge our families for their patience and support as we worked on this project.

We also acknowledge the many patients and their families who have helped us understand what they want to know about caring for their child with cerebral palsy and encouraged us to write this book.

Finally, we acknowledge the help and support of the Nemours Foundation, the Nemours / Alfred I. duPont Hospital for Children, and CEO Roy Proujansky, MD, whose support has been crucial to this project.

Steven J. Bachrach, MD
Freeman Miller, MD

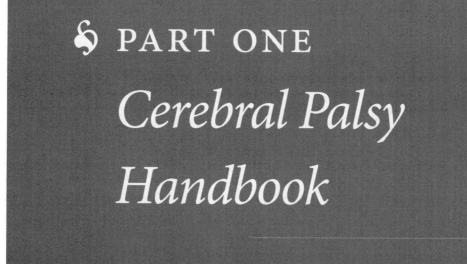

PART ONE

Cerebral Palsy Handbook

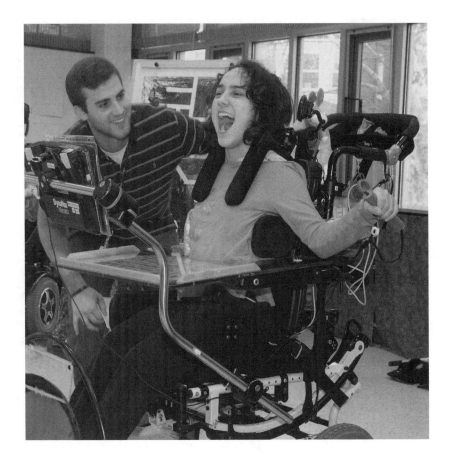

1

What Is Cerebral Palsy?

CEREBRAL PALSY is a collection of motor disorders resulting from damage to the brain that occurs before, during, or after birth. The damage to the child's brain affects the motor system, and as a result the child has poor coordination, poor balance, or abnormal movement patterns—or a combination of these characteristics.

Cerebral palsy (CP) is a *static* disorder of the brain, not a progressive disorder. This means that the disorder or disease process will not get worse as time goes on. Nor are the motor disorders associated with cerebral palsy temporary. Therefore, a child who has temporary motor problems, or who has motor problems that get worse over time, does not have cerebral palsy. Children with cerebral palsy may have many other kinds of medical problems. Most of these problems are related to the brain injury. They may include epilepsy, intellectual disability, learning disabilities, and/or attention deficit–hyperactivity disorder. In addition, the child with cerebral palsy may also have limitations in vision, hearing, speech, feeding, swallowing, or breathing. (See Chapter 3 for more details.)

Congenital cerebral palsy (or cerebral palsy that exists from birth) is responsible for the largest proportion of cases of cerebral palsy. For a small percentage of children, injuries sustained during the birthing process or in early childhood may be considered the cause of cerebral palsy. When motor disorders appear after age 5, they are slightly different from the motor disorders of cerebral palsy and are usually diagnosed as they would be in an adult, as stroke or traumatic brain injury.

Cerebral palsy is the most common permanent disabling condition of childhood: of every 2,000 infants born, 5 are born with cerebral palsy. This incidence has remained constant for many decades, despite advances in obstetrical and pediatric care that have dramatically lowered the infant mortality rate. Although improvements in medical care have decreased the incidence of CP among some children who otherwise would have developed the disorder, medical advances have also resulted in the survival of children who previously would have died at a young age, and many of these children survive with an impairment or a disability such as cerebral palsy.

Some causes of CP that used to be common, such as bacterial meningitis, have almost been eliminated in this country through the use of vaccines to prevent these infections. The treatment of newborn jaundice has almost entirely eliminated kernicterus, a form of brain damage that caused athetoid CP years ago. In recent years there has been an increased focus on preventing neurological injury in children born with severe asphyxia (lack of oxygen) through the use of hypothermia. Hypothermia is achieved by cooling the whole infant or just the infant's head. This has been shown to help prevent neurological disability in some but not all such infants. Another treatment under investigation is giving cord blood as a transfusion to a child who has suffered a brain injury in order to minimize the long-term effects. At this time, we do not know whether giving cord blood will be a useful treatment.

What has also changed is the *type* of cerebral palsy that is most prevalent in the developed Western world. In the 1960s in the United States, 20 percent of all children with cerebral palsy had *athetoid* cerebral palsy, a type of CP caused by *hyperbilirubinemia* and characterized by slow, writhing involuntary movements. Today only 5 to 10 percent of children have this type of CP, and 80 to 90 percent have spastic CP. The decrease is mainly due to advances in the treatment of hyperbilirubinemia. At the same time, *spastic* cerebral palsy, characterized by rigidity in muscles, which causes stiffness and restricted movement, has become more prevalent because intensive care for newborns has resulted in higher survival rates for very small premature babies. These babies are at high risk of developing spastic cerebral palsy: between 5 and 10 percent of premature infants under 1,500 grams (3 lb. 5 oz.) who survive have cerebral palsy.

What causes cerebral palsy?

When cerebral palsy was first described in the 1880s, it was believed to be caused by a lack of oxygen for the infant at birth. We now know that this is the cause in only a small minority, approximately 10 percent, of children with CP. In the great majority of cases, CP is caused by damage to the brain during fetal development, well before the birth process begins. Although the cause of this damage frequently is not known (the medical term for "unknown cause" is *idiopathic*), we know from modern imaging techniques (computerized tomography and magnetic resonance imaging) that some cases of CP are caused by strokes or hemorrhaging in the brain in the late stages of fetal development. Others are caused by abnormal development of the brain in the early stages of fetal development (called a *malformation* or *birth defect of the brain*). The brain damage that leads to CP can be caused by:

A viral infection during pregnancy, such as cytomegalovirus (CMV) or rubella
Hydrocephalus, either before or after birth
A blood clot in the fetus's brain causing a stroke while in utero
Bleeding into the brain: while in utero, this could be due to a bleeding disorder; after birth, this can be seen as a complication of extreme prematurity.
Abnormal development of the brain during the first trimester of pregnancy
A prolonged period of asphyxia (lack of oxygen) from, for example, abruptio placenta, when the placenta tears away from the uterine wall during labor, cutting off the baby's blood supply
Bacterial meningitis after birth
Head trauma from shaken baby syndrome (child abuse) during the first year of life

Lead poisoning during the first two years of life

A chromosomal (genetic) defect: Until recently, 1 to 2 percent of cases of CP were linked to chromosomal mutations, and these were usually familial cases (such as two children in the same family with CP). Recent genetic studies of sporadic cases (meaning no family pattern is found) using what is called "exome sequencing," a technique for sequencing the genes in a chromosome, have shown that 14 percent of cases likely are caused by a single gene mutation. This field of study is developing rapidly, and these numbers will likely change, though the basic message will likely continue to be that genetics plays a role in the development of CP in some children. It may well be that a combination of risk factors act as a trigger for CP in some children with a genetic susceptibility to developing CP.

Idiopathic (no known cause of damage to the brain during pregnancy): new knowledge, such as that gained from genetic testing and imaging techniques, has revealed underlying abnormalities and is reducing the number of cases with CP in this category. There are fewer cases now than in the past in which we do not understand the cause.

There is no way to predict which children's brains will be damaged by one of these factors or what the extent of the damage will be. However, none of these factors always results in brain damage, and even when brain damage occurs, the damage does not always result in CP. Some children may have an isolated hearing loss from their meningitis, others will have severe intellectual disability, and some will have CP (either alone or combined with these other problems).

There is a much higher risk (20 to 40 times higher) of CP in children born prematurely than in children born at full term. The most recent understanding of the cause of CP associated with prematurity is that something (possibly an infection in the amniotic fluid, which surrounds the fetus in the womb) sets off an inflammatory reaction in the brain of the fetus, and this inflammation causes the brain damage resulting in CP. While this theory has not been fully proven, some experimental evidence supports it. This inflammation may also be the cause of premature labor in many cases, which may explain why CP and prematurity often occur in the same child.

What are the different types of cerebral palsy? Cerebral palsy is classified by the type of movement problem (spastic, athetoid, hypotonic, or mixed) and by the body parts involved (legs only, one arm and one leg, or all four limbs). Motor ability and coordination vary greatly from one child to another, and few statements hold true for *all* children with CP. Thus, generalizations about children with CP can only have meaning within the context of the subgroups described below. That's why subgroups are used in this book whenever treatment and outcome expectations are discussed. Most professionals who care for children with CP are familiar with these diagnoses and use them to communicate about a child's condition.

Spasticity refers to the inability of a muscle to relax, while *athetosis* refers to a writhing movement of a muscle that cannot be controlled by the individual.

Dystonia is a movement disorder resulting in a twisting movement of a limb that is often very uncomfortable; it is often hard to separate from athetosis. Infants who at first are *hypotonic*, or very floppy, may later develop spasticity. *Hemiplegia*, also called *unilateral* (one sided) CP, is cerebral palsy that involves one arm and one leg, both on the same side of the body, whereas *diplegia* primarily involves both legs. *Quadriplegia* refers to a pattern involving all four extremities as well as trunk and neck muscles. (Both diplegia and quadriplegia fall into the category of bilateral CP.) Generally, a child with quadriplegia does not walk independently. Another category is *ataxia*, which refers to balance and coordination problems.

Although almost all children with cerebral palsy can be classified as having hemiplegia, diplegia, or quadriplegia, there are significant overlaps. These overlaps have led to the use of additional terms, some of which are confusing. Occasionally you'll encounter terms like *paraplegia, double hemiplegia, triplegia,* and *pentaplegia*; these classifications are also based on the parts of the body involved. For simplicity, however, the discussion of CP in this book is limited to the three broader categories.

The word for the dominant type of movement or muscle coordination problem is often combined with the word for the component that seems to be most problematic for the child. The result is a more specific descriptive term. For example, the child with *spastic diplegia* has mostly spastic muscle problems, and mainly his legs are affected, although his arms may be affected to a certain degree. In the child with *athetoid quadriplegia*, on the other hand, both arms and legs are involved, primarily with athetoid muscle problems, but he or she often also has some ataxia and spasticity.

To summarize, we can classify different kinds of cerebral palsy according to the type of movement the child makes or to the part of the body that is most involved, or both:

By type of movement

Spastic	too much muscle tone
Athetoid	uncontrolled muscle movements
Hypotonic	decreased muscle tone (not enough tone)
Ataxic	balance and coordination problems
Mixed	mixture of two or more of the above

By involved body parts

Hemiplegia	one arm and one leg, on the same side of the body
Diplegia	predominantly both legs (arms also involved)
Quadriplegia	all four extremities

And more recently, by side of body involved

Unilateral	involving one side of the body
Bilateral	involving both sides of the body

Other terms used to define specific problems of movement or muscle function include *dystonia, tremor,* and *rigidity*. The words *severe, moderate,* and *mild* are also often used in combination with classification terms for both anatomical pattern and motor function (*severe spastic diplegia*, for example), but these qualifying words do not have any specific meaning. They are subjective words, and their meaning varies depending upon the person who is using them. Therefore, a more objective classification system has been developed so that a given word will mean the same thing to everyone. This system is based on the child's ability to move, or his or her motor ability. This system is called the Gross Motor Function Classification System, or GMFCS. There are five levels of GMFCS, and it is used for children at least 4 years of age. This system was initially designed to predict the outcome of the child's motor disability, and it works reasonably well for children aged 4 to 5 years and above. However, the outcome is much less predictable for children younger than 2 to 3 years of age. This general classification system is as follows (see also page 8):

GMFCS I   Walks without major limitations but not completely normally
GMFCS II   Walks without any device or assistance but has problems keeping up with peers or on uneven ground or stairs
GMFCS III   Requires a walker, a cane, or crutches for most walking
GMFCS IV   Is mostly in a wheelchair, may do standing transfers, may use a walker for exercise, requires assistance with transferring from the wheelchair
GMFCS V   Requires a wheelchair for all transport, and is dependent or requires full support to transfer from the wheelchair

What are the right words to use when referring to children with cerebral palsy?

Cerebral palsy is the term used to describe the motor impairment resulting from brain damage in the young child, regardless of the cause of the damage or its effect on the child. *Impairment* is the correct term to use to define a deviation from normal, such as not being able to make a muscle move or not being able to control an unwanted movement. *Disability* is the term used to define a restriction in the ability to perform a normal daily activity that someone of the same age is able to perform. (For example, since a typical 3-year-old can walk independently, a 3-year-old child who is not able to walk has a disability.) *Handicap* is the term used to describe the condition of a child or adult who, because of the disability, is unable to play a role in society appropriate to his or her age and environment.

A 16-year-old who is unable to prepare his own lunch or brush his teeth is handicapped. But a 16-year-old who walks with the assistance of crutches, attends a regular school, and is fully independent in daily activities is disabled, not handicapped. Thus, a person can be impaired and not necessarily be disabled, and a person can be disabled without being handicapped. To summarize: *impaired* means deviating from normal; *disabled* denotes restricted ability to perform normal activities of daily living; and *handicapped* means being unable to play an age-appropriate role in society.

These definitions have been expanded by the World Health Organization (WHO) and changed somewhat to also focus on the environmental aspects of participation in daily function and life activities. The new definitions take into account the individual's impairments, what he or she wants to accomplish,

GMFCS between 6th and 12th birthday: Descriptors and illustrations

GMFCS Level I

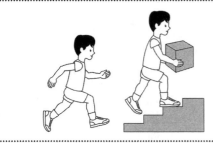

Children walk at home, school, outdoors and in the community. They can climb stairs without the use of a railing. Children perform gross motor skills such as running and jumping, but speed, balance and coordination are limited.

GMFCS Level II

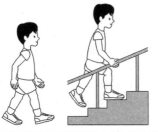

Children walk in most settings and climb stairs holding onto a railing. They may experience difficulty walking long distances and balancing on uneven terrain, inclines, in crowded areas or confined spaces. Children may walk with physical assistance, a hand-held mobility device or used wheeled mobility over long distances. Children have only minimal ability to perform gross motor skills such as running and jumping.

GMFCS Level III

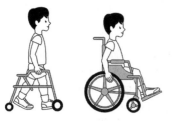

Children walk using a hand-held mobility device in most indoor settings. They may climb stairs holding onto a railing with supervision or assistance. Children use wheeled mobility when traveling long distances and may self-propel for shorter distances.

GMFCS Level IV

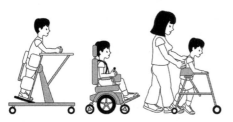

Children use methods of mobility that require physical assistance or powered mobility in most settings. They may walk for short distances at home with physical assistance or use powered mobility or a body support walker when positioned. At school, outdoors and in the community children are transported in a manual wheelchair or use powered mobility.

GMFCS Level V

Children are transported in a manual wheelchair in all settings. Children are limited in their ability to maintain antigravity head and trunk postures and control leg and arm movements.

GMFCS descriptors: Palisano et al. (1997) Dev Med Child Neurol 39:214-23
CanChild: www.canchild.ca

Illustrations Version 2 © Bill Reid, Kate Willoughby, Adrienne Harvey and Kerr Graham, The Royal Children's Hospital Melbourne   ERC151050 and the environmental limitations imposed by the surroundings. The goal is to define inherent limitations of the affected person and options for overcoming those limitations with assistance from others or adaptations to the environment. A detailed International Classification of Functioning, Disability and Health (ICF), of the WHO, can be used to assess an individual. This is available as a public document on the websites of a number of organizations.

In the past there was a lack of awareness and sensitivity among the general public with respect to the words used to describe people with disabilities. Over the past decades, however, increasing attention has been paid to such language, and recently a great deal of attention has been given to issues of education, employment, and public access for individuals with disabilities. Because of this evolving awareness and respect, it is no longer acceptable to refer to individuals by their disability ("the epileptic," "the spastic," or "the intellectually impaired child"). The current acceptable terminology stresses the *individual person* and then mentions the disability that the person has: "a girl with spastic diplegia" or "a boy with cognitive limitations." Clearly, this language acknowledges that there is much more to a person than his or her disability. The term *mental retardation* is no longer acceptable; we now refer to a child as having *cognitive limitations* or *intellectual disability*. In this book, we have chosen to use respectful language that presents information in a way that can be understood by the general reader.

What medical problems will my child encounter? The following list presents the medical problems most often associated with cerebral palsy. The neurological problems (and other medical problems) are discussed in detail in Chapter 3, and the orthopedic problems are discussed in Chapters 5, 6, and 7.

Neurological problems	*Orthopedic problems*
Cognitive limitations	Scoliosis
Learning disabilities	Hip dislocation
Attention deficit–hyperactivity disorder (ADD or ADHD)	Contractures of joints
	Discrepancy in leg length
Seizure disorder (epilepsy)	Foot deformities
Visual impairment	
Swallowing difficulties	
Speech impairment (dysarthria)	
Hearing impairment	

Secondary effects
Communication disorder
Drooling
Poor nutrition
Depression
Fragile bones and frequent fractures
Dental cavities
Constipation

What are some
disorders that look
like cerebral palsy but
are in fact a different
problem?

Children with different kinds of physical disabilities can have many problems in common, especially in interacting with family members and society. Although the physical and medical difficulties of children with disabilities vary widely, some of the characteristics of various disorders *resemble* those of cerebral palsy. It isn't until after closer examination that the medical issues turn out to be quite distinct.

Children with spinal cord dysfunction, for example, face medical problems such as a lack of feeling in their skin and a lack of bowel and bladder control, which differ markedly from the medical problems faced by children with cerebral palsy. Spinal cord dysfunction may be a result of spinal cord injury, spina bifida (a defect in the formation of the spinal *column*), or a congenital spinal cord malformation (a defect in the formation of the spinal *cord*). Other children who may look similar to children with cerebral palsy are children with temporary motor problems resulting from closed head injuries, seizures, drug overdoses, or some brain tumors. The medical issues for this group of children differ from the medical issues for children with cerebral palsy in that their injuries can occur at any age, and the severity of the problems caused by these injuries changes over time.

Disorders that are primarily of muscle, nerve, and bone are not cerebral palsy. Such conditions include muscular dystrophy, peripheral neuropathies such as Charcot-Marie-Tooth disease, and osteogenesis imperfecta. All of these conditions are associated with specific medical problems.

Children with progressive neurological disorders (such as leukodystrophy and Tay-Sachs disease) also have medical needs that differ from those of children with cerebral palsy. Some children with chromosomal anomalies (for example, trisomy 13 and 18) or congenital disorders (hereditary spastic paraplegia, for example) may appear similar to children with cerebral palsy; others, such as children with Down syndrome, appear very different but may have some issues in common with children who have cerebral palsy. They also have problems that are unique to children with that specific disorder.

Can cerebral palsy be
prevented?

When a physician diagnoses a baby with CP, the mother and father often feel guilty and wonder what they did to contribute to their child's disorder. While it is certainly true that good prenatal care is an essential part of preventing congenital problems, these "birth defects" often occur even when the mother has strictly followed her physician's advice in caring for herself and the developing infant. Since the cause of many cases of CP still is not understood (see pages 4–5), prevention in those cases is not yet possible. However, when there are specific known causes, the possibility of prevention exists.

Infections such as rubella (German measles), toxoplasmosis (a disease caused by the invasion of parasitic microorganisms), and the virus known as cytomegalovirus (CMV) can cause brain damage in the fetus. Rubella can be prevented by immunization (a woman should be immunized *before* becoming pregnant), and the chances of becoming infected with toxoplasmosis can be minimized by not handling the feces of cats and by avoiding raw or undercooked meat. There is no immunization for CMV. Bacterial meningitis can cause severe brain damage in young infants after birth and is caused by a number of different bacteria. One of the major changes in pediatrics in the past 40 years has been the almost complete eradication of bacterial meningitis due to immunizations against *Haemophilus influenzae* type B and pneumococcus, which previously caused many deaths and left those who survived with severe disabilities.

Premature infants are at a much higher risk for developing cerebral palsy than full-term babies, and the risk increases as the birthweight decreases. Between 5 and 10 percent of infants weighing less than 1,500 grams (3 lb. 5 oz.) at birth develop cerebral palsy, and infants weighing less than 1,500 grams are 40 times more likely to develop cerebral palsy than infants who are born at full term weighing more than 2,500 grams (5 lb. 8 oz.). Many premature infants suffer bleeding within the brain, called *intraventricular hemorrhages* or *intracranial hemorrhages*. The highest frequency of hemorrhages is found in babies with the lowest weight; the problem is rare in babies who weigh more than 2,000 grams (4 lb. 6 oz.). This bleeding may damage the part of the brain that controls motor function and thereby lead to cerebral palsy. If the hemorrhages result in destruction of normal brain tissue and the development of small cysts around the ventricles and in the motor region of the brain (a condition called *periventricular leukomalacia*), then the infant is more likely to have CP than an infant with hemorrhages alone. While we do not yet know the cause of premature labor, available treatments sometimes succeed in stopping such labor or at least delaying delivery of the infant for a while. Prevention of early delivery, along with medicines to help mature the lungs, may prevent some of the severe medical and neurological problems associated with premature birth.

What circumstances in the birthing process might cause a newborn to have cerebral palsy? In the nineteenth century, William John Little, MD, described cerebral palsy and stated that in most cases the condition was due to birth injury. Sigmund Freud, MD, who was a prominent neurologist before he created the field of psychiatry, also investigated the causes of cerebral palsy. Dr. Freud thought that the condition was due to something that occurred before the child's birth. He argued that the breathing problems seen at birth were often due to an abnormality present in the baby's brain before birth, rather than breathing problems causing brain damage. Freud's view was ignored for nearly a century, but recent research has lent support to the idea that cerebral palsy is most often a result of a congenital abnormality, rather than an injury sustained at birth.

The birthing process can be traumatic for an infant, however, and injuries occurring during birth do sometimes cause cerebral palsy. Modern prenatal care and improved obstetrical care have significantly reduced the incidence of birth injury, but it is unlikely that it will ever be completely eliminated.

There are no specific events that, if they occur during pregnancy, delivery, or infancy, always cause cerebral palsy. One large study, for example, indicated that more than 60 percent of all pregnancies have at least one complication and that most of these complications cause no problems. For instance, 25 percent of all the newborns in the study had the umbilical cord wrapped around their necks, and 16 percent passed meconium (had the first bowel movement) at the time of birth. Fortunately, these common "birth events" and the development of CP have only a small correlation.

On the other hand, newborns in this study with very low Apgar scores for a prolonged period (scores of less than 3 at 20 minutes) had a risk of developing cerebral palsy that was 250 times greater than that of infants with normal Apgar scores. (An Apgar score is an assessment of the condition of a newborn baby by scoring respiratory effort, heart rate, color, muscle tone, and motor reactions, usually at 1 and 5 minutes after birth.) An Apgar score of less than 3 at 20 minutes after birth suggests that the infant suffered severe asphyxia during birth (asphyxia is a lack of sufficient oxygen to the brain). Half of the infants who suffered severe asphyxia during birth and survived did *not* develop cerebral palsy, however.

When CP is diagnosed in childhood, it is often found that the child suffered asphyxia at birth. The asphyxia, however, is often considered the *symptom* of an otherwise sick baby with a neurological problem, not the primary *cause* of CP. In a number of studies, about 9 percent of children with CP were thought to have CP directly and exclusively related to asphyxia at delivery. In 91 percent of the babies, brain damage was the result of other causes unrelated to their birth experience (many of which are listed above in this chapter). This is apparently why the incidence of CP in undeveloped and poverty-stricken countries, where infant mortality is very high, is the same as in northern Europe, where infant mortality is the lowest in the world. It may also explain why modern obstetrical care, including fetal monitoring and a high rate of cesarean section, has lowered infant mortality rates but not the incidence of cerebral palsy.

What might cause a child between birth and the age of 2 to 3 years to develop CP?

During infancy and early childhood, a child is completely dependent on others for his or her safety and protection, and shielding a child from injury is one of the most important responsibilities of a child's caregivers. An injury like asphyxia damages the brain in a variety of ways, and it is the leading cause of CP in this age group. Asphyxia is most commonly caused by poisoning, nearly drowning, and choking on foreign objects such as toys and pieces of food (including peanuts, popcorn, and hot dogs).

The brain may also be damaged when it is physically traumatized as a result of a blow to the head. A child who falls, is involved in a motor vehicle accident, or is the victim of physical abuse may suffer irreparable injury to the brain. One form of child abuse is the shaken baby syndrome, in which the caregiver tries to quiet the baby by shaking him but shakes him too vigorously, causing the infant's brain to strike repeatedly against the skull under high pressure. This kind of abuse can damage the brain.

Severe infections, especially *meningitis* or *encephalitis*, can also lead to brain damage in this age group. Meningitis is inflammation of the meninges (the covering of the brain and the spinal cord), usually caused by a bacterial infection. Encephalitis is brain inflammation that may be caused by bacterial or viral infections. Either of these infections can cause disabilities ranging from hearing loss to CP and severe intellectual impairment.

How does a physician diagnose cerebral palsy?

Many of a child's normal developmental milestones, such as reaching for toys (3 to 4 months), sitting (6 to 7 months), and walking (10 to 14 months), are based on motor function. A physician may suspect cerebral palsy if a child is slow to develop these skills. In making a diagnosis of cerebral palsy, the physician takes into account the delay in developmental milestones as well as physical warning signs such as abnormal muscle tone, abnormal movements, and persistent infantile reflexes.

Making a definite diagnosis of cerebral palsy is not always easy, especially before the child's first birthday. In fact, diagnosing cerebral palsy usually involves a period of waiting for the definite and permanent appearance of specific motor problems. Most children with cerebral palsy can be diagnosed by the age of 18 months, but this is a long time for parents to wait for a diagnosis, and it is understandably a difficult and trying period.

Making a diagnosis of cerebral palsy is also difficult when, for example, a 2-year-old has suffered a head injury. The child may appear to be severely injured in the period immediately after the trauma, and three months after the injury he may have symptoms that are typical of a child with cerebral palsy. But one year after the injury the child may be completely recovered, with no sign of cerebral palsy. Although he has a scar on his brain, the scar is not permanently impairing his motor activities. During the year between the injury and the diagnosis of no permanent injury, the parents will have a difficult time waiting. No matter how frustrating this period of waiting and observing is, however, it must pass before the diagnosis can be made.

Do x-rays or other tests help in the diagnosis?

In making a diagnosis of cerebral palsy, the most meaningful aspect of the evaluation is the physical evidence of abnormal motor function, such as too much or too little muscle tone, hyperactive reflexes, and persistent infantile reflexes that should disappear by around 6 months. A diagnosis of cerebral palsy cannot be made solely on the basis of an x-ray or a blood test, though the physician may order such tests to exclude other neurological diseases that could cause similar symptoms.

Blood tests and chromosome analysis are helpful in diagnosing hereditary conditions that may be the cause of the abnormal motor function. It is important to diagnose these conditions for the child's sake, to understand the cause of her problems and the possible prognosis. It is also important for the family, because it may influence the parents' decision whether to have more children. When the tests indicate that a child's condition is inherited, family members often benefit from genetic counseling. As mentioned earlier in this chapter, children who have CP without a known cause are now often tested for genetic abnormalities, and a chromosomal mutation, or an abnormality known as copy number variants (CNVs), is now frequently found, though the mutation may or may not be the cause of the CP. This type of abnormality is often new, meaning it was not present in the parents but developed in the chromosome of the new baby. Magnetic resonance imaging (MRI) or computerized tomography (CT) scans are often ordered when the physician suspects that the child has cerebral palsy. These tests may provide evidence of a malformation of the brain (such as lissencephaly), an intrauterine stroke, periventricular leukomalacia (PVL), hydrocephalus, or a bleed into the brain.

Seeing these abnormalities on the MRI of a child who has abnormal tone lends support to the diagnosis of CP and sometimes may explain the nature and timing of the brain injury. Sometimes these scans show evidence of a progressive neurological disease, which means the child has a disease other than CP. Sometimes the scan appears normal. A normal scan tells us that the structure of the brain appears normal. However, the function of the brain at the level of connections between nerves may still be abnormal, so a normal scan does not mean that the child has no problems. An abnormal neurological exam (such as abnormally high or low tone) and delay in the child's development are the best indicators of neurological problems. These scans, even when abnormal, also cannot predict how a specific child will function as he or she grows. Thus, children with normal scans may have severe cerebral palsy, and children with clearly abnormal scans may have only mild physical evidence of cerebral palsy. A child with an abnormal scan might appear normal until she begins school, for example, when significant learning problems may surface.

As a group, children with cerebral palsy do have brain scars, cysts, and other changes that show up on scans more frequently than in children without cerebral palsy. Therefore, when an abnormality is seen on a CT scan of the brain of a child whose physical examination suggests he may have cerebral palsy, it is one more indication that the child is likely to have motor problems in the future.

My infant has just been diagnosed with cerebral palsy. What can I expect for her future?

The first questions usually asked by parents after they are told their child has cerebral palsy are, "What will my child be like?" and "Will she walk?" Predicting what a young child with cerebral palsy will be like or what he or she will or will not do (this prediction is called the *prognosis*) is very difficult. Any predictions for an infant under 6 months of age are little better than guesses, and even for children younger than 1 year it is often difficult to predict the severity of CP. By the time the child is 2 years old, however, a qualified physician can usually but not always determine whether the child has hemiplegia, diplegia, or quadriplegia. Based on this involvement pattern, some predictions can be made.

Remember, children with cerebral palsy do not stop activities once they have begun them. Such a loss of skills, called *regression*, is not characteristic of this disorder. If the child is sitting by herself, pulling herself up to a standing position and walking along furniture, speaking words that are understandable, or self-feeding and then loses these motor skills over time, regression has occurred. If regression does occur, a different diagnosis for the child's problems should be sought.

For a child to be able to walk, some major events in motor control have to occur. A child must be able to hold his head up before he can sit up on his own, and he must be able to sit independently before he can walk on his own. It is generally assumed that if a child is not sitting up by himself by age 4 or walking by age 5, he will never be an independent walker. But a child who starts to walk at age 3 will certainly continue to walk. It is even more difficult to make early predictions about speaking ability or cognitive ability than it is to predict motor function. Here, too, evaluation is much more reliable after age 2, although a motor disability can make the evaluation of intellectual function quite difficult. Sometimes "motor-free" tests, which can assess intellectual ability without the child using his hands, are administered by psychologists who are experts in this type of testing. Overall, a child's intellectual ability, far more than his physical disability, will determine the long-term prognosis for independent living and being self-supporting. In other words, intellectual disability is far more likely to impair a child's ability to function in the world than is cerebral palsy.

What can my doctor tell me about my newborn's neurological problems?

As a parent, you're naturally concerned when your newborn has problems. Although your child's physician needs to evaluate your child's condition and prognosis and discuss this with you, the long-term outcome of cerebral palsy cannot be reliably predicted. Remember, although an increased risk of CP can sometimes be identified at birth, an actual diagnosis of cerebral palsy cannot be made at birth, and certainly the extent and severity of involvement that an individual child might eventually have is impossible to assess at birth.

Some neonatologists (doctors who specialize in the care of newborn infants) may avoid discussing the infant's problems in detail with the parents. They do this because they are aware of the normal interaction and bonding that occurs between the newborn and parents, and they don't want to do anything to interfere with that healthy interaction. The presumption of a bleak future for a child sometimes causes parents to withdraw from the child, and this can have a significant negative effect on the child.

Physicians usually communicate their concerns in terms of the child's symptoms, such as muscle problems, and prepare parents for the possibility of neurological damage. Clearly, it is part of the physician's role to inform parents, but the variability of outcome makes it virtually impossible for the physician to predict the future, and so the physician must weigh the need to inform (and the imprecision of the information that is available) against the need for the parents to have hope for, and become close to, their child.

Given all these uncertainties, what kind of medical treatment should a sick newborn receive?

When a child is 2 to 3 years old and has a severe disability, parents may begin to wonder whether treatment should have been less aggressive during those first few years. Given the tremendous uncertainties in outcome, physicians and parents often choose to treat newborns and preserve life with the hope that the outcome will be a good one. There are clearly exceptions, such as when the baby has a known chromosomal defect (such as trisomy 18), in which a poor prognosis is known and very aggressive treatment may be futile. However, in the majority of cases, neither the doctor nor the parents know what the outcome will be, and they must do the best they can with the limited information they have.

Often the prognosis is based on information from studies of a large number of babies with similar birthweights. The likelihood of an individual baby's having cerebral palsy or cognitive impairment (expressed as a percentage) is derived from these studies. Nevertheless, it is impossible to know whether an individual infant will be among the 70 to 90 percent that have a good outcome or the 10 to 30 percent with a poor outcome.

The role of the physician is to gather as much information about the child's condition as possible and convey this information to families, along with the best information available about chances of outcome. The role of the family is to participate in the decision-making process, especially when decisions must be made about further aggressive treatment. Ultimately, treatment decisions are medical ones, but they should be made with input from the family. The relationship between physician, patient, and family should be one of mutual respect, with each member of the "team" working toward what is good for the patient. Only with an open exchange of information and communication is this possible.

The problem is trying to figure out what is best for the child. At the time the decisions must be made it is often very difficult to know what will ultimately be best. A decision to treat aggressively usually involves the use of sophisticated technology, although the availability of such technology does not mean that it must always be used, and there are clearly times when it is more humane to withhold or withdraw aggressive treatment. These are never easy decisions to make. Clergy, social workers, ethicists, and other health care workers who have come to know the patient and family often help in making decisions. Many hospitals have an ethics committee, and family members or members of the health care team can request a consultation when a difficult decision is being made and extra advice is needed.

As parents reflect back over previous treatments, they should remember all these uncertainties and focus on the fact that decisions were made based on the best information available at the time. Focusing on decisions that in hindsight are thought to have been wrong is not beneficial to anyone. Similarly, the treatment plan should be a flexible one, and parents and medical specialists should not be afraid to alter the course as new information becomes available.

As parents, how can we work with doctors to set realistic goals for our child?

When it comes to expectations and questions of what the future holds for the child with CP, a combination of optimism and realism is probably your best bet. Consider that the parents of a 3-year-old without a disability who hope and expect that the child will go to college and law school, enter politics, and eventually become president of the United States have a vision for their child that combines realism and fantasy. Rather than map out a child's career path in this way, it would be far better for parents to care for the child as a 3-year-old—not as a college student or as a budding politician. It is equally important for the parent of a child with a disability to understand the child's present and likely future abilities and to develop a set of realistic goals to live by.

Occasionally, difficulties in communication arise when parents, educators, and medical care providers discuss the child's present abilities. It's often a challenge to improve communication so that everyone involved in the decision-making process is heard. People who are involved in making difficult decisions in an emotionally charged atmosphere must know that they will have a chance to express their opinions regarding the child's treatment and that these opinions will be taken seriously. Parents know their child best, but their judgment may be clouded by unrealistic expectations; physicians need to help parents develop realistic goals without quashing their hope. Sometimes parents don't have *high enough* expectations for their child, and in this case doctors need to provide encouragement to the parents to help them help their child achieve everything that he or she is able to.

An attempt to define future expectations is usually most important in the teenage years and beyond, when function is better defined and the future looks clearer to everyone involved. However, if all the parties keep their sights set on the primary goal—helping the child function at his or her maximum ability—then a team spirit is often a natural result.

What advice can help families cope with having a child with cerebral palsy?

The way a family experiences a diagnosis of cerebral palsy in their child varies widely. Here are three parents and one young adult with CP who have agreed to share their experiences and thoughts with our readers.

Creating balance in your life when you have a child with cerebral palsy or any other chronic health condition can be difficult. Ever since my daughter's diagnosis of CP eight years ago, I have struggled with the ongoing tension between wanting to seize opportunities to encourage her greatest improvement and not making our life all about therapy and treatment. For many years when she was very young, there was great uncertainty about her developmental path, and during this time it was difficult for me to find much balance in daily life. As her primary caregiver I kept seeing all of the activities and peer interactions she was missing out on, and I felt I needed to fight harder and "shout louder" against her CP and the confusing tide of signals her brain was sending her muscles. I figured it was better to sacrifice parts of my daughter's childhood and a few years of mine and my husband's life than to miss what I understood were "critical opportunities" to help her have the best possible future.

The difficulty in creating a balanced lifestyle when a child has had a brain injury or disturbance in brain development often relates to the confusion of dealing with an unknown future. This is because no one can tell you with certainty how much potential for change your child has. During my daughter's toddler years I felt as if I were in a race without a finish line, wondering how many areas of development I could support to keep her development as close to that of her same-aged peers as possible. As she got older, however, I slowly let go of this thinking as I saw that my daughter continued to fall further behind even as I pushed the daily limits of her energy and the energy of our family. You may be in a similar position. You may often feel as if there are not enough hours in the day to meet your own basic needs or your child's and your family's basic needs. People may tell you that "you must take care of yourself," which sounds like a nice idea that you will get to some day in the far-off distance. There are, however, a few tips and tricks that may shift your approach to caring for your child and free up some of your emotional and mental energy and maybe even some of your time.

Responding to a CP Diagnosis

In order to fully implement some of these simple strategies, it is helpful to understand why CP is so difficult to manage and to evaluate the ways you are coping with your child's CP diagnosis. With many health conditions a diagnosis offers guidance to parents about what they can expect as their child grows. This information allows parents to begin to set down emotional roots, start to cope with their child's present symptoms, and prepare for known future conditions. A diagnosis like cerebral palsy is different because the developmental path is often unclear and will vary from one individual to another. The diagnosis of CP allows families to access services and health benefits and provides them with a name for their child's symptoms, but it does not offer parents the road map they desire. This uncertainty can create extraordinary emotional strain, as well as anxiety and confusion, for the parents, who are unsure of what changes they can help foster in their child and what circumstances they will ultimately need to accept.

Here are some examples of how parents may respond to a CP diagnosis:

1. Blame themselves.
2. Deny that their child is having difficulty.
3. Aggressively fight the diagnosis and symptoms through constant and intensive therapy planning. (This is not always a bad thing, but balance is important.)
4. Constantly search the Internet for new and experimental treatments.
5. Repeatedly ask others—doctors, therapists, and other parents—to make predictions about their child.

These are understandable and normal ways of coping with the diagnosis, but each of them has pitfalls. As an example, you may spend so much time searching for answers on the Internet that your relationship with your spouse begins to suffer. Or you may find unreliable hope in a remedy found online that will cost your family lots of money and disappointment.

This journey isn't easy, and it's different for everyone. But we all face fears and even guilt, and these lead us to try to do whatever we can to help our children. Be easy on yourself, and if you feel you have been pushing too hard, know that it's ok. As parents we do the best we can with what we know, understand, and realize at any given time. Those of you who are feeling out of balance may find the following list of insights and tips helpful in thinking about how to approach caring for your child:

1. *Pay attention to how much intellectual and personal energy you are spending finding answers for your child.* Be sure to carve out times during the day to simply be with your child, other family members, or spouse without thinking about CP or without focusing on how your child is moving, speaking, walking, etc.

2. *Don't sacrifice reason and good sense to help your child.* Before trying a

new therapy, make a list of the sacrifices the treatment will require you and your family to make. Weigh the emotional and financial costs and the physical, safety, and unknown risks the treatment will present against the possible benefits for your child. Remember that a treatment without any known risks is not necessarily risk free. Discuss these issues with your child's medical team and other people you trust. Set time commitment and financial limits and discuss expectations.

3. *Your child will have his or her own developmental timeline.* When you compare your child with same-aged peers, you may subliminally approach your child with disappointment, and your child may perceive this as meaning she or he is doing something wrong. Focus on the positive points, the things that are working and the small, incremental steps that lead to putting larger developmental pieces together.

4. *Assess and honor your child's physical and cognitive energy limits each day.* These may change daily. You know your child best. Don't be afraid to speak up if you think what is best for your child is different from what the experts advise.

5. *Be aware of what is driving your approach to your child's therapy or developmental support program.* Be honest with yourself and look out for guilt, fear, and hopelessness, which may be motivating you to push your child and other family members in unhealthy ways. For many parents the realization that one's motivations may not align with what is best for one's child is part of the emotional journey that is a necessary step on the way to accepting the CP diagnosis. Remember, it's your child who ultimately has to participate in the therapy and integrate all of the information that comes from your therapy planning. Looking back, I understand that I was driven to find better ways of helping my child because accepting the status quo wasn't equating with the progress I envisioned. I felt that I couldn't stand idly by, watching and waiting. I had to do whatever I could to potentially make her path easier.

6. *Creating a balanced schedule becomes easier as your child's developmental picture becomes clearer.* Over time, as you and your professional team have a chance to observe your child, you will have a better understanding of how to focus your time and which therapies and treatments work best for your child.

7. *Focus on what your child does well and what he or she likes.* Integrate interests with opportunities for development. Maya loves horseback riding, and because it doesn't feel like therapy to her, it provides both enjoyment and therapeutic benefit. The riding facility we go to compares therapeutic horseback riding to sneaking broccoli into cookies, and I couldn't agree more!

8. *There is no secret cure for CP, and when there is a major treatment breakthrough it won't be a secret.* I am not discouraging you from trying to create a program that works for your child, but just be sure to give other aspects of your life and your child's life attention as well.

Over the past eight years it has become much easier to accept that my daughter has a disability. I now spend much less of my time and energy thinking about how to make her CP symptoms go away and focus more on helping her plan and achieve her individual goals in a time frame that is best for her. I feel optimistic and hopeful rather than hurried and guilty. I look for smaller developmental changes, still hoping for the larger ones but perhaps not counting on them. I celebrate her triumphs with her. We spend much more time laughing and having fun. Looking back, I cannot say that I would have approached her diagnoses differently, but I wish I had chosen an easier route. I believe that in order for me to arrive at the place of acceptance where I am now, I had to experience and accept the limits of my power. I learned to accept what I reasonably could not change, yet I still remain open to and hopeful for new possibilities and technology that may increase my daughter's participation in life. To my surprise, I also learned that often my daughter will spontaneously put together new skills during prolonged breaks from therapy, at times when we are focused on enjoying life instead of obsessively tuning into things such as how she is using her hands or holding her head.

Coming to terms with a diagnosis like CP is not always about grief. Sometimes it's about celebrating our children's victories and talents and making sure that they have the necessary support at home and in society to allow those strengths to come forward and be shared with the world.

MICHELE SHUSTERMAN, parent of a child with CP and founder of the resource website and blog *CP Daily Living*

For a parent or a primary caregiver of a special needs child, the to-do list never ends. If anything, it just gets longer. But it will get easier. Staying organized and having good communication with all the care providers involved will make life easier and save you time. I find it very handy to have an agenda. There is an administration behind every special needs child. You will become the advocate, secretary, social worker, nurse, lawyer, driver, therapist, and parent.

The circumstances differ from family to family. Some parents take their premature babies home after a long hospital stay. Some just never meet their milestones. Others may suffer an illness or an accident. All of these events will change a family forever. The unknown is never easy. Some families take longer to adjust, and others may adjust more quickly. Each special needs child is unique. Some may need skilled nursing support, some may not. Some need medical equipment, some just need extra time for their care. Parents and caregivers adjust as they come to understand what their new future will be like.

As a parent of a special needs child I continue to learn. It took me two years to understand all of my child's needs. Maybe I just didn't understand, or I was not ready to accept, the future ahead of us. I thought that the things we were going through were normal. This was life as a parent of a child with cerebral palsy. One day, after an ER visit, I got a call from a physician. He asked how my child's hospital visit had been. I said I didn't understand why we had to see so many residents.

He was kind enough to explain to me that my child was considered medically complex and what that meant to the medical community. My child was a challenge and a learning experience for any doctor. My early memories are of his neurologist telling me that my best resources would be other parents. He was right.

Ten years later I have seen the evolution from doctors caring for my child to me caring for my child. The communication has changed for both of us. I am more knowledgeable, and I now understand medical terminology. You will learn not to panic or think you can't manage. Now I make a 48-hour schedule for treatments, make phone calls to the on-call doctor, and send e-mails out to his doctors.

Some children require skilled nursing care, which is determined by the child's skilled needs and by recommendations from the child's team of doctors. The number of hours provided vary from state to state and also from case to case. For some families, nursing must be in place before the child is discharged from the hospital. You may need more than one agency to cover all the hours and shifts. The agency will give your child a case manager, who will be a great support person for you and your child. The case manager will also follow up on all the doctors' orders. It is crucial that everyone providing care follows the same care plan. Health care providers supplied by an agency have basic skills. They are licensed and certified. It is the agencies they work for that must check their credentials, certifications, and training. A parent cannot give medical orders to the nurses. Nurses can only follow direct orders from the doctor. If a specific care plan needs to be changed, either a follow-up visit with the doctor or a phone call must take place so that the doctor can order the changes to the care plan. Nurses cannot provide care that is not specified in the care plan. However, you as the primary caregiver can educate the nursing staff about the child's home routine.

With home care, it takes time to find the right people. Keep in mind that you need a team of people and the right staff to care for your loved one. It's very important that families treat the nursing staff as guests in their home. Families must be aware that their home environment is someone's workplace. Treat them with respect. Nurses know they are guests in your home and will treat your home with respect. Have a communication book that includes any information you may want to know, such as a bowel movement chart, a chart that all care providers, including family members, can follow. Your child will thank you. Give the nurses a chance to learn your child's routine. Sometimes it can take one person more time than another to learn your child's routine and schedule. Any person with a special need requires structure and a scheduled routine. This way they will know what is next and what to expect. If you don't have the resources for a big home, don't worry. Sometimes we can just move our children into the dining room. This will eliminate steps and put them closer to the front door. In case of an emergency, they most definitely will be part of the family. This will also keep all family members involved and not isolated. For privacy, you can put up a room divider or some curtains. Plastic cubbies can help keep their supplies organized, and you can remind people to put everything back in its place so that everyone knows where to find things. Ask nurses to let you know when supplies are running low and not to wait until you are out of something. This way you can reorder and have supplies delivered or picked up on time. Keep your child's bed in the middle of the room; this will relieve stress from always using and pulling on the same extremities. It is best practice to work from all sides. Most fractures for special needs children happen during routine care. Your child's doctors will help you with medical equipment. An electric hospital bed sometimes is a must. It can help to elevate a person's head and also help the care providers avoid back injury.

The primary caregiver must be the key person making phone calls, filling out forms and applications, and checking the mail for important documents. It's very important to keep letters with their original envelopes, and to keep copies of e-mails, and to follow up on everything in a timely manner. You should have an agenda—it will be very helpful to you. Use it for appointments. You can also use it as a log, as well as a place to keep important information, including all important numbers that you need for your child's care and needs.

Keep an archive of important documents, such as discharge summaries and doctors' letters that are important for your child's services. Make sure you are getting updated letters every year. You will need them for your child's services. Also keep your child's Individualized Education Program (IEP) handy. School papers are also very important for their services. It is also important to save your monthly finances and pay stubs.

Make sure you know what local governmental offices are located in your area; sometimes they are determined by your zip code. You may need services one day. Keeping all your documentation on file will help make any process much easier.

Look for nonprofits that help special needs children and their families. Insurance companies consider some therapies and equipment a convenience to the caregiver, and not a medical need for the child, and therefore won't pay for them. This is when nonprofits can be very helpful to families. Many of them have an age limit, either 18 or 21 years of age. Make sure you are familiar with your local Disability Law office; they are a great resource.

From one special needs parent to another: There will be times when your feelings will be at a crossroad; all your feelings are valid. Maybe you just need to step away and have a cup of tea. Or call a good friend. Our life is a roller coaster, sometime happy tears, worried tears, or I-just-don't-know-why tears. Share your story. Together we can only try to change the world. But we can definitely impact our communities and our local officials, from governor to senators and representatives in Congress.

Dedicated to my beautiful children: to my firstborn, Selene, who has walked this journey with us, and to Christopher, my sweet boy, who continues to teach me how it really is every step of the way. Never stopping, and believing that we all have the right to a life of Love, Dignity, and Respect.

NANCY LEMUS, Parent and Advocate

Some of the challenges experienced by a teenager and young adult with CP are well described by Josh and by his mother, who submitted the following about that phase of his life:

A Young Man's View
I'm Josh. I'm 24 years old and I have cerebral palsy. I have been living on my own for the past three years. Now that may not seem like much, but when I was born they didn't know if I was going to survive. I'm a fighter. I've had 12 surgeries and spent the first five years of my life seeing one doctor after another and physical therapists for hours at a time. It's been a long and winding road for me to get where I am, but I think I am going in the right direction. I've decided to tell you about the time of my life between 13 and now. It was a very traumatic and changing time for me. I guess the best way to start this narrative is with one word: *nothing*. Nothing is what I did between the ages of 13 and 18. I mean I went to school, graduated with a 2.96 gpa, and the only reason it was that high was because of my test-taking abilities. I never did any homework or studied. I got the grades that I got by paying attention in class. Now that I look back on it, I think it was a mistake. If I had done my homework, I would have graduated on the honor roll.

The events that have gotten me where I am started before I graduated. High school was mostly about being pushed around and called names by the other kids, dodging being thrown into lockers, and being called "tard." But my freshman year of high school I had a teacher for World Civ by the name of George M. Mr. M is a very unique teacher. He has since become the principal of that high school. He made me want to be in his class. I will never forget the day I decided I wanted to be a teacher. It was the day before my very last orthopedic surgery. Mr. M decided that before he started class we would have a party for me. So we're sitting there talking and eating snacks and I said to myself, "This is what I want to do. I want to make other people feel the same way I do right now." I can say that is the exact moment that I wanted to be a teacher.

Let's flash forward to my first year of college. I had just gotten accepted to a five-year program that would end with me having a master's in education. I wasn't ready for college. I decided I'd rather smoke pot than go to class. So I flunked out. Then I thought that I wanted to be an artist, so I applied to the School of Visual Arts for photography. I was accepted. When school started, I became very depressed. There were days when I didn't get out of bed until five in the afternoon. I didn't want to do anything. So needless to say, after two semesters I flunked out again. That was the end of my college days. My parents brought me home. I continued to be depressed and didn't know what to do with my life.

When I got home, that's when it got hard. My parents and I were not getting along, I wasn't doing anything, and I was just wasting away. At first I tried to work at a convenience store, but I wasn't able to stock the shelves or clean fast enough. Then I worked as a computer consultant, and I kept that job for a total of five months, when they told me they wanted someone with more graphic design abilities. I think that was just a nice way of firing me. My parents decided that I had to do something. So they insisted that I enroll in the local community college, and I stayed there and received computer certification. My mother drove me to and from school every day, and I did complete that certification. I was somewhat proud. But I still had not reached my dream of being a teacher.

That was when my parents and I decided that I couldn't live with them anymore. I decided to move into Center City. I come from a very fortunate family, and my parents were nice enough to help me with my rent. They have been helping me for the past three years. It seemed that the only way I was going to be able to find a job in such a big city was with some help, so I went to OVR, the Office of Vocational Rehab. Through OVR I was introduced to Liberty Resources.

Liberty Resources is a CIL (Center for Independent Living). At Liberty Resources, adults with physical and neurological disabilities are given opportunities that would otherwise be difficult to get—specifically, job training. A very large portion of Liberty Resources is called the Workplace Academy. It is a group of classes specializing in workplace skills and etiquette. Through OVR I was enrolled in a few of these classes. While I was waiting for these classes to start, I went in and talked to the director about what I could do to keep myself busy until I started my classes. She and I decided that I could do some volunteer work. I decided to ask her if I could teach. I explained to her that I have computer certification and that I would have no problem helping teach the computer classes they offered there. I've been volunteering at Liberty for the past seven months. There has been talk of a permanent teacher's aide position.

It may have taken me a while, and I've taken many different roads, but I think I am on the verge of reaching my goal of being a teacher and fulfilling my ambitions. I can only tell you that I think I've learned that it is important to take a risk in life. I have been fortunate to be exposed to many different people and things in my life. I guess you can say we grow when we grow up. I now work and help many people with many challenging disabilities. Sometimes I still get angry with people for not seeming to accept my cerebral palsy, but I now realize that is their issue, not mine. Again, I say take a risk and reach for your dreams. I'm still reaching.

A Mother's View

When Josh started middle school at the age of 13, he was full of hope and so were we. He was totally mainstreamed, which we had fought for because we felt he belonged in that situation. He was smart, intelligent, and very eager to learn. I should say that throughout his entire school years he was thrown in and out of special ed, mainly because of behavior and insubordination. When he liked a subject, his star shone brightly. When he liked a teacher, he did the same. He was a very sociable guy and loved to talk . . . and debate. He was small for his size, so he was constantly being challenged by bigger boys. He was a bully's dream. Because of his limp and his somewhat bent-over appearance, he was constantly the target and butt end of jokes and taunts. He came home every day after school either crying or complaining about something or someone. His grades began to slip and he stopped doing his work. All he wanted was to be accepted by his peers, and it was a very sad time for him and us. His usual gregarious personality became sullen, he never smiled any more, and we became worried about him. He was seeing a psychologist, which took the pressure off of us, but to no avail. Right before his thirteenth birthday and bar mitzvah, he had an emotional breakdown and was placed at Child Guidance Hospital for 30 days. That time caused much stress and fighting in our lives, for Joshua, his parents, and his siblings. After coming out of Child Guidance, he went back to middle school and again was taunted by the children. He was tripped in gym class, broke his knee, and needed to be in a cast for eight weeks. The day his cast came off, he was tripped again, and that was the last straw. I went to his school with my "dukes up," prepared for a big fight. We got no cooperation from the public school, and my husband and I decided to take him out of public middle school. He was in the eighth grade. We searched for all types of schools and finally made the decision to send him to a private school about 20 minutes away. The only compromise we had to make was that they insisted he repeat the seventh grade as he really hadn't done much work. We agreed. He really liked the school and started out doing very well. He was being academically challenged, but he was still acting out because he so desperately wanted to be accepted. But he was liked at this school, and we loved their philosophy. He was treated kindly and with respect and accepted for his differences. He was even on the school basketball team. He suited up and played sometimes. It was a great boost to his morale. He made friends and flourished. He was happy. And so were we.

Then he decided that he wanted to go to a public high school, and I feel it was the beginning of a great depression. He barely did any work the entire four years of high school. If he liked the teacher, he was fine. He battled kids every day who called him names and taunted him. He was thrown into lockers, bullied, and at times would act out in school. He did have some teachers who protected him; a few students too. After graduating he tried college but flunked out because of not going to class. We brought him home, and he signed up for computer certification. Loving computers, he succeeded and flourished. He had several jobs, but they didn't last, because he had a problem with authority. Finally, his cousin found out about a place called Liberty Resources, which is a nonprofit organization that helps people with disabilities function in the real world. It was a wonderful experience for Josh, as he loved the people there and they were willing to give him a chance. He took more computer classes and also classes to help him look for, get, and keep a job. At this point, he is teaching computers to other disabled adults and loves his role as a teacher's assistant. He is waiting to hear whether they will hire him permanently. A great lesson was learned here. If you persist and try hard, you can turn your life around and do something productive with your life, no matter what . . . we are very proud of the wonderful job and effort our son is providing for himself and others. Growing up for anyone has its bumps and peaks and valleys, but growing up challenged can also provide the person with a desire to succeed. Our son Joshua has done just that.

The next chapter describes the general patterns of typical pediatric development. These patterns provide a basis of comparison for parents whose child has problems associated with cerebral palsy. By comparing their own child's development with that of the child whose development is proceeding as expected, parents whose child has CP can sometimes be comforted by seeing that their child is developing along certain avenues just as he or she is expected to do. If, on the other hand, the child is experiencing developmental delays, parents can bring the problems to the attention of their child's physician, who can then work with the parents to determine the best course of action.

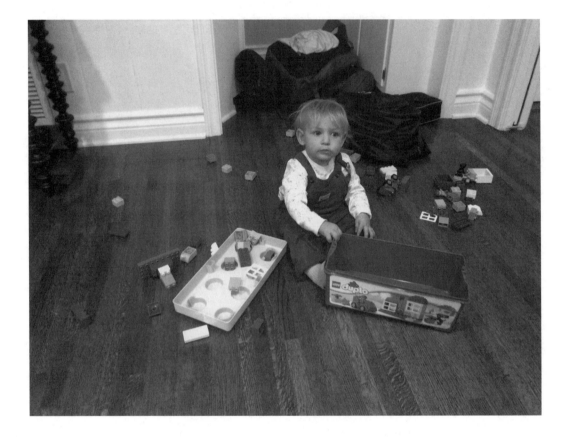

§2
An Overview
of Early Child Development

WHEN WE TALK about the changes that an individual goes through while maturing from infancy into being a toddler, a child, an adolescent, and, finally, an adult, we sometimes use the words *growth* and *development*. When we use the word *growth*, we are referring to an increase in physical size, but when we talk about *development*, we mean an increase in control over body movements. In this chapter, we will be focusing on this second aspect of the maturation process.

A newborn infant responds primarily in an involuntary, or reflexive, way to his or her environment, but over the next few years a combination of physical growth and learning experiences will enable the child to participate actively in the world. The child will learn to run, talk, and think creatively, and this development will occur step by step, in a sequential fashion.

Many parents have their own ideas about "normal development"—that is, what a "normal" child should do at any given age. This perception is based on common family experiences, on what the parents have read in parenting books, and on the advice they have received from pediatricians and other professionals. While most books caution parents about comparing their child's development with the "norms," it is only natural for parents to consider their child as either advanced or delayed according to their perception of "normal."

It's important to keep in mind that each baby develops in his or her own way. Although there is a sequential unfolding of developmental milestones, most parents, educators, and professionals who spend time around children know that different children develop at different rates. These developmental differences may be due to an inborn "inner nature," which is influenced by the environment in which the child grows. Clearly, however, there are some children whose development is delayed to the point where the parents begin to worry, and some children's development differs from the range of norms in a way that interferes with an orderly acquisition of skills.

The growth and development of infants born with disabilities or chronic or life-threatening illnesses may be erratic, showing normal patterns of development in some areas but not in others. It is at these points of perceived delay that parents need to become concerned, seek professional advice, investigate the problem, and, if necessary, obtain remedial help for the child. While their infant is maturing, it's worthwhile for parents to keep in mind some general principles of development. This will make them more likely to recognize when their child may need some help.

First, parents need to view development as a continuous process from conception to maturity rather than as a series of milestones. Before such markers are reached, a child proceeds through many stages of development, and as a parent you need to observe not only *what* a child does but *how* he does it. It is important to know that development depends on the maturation of the nervous system. No amount of practice or coaching can make a child learn a skill that his brain is not yet capable of directing.

While the *sequence* of development is the same for all children, the *rate* of development varies from child to child. For example, a child learns to sit before he walks, but the age at which different children learn to sit and walk varies considerably. Certain so-called primitive reflexes need to be lost before voluntary movement can develop. (In children with severe motor disabilities, these primitive reflexes are likely to persist beyond the usual age and may, in fact, impede normal development.)

Finally, the direction of development is *cephalocaudal*, that is, from head to toe. The child must be able to control his head before he can control the spinal muscles; ultimately he will gain control of the extremities as he progresses through the developmental stages and begins walking.

Remember that developmental "norms" are not absolutes. Your child may acquire individual skills earlier or later than other children. In children with cerebral palsy, neurological problems accompany the primary motor disability. In fact, many of the problems associated with CP (such as intellectual disability, communication or learning disorders, disturbances of hearing or vision, emotional problems, seizures, and orthopedic complications) have a greater effect on development than the primary motor dysfunction does. This does not mean that each and every child who is diagnosed with cerebral palsy is going to experience difficulties in all areas of development. Nor does it mean that your child, or any child with CP, will experience any or all of the associated dysfunctions. But as a parent, you need to educate yourself about delays in development and potential difficulties in various parts of the body and be ready to investigate if you become concerned. This chapter will help you do that.

What specific skills do children generally master during development?

Early child development involves gaining mastery of four major types of skills: gross motor, fine motor, communication, and social. Development in these areas occurs simultaneously to prepare the child to meet physical, social, linguistic, and emotional demands. Gross motor skills such as posturing, locomotion, and coordination require the use of large muscles to sit, crawl, stand, walk, and run, as well as other activities (table 1).

Fine motor or adaptive skills include manipulative skills, such as those used for feeding and dressing, skills that are necessary to interact effectively with the environment. Fine motor activities involve the use of small muscles in the fingers and hands in tasks such as picking up small objects.

Communication skills are the capacities needed to understand others and express oneself. Communication skills are both verbal and nonverbal and are used in understanding both simple and complex instructions. This area encompasses the development of receptive language, the ability to receive and process information and understand its meaning. Communication also in-

Table 1. Overview of Developmental Milestones

Age	Gross Motor	Visual/Fine Motor	Language	Social
1 month	Prone, lifts head	Hands usually fisted; stares at objects	Soothes to voice	Regards face
3 months	Supports chest in prone position	Grasps placed rattle; follows slow-moving objects with eyes	Coos/laughs	Smiles easily, spontaneously
6 months	Rolls and sits well, without support	Reaches and grasps, transfers hand to hand	Babbles; plays peek-a-boo	Fear of strangers; smiles at self in mirror
12 months	Walks alone	Pincer grasp of raisin	Says "mama,""dada," + 2 other words	Shy, but plays a game, gives affection
18 months	Walks up steps	Stacks 3 blocks; manages spoon	Points to named body parts; follows simple command	Helps with simple tasks; imitates play
24 months	Alternates feet on stairs; kicks ball	Stacks 6 cubes; turns book pages	At least 50-word vocabulary; understands 2-step commands	Washes/dries hands; helps get dressed
30 months	Jumps with both feet	Holds pencil in hand, not fist	Uses pronouns "I,""you," "me" correctly; states full name	Plays tag; asserts personality
36 months	Balances on 1 foot, 5 sec rides tricycle	Imitates block bridge; buttons	Recognizes 3 colors	Plays with children, takes turns

Source: Adapted from *The Harriet Lane Handbook,* 20th ed. (Philadelphia: Elsevier, 2015).
Note: It is not uncommon for a child to lag behind in one area and be advanced in another. However, there are generally accepted limits for what is considered "normal development."

cludes expressive language, the ability to transmit information. Social skills are the skills required to interact with other individuals.

What are some signs of developmental problems?

Significant delays in early child development are "red flags" that should prompt parents to discuss their concerns with the child's doctors (table 2). Significant delays in gross motor development include the inability to hold the head up securely by about age 3 months, to sit independently when placed in a sitting position by 10 months, or to walk independently by 18 months. Warning signs of fine motor problems include the inability to bring hands to midline (to center the hands in front of the body) or objects to the mouth by 6 months. A child who persistently keeps her hands fisted should also be checked. Babies generally pass out of the hand-clenching stage by 3 to 4 months of age. Persistence of this posture will interfere with both fine and gross motor development, and any child who consistently keeps her hands clenched should be examined for underlying abnormal neurological tonal imbalance.

Delays that are a cause of concern in language development include lack of babbling, making raspberries, or cooing by 8 months, no intelligible words by 15 months, and no two-word distinct combinations by 2 years. Any child with these types of language delays should be examined for problems with

Table 2. Developmental Red Flags

Milestone	"Normal"	Concern If Not Acquired By
Gross Motor		
Head up/chest off in prone position	2 months	3 months
Rolls front to back, back to front	4–5 months	6–8 months
Sits well unsupported	6 months	8–10 months
Creeps, crawls, cruises	9 months	12 months
Walks alone	12 months	15–18 months
Runs; throws toy from standing without falling	18 months	21–24 months
Walks up and down steps	24 months	2–3 years
Alternates feet on stairs; pedals tricycle	3 years	3½–4 years
Hops, skips; alternates feet going down stairs	4 years	5 years
Fine Motor		
Unfists hands, touches object in front of them	3 months	4 months
Moves arms in unison to grasp	4–5 months	6 months
Reaches either hand, transfers	6 months	6–8 months
Pokes forefinger; pincer grasp; finger feeds; holds bottle	9 months	1 year
Throws objects, voluntary release; mature pincer grasp	12 months	15 months
Scribbles in imitation; holds utensil	15 months	18 months
Feeds self with spoon; stacks 3 cubes	18 months	21–24 months
Turns pages in books; is steady cup drinker; removes shoes and socks	24 months	30 months
Unbuttons; has adult pencil grasp	30 months	3 years
Draws a circle	36 months	4 years
Buttons clothes; catches a ball	4 years	5 years
Language		
Smiles socially when talked to	6 weeks	3 months
Coos	3 months	5–6 months
Orients to voice	4 months	6 months
Babbles	6 months	8 months
Waves bye-bye; says "dada," "mama" indiscriminately	8–9 months	12 months
1–2 words other than "dada"/"mama"; follows 1-step command with gesture	12 months	15 months
7–20 words; knows 1 body part; uses mature jargoning	18 months	21–24 months
2-word combinations; 20 words; points to 3 body parts	21 months	24 months
50 words; 2-word sentences; pronouns (inappropriate); understands 2-step commands	24 months	30 months
3-word sentences; plurals; minimum 250 words	36 months	3½–4 years
Knows colors; asks questions; multiple-word sentences (tells story)	4 years	5 years
Social		
Regards face	1 month	1–2 months
Recognizes parents	2 months	2–3 months
Enjoys viewing surroundings	4 months	5–6 months
Recognizes strangers	6 months	7–8 months
Reciprocal games: so big, pat-a-cake	9 months	12 months

hearing. In addition, a young infant who is not easily startled at loud sounds, a 6-month-old who does not turn toward a voice, or a 1-year-old who does not appear to respond to her name when called requires a hearing evaluation. Questions or concerns about an infant's vision should be raised if by approximately 3 months of age the infant does not focus on a person's face or follow moving objects or people with his or her eyes. If a child has random eye movements (nystagmus), the parents should call the child's pediatrician.

"Red flag" concerns about social and emotional development are often more difficult to identify than physical ones because cultural, ethnic, and familial expectations about a child's emotional makeup and temperament vary widely. However, we can say that if an infant by several months of age does not smile when talked to by family or friends, that infant ought to be examined. The same applies to an infant who in the first six months of life appears to stiffen when held or is extraordinarily "unhuggable." Such a child is distinctly different from a motor-impaired child with tonal abnormalities; the latter is physically unable to hug, whereas the former is capable of reciprocating a hug or an endearing gesture but appears totally uninterested in doing so. Children generally enjoy making eye contact with parents and others with whom they are comfortable. A child at any stage of development after the first several months of infancy who cannot make or who actually appears to avoid making eye contact with familiar people should be examined for a potential social or emotional problem.

Concerns about developmental delays should be discussed with your child's physician. Depending on your child's age and other factors, several options are available, from a full neurodevelopmental evaluation to a watch-and-wait-and-see approach. Often your doctor can reassure you that your child's progress is within the range of normal development.

Birth to One Year

The first year of life is filled with advances in all aspects of development. Parents expect their baby to progress on to walking (or close to it), talking (one or more words), and semi-independence in feeding skills (introduction of cup, holding of spoon). For many parents of children ultimately diagnosed as having cerebral palsy, the first year of life may be the beginning of their realization that their own child's development "is not quite right." They notice that their child's progress is not exactly what their parents, friends, experiences with other children, or consultation with baby books have led them to expect.

What follows is a discussion of the first-year milestones, based on norms of child development. We do not mean to imply that your child's development should adhere to these norms. Remember, each child develops at his or her own rate, all the while following a sequential pattern. There is a wide range of "normal," from the very precocious child, who rolls over, sits up, crawls, and walks and talks at a much younger age than the average, to the child who does all these things later than most other children do.

The following discussion should be used as a guide, then, for becoming aware of patterns of development. These discussions may alert you to a problem in your child's overall development or to a problem in one of the areas of development, at which point you may want to discuss the problem with your child's physician. What follows may also enhance your knowledge of what your child may be capable of at a given stage, thereby helping to guide your interaction and play time with your child.

During the first four weeks of life (the neonatal period) the infant's gross and fine motor movements are primarily reflexive. That is, they are controlled by persistent automatic responses to situations and stimuli. The newborn baby lies primarily in a flex position (the so-called fetal position), keeps his hands in tight fists, and has little head control when held in a sitting position. Lying on his stomach, a newborn may be able to turn his head from side to side, and during the first four weeks he will begin to be able to lift his head briefly.

Newborn infants can briefly fix their eyes on an object in their line of vision (that is, an object held in the direction their eyes are facing). They focus best on objects that are about 8 to 14 inches away. It is not unusual for a newborn to sleep for about 75 percent of a 24-hour day. Newborns go through several states of arousal, including lying quietly, being intensely active, and crying—seemingly inconsolably—for what seem to be long periods of time. Infants can require as many as eight feedings a day, or an average of one feeding every three hours (but rarely is a newborn's feeding schedule so predictable, as any mother will tell you). Babies often don't seem to react much to noises when they are "sleeping right through things," but in fact most babies will react to loud noises by acting startled, or by changing their "arousal state." While it is difficult to describe a newborn infant's social or emotional development, it does seem that infants respond to human voices more than to other noises. And most newborns soon begin to show visual preference for a human face.

By the second month, or between 4 and 8 weeks of age, infants become more socially interactive. By approximately 6 weeks the so-called social smile emerges. Generally by the eighth week of life an infant will return a person's gaze and give the appearance of smiling or even of giggling. There are also significant developments in gross and fine motor skills. Specifically, when placed on her stomach, an infant of between 4 and 8 weeks of age can begin to lift her chin off a flat surface, so that her face is at a 45-degree angle from the flat surface. When the infant is pulled to a sitting position from lying down, the infant's head does not lag quite as much as it did in early infancy. The hands generally are still persistently fisted, but infants may begin to study their own hand movements (often looking quite "serious" while doing this). Eyes that previously wandered and occasionally crossed may appear to focus and in fact begin to follow an object briefly in a limited range.

Children between 4 and 8 weeks may be able to express distress or delight and be soothed by a familiar person's touch. Some children by 8 weeks will in fact appear to listen to voices and actually to coo in response (most specialists call this "pre-cooing," to distinguish it from the various pitched squeals that older infants make).

At 3 months, or around 12 weeks, the infant may produce a series of gurgling and cooing sounds. The baby's fingers usually begin to relax, and fisting is no longer commonplace. A 3-month-old generally can make sustained so-cial contact in the sense of smiling easily and spontaneously, and barring any visual problem, an infant of this age can follow slow-moving objects. Some infants may in fact begin to recognize and differentiate family members from strangers. There is much greater head control as the infant is pulled up from a lying to a sitting position.

Placed on her stomach, a 3-month-old can lift her head and chest with her arms extended. Infants at this stage may begin to swing at or reach toward (and miss) objects. There is a general diminishment of the so-called primitive reflexes, and the infant may actually make defensive movements or selective withdrawal reactions. By the end of the third month, the infant's suck-and-swallow feeding from either bottle or breast is coordinated to the point of seeming effortless. Those who choke, gag, cough, and sputter, or who do not appear to have mastered their breathing and eating patterns, or who persist in making seemingly odd, high-pitched, or guttural sounds while eating should be seen by a physician.

Somewhere near 4 months of age, infants begin to roll (front to back, back to front). A 4-month-old will react to sound and may turn to a familiar voice; the infant in the crib hears her mother's voice, for example, and turns in her direction before she comes into sight. The infant's ability to follow movement visually in all directions should be more accurate and active.

By 6 months the infant's language has developed from pre-cooing to coo-ing and then to continuous vowel sounds. True babbling (vowel-consonant combinations expressed repetitively, such as "ma-ma-ma-mama") emerges. The 6-month-old may truly begin to show fear of strangers and appear shy. In addition, a personality emerges, as the baby begins to show likes and dislikes for certain positions, sounds, and foods (by now most children will have added cereals and various purees to bottle or breast).

By 7 months most infants can bear some weight on their legs when held up-right, should be able to sit without support, and may even be able to pull them-selves to a standing position from sitting, as well as get into a sitting position from the stomach. At this age, a child may try to grab a toy that is placed out of reach, hold a block or rattle in one hand, and rake up small objects such as raisins with his fist. An infant between 7 and 8 months is able to grasp objects with his thumb and forefinger and to "isolate his forefinger," meaning that he can poke at objects with his index finger.

The infant may begin to crawl at this age, as she pulls herself forward with her hands and slithers on her belly, pulls up on her knees to crawl, or moves forward in some modified style, often called "commando crawling" (since it imitates the movement of a soldier crawling on his arms in a crouched posi-tion). By 9 months the infant begins to play games such as pat-a-cake or wav-ing bye-bye.

An infant between 7 and 8 months of age should definitely be able to turn in the direction of a loved one's voice and may begin to respond to the sound of her own name. Language continues to be a progression of repetitive consonant-vowel sounds, and distinct "mamas" and "dadas" begin to be heard, although not necessarily referring to the child's mother or father. By 8 months most children look for a dropped object by playing "over-the-edge," and many infants of this age begin throwing things off the highchair. An infant between 7 and 8 months of age may truly begin to develop "stranger anxiety," although this aversion to strangers may in fact have been surfacing for several months.

By 10 months an infant's gross motor development should include crawling backward and forward using reciprocal movements; assuming the sitting position and sitting with the back straight; and pulling himself up to a standing position. There are certainly 10-month-olds who can stand with or without support, and there are children who by the end of the tenth month stand with little support. Infants at this age also tend to explore in a poking fashion, beginning to master what developmental specialists call the "pincer grasp," in which the thumb and index finger meet in a way that allows significant control of an object.

At 10 months, infants are interested in fitting things together, and some may enjoy splashing in water and messing up their food. Searching for hidden objects, enjoying peek-a-boo and pat-a-cake games, and inviting a parent or other friendly person to play are all characteristic of a 10-month-old. The baby's language continues to progress, perhaps to the point where the baby can say "dada" or "mama" discriminately and understand the word "no" (although she may choose not to obey it).

By the end of the first year of life most infants can stand alone, and most take a step or two without holding on to anything for support. Many 1-year-olds walk in some combination of standing, "cruising" along furniture, and taking independent steps. Reaching becomes much more accurate as a child searches for objects that are farther away. Objects held in the two hands can be brought together purposefully (banging cymbals, for example), and the infant can purposefully release an object from his grasp.

At age 1 the infant begins to distinguish himself as separate from others (matching objects that are his), seek approval and avoid disapproval, and most likely understand the meaning of "no" more fully. Some 12-month-olds also cooperate in dressing and understand a one-step command when it is accompanied by a gesture such as "Give me that toy." Spoken language at a year is highly variable and may include "mama" and "dada" as well as one or two other single words. One-year-olds freely show affection and also show attachment to favorite objects, such as stuffed animals or blankets.

How may the development of a child with cerebral palsy differ from this?

Developmental delays are anticipated for the child with CP. These are perhaps most easily recognized when the child does not reach milestones when expected. The child with cerebral palsy most often does not accomplish gross motor tasks at the same rate as the child without CP. Differences in the pattern of movement may be seen as well. Due to increased tone, or spasticity, a child with CP may not be able to fully separate the movement of his head from the movement of the rest of his body, so that limbs feel and look stiff when he rolls, attempts to sit, or tries to walk. The child who is "floppy" or who has low tone may not be able to generate the forces necessary to hold his head up or roll in a smooth pattern. This child may slump when seated or placed to sit and may buckle or collapse at the knees when attempting to stand.

In terms of fine motor skills, small muscles in the hand that are used to manipulate objects are often affected by tone imbalances in children with cerebral palsy. In children with spasticity, or increased tone, impairment may begin at the shoulder, with the inability to extend the arm to reach for an object. The hand itself may be less controlled in fine regulation of movement, making it difficult for the child to reach and grasp. In children with an athetoid component, the "fine tuning" required to coordinate reaching, grasping, and releasing may be missing.

The child with a known or emerging hemiplegic pattern may prefer to use one hand over the other. Parents may think that their child is a "lefty," when in fact the function of the child's right hand is affected by the cerebral palsy. Hand preference usually doesn't emerge until about 18 months, so if your child does not use both hands equally when he or she is younger than 18 months, you should mention this to your child's doctor.

Language development and problem-solving abilities are not necessarily affected in the young child with cerebral palsy, although language delay and intellectual disability do sometimes accompany cerebral palsy. You need to be aware of normal milestones and bring to the doctor's attention any behavior that is significantly behind what you perceive to be normal for a child of this age.

Many children with cerebral palsy are active and very social in the first years of life. A child with physical limitations, just like other children, seeks and needs verbal and physical affection in order for his personality and identity to develop. Visually impaired children, for example, often need more touching and verbal feedback than other children, since they can't rely on their sight to pick up a parent's soothing expressions.

You may find, however, that your child is less "huggable" and cannot return your embraces, but you shouldn't necessarily view this as your child's choice. A very small percentage of children with cerebral palsy exhibit autistic-like tendencies in the first year of life. These children appear to be in a "world of their own," neither seeking nor returning affection, eye contact, or social contact. This behavior should be brought to the attention of the child's physician, and therapy may be initiated to help stimulate the parent-child interaction.

Ages One to Three

The child entering his or her second year truly becomes a toddler, with significant strides made in the area of locomotion—getting around, walking, and "getting into everything." Over the next several years the child begins to develop a sense of self-mastery and tries to understand her "fit" in the world around her, composed of parents, siblings, and perhaps an emerging peer group.

Many parents describe the period between 12 and 15 months as one of the most pleasurable in the raising of their children. Language is beginning to emerge, a sense of curiosity is exploding, and the physical ability to get around has developed to the point where the child is truly exploring his environment. By 15 months, most children are walking without support (although they may hold their arms up, in a high position) and beginning to creep upstairs (and therefore need to be watched carefully). Fine motor skill increases as an infant is able to solve simple games, successfully nest, or stack, objects inside each other, and grasp a crayon with enough coordination to make a mark on a piece of paper.

While the child may make known the vast majority of her needs by pointing and gesturing, many children 15 to 16 months old have a spoken vocabulary of four to six words. Often, parents describe jargon that actually has the rhythm and flow of speech, but with very few intelligible words. A 15-month-old can follow simple commands and should have a clear understanding of the concept "no." Socially the infant is much more available: he often hugs his parents spontaneously and reciprocates affection, either by blowing kisses or by responding to commands such as "give mommy a hug." Hiding objects and throwing them continue to be a favorite pastime as the child develops a sense of difference between an inanimate object and himself. The child also understands the concept of retrieving an object—although often it is the parent, not the child, who retrieves it.

The parent-child interactions that emerge at 15 months continue to develop as the child reaches 18 months of age, including hugging and reciprocal affection involving parents, siblings, and inanimate objects (the child begins to lug around her favorite doll or other toy). Children now are also more capable of feeding themselves (mastering a spoon and generally a "sipee," or spouted cup) and may seek help or consolation when in trouble and look to others for entertainment or amusement. Walking should be more steady by this time. Many 18-month-olds have mastered the ability to seat themselves in child-sized chairs, throw a ball in response to "Let's play catch," and make towers of cubes.

At this age, many children love to scribble (although in an imitative fashion) and prefer to use either the left or the right hand to do most things. Although hand preference may begin to appear at age 18 months, it usually does not fully emerge until about age 2. The average 18-month-old's spoken vocabulary is composed of 7 to 20 words, a mixture of understandable words and gibberish. Most 18-month-olds can identify one or two familiar objects by pointing to pictures, and they can identify several parts of the body. While it is somewhat early for the "terrible twos," 18-month-olds may begin to show their temper by either playfully or willfully refusing to comply with what a parent asks of them.

By age 2, most toddlers are very assertive and independent. While the terrible twos don't strike with the same intensity in all children, it is perfectly normal for 2- and 3-year-olds to refuse to comply with demands and to test the boundaries their parents have set. While this may be incredibly frustrating at times, parents need to remember that the child is becoming a person, with a mind of her own.

The 2-year-old has begun to run well (only infrequently falling), kick a large ball, walk up and down stairs one at a time while holding on to a railing, and open and close doors. His fine motor abilities have expanded to include circular scribbling with a crayon, helping to dress and undress himself, feeding himself with less spilling, and successfully drinking from a sip cup. Children of this age begin to be able to name body parts, associate use with objects, and listen to stories. They can identify more pictures. In terms of spoken language, the average 2-year-old has at least 200 to 250 words in her vocabulary and can form two-word sentences, although the voice pattern will be somewhat broken in rhythm when compared with adult speech. Most 2-year-olds begin to make known their toileting needs. Issues of toileting sometimes become a large struggle in the quest for independence.

As a child progresses to age 2½ , he starts to master coordination, including jumping up and down and walking backwards. Pencil or crayon grasp is also much more steady. Most 2-and-a-half-year-olds refer to themselves as "I" or "me" and know their first and last names. Spoken vocabulary starts to expand and may include repetition of simple nursery rhymes. Between ages 2 and 3, children become much more "helpful" (for example, they will help put toys away), and they demonstrate some imagination (they "pretend") when playing with objects or other people.

By 3 years of age children can go up and down stairs alternating feet, ride a tricycle, stand on one foot, and attempt to throw a ball overhand. Feeding is much neater, most buttons can be negotiated to the point of unbuttoning, and shoes and socks can be pulled on. They may engage in some simple tasks of body grooming, such as washing and drying their hands and imitating combing their hair. Three-year-olds begin to play simple games with other children. They should begin to know their age and differentiate between the sexes, count to three, and be able to use sentences of three or more words. Most 3-year-olds can name several colors and understand three prepositions (most likely *under*, *over*, and similar prepositions) and are extremely curious, asking endless questions.

Parents can expect 3-year-olds to have some awareness of a dangerous situation (they may say "That's hot," for example). By age 3, with some help, most children start to use the toilet, although the age when bodily functions are mastered varies greatly from child to child. In general, as compared with the 2-year-old, the 3-year-old is slightly more cooperative and eager to please. Sharing and turn taking become more acceptable.

Three-year-olds may be much more fearful than 2-year-olds, however, and may express displeasure at new situations. Many have difficulty separating from their parents at bedtime. Fortunately, most 3-year-olds can also better understand explanations for the cause of their fears. Their average vocabulary is somewhere between 800 and 900 words, with four-word sentences and the ability to tell simple stories and understand actions. By the end of the third year, as the child progresses to preschool, many parents say they have lost their "baby" and now have a "little person" capable of thinking and talking his way through situations.

My toddler has CP. How might his development differ from this?

Generally, children with increased tone (spasticity) experience delays in walking. A general rule is that children who sit unsupported by age 2 will most likely be walking (with or without braces or assistive devices) by age 4. Most "tight" children may appear to roll on time, or close to it (due to excess tone, they may actually "flip"), but then make no further developmental progress for many months, not crawling or pulling themselves to a standing position until well after their first birthday. Hypotonic, or "floppy," children may actually stand with support (they may cruise around the coffee table) close to the appropriate age, but they have long lags before developing enough stability in the trunk to walk independently.

In children with cerebral palsy there are often delays in small, or fine, motor development. In the toddler years, this is typically seen in their feeding and dressing skills. The child may not be fully able to grasp objects between thumb and index finger and therefore may have to rely on clumsier, raking movements to grasp objects. Holding a bottle may be difficult, and steadiness with cup drinking may be delayed or impossible. Both snapping snaps and tying knots rely on smooth, fine motor control and good hand-eye coordination, so a child with cerebral palsy whose control is affected may have difficulty dressing herself. The ability to grasp a pencil, generally in place by age 2 or 3, may elude children with CP.

Children with severe cerebral palsy also experience delays in language and problem-solving abilities. In the toddler years, such delays might show themselves in the child's limited vocabulary or in his inability to combine words into phrases or sentences. Children with cerebral palsy may understand what they are being asked to do but be physically limited in their ability to carry out these tasks. Thus, the child may appear dull because he doesn't respond, when what's really going on is that he is physically unable to carry out the task.

In standard IQ tests for the 1- to 3-year-old, much of the material involves tasks requiring the child to use motor skills and to perform in response to commands. The results of such a test for the child with CP may be misleading; for example, the child's language skills may be underestimated if his disability prevents him from forming words. We recommend that parents have their child tested by professionals who are skilled in interpreting results of "standard IQ" tests in children with cerebral palsy, with an emphasis on nonverbal performance standards. This kind of specialized testing may not be available in the school diagnostic setting. In this case, outside (independent) evaluation should be sought to obtain an accurate picture of the child's abilities.

The world of a 1-, 2-, or 3-year-old involves play and the beginning of social interaction. At first a child just plays alongside other children (this is called *parallel play*) or imitates what another child is doing (*imitative play*), but later on she will begin to play *with* other children, in *interactive play*. A youngster with a significant motor disability is physically unable to keep up with active toddlers and must be encouraged to persist in activities to help foster social skills such as taking turns and sharing. Circle games, storytelling, acting out characters, sing-alongs—all are examples of less physically demanding activities that can help the child with cerebral palsy, with or without cognitive limitations, learn social skills.

Are there any guidelines for toilet training?

By the time a child is 2 years old, most parents are anxiously anticipating the start of toilet training and the end of diapering. But a child must be temperamentally, physically, and cognitively ready to accept toilet training in order to have any success at the task. Daytime bladder control can usually be achieved by 32 months (the range is from 18 to 40 months), and bowel control by 29 months (with a range from 16 to 48 months). Most experts (and parents looking back on the experience) agree that the best approach to toilet training is a fairly casual, nonconfrontational introduction to the process. Indications of readiness include a child's ability to understand that he is "wet" or "soiled" and an ability to communicate this information, through gesture or word, to the caregiver.

A child probably cannot voluntarily control the functioning of bowel or bladder until age 18 months. Before that age, or for a child who is intellectually disabled, toilet training is more a reflexive act than a cognitive act. The child who is put on the potty chair will sometimes by coincidence relax her sphincter tone and produce a bowel movement, but this is very different from voluntarily directing her muscles to relax so she can evacuate her bowels.

How does a child's cerebral palsy affect toilet training?

Training the child with cerebral palsy may involve several difficulties. A child may be physically unable to sit on a toilet seat, for example, and therefore will have a difficult time getting urine or a bowel movement into the bowl. This problem is best remedied by using one of the many adaptive potty seat systems available. A physical or occupational therapist can provide guidance in the selection and purchase of these systems.

Many children experience a fear of losing a part of their body as they see their bowel movements flushed away. Although most children come to terms with this in a matter of a few weeks, some children continue to imagine that part of them may be "flushed away." This fear may be accentuated in the child with CP, whose unsteadiness on the potty may lead to falls. Unsteadiness during elimination can be very scary to a young child. To overcome this, usually all that is needed is reassurance by the parents that all is well and that they will not let the child be harmed or flushed away. A child with a persistent fear of toileting may be helped by a physician or a behavioral therapist.

The child with cerebral palsy and intellectual disability poses an additional challenge regarding toileting, in that the child may not understand the need to eliminate in a bathroom setting. These children often respond best to a program that incorporates "clock timing," whereby the child is placed on the toilet upon waking in the morning and half an hour after each meal every day. Parents can ask the physician or other health care provider to give them a detailed description of this method of toilet training, sometimes called *habit training*.

How do I handle my child's temper tantrums?

All children go through periods of having temper tantrums, most commonly in the second year of life. Most tantrums arise from frustration or the inability to communicate wants or needs through words and gestures. Some tantrums seem to arise out of the blue, apparently unprovoked, and may simply be a child's way of testing his parent's or caregiver's limits. Parental response to tantrums should allow children to regain their sense of self-control.

Physical punishment rarely has an effect on tantrum throwing. Physically punishing the child may bring that particular tantrum to an end, but the long-term pattern of throwing tantrums will not be broken by spanking. Rather, the parent should attempt to distract the child and get him or her involved in a more appropriate or more easily handled activity. If this fails, then isolating the child in a "time out" situation will usually be effective in sending the message that the given behavior is unacceptable.

Setting limits is accomplished by displaying a mixture of consistent disappointment in unacceptable behavior and praise for acceptable behavior. Rewards are also useful, as are behavior systems such as "point cards," which award prizes or special time once goals are reached. Rewards can serve as meaningful reminders to children that they *can* behave and they *can* stop throwing tantrums, if they want to.

How does cerebral palsy affect temper tantrums?

As a parent of a child with physical limitations, you must realize that your child is just as prone to temper outbursts and tantrums as any other child. Certainly tantrums may arise from a child's frustration surrounding his inability to be understood, especially when receptive abilities (understanding language) exceed expressive capabilities (speaking or communicating). Extra time may be needed to figure out your child's communicative intent—to "crack the code" of what he is frustrated about. However, escalation of behaviors to get your attention may cross the line into harm to self or others. You need not feel guilty for imposing appropriate limits on your child or for discussing intolerable behavior with him. Applying consistent, loving rules is the best approach when children act up. Should the child's behavior become harmful to him or to others, you may want to seek professional counseling for the child.

What about sleep disturbances?

One of the most sought-after developmental milestones in any home is the child's ability to sleep through the night. Almost three-quarters of all infants will sleep at night without interruption for six or seven hours by 6 months of age. When a young infant wakes up during the night, it is usually because he or she is uncomfortable—hungry, wet, or badly positioned—and needs someone to respond or soothe him or her back to sleep. In the second year of life, some children develop problems getting to sleep, often because of anxiety over separation. Setting routines and rituals (reading a story, having a regular bath time, drinking a cup of juice or milk) often goes a long way toward soothing a child with separation issues at sleep time.

How can CP affect sleep?

For children with a physical disability, fear of separation may be compounded by a sense that they are helpless to get up and reach their parents. Should your child's anxieties become intense, you may need to reassure your child that you check on him frequently while he sleeps. Because some nighttime awakening can be due to the need for position changes in children with CP (due to muscle tone imbalance), repositioning your child and comforting him may be helpful. Using an intercom or a baby monitor may be helpful, because it allows your child to realize that you will hear him and be able to respond should he need you in the middle of the night.

Should I be concerned about my child's masturbation?

Exploration of the body, including the genital, or "private," areas, is a natural, healthy occurrence in children of all ages. While many theories and cultural or religious biases exist to explain or condemn masturbation, most developmental experts agree that discovery of the genitals and manipulation of them for pleasure is a natural process, occurring in all children regardless of physical or mental limitations. Perhaps the best approach for parents of a young child (age 3 to 4) is to ignore the behavior. As children get older, they can be told that certain parts of the body are private and should be touched by them in a private place such as the bathroom or bedroom, not in front of playmates. Most children in the preschool years do not make the mental connection between masturbation and sexual pleasure. That is, they may touch themselves out of habit, perhaps as a way of self-soothing, but they are not consciously teaching themselves to achieve sexual satisfaction.

How parents react to masturbation in an older child is often colored by the parent's own feelings, cultural practices, or family experiences. There are no data to suggest that masturbation leads to or comes from perverted thoughts or is associated with sexual aggressiveness. Parents should discuss with their children the concept of taking care of bodily functions in private. In addition, parents should instruct children that there are inappropriate social settings for masturbation. If necessary, guidance can be sought from a pediatrician or a developmental counselor.

Ages Four to Six

Somewhere around the fourth year of life, children develop the ability to play with several children in a cooperative setting, and they are able to share with others more readily. The vast majority of 4-year-olds are toilet trained and can feed themselves and generally amuse themselves in a situation that is structured and supervised by adults. In terms of language, they are able to use plurals, different tenses (distinguishing present and future, for example), and opposites, and they can tell stories. Children at this age are capable of dressing and undressing with supervision and can copy simple shapes, draw stick figure people, and imitate simple block designs. The child can now throw a ball overhand or underhand and climb in a coordinated way.

A 4-year-old may be much more verbal about his fears, but he will probably separate more easily from his mother than will a younger child because he can understand that his mother will return. Four-year-olds are generally less eager to conform and please than children at 3 years of age because the desire to assert their own will reemerges, although not usually as strongly as during the "terrible twos." Four-year-olds tend to understand special friendships and seek out play eagerly. Language develops rapidly to the point where four- and five-word sentences are used, simple words can be defined, and stories are listened to enthusiastically. Many 4-year-olds can follow multiple-stage, rapid-fire commands, know at least four colors and the difference between night and day, and recognize some capital letters as well as shapes.

The 5-year-old can skip, kick a ball several feet, and run and jump. This is the age when children begin to ride a bike with training wheels. Five-year-olds can hold a pencil using the thumb and index and middle fingers (as an adult does), can eat with a knife and fork, and know how to spread butter. Tying shoes is still difficult for a child at this age, and the child may still reverse letters and numbers. The child's knowledge expands to include names of siblings (and often their ages) as well as the child's own address and phone number and basic colors and shapes. A 5-year-old's language may include five- and six-word sentences.

Social interaction is better developed. Most 5-year-olds want to be "good," and they actually seek adult approval. Small group play is generally favored, but 5-year-olds also enjoy "team" games and sports. Fears resurface: the child may worry about separation from his parent, lightning and thunder, or becoming lost. Generally, however, 5-year-olds "go with the flow" and can be led back from their fears with gentle reassurance, since they have the ability to understand past, present, and future and to understand that separations will not be permanent.

The seventh year of life, between age 6 and age 7, is often one of significant transition, falling between the preschool and school years. Many children at age 6 are easily excitable and tend to show off and act silly, with occasional spells of more mature behavior. The inconsistency in behavior is probably the result of trying to fit themselves into the tasks of schooling and new regimentation. Six-year-olds are ready to attend a full day of school but still need a good deal of physical activity to burn off excess energy. They are notorious for procrastinating but form friendships easily and readily take part in enjoyable activities.

Most 6-year-olds can describe how several objects are different or alike, begin to have an understanding of the concept of time, and know the alphabet. While a 5-year-old can count aloud to 20, a 6-year-old understands the concepts of numbers up to 10, knows all the primary colors, and understands simple money concepts. Gross motor skills are much smoother, as balance emerges along with true physical independence in purposeful activities. In the fine motor sphere, around 6 years of age the child begins to develop skill at grasping a pencil like an adult, although he or she will press fairly hard while writing.

Six-year-olds are generally independent in self-care and are able to handle simple household tasks. The average vocabulary consists of approximately 1,500 to 2,000 words, but the *receptive* fund of knowledge (words whose meaning the child understands, as demonstrated by pointing to pictures) may be much greater: 10,000 to 13,000 words. Language is now used in a much more social way, to include others and to express ideas, especially by children who have early school experiences and who have come to understand that words are listened to, while gestures are often ignored.

How might the development of a child with CP be different from this?

The child with physical limitations may have a hard time keeping up with the explosion of physical activity that occurs during the preschool years. Verbally talented youngsters with cerebral palsy may begin to express their frustration over this and may even begin to ask, "Why me?" Parents can provide alternative activities for the child, such as swimming, adaptive horseback riding, and participation in Special Olympics. Despite these outlets, the preschool child with CP may realize that his disability may restrict him from fully participating in activities. Bicycle riding may be difficult, coordinated self-feeding next to impossible, and handwriting unintelligible. Occupational therapists can help by recommending adaptive equipment such as computers and special eating utensils.

Daily living activities such as bathing and toileting may become more cumbersome during these years, as the child grows physically larger and may have difficulty positioning himself for these tasks. Bath chairs, potty chairs, home lifts, and van modifications are often helpful. Most gross and fine motor skill patterns are set by this time, so the aims of therapy are to maximize the child's potential in his or her environment through adaptive equipment modifications.

The child who had expressive speech and language delays prior to the preschool years may now obviously appear to be a slow talker compared with his peers, who tell stories and engage in more adultlike conversation. Children whose speech is hampered by tone or a difficulty in articulating words can learn to communicate more effectively during the preschool years by using a combination of signing and communication boards and computer-assisted devices. A common misconception is that a child who is taught sign or picture language will then "forget" how to talk or become too lazy to use spoken words. Actually, alternative means of communication often provide these youngsters with an avenue for expression, and this helps relieve their frustrations over not being understood. When the child is able to speak, the child's speech will progress along with the other means of communication.

At this age the sense of self, or identity, emerges, adding to children's security in themselves, their family, their school world, and their peer world. Children with severe motor disabilities may experience a sense of loss at their inability to mix with others and may withdraw or, conversely, act out. Parents can help their child feel as if she belongs by fostering a "can do" attitude regarding their child's desire to be with others. Children need group experiences in outings, scouting organizations, church groups, and elsewhere as they pass from preschool into the elementary school years so that the foundation for personal growth and exploration is set. Put more simply, a child with physical limitations should not be protected from or excluded from age or cognitively matched social experiences just because his parents feel he is different and might be sensitive to mixing with other, perhaps more able-bodied children. Parent support groups and other resources often offer suggestions for activities suitable for children with motor disabilities, and these should be explored. If summer camp opportunities exist, they should be pursued (even at this age), since they are usually nonthreatening for the child.

Ages Six to Twelve

As the child grows older, he not only matures physically but is expected to perform in a school setting. From age 6 to age 12 children attend elementary school, where they are exposed to the "rules of learning" and the whole idea of a social world outside the family and immediate neighborhood friends. Seven- and 8-year-olds are generally fairly anxious to please—they may even be somewhat perfectionist in this sense—and also fairly self-confident. The younger 7-year-old will be somewhat sensitive to praise and blame, concerned about right and wrong. A sense of humor in most children emerges by about the eighth year of life. Eight-year-olds are thought to have the capacity for self-evaluation. Participation in group activities, including team sports, becomes important, and participation in organized activities is often extremely important to this age group.

Eye-hand coordination improves at this age, and by 7 years of age most children have learned the days of the week, can tell time, and are beginning to think in concrete terms. Handwriting skills are perfected, and the child can now correct something that doesn't "look right" on the written page. Seven-year-olds generally read and write between the first and second grade level. Written letters may occasionally be reversed, although this mistake generally disappears by 8 years.

Adult concerns about the child's learning abilities begin to surface as school tasks progress from word decoding and basic addition and subtraction to actual reading comprehension and applying math principles. Any developmental lag as it relates to a child's ability to understand directions may show up as academic or behavioral difficulties in the classroom; such a lag may be simply a learning inefficiency, or it may be a true learning disability. In either case, it needs to be closely monitored.

The 9-year-old's language ability differs from that of younger children. True sequencing, such as day, month, and year, as well as ordering of information, can be understood by the 9-year-old. Simple multiplication and division concepts also appear to make sense to most children at this age. Balance and coordination have progressed to the point where the child can stand on one leg, play follow the leader, and play backyard games such as kickball.

Significant sex differences begin to appear in the tenth year of life, as girls generally begin to appear more mature than boys, with some girls beginning to show physical signs of sexual maturation. Most 10-year-olds understand rules and will follow them. Lasting friendships are formed that replace the earlier, temporary "play friends." Ten-year-olds begin to understand simple fractions, including parts of an hour, and are able to understand the concept of higher numbers and possibly begin to think in abstract terms.

The ability to think abstractly fully surfaces in the preadolescent youth (11 to 12 years of age). Preadolescents begin to reason through problems and situations, understand social and political issues, and perhaps even form an opinion on family matters. Preadolescents are joiners of groups and clubs. At this point in development girls begin to fall behind in physical strength, although they are generally taller than boys for the next several years.

How might the development of a child with CP differ from this?

The increasing hand-eye coordination that occurs in the school-age years may be significantly limited in the child with physical disabilities, and the ability to write legibly may be hampered by fluctuations in tone (increased or decreased) in children with cerebral palsy. Many children find the computer tremendously helpful in compensating for difficulties with writing. The computer may be especially helpful for the child with athetoid movements, for whom an adapted keyboard may make a significant difference in communication skills.

Differences in physical ability, particularly at team sports, become clear among school-age children. A child's self-esteem is often derived from his perception of how others view him. For this reason, children with cerebral palsy need to receive continued reassurance that they can master some physical activities. Even children with significant disabilities can engage in supervised adaptive aquatics and bowling and modified dance routines.

The child with hemiplegia has some unique fine and gross motor limitations that may become strikingly evident in the school years. *Hemiatrophy* (poor development of musculature and bone structure) on the side of the involved limb may appear more obvious as the child's growth spurt begins. The child may be unable to keep up in activities such as physical education, climbing, and throwing or batting a ball. Adaptations made for doing things (such as using Velcro or loops instead of buttons) may function well but may make the child self-conscious; she may wonder why she can't button her clothes. Sometimes it's helpful to buy the child clothes like those her classmates are wearing, explaining that hers are specially tailored for her.

Many children with hemiplegia can use their uninvolved side for writing and for performing most fine motor tasks, so the child can do most activities of daily living, such as dressing, eating, and toothbrushing, without assistance from parents. Subtle learning difficulties and true learning disabilities will surface during the school years. Parents need to determine whether the child is performing less well than expected because of anxiety (the child may be wondering why he is different, causing his attention to wander from schoolwork) or because the child might truly be unable to master higher academic concepts due to a learning block or disability. (A learning block may be global, meaning that all areas are affected, or it may be specific to one academic area.) The child may be performing poorly in school because she is intellectually limited compared with her classmates. Psychological testing can help sort these issues out, and more accurate class placement and utilization of special education resources help such children reach academic goals.

From age 6 to age 12, the child with cerebral palsy may perceive himself to be different and begin to isolate himself from social situations so he doesn't feel hurt when others make comments or exclude him from team play. These are the years when parents can have the most profound impact on the child's emerging identity. Frank discussion—being honest about the child's limitations—is probably best, although overpraising for a job well done can occasionally bolster a child's self-esteem. Even children with severe cognitive limitations respond to praise and reward and detect even the slightest amount of parental criticism or disapproval. For the child with cerebral palsy the school-age years may be a time when the family chooses to seek counseling or to re-activate themselves in family support groups to obtain new strategies to bolster their child's positive sense of self.

Ages Thirteen to Eighteen

The adolescent years are years of physical and sexual maturity and intellectual and social expansion. Increases in height and weight occur earlier in girls than in boys. The so-called growth spurt in girls may begin from age 10 to age 11 and generally is nearly completed by age 13 to age 14. In contrast, boys begin rapid growth between 13 and 15 years of age. Sexual maturation is a gradual process in both sexes. In girls, sexual maturity is accompanied by the growth of pubic hair, widening of the hips and pelvis, and development of mature breasts with projecting nipples. Boys grow pubic as well as body and facial hair, and the penis and testes grow and mature.

Along with the physical changes of sexual maturation comes the ability to produce children—the stage of maturation defined as puberty. Puberty in girls is defined as beginning at *menarche*, the first menstrual period. No such clear beginning for puberty is noted in boys, but most pediatricians would agree that growth of the testes in the scrotal sac and growth of the penis are signs that puberty has begun.

Gains in height, weight, and physical sexual maturity are only some of the changes that occur in adolescence. As every person who has ever been through adolescence, and every parent who has raised teenagers, will tell you, these years are among the most confusing for a young person searching for his or her identity. Psychologists have long considered adolescence a period of potential turmoil. From being completely dependent on the family, the individual begins to turn increasingly to friends, and the evolution of his own identity continues. All individuals, whether able-bodied or physically limited, can experience anxiety and mood changes as they try to make sense of their adolescent world.

How might cerebral palsy affect the adolescent?

Discussions of adolescence in children with cerebral palsy are few and far between, probably at least in part because the focus for many years has been on physical maturation rather than on psychosocial development (see Chapter 4). Some children with cerebral palsy experience precocious puberty, a hormone-induced early onset of sexual maturation. The child's body undergoes all of the aforementioned physical changes prematurely. In girls, breast development and pubic hair can appear at a young age (even in the infancy or toddler stages). In boys, enlargement of the penis and testes can occur at very young ages as well.

Signs of precocious puberty should be brought to the physician's attention so that underlying causes can be investigated. The changes of puberty normally occur under the control of the pituitary, or hypothalamic, and gonadal glands. The more unusual causes of precocious puberty include endocrine (hormonal) imbalance, lesions or disturbances of the central nervous system, and genetic syndromes. Generally, however, precocious puberty in the child with cerebral palsy is not due to a rare disease. In typically developing children, 50 to 75 percent of precocious puberty exists without other pathological findings. Perhaps the brain lesion or injury associated with CP also contributes to the disordered hormonal signal that triggers early sexual maturation.

While some children with cerebral palsy undergo precocious puberty, others may experience delayed sexual maturation well into their teens or early twenties. Some girls with CP never menstruate. The reason for delays or absences is unclear. The vast majority of adolescents with delayed puberty will, however, eventually achieve sexual maturation. In girls who have severe physical disabilities, the delayed or absent menstruation can be an advantage for reasons of hygiene. Generally, a major medical exam is undertaken only if a girl reaches age 13 or 14 without breast buds (breast buds generally develop one and a half to two years before the onset of periods). It may be helpful to consult with your child's physician as the teenage years approach. If necessary, a specialist in puberty, such as an endocrinologist, may be asked to help evaluate the delay.

Support groups, social activities with peers, and a supportive school and home environment can be crucial to the adolescent's emotional well-being. Counseling should be sought if suicidal, hopeless, or self-abusive or self-injurious behavior (including substance abuse) surfaces during this time. Parents may also experience much joy as they watch their youngsters turn into young adults. Praise for jobs accomplished, academic achievement, and exploration of new ideas is always helpful to a teen's self-esteem when it comes honestly from a parent.

Career counseling for potential academic pathways should begin early in adolescence. The teen who has cerebral palsy and good cognitive ability might be guided to a college preparatory academic curriculum or to job training such as apprenticeships. The teen needs to know that his or her physical limitations don't have to block the pathway to personal growth in academic or employment pursuits. For teens with cerebral palsy and some cognitive limitations or intellectual disability, emphasis should be placed on mastering daily living skills. Employment opportunities, including "sheltered workshops," can be offered to help the adolescent make the transition from a school to a work environment.

In this chapter we have seen the variability within normal child development as well as the variety of effects cerebral palsy can have on development. Most importantly, we have seen the marvelous uniqueness that is part of each child.

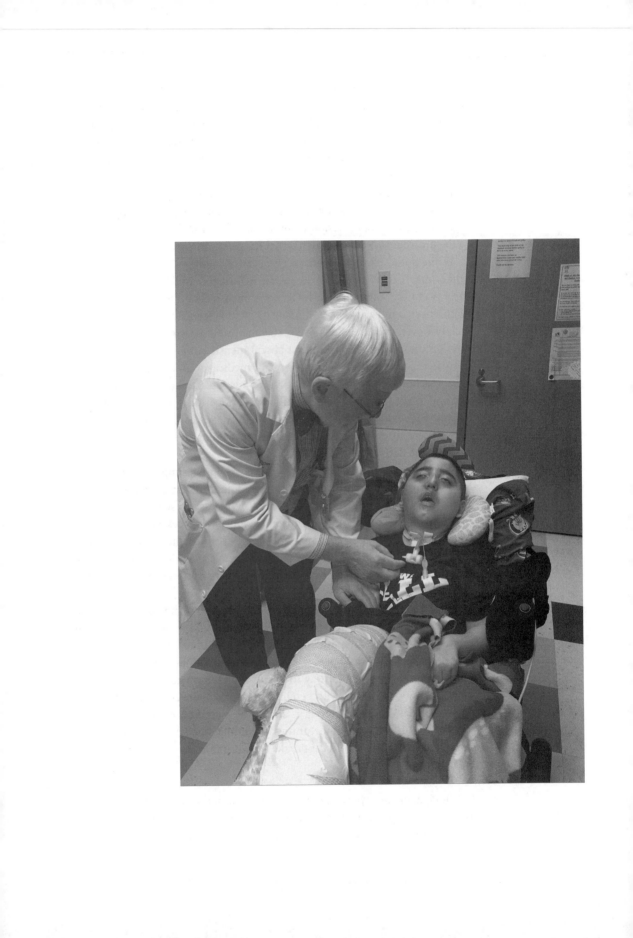

§ 3

Medical Problems Associated with Cerebral Palsy

BECAUSE cerebral palsy is a condition caused by damage to the brain, many of the other problems that children with cerebral palsy have are also neurological. Children with CP may also have orthopedic problems—problems that affect the spine, bones, joints, muscles, or other parts of the skeletal system. And they may have problems that are considered to be "secondary" to the neurological and orthopedic problems. One example of a secondary problem associated with CP is poor nutrition, which can be seen when the child with CP has difficulty in chewing, swallowing, or both.

For some children, the physical impairment caused by cerebral palsy will be a relatively minor issue. For example, for a child with CP who is able to walk and who has few physical limitations but has severe cognitive impairment, the focus of care will be on the cognitive disability rather than on the cerebral palsy.

In this chapter we consider the neurological and secondary problems associated with cerebral palsy. (The orthopedic aspects of CP are covered in Chapters 5 through 7.) Neurological problems associated with cerebral palsy include:

Seizure disorder / epilepsy	Behavior problems
Cognitive impairment	Visual impairment
Learning disabilities	Hearing impairment
Attention deficit–hyperactivity disorder (ADD or ADHD)	Speech impairment
	Feeding difficulties
Hydrocephalus	

The secondary effects of cerebral palsy include:

Poor growth	Sleep disorders
Poor nutrition	Upper airway obstruction
Aspiration pneumonia	Communication disorder
Gastroesophageal reflux	Tooth decay and gum disease
Fragility fractures/osteoporosis	Hernia
Constipation	Bladder control problems
Drooling	Poor temperature control

Primary Care Issues

What is the role of the doctor in caring for the child with cerebral palsy?

The primary care physician (the pediatrician, family medicine physician, internal medicine–pediatrics physician) is the doctor who provides preventive care and continuity of care over time, no matter how complex. The primary care physician should play a central role in caring for a child with a developmental disability such as cerebral palsy and should remain in contact with the family as the child matures through the years. Thus, the primary care physician should play the same role he or she plays for any pediatric patient. The child with cerebral palsy should receive the same care from his or her primary care physician that every other child does.

Why does my child need regular checkups if she is already seeing a specialist?

While many of the concerns related to CP (such as seizures and orthopedic problems) are addressed during a visit to the specialist, preventive care and other primary care issues need to be reviewed when your child visits his or her primary care doctor. The American Academy of Pediatrics (AAP) recommends preventive child care visits for health promotion and disease prevention at ages 3–5 days, by 4 weeks, at 2 months, 4 months, 6 months, 9 months, 12 months, 15 months, 18 months, 24 months, and 30 months, and then annually from 3 years of age until 21 years old. The primary care physician (PCP) follows guidelines for supervising the health of infants, children, and adolescents with cerebral palsy in many ways at each well visit. The PCP monitors physical growth and nutritional status (by measuring and recording the child's height, weight, head circumference, and blood pressure), assesses development and behavior (especially in areas other than the motor area, which is expected to be delayed in cerebral palsy), and administers immunizations, while providing counseling on such issues as safety and accident prevention. Also during these visits, the PCP provides vision and hearing screening, both of which are extremely important, particularly for children with an increased risk of sensory deficits, such as children born prematurely. If there is any concern about vision or hearing or medical risk factors for hearing and vision problems, such as a history of prematurity, the child should be referred for further assessment to a pediatric ophthalmologist for vision testing and an audiologist for additional hearing evaluation, regardless of his or her age. If there are no concerns, vision and hearing screening should start around age 3 or 4. If the child is unable to complete the vision and hearing screenings, the child should be referred to a pediatric ophthalmologist and/or audiologist. In addition, every newborn should receive a hearing screen, which often takes place in the hospital prior to discharge. (There is more information about vision and hearing testing later in this chapter.)

The primary care physician's role in providing guidance to both caregiver and child with CP evolves over the years and will be tailored to the family based on the child's abilities and needs and the family's care goals. The PCP can provide general guidance on parenting concerns such as sleep and diet. Providing parents of toddlers with guidance about accident prevention is most important. Behavioral issues gain importance for the preschool and school-age child, and issues involving sexuality and independence must be addressed for the adolescent and young adult. This role of the primary care physician has been defined as providing a medical home.

What is a medical home?

A medical home is not a physical place but a philosophy of practicing comprehensive primary care that addresses a child's medical and nonmedical needs.

Even when the child is being seen by various specialists, the primary care physician should guide and coordinate care, serving as the leader of the child's medical home within the office setting. The needs of children with cerebral palsy can be better met when their PCP uses the concept of the medical home. The medical home is widely accepted by many medical associations as the optimal model for delivering comprehensive primary care. It considers the unique needs of each patient and family and aims to maximize a patient's health outcomes through safe, effective, quality care.

The AAP believes that every child deserves a medical home, where care is patient and family centered, accessible, continuous, comprehensive, coordinated, compassionate, and culturally effective. At the center of the medical home is the primary care provider, who acts as a medical coordinator and helps facilitate care with other specialists and with therapeutic, educational, or community services the child may need. Having a strong, long-term relationship with the family puts the PCP in a position to help the family navigate the medical options and make informed decisions about their child's care. Families often have a hard time processing medical language and recommendations. The PCP who knows what the family understands is able to explain concepts in a way that helps bridge the gap in knowledge, enabling the family to make educated and informed decisions regarding their child's care.

The primary care physician remains an advocate for the child within the medical care system and provides continuity of care. Pediatricians care for children from birth until adulthood, often until 18 to 21 years of age, depending on the practice. Internal medicine–pediatrics physicians and family medicine physicians follow patients from birth throughout their life course. The PCP helps the family find an appropriate physician to transition care to, when needed. Regardless of setting, when a child becomes an adult (18 years old in most states), PCPs should transition to an adult model of care, according to which the patient gives consent for treatment and takes ownership of medical care, unless a guardian serves in this role due to the patient's cognitive impairments.

Many children's hospitals now have programs to help with transitioning pediatric care to adult clinicians (primary care and specialists), so the primary care physician may refer the child to a "transitions" program. As the adolescent approaches adulthood, parents must also consider preparing their young adult to leave home and begin functioning in the adult world. Many young adults continue living at home, but some people with cerebral palsy can achieve full independence. For others, a sheltered setting or an institutional setting is more appropriate. In addition to assisting with transitioning medical care, a transitions of care provider can help the family with life planning for the child with cerebral palsy, including the most appropriate place for a child to live. More information about transitioning care and adulthood can be found in Chapter 8, on the adult with cerebral palsy.

What is a care plan?

Every patient can benefit from a medical summary, also known as a care plan, which includes the patient's pertinent current and past medical history, as well as his social history. For children with cerebral palsy, the care plan should contain the names and contact information of all the subspecialists the child sees, current goals of care, and any specific interventions or medical technology the child requires. A care plan can also contain an emergency plan with detailed instructions for other caregivers should anything happen to the child's primary caregiver. At every office visit, the primary care physician should review the care plan to ensure that the information is accurate and that goals of care are being met and updated. While not specifically a care plan, families may find the MyHealth Passport, created by the Hospital for Sick Children in Toronto, Ontario, a useful tool for organizing their child's medical information. It can be found at https://www.sickkids.ca/myhealthpassport/. There are many different types of passports to choose from. Ideally a health care provider will help you create one. The developmental disability passport may be most relevant for children with cerebral palsy.

Should my child with cerebral palsy receive the same immunizations as other children?

Yes. In the United States today, infants and young children are routinely immunized against diphtheria, *Haemophilus influenzae* type B, hepatitis A, hepatitis B, influenza (flu), measles, mumps, pertussis, polio, pneumococcal disease, rotavirus, rubella, tetanus, and varicella (chickenpox). Thus, by the time the child has reached 4 years of age—whether or not the child has CP—he or she should be protected against all these diseases. Adolescents are regularly immunized against human papillomavirus and meningococcal meningitis and given boosters against diphtheria, pertussis, and tetanus.

Each year the Advisory Committee for Immunization Practices, a group of medical and public health experts, develops recommendations on how to use vaccines to decrease vaccine preventable disease in a safe and effective way. These recommendations guide the updated vaccine schedule, revised annually. More trusted information about vaccines can be found on the Centers for Disease Control (CDC) website. Families can find information about the vaccine schedule at http://www.cdc.gov/vaccines/schedules/easy-to-read/index.html. Many families find it helpful to review the Vaccine Information Statements (VISs), which explain the benefits and risks of each vaccine, before taking their child to be vaccinated. A VIS on each vaccine can also be found on the CDC website at http://www.cdc.gov/vaccines/hcp/vis/index.html. Any questions you have about vaccines should be discussed with your child's primary care physician.

The child with CP should receive all these immunizations, as should premature infants, and at the same age as other children. In addition, strong consideration should be given to administering the influenza vaccine each winter to children with CP, especially those who cannot walk. (Someone who spends most of the time in bed or in a wheelchair is likely to get sicker from influenza than someone who is up walking, because such a person doesn't breathe as deeply as an active person does.) If you are planning to travel outside the United States with your child, review the "Traveler's Health" page on the CDC website (http://wwwnc.cdc.gov/travel) and talk to your child's doctor to determine whether your child will need special immunizations for the trip.

Are there some immunizations my child with cerebral palsy may need that other children may not need?

Some children with cerebral palsy who are born significantly premature or have chronic lung disease, an anatomic abnormality in their lungs, neuromuscular disease, or congenital heart disease may qualify for Synagis in their first one or two years of life. Synagis is an antibody against the respiratory syncytial virus (RSV) that is given monthly during RSV season. RSV can cause a serious respiratory tract infection during the late fall, winter, and early spring. Your child's primary care physician can determine whether your child qualifies for Synagis.

Children with cerebral palsy who also have cochlear implants, chronic heart disease, chronic lung disease, sickle cell disease, or chronic renal failure or who are immunosuppressed may need pneumococcal polysaccharide vaccine (PPSV23) when they turn 2 years old. PPSV23 gives additional protection against other types of pneumococcal bacteria for this special set of children who are not protected by pneumococcal conjugate vaccine (PCV13), which almost all children receive. There may be other medical problems that PPSV23 protects against. Your child's primary care physician can discuss this with you.

Are there any vaccines that should be avoided because my child has CP?

No, unless your child also has uncontrolled seizures or a progressive neurological condition. By definition, CP is a *nonprogressive* condition. The vaccines previously considered controversial were the vaccines against pertussis (whooping cough) and measles. Prior to the 1990s, there was concern that the pertussis component of the DPT (diphtheria, pertussis, and tetanus) vaccine, which currently is not routinely used, contributed to neurological problems in some children. While a number of studies published in the 1990s suggested this was unlikely, a new form of the pertussis vaccine (known as acellular pertussis vaccine) , which was not made from the bacteria itself as the original vaccine had been, was manufactured. This new DTaP (diphtheria, tetanus, and acellular pertussis) vaccine has been found to have fewer side effects than the original DPT vaccine, including less frequent fever and febrile seizures. However, children who have uncontrolled seizures or a progressive or unstable neurological disease (a disease that is ongoing and causing loss of function) should not receive the pertussis component of the DTaP vaccine until a treatment plan has been established and the condition has stabilized, as recommended by the Advisory Committee for Immunization Practices.

What about concerns about the measles-mumps-rubella (MMR) vaccine and autism? While the cause of autism is unknown and is currently being researched, many physicians suspect that genetics plays a role. MMR vaccine does not. In a child who is somewhat debilitated or is bed bound, the risk from pertussis or measles (or any of the illnesses that these immunizations prevent) is far greater than the risk from the immunization. Any of these illnesses can result in hospitalization and, in severe cases, death.

There is a small subset of children who should not receive certain vaccines for other reasons, such as those who have a severe immunodeficiency, those who are pregnant, or those who have experienced a rare but severe allergic reaction (anaphylaxis) to a previous vaccine. The Vaccine Information Statement for each vaccine describes what disease the vaccine prevents, the benefits and risks of the vaccine, and why someone should not receive that particular vaccine or should wait to receive it. You should always discuss any questions you may have about vaccines with your child's doctor.

How is vaccine safety monitored?

The Vaccine Adverse Events Reporting System (VAERS) is a national vaccine safety monitoring program that collects reports about illnesses or adverse reactions that occur after a vaccine is given. The vast majority of reports describe a mild adverse experience such as fever, crying, mild irritability, or local reaction. You child's clinician can file a report to VAERS even if there is uncertainty about whether the vaccine caused the adverse reaction. By monitoring these reports, VAERS can help identify any new safety concerns that may arise and help ensure that the benefits of vaccines continue to be much greater than the risks. You can learn more about VAERS by calling 1-800-822-7967 or by visiting the website, at https://vaers.hhs.gov/index.

What are the provisions of the National Childhood Vaccine Injury Act?

In 1986 Congress passed a law that funds a program called the National Vaccine Injury Compensation Program to compensate parents of children who may have been injured by certain vaccines. The purpose of the law is to keep parents whose children were injured by a vaccine from having to go through the court system to sue an individual physician or manufacturer of the vaccine. Instead, the government pays the family for expenses related to the vaccine injury and loss of future earning ability. There are specific symptoms that qualify a family for compensation under this law if the symptoms occur very close to the time of immunization. If you believe that your child was injured by an immunization, you can learn more about the program and about filing a claim by calling 1-800-338-2382 or by visiting the website at http://www.hrsa.gov/vaccinecompensation/index.html. It is important for families to understand that reporting an adverse event experienced after a vaccine to VAERS is not the same as filing a claim with the Vaccine Injury Compensation Program.

Epilepsy / Seizure Disorder

What are seizures?

A *seizure* is a sudden burst of abnormal electrical activity in the brain that interferes with normal brain functioning. It can cause involuntary (uncontrolled) movements and/or behavior changes and a change in awareness. *Epilepsy* is a group of disorders characterized by recurrent seizures. Epilepsy is not a disease.

What causes a seizure?

In many cases of epilepsy, no cause for the seizure is ever found. Where causes are known, they may include the following:

- *Gestational.* Harm to the fetus by an insult to the brain such as a viral infection of the mother or bleeding in the brain of the fetus. Abnormal brain development can occur during this time.
- *Genetic.* A change in one of the many genes that control how neurons behave. Frequently, neither parent has a recognized history of epilepsy.

- *Metabolic.* Problems that can occur when certain natural chemical functions in the body are abnormal.
- *Infectious.* The aftereffects of *meningitis,* an infection in the covering of the brain or spinal cord, or *encephalitis,* an infection in the brain.
- *Traumatic.* The result of severe head trauma from events such as a fall, child abuse, a sports injury, or a bike or car accident. The injury can cause scarring in the brain.
- *Neoplastic.* Brain tumors, leukemia, or other cancers.
- *Vascular.* A problem with the veins or arteries in the brain.
- *Intraventricular hemorrhagic.* A bleed in the brain often related to prematurity.
- *Asphyxial.* A lack of oxygen and blood flow to the brain.
- *Toxic.* Ingestion of lead, alcohol, or other substances that are toxic to the brain.

Cerebral palsy is also associated with scarring or some form of brain abnormality, and all the causes of epilepsy listed above could also cause CP. Therefore, CP is often associated with seizures, meaning that both CP and epilepsy are often present in the same child, though either can be present without the other.

How common are seizures?

In the general population, the incidence of epilepsy is 0.5 to 3 percent. Among children with cerebral palsy, however, the incidence is approximately 30 to 50 percent. Epilepsy is more common in the child with spastic quadriplegic or hemiplegic forms of cerebral palsy. Complex partial seizures are the most common type of seizures in the person with cerebral palsy.

How are seizures and epilepsy diagnosed?

Seizures are usually diagnosed by health care providers who specialize in neurology, including neurologists (doctors who specialize in disorders of the brain), pediatric nurse practitioners, clinical nurse specialists, or physician assistants, though they can be diagnosed by any health care provider familiar with the condition. The diagnosis is based on the child's *history, physical examination, neurological examination,* and *diagnostic tests.* The *history* includes facts about your child's problems and condition. Information obtained about the seizure event includes the timing of the event, warning signs before the event, parts of the body involved, the child's awareness during the event, loss of bowel or bladder control, the length of the event, the presence of weakness on one side of the body after the event, the child's appearance once the event is over, the child's memory of the event, and the presence of fever or illness at the time of the event.

The history of the seizure is important as it may give clues to a *preexisting neurological condition,* a condition of the brain or the central nervous system (CNS) that was present before the seizure occurred. In a *physical examination* the health care provider observes, listens to, and examines your child. The *neurological examination* tells the provider how certain parts of the brain function. *Diagnostic tests* are performed to help the provider determine a possible cause for your child's seizures or the type of seizures.

What kinds of tests
are performed when
someone is being
evaluated for seizures?

Diagnostic testing can help make the diagnosis of seizures or epilepsy. The testing may help the neurology care provider discover whether there is a problem in your child's brain or a reason for your child's seizures.

An *electroencephalogram* (EEG) looks for abnormal brain activity by recording the brain's *electrical activity*, or the signals that go from one cell to another. Some EEG departments use video cameras to also record your child's physical activity during the EEG recording. The EEG is often done first when your child is awake and then when he or she is asleep. You will be asked to deprive your child of sleep the night before the test, for example, by keeping him up until midnight and then waking him at five. You will then be instructed to keep your child awake until arriving for the test. You will be asked to prevent your child from taking a short "power nap" in the car on the way to your EEG appointment, because this may affect his ability to fall asleep during the EEG. It is very helpful to record sleep on the EEG. Infants' and young toddlers' EEGs are usually scheduled around naptime, if possible. The parent is asked to bring a bottle if the child is bottle fed. The EEG test takes about 60 to 90 minutes.

Sometimes a longer tracing of the brain activity (lasting 24 to 72 hours) is necessary. In such cases an *ambulatory EEG* is performed during the child's normal waking and sleeping hours. The child is set up with the EEG and then goes home. When it is important to *capture* an event on a video camera while the EEG is running, a *long-term overnight video EEG* is done. It can be a single overnight test or last up to several days. Your child is admitted to the hospital for this test. It is important to know that a child can have a normal EEG (no seizure activity on the EEG) and still have epilepsy.

Brain-imaging techniques, such as *computerized tomography* (CT scan), *magnetic resonance imaging* (MRI), *positron emission tomography* (PET scan), and *single photon emission computed tomography* (SPECT scan) of the brain, to name a few, may also be used. These tests give information about the structure and activity of the brain. The CT and MRI show physical structures of the brain, whereas the PET and SPECT show metabolic activity in the brain. In children who have both cerebral palsy and seizures, the chances of finding an abnormality on the test are increased. The most common abnormality is cortical atrophy (or shrinkage) of the brain's gray matter. No specific treatment is available for most of the abnormalities that are found in a child with cerebral palsy.

The child's neurology care provider may order further tests, such as blood and urine tests, nasal and mouth swabs, lumbar punctures, etc., to determine the reason for your child's problem.

What are the different
kinds of seizures?

Seizures can be either partial or generalized. *Partial seizures* occur when the bursts of abnormal electrical activity occur in one part of the brain. If the abnormal activity occurs on the right side of the brain, you may see movement on the left side of the body. If the abnormal activity occurs on the left side of the brain, you may see movement on the right side of the body. Partial seizures can cause *motor* symptoms such as jerking, twitching, or shaking; *somato-sensory* symptoms such as a change in the way things look, sound, smell, or taste; *autonomic* symptoms such as becoming pale or flushed; or *psychic* symptoms such as fear, anger, hallucinations, or déjà vu (reliving an experience one had in the past). Sometimes after a partial seizure is over the child has a weakness of one side of the body that can last up to 24 to 48 hours. This is called a *Todd's paralysis*.

A *simple partial seizure* occurs when the abnormal activity in the brain occurs in one part of the brain but consciousness is not affected. Therefore, the person is aware during the event and can carry on a conversation but cannot control the symptoms that occur.

Complex partial seizures, once known as psychomotor or temporal lobe seizures, occur when the electrical activity in the brain occurs in one part of the brain but consciousness is also affected. No complete loss of consciousness occurs, however. Complex partial seizures can have all the symptoms that simple partial seizures have, but the child is also confused, disoriented, or unresponsive. The child may hear you talk but cannot answer you. He or she may be unable to follow directions. The child may move or wander around and mumble. After the seizure is over, the child may be aware that the seizure occurred or have no memory of the seizure.

An *aura* is a "warning" some people have before a seizure. It can be a smell, a feeling, a visual change, or something else. This aura is considered a type of simple partial seizure.

A *generalized seizure* occurs when the abnormal electrical activity in the brain occurs over the whole brain at one time. The entire body is affected equally (both sides), and there is a complete loss of consciousness. During this type of seizure the child cannot talk or respond and is unaware of his or her surroundings, and the child has no memory of the seizure afterward. There may be a loss of bowel or bladder control during this type of seizure. There are many types of generalized seizures.

Seizures can progress from a simple partial seizure to a complex partial seizure and then to a generalized seizure, but they cannot go in the reverse direction. *Absence seizures*, once known as "petit mal" seizures, occur for brief periods in which the child will suddenly stare, be unaware of where he or she is, and be unable to talk or respond. There can be *automatisms*, such as eye fluttering and movements of the mouth or fingers. These seizures can last up to twenty seconds. They can occur many times a day. The child always returns to his or her previous activity after the seizure is over, unaware of the seizure.

Tonic seizures cause the child's body to become stiff and rigid. There may be slight tremors or fine shaking. If standing, the child will fall to the ground. A *postictal state* can occur after this type of seizure. This is a period of time when the child may sleep.

Tonic-clonic seizures were once known as "grand mal" seizures. The child's body stiffens and then jerks in a rhythmic pattern. Breathing can become shallow during this type of seizure. If standing, the child will fall to the ground.

Myoclonic seizures are very quick, forceful muscle jerks that the child cannot control. They often involve the arm or face but may also involve the whole body. A myoclonic seizure looks like a quick startle. These seizures are not triggered by any type of event, such as a loud noise, light, or a sudden movement.

Akinetic seizures are also known as drop attacks, because the child suddenly and forcefully drops to the ground. The child then immediately gets back up. Children who have these types of seizures may sustain head or face injuries from the sudden fall, so it is recommended that they wear a helmet to lessen the chance of injury.

Atonic seizures result in a sudden loss of muscle tone. The child suddenly drops, or "melts," to the ground and is limp for a period of time. Children who have these types of seizures also may sustain head or face injuries from the fall, so it is recommended that they wear a helmet to lessen the chance of injury.

Infantile spasms are a rare type of generalized seizure. They look like a sudden jerk or startle. The seizure episode can range from a sudden head jerk to an episode that affects the whole body. These seizures usually occur in clusters and are very brief. They usually occur before 12 months of age, peaking at about 4 to 6 months of age. These seizures are a neurological emergency. There are three types of infantile spasms:

- *Flexor spasms* are abrupt flexing or bending spasms of the neck, trunk, arms, and legs. They are often called *jack-knife seizures* or *salaam seizures*. It looks as if the child is suddenly bending in half.
- *Extensor spasms* are the least common. They are abrupt extension or straightening spasms involving movement of the neck, trunk, arms, and legs. They are often called *cheerleader spasms*.
- *Mixed spasms* are the most common. They usually include flexion of the neck, trunk, and arms and extension of the legs.

What are epilepsy syndromes?

Epilepsy syndromes are a group of clinical features related to age of onset of seizures, seizure type or types, neurological signs and symptoms, and a family history of epilepsy.

When an epilepsy syndrome is diagnosed, the neurology care provider is better able to choose the best course of treatment (an antiepileptic drug or other treatment), describe how easy or how difficult it might be to control seizures in the child with epilepsy, and explain the expected outcome for the child. The provider can help the family with referrals to the appropriate providers, such as a geneticist (who manages children with hereditary conditions or congenital malformations) or a developmental pediatrician (who manages children with developmental problems), for additional care.

What can trigger a seizure?

Many factors can trigger a seizure in a child who already has a seizure disorder. *Illness*, especially when accompanied by fever, can cause an increase in the number and severity of seizures. It is important to treat illness as directed by your child's health care provider. *Lack of sleep* can be a triggering event for some people with seizures. If a child needs eight hours of sleep a night but gets only five or six hours for one or two nights, the child may experience an increase in the number of seizures. It is important for your child to get adequate nightly sleep. *Stress*, which can result in a lack of sleep, can cause an increased number of seizures a day or so after the event. Stress can be good stress (Christmas, birthdays, a trip to an amusement park) or bad stress (death in the family, divorce). The cause of the seizures may not be the stressful event itself but rather the lack of sleep that may occur during this time. For a small number of children with a specific type of epilepsy called *reflex epilepsy*, their seizures are triggered by certain *stimuli* in the environment. For these people, music, certain sounds, reading (rare), and flickering lights can be triggers. Nightclub and arcade lights, video games, television, amusement attractions, and traveling in cars (sunlight through trees, headlights) are common sources of flickering lights. These are only some of the common triggers for seizures.

These triggers are not the cause of your child's seizure disorder, but they can cause an increase in the number and severity of seizures in a child who has epilepsy.

What is status epilepticus?

Status epilepticus is described as a seizure that lasts 30 minutes or longer. It can also occur as a series of short continuous seizures in which the child does not regain consciousness between seizures. This is a medical emergency. *If your child has a seizure that lasts five minutes or longer or repetitive seizures (one after another), call 911 or emergency services in your area.* Rectal (into the rectum) Diastat (Valium) can be given for a seizure that lasts longer than 5 minutes. *The first time you administer Diastat to your child, call 911 or emergency services to have your child seen in your local emergency department for evaluation.* Any time you are concerned about the safety of your child during or after a seizure, call 911 or emergency services. Other medications that can be used for prolonged seizures are intranasal (into the nose) Versed (midazolam) or Klonopin (clonazepam) dissolving wafers, which can be placed under the tongue or in the cheek. You will need an order from your neurology care provider for one of these three medications, so you can have them ready at home for emergency use.

What is a febrile seizure?

Febrile seizures are seizures that occur in young children (from 1 month to about 7 years of age) who have an elevated temperature. These seizures are not associated with a central nervous system infection. They are not treated with an antiepileptic drug. The febrile seizure usually occurs within the first 24 to 48 hours of a fever, often as the temperature rises. They are more common in boys than in girls. Febrile seizures are not a type of epilepsy. However, some children with febrile seizures do go on to develop epilepsy in later years.

What is it like for the parents or caregivers when the child is having a seizure?

It is very frightening for the parent or caregiver the first time they see the child have a seizure. They may think the child is going to die. The more educated parents are about seizures, the better they will respond. They should be instructed that most seizures are over in less than five minutes. The neurology care provider will teach the family seizure precautions and first aid for seizures (discussed below). Most parents and caregivers eventually overcome their anxiety about seizures. It is important for the parent and caregiver to try to remain calm during the child's seizure.

What is it like for the child who is having a seizure?

The child may or may not be aware of the seizure, but he or she will not be able to control the symptoms. During a simple partial seizure, the child will be aware of the seizure, and he or she will have memory of the seizure after it is over. During a *complex partial seizure*, the child may or may not be aware during the seizure, and he or she may or may not have memory of the seizure when it is over. During a generalized seizure the child will have a total loss of consciousness and will be unaware during the seizure, and he will have no memory of the event once it is over.

The seizure itself is not painful, but depending on what type of seizure the child is having, the child may be injured. The child's reaction after the seizure ends will depend on how the people around him react during the seizure. To help with the child's anxiety about the seizure, it is best to teach the child about the seizures and what they look like.

How are seizures treated?

There are various options for treatment of seizures. *Pharmacological treatment* consists of antiepileptic drugs (AEDs), and *nonpharmacological treatments* include special diet, the vagus nerve stimulator, and epilepsy surgery. Some families have elected to treat seizures with *alternative therapies* such as herbal preparations and supplements. Medical marijuana is also being used for the treatment of epilepsy, but so far there is not adequate evidence that it works. The decision to treat should be made after discussion with your child's neurology care provider.

AEDs raise the seizure threshold by decreasing the electrical impulses of the cells in the brain to try to stop the seizure from occurring or from spreading. It may help to picture the seizure threshold as a brick wall: the medication builds up the brick wall (raises the seizure threshold) to prevent the seizures from getting through. The triggering factors for seizures (such as illness, lack of sleep, stress) can break down the wall (lower the seizure threshold), resulting in a seizure. The primary goal of therapy is to have complete seizure control with no medication side effects. If this goal is not attainable, then the secondary goal of therapy is to reduce the number of seizures, decrease the frequency of the seizures, decrease the duration of the seizures, and/or decrease the side effects of the AEDs. There are numerous AEDs that your health care provider can choose from when treating your child's seizures. Each AED will have two names. The drug company's brand name for the drug is the *trade name,* and the chemical name of the drug is the *generic name.* Your neurology care provider will try to treat your child's seizures with *monotherapy,* that is, by using a single AED. However, sometimes *polytherapy*, the use of several AEDs, is necessary. For successful therapy, the AED should be taken properly by following the correct schedule and taking the correct dose. Your child should continue on medication even when he becomes seizure free. Your child should never stop taking AEDs abruptly, because this can sometimes result in a sudden increase in seizures, or even status epilepticus. Your neurology care provider will provide you with further information about the medication your child will be taking. In addition, the care provider will tell you if and when it may be possible to slowly come off medication.

Depending on the AED your child is taking, he or she may need to get *blood levels* checked. This is the measurement of the amount of the drug that is in the body. It can take one to two weeks for the medication level to rise in the blood and then level off; this is called the *steady state*. AEDs have *peaks* (the highest level in the blood) and *troughs* (the lowest level in the blood). Drug levels are usually drawn as trough levels, first thing in the morning, before the morning dose of medication, close to the time of that morning dose. Peak levels are drawn when side effects are a problem for the child. The *therapeutic range* is the range of the level of the AED in the blood, determined during drug trials that gave the majority of people good seizure control with minimal side effects. Your child's medication dose may be changed depending on the result of the blood levels.

The *ketogenic diet* is sometimes used to help control seizures. This diet is a rigid, carefully calculated diet that is high in fat and low in carbohydrates and contains an adequate amount of protein. The amount of fat in the diet is usually three to four times the amount of carbohydrates and protein combined. This diet keeps the child in a fastlike state, so that the body burns fat, instead of carbohydrates (sugars and starches), for energy. A strict calorie and fluid intake must be followed when on this diet. Nutritional deficiencies (vitamin deficiencies) can develop in some children on the ketogenic diet. A neurology care provider and dietitian who are well educated in the diet must manage this diet. The dietitian will also be sure that the child gets the proper vitamins and nutrients while on the diet. You should never attempt to try this diet on your own without the help of the proper professionals.

The *modified Atkins diet* (MAD) is also used to help control seizures. It is still very strict, but not as strict as the ketogenic diet. Carbohydrates are limited, there are fewer fats, and there is more protein in the MAD than in the ketogenic diet. Proteins and calories are not restricted, and the family does not have to weigh foods on a gram scale, but it is still necessary to measure food portions and keep track of daily carbohydrates. Once the family learns the diet, there is less dietitian support. Nutritional deficiencies can develop in some children using the MAD. A neurology care provider and dietitian who are well educated in the diet must manage the diet. You should never attempt to try this diet on your own without the help of these professionals.

The *low glycemic index* (LGI) *diet* is the least restrictive of the diets to help control epilepsy. This diet is not used very often. The *glycemic index* (GI) measures how quickly a carbohydrate increases the blood sugar level in the body.

The LGI diet is even lower in fat and higher in carbohydrates than the MAD. There is no restriction of protein with this diet. The family has to learn how to balance meals in terms of proteins, fats, and carbohydrates. The family must have a good understanding of the glycemic index to follow this diet. Once the family learns the diet, there is less dietitian support, as with the MAD. And as with the other two diets that treat epilepsy, nutritional deficiencies can develop in some children using the LGI. A neurology care provider and dietitian who are well educated in the diet must manage the diet. You should never attempt to try this diet on your own without the help of these professionals.

The *vagus nerve stimulator* (VNS) can also be used to try to control seizures. This is a small device that is surgically placed under the skin and muscle in the left chest area with wires that thread under the skin and wrap around the vagus nerve, in the left neck area. The vagus nerve is a link to the brain. When this nerve is stimulated by the device, the stimulation reaches the base of the brain, which in turn can sometimes help to control seizures. The device stimulates the vagus nerve at preset intervals throughout the day. The family is also given a special, very strong magnet that can be passed over the device in the chest to give an extra "dose" of stimulation to prevent or stop a seizure.

Epilepsy surgery is performed in some people when all other methods fail. To be a candidate for this surgery, the individual must have a *focus*, a specific spot from which the seizures originate. Epilepsy surgery involves removing the part of the brain identified as the area that is producing the seizures. (See Part 3 for more details.)

Many people use *alternative therapies*, such as *herbal preparations* and *supplements*, to treat medical problems. A number of herbs have been labeled as being effective in controlling seizures; however, none are recommended for use in children. An important fact to keep in mind is that herbal preparations and supplements are also medications, and as such they have potential side effects. These preparations can interact with the body and with other medications the individual may already be taking.

What are the first aid procedures for seizures?

The main things to do when a child is having a seizure are to prevent injury to the child and to monitor the seizure. It is important to remain with the child during the seizure. It is also important to make the environment safe during a seizure by moving sharp objects and furniture out of the way if possible. Once the seizure is over, do not rush your child to stand up, walk, drink, or eat something until he is fully awake.

For generalized seizures:

- Stay with the child during the seizure.
- Gently lower the child to the floor if the child is not already there.
- Position the child on his or her side.
- Support the child's head so it is in straight alignment with the child's body. You can use a jacket, towel, small pillow, or your hand to do this.
- Do not put anything into the child's mouth (including a finger or hard object).

- Loosen any tight clothing around the neck, chest, and abdomen.
- Do not restrain the child.
- Move furniture and sharp objects away from the child if possible.

Once the seizure is over, the child may sleep for a period of time. Once awake, the child can resume previous activity.

For complex partial seizures:

- Stay with the child during the seizure.
- Do not restrain the child.
- Speak softly.
- If the child is walking, place your hands on the child's shoulders from be-hind and gently guide the child away from a dangerous situation.
- If the seizure becomes a generalized seizure, follow the first aid guidelines for a generalized seizure.

Once the seizure is over, the child may sleep for a period of time. Once awake, the child can resume previous activity.

For absence seizures:

- Stay with the child.
- Do not restrain the child.
- Reorient the child to the surroundings, if necessary, after the seizure is over.

Sometimes when a seizure starts, there is no way to stop it without special medications. Many physicians recommend giving Diastat (Valium) rectally if a child has a seizure that lasts five minutes or longer. The Diastat comes pre-measured in a rectal syringe. This medication usually stops a seizure within five to ten minutes. *Call 911 or emergency services in your area if the seizure does not stop with Diastat, if a seizure lasts longer than five minutes and you don't have Diastat to give, if seizures occur one right after another, or if your child has breathing difficulties once on his side.*

What are some important seizure precautions?

To keep your child safe, some precautions are necessary for the child who has epilepsy:

Water. Your child should take showers instead of baths if she is able and old enough. Be sure your bathtub drain works well. If your child is taking a bath, you must be present and watching at all times to prevent drowning if a seizure occurs (a child can drown in a half inch of water). When in the bathroom, your child should not lock the door. Your child should never take a shower or bath when home alone.

Swimming. Your child should never swim alone. Your child must have one-to-one supervision by an adult when swimming. If a seizure occurs while the child is in the water swimming, the adult should get the child out of the water immediately. Contact your health care provider if a seizure occurs while your child is in the water.

High places. If your child's seizures are not controlled, he should not be climbing in high places (rope climbing, mountain climbing, rock climbing, parallel bars, jungle gyms). If your child is playing on park equipment, be sure there is soft ground beneath and appropriate adult supervision. On amusement park rides, your child must be securely strapped into the ride and should not ride alone. If your child has active seizures, he or she should not go on high-risk rides such as roller coasters.

Heat. When cooking at home, be sure the pot and pan handles are turned inward, to the center of the stove. If your child is near the stove, be sure an adult is present. Your child should never use the stove when home alone. It is okay for your child to use the microwave. Be careful with hot or boiling water. At a campfire or a bonfire, be sure your child is far enough away from the fire so that if a seizure occurred, your child would not fall into the fire.

Mechanical equipment. If your child's seizures are not controlled, he or she should not be near or use electrical or mechanical equipment such as a lawnmower, electric saw, or leaf blower. Even children with controlled seizures should only use this type of equipment under the supervision of a responsible adult.

Horseback riding. If your child rides a horse, he or she must wear a fitted helmet at all times. Check with your health care provider before you allow your child on a horse.

Bike riding or skating. When bike riding or skating, your child should wear a fitted helmet at all times and should not perform these activities on busy streets.

Sports. Some sports have the potential for serious injuries. *Always check with your PCP or neurology care provider before your child participates in any sport.*

Other activities. If your child would like to engage in an activity that is not discussed above, check with your PCP or neurology care provider before allowing your child to take part.

Should my child attend school?

Your child should continue in day care or school if possible. Some epilepsy diets or medications may need to be given while your child is in day care or school. Ask your neurology care provider to help you get the proper paperwork for this to happen. In regard to special diets for epilepsy, the school staff will need to be educated about the diet. Your child's classmates, teachers, and school nurses can be taught about your child's seizures as well. If your child has a seizure at school, he or she can return to class when the seizure is over (if able), after resting for a time. A *seizure action plan* developed by your neurology care provider should be kept at the school nurses' office. The action plan will give specific instructions for the school staff to follow if your child has a seizure while at school.

Are there any changes in seizures during adolescence?

During adolescence there can be a change in your child's seizures. This sometimes happens because of the hormonal changes that occur in the body during puberty. Seizures may worsen during this time. In females, there may be an increase in seizures right before, during, or just after menstruation. In addition, the chemical changes in the body cause the body to metabolize AEDs more quickly as a child matures and becomes an adult. Therefore, as a child enters puberty, an adjustment in the dose of his or her medication may be necessary.

What health management is necessary for my child with seizures?

It is important for your child to get the necessary vitamins and nutrients. Your child should take a daily multivitamin with minerals while on AEDs. Preteen girls to adult women may also need folic acid while on AEDs. Your child should be on a regular sleep schedule and get at least eight hours of sleep each night. Your child should be taking his or her AEDs on a regular daily schedule. In addition, your child should continue regular routine follow-up care with your child's primary care provider. If your child becomes ill, contact your child's PCP. Contact your child's neurology care provider if you have any questions or concerns about your child with seizures.

What should I do if my child with seizures becomes ill?

All children get sick from time to time. They develop ear infections, strep throat, and other viral or bacterial infections. For the child with epilepsy, it is possible that seizure activity will increase when he or she is ill. Be sure to contact your PCP if your child becomes ill, especially if the child experiences fever, vomiting, or diarrhea. As already discussed, fever can increase the frequency of seizures. Vomiting or diarrhea can affect the absorption of AEDs.

Some medications, such as antibiotics and antihistamines, can interact with certain AEDs. Some may affect the absorption of various AEDs. Others may lower the seizure threshold in the brain. It is important for you to know which medications your child on an AED can and cannot take. If you need further information about the medication your child is taking for other medical conditions, contact your child's PCP.

If your child on an epilepsy diet becomes ill, be sure to get sick day instructions by contacting a dietitian knowledgeable in the diet or the neurology care provider who specializes in these diets.

Where can I get further information about seizures?

You can get further information about your child's seizures from your child's primary care provider or neurology care provider. You can also obtain further information about epilepsy and your child's seizures by contacting the Epilepsy Foundation at 1-800-332-1000, or check out their website at www .epilepsy.com. The website will be able to tell you how to contact the local chapter in your area.

Cognitive Impairment, Learning Disabilities, and ADHD

I've heard the term "developmental delay" used. What does it mean?

Developmental delay is a descriptive term that refers to a lag in developmental milestones in an infant or young child. This delay could occur in just one area of development, such as motor skills, which could be seen in a child with cerebral palsy, or just language skills, which could be seen in a child who has a hearing deficit. Alternatively, there could be a delay in all areas of development, including cognitive and physical development, which is known as *global developmental delay*. If a global developmental delay persists beyond age 4, a formal psychological evaluation should be conducted to assess the child's cognitive function.

What is cognitive impairment?	*Cognitive impairment* is a barrier to the cognition, or thinking, process. The term may describe deficits in global intellectual performance, as with intellectual disability; specific deficits in cognitive abilities, such as learning disorders or dyslexia; or drug-induced cognitive or memory impairment, such as that seen with alcohol or barbiturate use.
What is intellectual disability?	*Intellectual disability* is below average intellectual functioning as measured on a standard test of intelligence. It reflects deficits in cognitive functioning, or thinking skills, and adaptive behavior, or one's ability to adapt to the environment. Average intellectual functioning is measured by an IQ of 100; intellectual disability is defined by having an IQ below 70.
What are the different categories of intellectual disability?	There are four categories of intellectual disability. They are: (1) mild, defined as an IQ between 55 and 69; (2) moderate, defined as an IQ between 40 and 54; (3) severe, defined as an IQ between 25 and 39; and (4) profound, defined as an IQ below 25. Someone with mild intellectual impairment is considered to be educable, meaning he can go to school and learn basic skills, such as simple reading and math. Someone who has moderate intellectual impairment is considered able to learn a job that does not require a lot of thinking, but rather more hands-on skills.
What are the implications of these categories?	People with severe or profound intellectual impairment (about 5 percent of all those with intellectual impairment) cannot function outside the home. That is, they cannot hold a job or live independently, and they will need life-long supervision by their families or a residential facility or agency. Those with moderate impairment (about 10 percent of the group) can be trained to do a job (usually a repetitive, unskilled task) while under supervision. They can care for themselves with supervision and often are able to live in a group home with supervision. Those with mild intellectual disability (85 percent of the total) can live independently. Eighty percent of them hold jobs that don't require high intellectual functioning and can live independently. More than 80 percent of these individuals are married.
What are the causes of intellectual impairment?	There are many possible causes, including all the factors that can cause brain damage of any sort. They include (1) factors that are present prior to or at the time of conception, such as genetic disorders, brain malformation, or metabolic disorders; (2) factors that affect the developing brain during pregnancy, such as alcohol, infections such as rubella (German measles), and malnutrition of the fetus caused by medical illness of the mother; (3) factors at the time of delivery, such as poor oxygenation of the brain, trauma, or infection; and (4) factors affecting the young child, such as lead intoxication, severe nutritional deficiencies, infections such as meningitis, and trauma from an automobile accident or child abuse. For more than 60 percent of people who have an intellectual disability, no cause can be identified.

Is there a difference between intellectual impairment and cerebral palsy?

Yes, there is a difference. Intellectual impairment or disability implies an impairment of cognitive and adaptive functioning, meaning a limitation of intellectual capabilities. Cerebral palsy implies an impairment of motor function, meaning that use of the muscles in the arms or legs is impaired. Someone can have CP and have normal intelligence, and someone can have intellectual impairment but have no physical impairment. Since cerebral palsy is also caused by a brain injury, intellectual impairment and cerebral palsy often but not always occur together.

Approximately two-thirds of people with cerebral palsy also have an intellectual disability. One-third of children with CP have mild to moderate intellectual disability, one-third have severe to profound intellectual disability, and one-third have a normal IQ, meaning normal intellectual function. Children with spastic quadriplegia are more likely than those with hemiplegia or diplegia to have an intellectual disability as well. Even children with CP who have normal intelligence, however, are at risk for learning disabilities or attention deficit disorder.

What is a learning disability?

By definition, children with learning disabilities have normal intelligence but have an impairment or disorder in one or more of the psychological processes involved in learning. As a result, their ability to listen, think, speak, read, write, spell, or do mathematical calculations is impaired. This means that despite normal cognitive potential, there is interference in learning abilities in subjects such as reading, writing, or mathematics or in the skills necessary for academic performance, such as thinking, listening, and speaking. This interference is due to a dysfunction of the central nervous system. Learning problems are often caused by perceptual difficulties or difficulty in processing information.

What is attention deficit–hyperactivity disorder?

Attention deficit–hyperactivity disorder (ADHD) is a disorder of the executive function of the brain, which allows a person to focus and organize. It is a developmental disability that occurs in approximately 5 to 10 percent of children overall, but it is more common in children who have CP (or any other disorder of the brain) and in children born prematurely. It is characterized by inattention, distractibility, and impulsivity, and it interferes with learning in the classroom and results in low academic achievement. There are three major types of ADHD: predominantly inattentive, predominantly hyperactive and impulsive, and the combined type. Sometimes, however, the symptoms are a side effect of a medication the child is taking (such as phenobarbital) or manifestations of a learning disability, anxiety, depression, or neglect.

Children with ADHD may fidget with their hands or feet when sitting, have difficulty remaining seated, be easily distracted, have difficulty waiting for their turn in a game, or have difficulty playing quietly. In the classroom they may talk excessively, blurt out answers to questions before the question has been completed, have a hard time following through on instructions, or fail to finish chores. They may shift from one uncompleted task to another, frequently lose things necessary for tests or activities at school or home, and engage in physically dangerous activities because they have not considered the possible consequences.

Many children with ADHD have poor social skills, resulting in difficulties making friends, playing with others, and sticking to the rules while playing games. In the classroom a child with ADHD may act out and become the class clown because he or she isn't able to pay attention to the teacher and to the work at hand. Children with ADHD may be singled out as disruptive or lazy, and this may lead to low self-esteem. Similar problems can occur in the family setting, as the child's poor social skills interfere with interactions in the home. In a child with cerebral palsy, who may be unable to move around or be physically impulsive, even though the child may have trouble paying attention, the disorder can be missed.

How are learning disabilities treated?

The major focus of the treatment is to ensure that the child gets into the proper educational environment. Appropriate management of learning disabilities includes a comprehensive, coordinated approach to educational, parental, and child issues. Parents and teachers must not incorrectly perceive the child as lazy, stubborn, or incorrigible. Reaching a thorough understanding of the child's learning abilities and disabilities, as well as developing an educational program that fits the child's specific learning style, is of paramount importance.

How is attention deficit–hyperactivity disorder treated?

Modification of the learning environment is the primary treatment. The optimal setting is a highly structured environment with minimal distractions and considerable small group or one-on-one instruction. To help the child manage organizational difficulties, she or he can be taught management techniques such as regular daily routines at home and in the classroom; short, concentrated work periods; and the use of calendars and communication books.

Many children with ADHD may also be treated with medications. Approximately 80 percent of children with ADHD will respond dramatically to stimulant medications. These include methylphenidate (Ritalin) and its long-acting forms, such as Concerta, and dextroamphetamine (Dexedrine) and Adderall or Vyvanse (which are mixtures of amphetamines and include a long-acting form). Other medications, such as atomoxetine (Strattera) and guanfacine (Tenex or Intuniv), which belong to a different category of medication than stimulants, have been found to be beneficial to some children with ADHD. However, medication alone is not sufficient. While the medications help improve the attention level and decrease the impulsivity of many children, the child with ADHD continues to face many social and learning problems. Teaching him specific learning strategies to address learning difficulties and counseling the parents and teachers to help shape more appropriate behavior are important parts of management. An individualized educational program is vital for the child with ADHD or learning disabilities.

What are the significant side effects of stimulant medications?

Many children show signs of insomnia (difficulty in getting to sleep) and decreased appetite, with resultant mild growth delay. In addition, some children develop a tic—a rapid, repetitive, stereotyped movement. While it is not believed that the medication causes tics, the medication may hasten the appearance of a tic that would eventually have appeared. The appearance of tics may be a reason to discontinue the stimulant medication. There is concern that the stimulant medication might lower the seizure threshold in children with seizure disorders and result in more difficult seizure control.

Hydrocephalus

What is hydrocephalus?

Hydrocephalus is an enlargement of the fluid-filled spaces in and around the brain known as ventricles, combined with signs and symptoms of increased intracranial pressure. It is caused by an imbalance in the production and absorption of cerebrospinal fluid (CSF), usually brought about by blockage in the normal circulation of this fluid. If the normal flow of CSF is blocked, the fluid backs up into the ventricles of the brain. The brain continues to produce CSF, however, causing the ventricles to enlarge and put pressure on the brain. Unless this pressure is treated, brain damage can eventually result.

What conditions cause hydrocephalus?

Sometimes the channel through which CSF normally passes from the third ventricle to the fourth is not properly formed. This is called *aqueductal stenosis*. Sometimes tumors or congenital malformations block the outflow of CSF. There is also a form of hydrocephalus that results when the CSF is blocked from being reabsorbed. This can result from meningitis, trauma, or bleeding within the ventricles of the brain. (This bleeding, called *intraventricular hemorrhage*, is a common cause of hydrocephalus in premature infants.)

How is hydrocephalus treated?

To correct the damaging effects of the fluid buildup, a surgical procedure is performed involving placement of a *shunt*, or tube. One end of the shunt is inserted into the ventricles in the head, and the other end is inserted into another cavity in the body. The purpose of the shunt is to bypass the obstruction and drain the cerebrospinal fluid into a place where the body can absorb it.

The most commonly used body cavity is the *peritoneal cavity*, the space inside the abdomen. This space can accept the daily fluid production and absorb it. The shunt inserted into this cavity is called a *ventriculo-peritoneal shunt*, or V-P shunt. A less commonly used option is to insert a shunt into the *jugular vein* or into the right atrium of the heart to allow fluid to drain into the bloodstream. These are known as *ventriculojugular shunts* or *ventriculoatrial shunts*. Another option is to insert the shunt into the pleural spaces around the lungs. This is called a *ventriculopleural shunt*.

Another option for the treatment of hydrocephalus is to perform an endoscopic third ventriculostomy. This procedure creates an internal bypass, allowing the fluid to escape the third ventricle. It is utilized in obstructive forms of hydrocephalus.

How is the shunt inserted?

A shunt is implanted during a surgical procedure performed under general anesthesia. This procedure is well tolerated and can be performed even on newborn babies. Once the anesthesia takes effect, a small incision is made in the scalp and a small hole is made through the skull. The shunt tubing is inserted into the ventricles; for a V-P shunt, tubing is then tunneled under the skin until it comes out through the incision in the abdomen, where it is inserted into the peritoneal cavity.

A valve, consisting of a bubblelike dome, is usually connected internally, within the tubing, which allows the functioning of the shunt to be assessed periodically. This dome can be accessed to provide information about the function of the shunt. It can also allow the medical team to measure the intracranial pressure and to remove spinal fluid. "Pumping" a shunt has not been shown to provide any useful information and indeed has been associated with shunt malfunction.

What are the possible complications from a shunt?

Sometimes shunts become clogged. When this occurs, the shunt has to be surgically repaired or replaced. Symptoms of shunt obstruction include persistent headaches and vomiting, as well as changes in mental status or increased irritability. A shunt can also become infected. Infection may remain confined to the shunt tubing itself, but infection can spread into the nervous system, causing meningitis (infection and inflammation of the *meninges*, or membranes that surround the brain), which is a serious condition that needs to be recognized and treated promptly.

Even with the most advanced technology, shunts are prone to problems, and it is likely that one or more surgical revisions will be performed following the initial placement of a shunt. About 50 percent of shunts will fail within two years of insertion, and more than 90 percent will fail within five years.

Behavioral Issues

What are self-injurious behaviors?

Self-injurious behaviors, or SIBs, are repetitious and chronic behaviors that a person inflicts upon himself or herself in order to cause physical harm. Some common forms of SIBs include biting oneself; pinching, scratching, or pulling on a body part; striking oneself (head banging or face slapping); repeated vomiting or rumination (self-induced vomiting); and severe pica (eating nonedible substances such as paint chips or dirt).

Many of these behaviors can be seen in the course of typical development in up to 20 percent of infants and preschool children. Such behaviors as body rocking, head rolling, and head banging often appear at around 8 to 9 months of age and disappear under typical circumstances by age 4. These behaviors almost always disappear as the child develops more sophisticated means of communication and stimulation.

Do these behaviors ever persist?

In people with developmental disabilities, self-injurious behaviors may persist for long periods and can result in serious tissue damage. SIBs that cause tissue damage have been described in 3 to 4 percent of children under 10 who have developmental disabilities, in 8 percent of 10- to 15-year-olds with developmental disabilities, and in 12 percent of people over 15 with developmental disabilities. These behaviors are most common in people with severe or profound intellectual disability.

Some specific but rare disorders are associated with such behaviors, especially the *Lesch-Nyhan syndrome*, which is caused by a gene mutation resulting in a specific enzyme deficiency. In the typical patient with cerebral palsy and severe intellectual disability, these behaviors may start as self-stimulatory activities and then be reinforced by the attention they attract from parents and caregivers.

I've heard of behavior management as a treatment for self-injurious behavior. How does it work?

Behavior management strategies are the primary treatment strategies for children with SIB. They may be used in conjunction with education and treatment with drugs. The key to any behavioral program is positive reinforcement for desired behaviors. Reinforcement increases the likelihood that the desired behaviors will occur and decreases the likelihood that the undesired behaviors will occur.

All too often, parents and other adults respond only when the child does something "wrong." This reaction, even if it takes the form of a scolding, provides attention to the child. If attention is motivating for the child (as it is for almost all of us), the end result will be that the child will repeat the behavior to get more attention. In contrast, when a child is playing quietly by himself, a parent often chooses that moment to do a chore or make a phone call, and so the child receives no attention or reward for this "good" behavior. Young children and those with developmental delays most often do not differentiate between attention obtained for "good" behavior and attention obtained for "negative" behaviors; for them, attention is attention, regardless of the behavior that caused it. Thus, they are likely to repeat the behavior that got them attention, even if it was "negative" attention.

In a behavior modification program, good behavior is rewarded, either with verbal feedback ("Johnny, I'm so glad to see you playing nicely with your sister") or with a concrete reward, like an ice cream cone or permission to watch a special show on television. Alternatively, this positive reinforcement might come in the form of a token that can later be traded for a desired reward. In contrast, a child who is having a temper tantrum should be ignored (not rewarded with attention) as long as he is not hurting himself. If a child is banging his head, the parent may need to move him to a carpeted floor, but the parent should do this with as little interaction and attention as possible.

Aside from behavior modification, what else can be done to manage SIB?

Sometimes behavior modification is not effective in treating SIB, especially when the behavior is maintained by internal cues rather than by social reinforcement. A number of medications have been used to treat SIB, with varying success. Some drugs commonly used to treat other conditions, including oral medications and local anesthetic creams, have been used with some success to treat SIB. It is sometimes necessary for a person to wear protective equipment to protect himself or herself from injury. Such protective equipment should be used as part of a program designed to increase adaptive behavior. For instance, helmets can be used to protect the head when head banging or head hitting is likely to occur. Elbow splints can be used to keep the person's arms extended and prevent head hitting, eye gouging, and hand biting. Gloves, padded clothing, and goggles can also be used.

Another treatment of SIB is more controversial than protective equipment. This is the application of aversive stimuli such as bitter substances, water mist, or mild electric shock to the skin. The use of these stimuli was more common in the past, typically in group home or institutional settings. Currently, they are sometimes used to a very limited degree when the person's behavior has not responded to other, conventional treatments and the individual is at high risk for injury from the behavior. This approach should be reserved for only the most serious situations and used only after the techniques have received approval from an outside agency or advisory panel not directly involved in the care of the child.

Besides SIB, what other behavioral concerns may arise in children with CP?

Children with CP (or any neurological impairment) may be more likely to have problems controlling their impulses, as well as difficulties with focus and attention that may have an impact on language, learning, and developmental progress. Just as in typically developing young children, defiance and noncompliance are common in children with CP. If parents of children with CP do not develop an effective system for managing these behaviors early on, they can persist into later years. Finally, children with CP may experience some anxiety, which behaviorally can result in repeatedly asking questions about upcoming events (for example, "Are we going to Grandma's today? . . . what time are we going to Grandma's? . . . is it time to go yet? . . . are we going at one o'clock? . . . what time are we going to Grandma's?"). A thorough evaluation by a mental health professional (a psychologist or clinical social worker) may be helpful in assessing the child's behavior in the context of overall intellectual functioning, individual temperament, and parent-child interaction. This will help determine whether the behaviors being observed are under the child's control or are more related to the child's developmental level or an underlying neurological condition.

How can such behavior be managed?

The first strategy is to structure the environment based on the child's developmental abilities. This means setting consistent limits at home and at school and using rewards that have meaning for that particular child. Very often, working with a professional who has experience with behavior management plans, such as a clinical psychologist or a board certified behavior analyst (BCBA), is helpful as you try to come up with a plan that works best for your family and your child.

Some children require medication to help regulate their behaviors because they are at risk of doing harm to themselves or others or are missing opportunities for developmental growth because of their attention difficulties. As previously discussed, stimulant medications are utilized to maximize focus (and often decrease hyperactivity) by stimulating the area of the brain that helps in attention regulation. Other classes of medications act as mood stabilizers, helping to modulate a child's reaction to his environment, while others can be used to prevent outbursts or impulsive behavior that could result in harm, as well as stimulate social awareness of consequences to actions. The use of medications for behavior management needs to be individualized and should be discussed with a physician familiar with their use in children with developmental disabilities. Not all medications used for behavior management in adults can or should be given to young children, because of different side effect profiles. The goal should always be judicious use of medication to maximize developmental progress without blunting the child's personality and spontaneity.

Visual Impairment

What are visual impairment and blindness?

The term *blindness* refers to diminished vision. Total blindness means that the person sees nothing, not even light. Total blindness occurs rarely. The term *blindness* has been replaced with *mild* (20/40 to 20/60), *moderate* (20/70 to better than 20/200), and *severe* (20/200 or worse) *visual impairment*. The visual acuity defining the level of impairment is based on corrected vision and is determined by the eye doctor.

Legal blindness is defined as a visual acuity of 20/200 or less in the better eye after the best possible correction, or a visual field of 20 degrees or less. This definition is used by the federal government and other agencies to determine eligibility for federal programs such as Supplemental Security Income (SSI).

In terms of the educational system, a child with a visual impairment is one whose visual limitations interfere with his ability to learn. There is no specific level of visual impairment a child must have in order to qualify for special educational services for the visually impaired. Eligibility will depend upon the state or agency providing services.

What kind of visual problems do children with cerebral palsy have?

Nearly half of all children with cerebral palsy have *strabismus*, commonly called "cross-eye," or misalignment of the eyes. Strabismus causes one of the eyes to turn outward or inward and/or to have a vertical problem. Strabismus may cause the brain to shut off input from the misaligned eye, resulting in visual loss in the misaligned eye (amblyopia).

Children born prematurely with a low birthweight are at risk for developing *retinopathy of prematurity*, a condition that in its severest form can cause blindness in one or both eyes. If the condition progresses to a certain stage, treatment is available that can significantly lessen the chances of severe visual impairment. The most common treatment is a laser treatment delivered to the retina or an injection of a medication into the eye. The treatments cause the abnormal blood vessels to regress.

Children with severe asphyxia (lack of oxygen) may also suffer from brain injury, causing visual difficulties, such as cortical visual impairment (CVI), along with other neurologic deficits.

Cortical visual impairment may occur in up to 70 percent of children with cerebral palsy. CVI is defined as deficient visual function caused by damage to the parts of the brain responsible for vision. Children with significant CVI typically display characteristic behaviors such as poor visual response, difficulty with complexity and novelty, improved visual function with movement, and unusual responses to visual stimuli, such as eccentric viewing. A child using eccentric viewing will reach for an object without looking at it, using peripheral vision instead of central vision to locate the object. It is not always clear why children behave this way. Some suggest that it may be because of a defect or blind spot in the central visual field.

Some children remain significantly impaired, while in many children visual function may improve over time. Some children may develop useful vision but have deficits with higher-level functions such as visually guided behavior and visual attention. Regardless of the level of function, interventions are directed at improving function so that children can use the vision they have to reach their full potential.

As many as 75 to 90 percent of children with CP may suffer from *optic atrophy* (a shrinking of the optic nerve due to damage), *nystagmus* (jerking movements of the eye in a vertical or horizontal direction), visual field defects (loss of an area of vision), or *refractive errors* (distorted or blurred vision secondary to nearsightedness and farsightedness and/or astigmatism).

What can be done for children with severe visual impairment or blindness?

Special educational techniques are vitally important to a child with severe visual impairment. The child may need to attend a special class in a regular school or may require special education throughout his or her educational career, depending on whether visual impairment is the only disability or just one of several disabilities. If visual problems are accompanied by other disabilities, such as intellectual disability, the visual impairment adds to the burden on the child and makes education that much more difficult. It is estimated that between 30 and 70 percent of children with severe visual impairment have other disabilities as well. Regardless of visual acuity, any child with normal cognitive and social skills can legally attend public school and expect to have the benefit of appropriate visual and educational aids. As discussed in Chapter 11, Public Law 94-142 requires that states provide a free and appropriate education to all children, whether or not they have a disability.

How is visual function assessed in the newborn or the child who is nonverbal and/or has developmental delay?

There are a number of ways to assess visual functioning in the newborn. *Optic-kinetic nystagmus*, a reflex normally present in newborns, can help the physician assess the pathways leading to the visual part of the brain. A drum with alternating black and white lines is rotated in front of the baby, with both of the baby's eyes opened or one eye patched. A positive reflex is indicated by horizontal jerks in the eye as the eye tries to follow and then pulls back, with the fast component being in the direction opposite to the rotation. This reflex can be seen in premature babies born as early as 30 weeks' gestation (after 30 weeks in the womb).

Other aspects of visual function can be measured by a baby's blink response to light, which develops at approximately 25 weeks' gestation. The pupils constrict in response to light at 29 to 31 weeks' gestation. Some discriminatory visual function appears by 31 to 32 weeks' gestational age. Tests using *preferential looking* (in which the baby chooses to focus on a more interesting or more appealing picture) can estimate the actual visual acuity of a newborn.

The techniques of *visual-evoked potential* (VEP), or visual-evoked response (VER), have also been used to assess the integrity of the entire system up to the cortex, but their usefulness is limited, because the exact site in the brain where the abnormal response occurs cannot be determined. A visual-evoked potential is an electrophysiologic test used in combination with a computer to assess the brain's response to visual stimuli, such as a flashing light or a checkerboard pattern. To test vision, the baby's responses are compared with those of children known to have normal vision.

Children who are nonverbal or who cannot cooperate for acuity testing may have instrument-based screening for risk factors for amblyopia. Instrument-based screening is an objective assessment of the refractive error of the eye (nearsightedness, farsightedness, and astigmatism) by using a handheld instrument in front of the child. The reading obtained will alert the health care provider to a refractive error, which could cause amblyopia. The child can then be referred to an eye care provider experienced in the care of children to determine whether further treatment is necessary. The advantage of this screening method is that no cooperation from the child is needed.

How is visual function assessed in young children who are verbal and able to cooperate for visual acuity testing?

The vision tests most commonly used for young children are a test using LEA cards and the HOTV game. LEA cards have pictures of objects familiar to children (such as a circle, an apple, or a house) and can be used to test near and distant vision. The child is asked to identify the pictures on the cards. In the HOTV game, a limited number of letters are used. In children who are older and know the alphabet, the familiar Snellen letters remain the standard test, using a chart with nine lines of letters measuring acuity from 20/10 to 20/200.

When should my child's eyes first be tested, and how often should they be examined after that?

All children receive screening of their eyes and vision at the newborn and well child examinations by the pediatrician or primary care physician. When there is any deviation from normal, a child with cerebral palsy, just like any other child, should have his or her eyes examined by a pediatric ophthalmologist or an eye doctor experienced in the care of children. Deviations from normal include poor vision, crossed eyes, roving eyes, or eyes that have an abnormal appearance. A child with developmental delay or a child who for any reason is not able to be screened by the pediatrician should have a complete eye examination by an eye doctor experienced in the care of children.

For children with significant physical risks, such as infants born prematurely with a very low birthweight, the initial eye exam is usually done in the newborn nursery by an ophthalmologist. Follow-up as recommended by the ophthalmologist is necessary to prevent permanent vision loss. The exam should include an evaluation of the way the eyes move (specifically looking for crossing of the eyes) and a sense of visual acuity, that is, how well the child is seeing and following with his or her eyes. If the child is referred to an ophthalmologist, the ophthalmologist will dilate the pupil with eye drops in order to examine for refractive errors (farsightedness, nearsightedness, or astigmatism) and to evaluate the retina and the internal structures of the eye.

How is strabismus treated?

There are three goals for any child with cross-eye. These goals are the same for any child, regardless of whether he or she has cerebral palsy. The goals are

(1) good and equal visual acuity in both eyes; (2) ocular alignment (meaning getting the eyes straight, for both cosmetic and functional reasons); and (3) being able to use both eyes together. Strabismus may be treated by correcting the visual acuity in each eye, either with glasses or by patching. An alternative to patching may be atropine drops, which blur the vision in the good eye to force the child to use the nonpreferred eye. Precautions are necessary because of the drops' possible side effects. The drops may not be an option for all cases of strabismus. This information will be discussed with you by the ophthalmologist.

Certain types of strabismus, such as intermittent drifting of the eyes, may respond to eye exercises. If a significant strabismus remains even after these therapies, then surgery is indicated. Parents should have a detailed discussion with the ophthalmologist who will perform the surgery.

What are the different forms of blindness, and which ones do children with CP have?

For a person to be able to see, several things must occur. First, the person must have a clear optical structure, meaning that there are no cataracts or opacities (conditions that block light) obstructing the vision of the eye itself. Second, the person must be able to focus on an object, which sometimes requires wearing corrective glasses. Third, the person's eye must be able to pick up the light and transfer it into energy to send the image to the brain. The retina picks up the light and transfers this light stimulus to the optic nerve, which then conducts the nerve impulse to the back of the brain. Finally, the brain must translate these electrical impulses into visual stimuli, which are then interpreted and acted upon.

In optic nerve atrophy, the third process described above is impaired. That is, the optic nerve itself is injured, and the light image is not transmitted properly. In cortical visual impairment, the ocular apparatus (the front of the eye, retina, and the optic nerve) is normal, but the brain, which should pick up the visual stimuli, is not working properly and cannot respond properly to the visual stimuli. In children with cerebral palsy, blindness can be a result of damage to the retina, the optic nerve, or the occipital lobe of the brain. Premature infants who were exposed to oxygen may suffer a severe form of retinopathy resulting in retinal detachment, which interferes with the reception of light by the retina due to damage to the photoreceptor cells and obstructs transmission of light to the optic nerve. Other children with cerebral palsy may have suffered a lack of oxygen or blood supply at birth or in the months thereafter, resulting in damage to either the optic nerve or the brain—or both.

Can head banging or rubbing the eyes cause blindness?

Repeated trauma from severe head banging can lead to a tear in the thin retinal surface, which will allow the membrane to detach. Once the retina is detached, it starves from lack of nutrients from its blood supply and rapidly degenerates. This process leads to blindness if not corrected quickly. For this reason, retinal detachment needs to be diagnosed and repaired promptly.

It is rare for permanent damage to occur from eye rubbing, however. While conjunctivitis and recurrent eye infections can be caused by constant rubbing, especially when dirt is introduced into the eye from the child's hands, eye rubbing will not cause blindness. It is common for children who have poor vision or who are blind to rub their eyes as a stimulating tactic (known as "blindism"). If the cornea of the eye gets scratched and an infection results, then the cornea can form an ulcer, and deep scarring can occur. Redness of an eye that does not improve or that gets worse over a 24-hour period should be evaluated and treated by a health care provider.

Hearing Impairment and Vestibular Disorders

Should my child be screened for hearing problems?

Severe to profound hearing loss affects 1 or 2 out of every 1,000 children. Inherited factors are thought to account for approximately 30 to 50 percent of children with hearing loss. Approximately 25 percent of childhood hearing loss is thought to result from environmental causes; in another 25 percent the cause is unclear. Approximately 15 percent of children with cerebral palsy have a hearing impairment.

The key to early detection of hearing problems is identifying children at high risk, including those with any of the following risk factors: (1) a family history of childhood hearing impairment, (2) congenital infections, (3) malformations that involve the head and neck, (4) a birthweight under 1,500 grams (3 lb. 5 oz.), (5) bacterial meningitis, (6) jaundice, or (7) severe asphyxia. Even if none of these risk factors are present, parents should bring any concerns regarding their child's hearing to the attention of their primary care physician. If the child does not act startled or turn his or her head toward loud noises, the physician may want to screen the child or recommend a more formal hearing test by an audiologist. Any failure of a newborn to "pass" a screening test for hearing should be followed up with formal audiology testing.

How is hearing tested?

Hearing is tested in different ways throughout childhood based on the child's ability to interact and participate in the test. The most commonly used test, the *behavioral audiogram*, is usually administered by a well-trained pediatric audiologist, who during the test will ask the child to respond directly to word or sound cues. For an infant younger than 6 months, hearing is gauged by observing the infant's responses to sounds of various intensities and frequencies; these responses include widening of the eyes, blinking, becoming quiet to pay attention, or turning the head toward the sound.

From age 6 to 24 months *visual reinforcement audiometry* can be used to test hearing. In this approach, a flashing light or animated toy is used to reinforce a response to sounds of controlled intensities and frequencies. When the child looks in the direction of a sound, a toy or bright light is presented on the same side as the sound stimulus to encourage the child to look again when he or she hears the sound.

Between the ages of 2 and 5 years, children are usually tested by a technique called *conditioned play audiometry*, in which they engage in a play activity such as putting a block in a box each time a sound is heard. Beyond the age of 5 years, testing is done in the same manner as for adults.

Tympanometry assesses middle ear pressure and eardrum mobility. Alterations in middle ear pressure due to Eustachian tube dysfunction can be seen. Ossicular abnormalities (abnormalities of the small bones in the inner ear) can cause an abnormally stiff or flaccid eardrum response. Eardrum mobility will be absent if there is fluid in the middle ear, a perforation, or a pressure equalizing tube.

A child who is developmentally delayed will be tested based on his developmental abilities rather than on his chronological age. For children who cannot cooperate or who give inconsistent responses, an *auditory brainstem response* (ABR) test is often used. This test measures the electrical signal generated in response to sound using electrodes on the scalp. It establishes a threshold of sound intensity below which the child cannot hear. Its limitations are that it primarily tests high-frequency sounds, sedation is often required to administer it, and it is more expensive than other methods of testing hearing.

An additional method of testing hearing, the *otoacoustic emissions* (OAE) test, measures the sounds produced by the outer hair cells of the cochlea (the auditory portion of the inner ear), which can be measured in the ear canal. The ability to detect these sounds indicates cochlear health and in most cases a normal hearing threshold. It is used as a routine screening test for newborns in most nurseries.

What are the different types of hearing impairment?

Hearing impairment is usually classified as one of two types, conductive or sensorineural. *Conductive* hearing loss occurs when a problem in the outer or middle ear prevents sound from being conducted normally into the inner ear and the auditory nerve. *Sensorineural* hearing loss occurs when there is damage to the inner ear or the auditory nerve itself. If both conductive and sensorineural hearing loss are present, the hearing loss is termed *mixed*.

How are the different degrees of hearing impairment classified?

Hearing impairment ranges from slight to profound based on the threshold (the minimum level) of sound the child hears. Table 3 identifies the kinds of assistance that will prove beneficial to people with various degrees of hearing impairment.

How are type and degree of hearing loss determined in children?

Once it is established that a child has a hearing loss, the next step is to determine the type and degree of hearing impairment. The degree of impairment is determined by testing, as noted above, and is based on the minimum level of sound the child can hear. Hearing can also be tested using *air* conduction (the child wears earphones, and sound is conducted down the ear canal to the middle ear) or *bone* conduction (the sound is conducted to the middle ear by vibrations against the skull). The air and bone conduction thresholds identify the hearing loss type.

How can children with hearing impairment be helped?

At the time of initial diagnosis a medical evaluation should look for underlying diseases, some of which may be treatable, as well as for genetic factors, which may affect other children in the family or future children. For most children with conductive hearing loss, medical or surgical intervention should restore most, if not all, of the hearing to normal. On the other hand, a sensorineural hearing loss is rarely treatable and almost always permanent. The child's hearing impairment in this case is treated through amplification with a hearing

Table 3. Ranges of Hearing Impairment

Level of Hearing Loss (Hz)	Description	Sounds Heard	Possible Needs
15–25 dB	Slight hearing loss	Hears vowels clearly	Preferential seating
25–40 dB	Mild hearing loss	Hears only some louder-voiced speech sounds	Hearing aid, lip reading, auditory training, speech-language therapy, FM system
40–65 dB	Moderate hearing loss	Misses most speech sounds at normal conversational level	All the needs listed for 15–25 dB and 25–40 dB, plus consideration of special classroom situation
65–95 dB	Severe hearing loss	Hears no speech sounds at normal conversational level	All the needs listed for 15–25 dB, 25–40 dB, and 40–65 dB, plus probable assignment to special classes, possible cochlear implantation
More than 95 dB	Profound hearing loss	Hears no speech or other sounds	All the needs listed for 15–25 dB, 25–40 dB, 40–65 dB, and 65–95 dB

aid. In the case of a mixed hearing loss the conductive impairment needs to be treated aggressively so as to minimize the hearing loss to only the sensorineural component, which can rarely be treated.

Children of any age, even infants, can successfully use a hearing aid, which is essentially made up of a microphone (to pick up the sound and amplify it to make the sound louder) and a loudspeaker (to deliver the amplified sound to the ear). The two most commonly used hearing aids in children are body-style hearing aids and behind-the-ear hearing aids. Even with these devices, however, hearing is still far from perfect. Hearing aids tend to amplify *all* sounds, including undesirable noises. Hearing aids don't clarify the sound; they simply amplify it.

For a child with a severe hearing impairment of the sensorineural type, there is almost always some degree of language delay, because so many of the auditory cues and experiences that are necessary to language development have been missed. Even after the diagnosis is made, learning continues to be a struggle for many children, especially those with a severe or profound hearing loss. Most children with sensorineural hearing loss benefit from early intervention programs designed for children with hearing impairments. In addition, special supportive services or special education may be necessary throughout the school years, particularly for children who have hearing impairment in conjunction with conditions such as cerebral palsy or intellectual impairment or if they also have visual impairment.

In select children with severe to profound hearing loss, cochlear implantation can be a treatment option. This is a surgical procedure in which a device is implanted into the deaf ear, allowing the hearing nerve to be directly stimulated electrically. It can be done as early as 7 months of age but typically is performed between 1 and 2 years of age. With intensive rehabilitation, these children will often develop normal hearing thresholds and speech and language on par with their peers. However, not all children with severe to profound hearing loss are candidates for cochlear implantation. For those who are not, alternative modes of communication must be developed, including cued speech or American Sign Language. Unfortunately, sign language may not be a practical option in a child for whom CP affects hand function.

What causes hearing loss?

By far the most common cause of conductive hearing impairment in children is middle ear disease, or otitis media. Other causes include congenital malformations of the middle ear or obstruction of the ear canal by cerumen (earwax). Sensorineural hearing impairment may be present at birth. If so, it may be inherited or it may be caused by a maternal infection or a drug, particularly one ingested during the first trimester, that interferes with the normal development of the inner ear. Acquired causes include a lack of oxygen at some time, head trauma, certain medications, high bilirubin levels (causing jaundice), and meningitis or mumps. Since many of these factors can also contribute to cerebral palsy, hearing impairment and cerebral palsy are often found together.

What is otitis media?

Otitis media is the medical term for a middle ear infection. It is a very common problem in children, second only to the common cold in frequency as the reason for illness-related visits to the pediatrician. Risk factors for developing otitis media include going to sleep with a bottle, being bottle fed as opposed to breast fed, male gender, environmental smoke, pacifier use, and day care attendance. It is estimated that more than 90 percent of all children have at least one such infection by age 5.

How is otitis media diagnosed?

Children with acute otitis media often complain of an earache. They may rub or tug at their ears, they may have drainage from their ears, and they may have a fever. Sometimes none of these symptoms are present, however. Upon examination of the ear and eardrum a physician sees a red, bulging, immobile eardrum. Such an infection is commonly treated with antibiotics. A virus can also cause ear infections, in which case antibiotics would be ineffective. Fluid in the middle ear may persist for weeks or even months following the acute infection.

What is serous otitis media?

A persistent accumulation of fluid in the middle ear that is not infected is a serous otitis media, or otitis media with effusion. This accumulation of fluid may make the child more susceptible to recurrent infections as well as hearing problems. The condition usually results from poor functioning of the Eustachian tube. The Eustachian tube normally equalizes pressure between the middle ear and the atmosphere and permits drainage of secretions from the middle ear. When this tube does not work well or when it is blocked, fluid can accumulate in the middle ear. This blockage most commonly arises when nasal tissues swell due to a cold or an allergy.

If fluid remains in the middle ear without being cleared, disease-producing bacteria and viruses can cause an active infection leading to acute otitis media.

Resolution of an acute otitis media can also result in persistent fluid in the middle ear long after the infection has been effectively treated with antibiotics.

How does serous otitis media affect hearing?

While the degree of hearing loss from serous otitis media can vary from mild to severe, the mild to moderate range of impairment is most common. It can cause obvious difficulty in hearing for a child who was hearing well before, or even greater loss of function for a child who already had some hearing impairment. Because serous otitis media is most common in children under 2 years of age, and because language takes shape during these first years of life, serous otitis media can interfere with the development of language, as this development is dependent upon hearing. There have been concerns raised that serous otitis media and hearing loss at this age can lead to long-term learning disabilities in children of school age, but this has not been proven.

What factors contribute to the development of recurrent otitis media with effusion?

Children under age 2 years are at the highest risk for the development of recurrent (or persistent) otitis media with effusion. The risk factors for developing otitis media with effusion include developing a first episode of otitis before 6 months of age, as well as those mentioned for otitis media. Children most commonly become infected in winter.

What other complications of otitis media are there?

One complication, known as *mastoiditis*, occurs when infection spreads from the middle ear into the mastoid bone and air cells behind the ear. This condition is sometimes treated successfully with antibiotics; successful treatment may require an operation, however.

An acute infection of the middle ear can also lead to perforation of the eardrum, which usually, but not always, will heal on its own. While perforation usually is not serious, it can lead to loss of hearing function and to susceptibility to cholesteatoma in the middle ear. *Cholesteatoma* is a condition in which surface skin cells in the external auditory canal grow into the middle ear space and form a benign tumor that can erode the small bones of the middle ear as well as the base of the skull. Rarely, acute otitis media can lead to meningitis, facial paralysis, brain abscess, or labyrinthitis (inflammation of the structures of the inner ear).

What is the treatment for acute otitis media?

The standard treatment for acute otitis media is antibiotics, which are available in many forms. In most cases the doctor prescribes one of the antibiotics that is effective in combating the three or four bacteria known most commonly to infect the middle ear. In some cases, however, the doctor wants to find out exactly which bacterium is primarily responsible for the infection. In those cases the doctor will insert a needle through the eardrum and extract a small amount of fluid from the middle ear to grow a culture. Whether a particular antibiotic is prescribed depends, among other things, on the resistance of the bacteria to that antibiotic, the part of the country where the child lives, the cost of the antibiotic, and the child's history of previous infections.

What is the treatment for serous otitis media?	Many medical treatments for serous otitis media have been tried, including steroids, antihistamines, and decongestants. None of these treatments has proved very effective, and even in children whose problem seemed to get better the condition recurred fairly quickly. Surgical placement of a pressure equalizing tube that sits in the eardrum is an option when serous otitis media is accompanied by hearing loss.
What about recurrent otitis media?	Recurrent otitis media is more difficult to manage. It can be treated with antibiotics or through surgical placement of a tympanostomy tube in the eardrum. Low doses of preventive antibiotics (called prophylactic antibiotics) may be prescribed, especially during the winter season, when the incidence is highest. However, concern about bacteria developing resistance to antibiotics that are used for a prolonged time has made this practice less common. Tympanostomy tube placement allows continuous drainage and provides ventilation of the middle ear space.
When are tympanostomy tubes used?	Tympanostomy tubes are recommended when antibiotic treatment of recurrent otitis media has failed. For persistent effusion, tubes are considered appropriate if the effusion is accompanied by hearing loss of at least 20 decibels and has lasted for at least three to four months. However, because opinions vary about when tympanostomy tubes are called for, it is best to consult your child's physician.
How are tympanostomy tubes placed in the ear?	Placing tympanostomy tubes in the ear, formally known as a *myringotomy*, is done under general anesthesia. The procedure is usually very brief, lasting approximately 10 minutes, and can almost always be done on an outpatient basis, with the child returning home once he or she has awakened and recovered from general anesthesia. Tympanostomy tubes remain in place in the eardrum for 6 to 12 months and usually fall out by themselves. They usually prevent middle ear infection and accumulation of fluid in the middle ear. When the tubes are present, water must not be allowed to enter the ear, since this can cause an infection. Thus, care must be taken when the child is showering or swimming, and earplugs are often recommended. If ear infections recur frequently once the tubes have been removed or have fallen out, the tubes are sometimes replaced. Some children get ear infections even with the tubes in place, and only topical antibiotics are required for adequate treatment in most cases.
How does the balance system work?	Balance relies on vision; input from the balance system, known as the vestibular system; and proprioception. Proprioception is the ability to sense the position, motion, and equilibrium of one's body. Balance is also affected by cognitive processing of these sensory inputs, which is called sensory integration. With CP, sensory integration can be over- or under-responsive.
What aspect of vestibular testing can be affected by CP?	Vestibular testing contains many components. Tests of posture and gait may show an abnormality in patients with CP.

What can be done to help with vestibular dysfunction?

Since balance is affected by vision, a patient with vestibular dysfunction should be seen by an ophthalmologist. This doctor can determine whether glasses or visual aids to optimize visual input are needed. Additionally, the patient may undergo vestibular rehabilitation therapy. This is an exercise program to help strengthen any remaining vestibular function and to help train the brain to use sensory information to improve balance and postural control.

Issues of Feeding and Nutrition

Does cerebral palsy affect height and weight?

For some children with cerebral palsy, growth is affected. They are much smaller than their same-age friends who do not have CP. In some children, cerebral palsy affects only weight; in others, it affects both weight and height. This is especially true for children with spastic quadriplegia, and much less true for those with hemiplegia or diplegia.

What causes this poor growth?

Several factors affect the growth of the child with CP, and not all of them are clearly understood. Primarily, poor weight gain is caused by an inadequate intake of nutrition. In addition, there apparently are some neurological factors that affect linear growth, primarily on the basis of hormones that come from the brain and that may be affected by the brain damage that caused the CP.

What causes poor nutrition?

Multiple factors interfere with good nutrition in children most severely affected by CP. Many children, especially those with spastic quadriplegia, have *pseudobulbar palsy*, which means that the muscles of the tongue and mouth are affected by CP. This interferes with the normal coordination of chewing and swallowing, and it causes problems with drooling and poor pronunciation as well. Many children with this constellation of problems also have a tongue thrust and a tonic bite, meaning that when something is introduced into the mouth, the jaws clench shut and the tongue pushes the food out instead of bringing it in and pushing it back toward the throat. These same abnormalities make it difficult to brush a child's teeth, so tooth decay and gum disease may develop. These conditions may compound the problem by making chewing food painful. In addition, many children with CP have tooth defects from birth that make chewing more difficult.

All of these factors make it difficult for the child to receive adequate intake of food and beverage. Meals may take more than an hour, with much of the food still not ending up in the child's stomach. The poor nutritional status resulting from an inadequate intake of essential nutrients can adversely affect weight gain, growth, and development.

What are the neurological factors that delay growth?

Even when their nutritional deficiency is corrected, some children fail to grow. This is especially true if the nutritional deficiencies are corrected later in childhood rather than in the first two or three years. While the neurological factors are not clearly understood, it has long been thought that damage to the brain affects those areas that produce various hormones, including growth hormone, which can lead to poor linear growth.

What can be done to stimulate the growth of a child with CP?

Little can be done about the neurological factors affecting growth. However, various methods are available for improving the nutritional intake of a child with cerebral palsy. Sometimes a change in feeding technique is enough. This might mean better seating (a more upright posture will help some children) or special techniques, such as holding the jaw forward. Other children might benefit from a change in food texture. For instance, many children with CP cannot swallow liquids or chew solid food but do well with pureed foods. And for children who simply cannot take large quantities of food, high-calorie supplements can help them gain weight. These might include very high calorie foods like butter, cream, or milkshakes or commercially available nutritional supplements. (See "Using Nutritional Boosters" in Part 2.) If the child cannot be adequately or safely fed by mouth, then a feeding tube may be recommended.

Can growth be prevented or slowed so that my child remains small and easier to care for?

Yes, growth can be suppressed by giving a child hormones at a young age, before he or she reaches puberty. This accelerates the child's growth and causes him or her to go through puberty early, so that the child's eventual height is less than it would have been if puberty had occurred naturally at a later time. However, hormonal treatment is a controversial issue because the hormones are potentially harmful to a young child. Strong and reasonable arguments can be made for each side of this argument. There are physicians (usually pediatric endocrinologists) who will administer this treatment to children. You should at least discuss this issue with your CP team if you are concerned that at his full adult size he will become hard to care for.

How is growth evaluated for the child with CP?

The primary care physician should measure the height and weight of the child with CP just as he or she would with any other child. For the child who is able to stand, a standing height is the most accurate. The doctor will try to get the child to stand as straight as possible. Weights should be measured on the appropriate scale for the age of the child: an infant scale for young children and a standard scale for older children. For the child who cannot stand, a recumbent (lying down) length is measured from the top of the head to the bottom of the foot with the ankle at 90 degrees. This measurement can be done on a special length board or on an examining table or bed. If a wheelchair scale is not available, the child's weight may have to be obtained while the caregiver holds the child. Growth charts show the normal growth for children in the United States from birth through age 20. These charts are divided into percentiles, which reflect the expected normal growth over time. These percentiles range from the 3rd to the 97th percentile. Anyone over the 97th percentile is overweight or unusually tall. A child who is under the 3rd percentile is underweight or unusually short—although, by definition, 3 percent of the normal population falls into this category.

Are there special growth charts for children with CP?

Growth charts for children with CP are divided by gender into the different GMFCS categories (I through V), which were described in Chapter 1. However, the information for the categories was gathered on children with CP who were fed in a variety of ways and with variable growth patterns, so it may not be helpful to evaluate your child's growth according to these charts. The information on these CP growth charts does not represent the ideal or even what should be expected for children with CP. Therefore, most clinicians continue to use the National Center for Health Statistics growth charts for typically developing children. For children who are very short for their age, which most often affects those in the GMFCS categories IV and V, the ideal weight is based on their height rather than on their age. Those with CP whose function falls into the GMFCS categories I through III would be expected to have a growth pattern similar to that of typically developing children.

How can a child who has contractures of the hip, foot, or ankle be measured?

Contractures make it impossible to fully extend the legs, and therefore it is nearly impossible to obtain an accurate measurement of length. There are several alternate ways to obtain a child's length. The forearm can be measured from the elbow to the tip of the longest finger. Femur length can be measured from the hip to the knee. Tibia length can be measured from the top of the tibia to below the anklebone, and knee height can be measured from the top of the knee to the bottom of the foot. All of these are height alternatives. Some, such as tibia length and knee height, can be put into an equation to estimate height. These values can then be plotted on a standard growth chart. For comparison over time, the same method of measuring should be used each time if possible.

Are there other ways to assess the nutritional status of a child with CP?

Triceps skinfold is a measurement of a child's fat stores. Triceps skinfold is helpful for monitoring a child's nutritional status, especially if the child has a weight and length below the 3rd percentile. A skinfold measurement within the normal range indicates good fat stores. The measurement is taken at the back of the upper arm at midpoint with a special caliper. The value is compared with those of other children of the same age and gender. This measurement can also be used to monitor nutritional status over time.

Mid-upper arm circumference (MUAC) is another measurement that may be used to identify malnutrition when weight and/or height are not available or are difficult to obtain. MUAC is the circumference at the midpoint of the upper arm. Changes in MUAC may indicate changes in body weight. For example, if MUAC decreases by 5 percent, it is likely that body weight has also decreased by 5 percent.

What if the child's weight is below the third or fifth percentile?

The growth of every child should be plotted on the growth chart during the early years of life. A weight or height that is consistently slightly below the 3rd or 5th percentile in a line parallel to the growth curve might simply mean that the child is growing normally and fits into the smallest 3 to 5 percent of children his or her age. However, if the child is "falling away from the curve," meaning that he or she is dropping down in percentile, then this usually calls for further evaluation. Triceps skinfold and weight to height ratios can also help determine whether further evaluation is needed. If more intervention is needed, your doctor may have you keep a diet record or get blood tests or x-rays, or some combination of these. Usually the initial evaluation is primarily a nutritional one, since the assumption is that a fall-off in weight is primar-ily due to inadequate nutrition.

If the problem is nutritional, what other evaluations are done?

If the physician feels that a child's fall-off in weight or poor weight gain is due to poor nutrition, then a detailed diet record is obtained. This may be done by the physician or a dietitian, who will assess what and how much the child is consuming, including calories, protein, fluid, vitamins, and minerals, and compare it with the child's estimated nutrient needs in order to grow and optimize health. If the physician feels that the child is not getting sufficient calories because of *oral motor dysfunction* (which includes poor chewing and swallowing, tongue thrust, tonic bite), then an evaluation by an occupational or speech-language therapist may be recommended. This evaluation includes a clinical visit in which the therapist watches the feeding of the child and tries to detect special problems. It may also include a modified barium swallow, an x-ray procedure that evaluates the ability of the child to eat and swallow food safely. Recommendations by the therapist to help deal with these problems might include better positioning or use of special techniques such as holding the child's jaw to help him swallow.

What is aspiration?

Aspiration is the process whereby food or secretions that are swallowed get into the lungs. Aspiration can result in acute infections of the lungs (aspiration pneumonia) or acute bronchospasm (wheezing), which may be diagnosed as asthma. Sometimes the child's only symptoms of aspiration are coughing dur-ing meals or sounding congested after meals. Some children show no symp-toms at all, at least early in life. If aspiration continues over many months or years, it can result in chronic damage to the lungs, eventually causing symp-toms such as a rapid respiratory rate or poor oxygenation. The child with CP may aspirate food into the lungs because of a lack of coordination in swallow-ing and a lack of a protective gag reflex. Some children even aspirate their own saliva. Many children who aspirate have no cough or gag reflex and show no obvious response to the aspiration until they become acutely ill.

How will I know if my child is aspirating?

The symptoms of aspiration of food may include coughing, gagging, choking, or difficulty breathing while eating or sounding congested after eating. Some children aspirate without showing any of these symptoms, however, because they have no gag reflex and the food gets into the lungs without producing any symptoms. Aspiration is suspected in such cases when the child suffers from repeated episodes of pneumonia. This is called *aspiration pneumonia*. A history of repeated episodes (two or more) of pneumonia should alert the physician to the possibility that the child is aspirating. Aspiration could be due to problems with swallowing or due to gastroesophageal reflux (when food comes back up the esophagus after reaching the stomach; see pages 91–94).

Are there tests that can show whether my child is aspirating?

A regular chest x-ray might show signs of chronic aspiration but often does not, as the signs become evident only after repeated episodes of aspiration. The test that provides information about the child's swallow and evidence of aspiration is the modified barium swallow. This test is done by a radiologist, usually with a speech or occupational therapist present to feed the child different textures to see how he or she swallows. It is also helpful to have a parent present to try to feed the child in the usual manner. In this test, the child is fed the way he is normally fed at home or at school, but a liquid element known as barium is mixed into foods of different consistencies, usually liquids, pureed food, and solid food. The child is then fed in the x-ray department, where the x-ray evaluation of the feeding in progress can be recorded on videotape and reviewed. Since the barium shows up on x-ray, it reveals where the food is going when the child swallows, whether into the esophagus and then the stomach (as it should) or into the lungs. Another possible source of aspiration, the child's own saliva, is investigated by means of a nuclear medicine test called a *salivagram* (see page 98).

What can be done if my child is aspirating food?	If the modified barium swallow shows aspiration primarily of one type of texture of food, then avoiding this texture of food will be recommended. For instance, if liquids are being aspirated but pureed foods are swallowed safely, then the recommendation can be made to thicken all liquids and not give any "thin liquids." (Liquids are usually more easily aspirated than pureed or solid foods.) The child can then continue to eat by mouth and simply avoid the foods that are hard for him or her to handle. Sometimes the modified barium swallow will show that a change in position or in feeding technique will stop the aspiration, and recommendations can be based on these findings.

If there is evidence that the child is aspirating everything he or she is eating, and if there has been a history of recurrent pneumonias or chronic congestion, then an alternative feeding method may well be recommended. A decision to use one of the alternative feeding methods is dependent on the child's and the family's lifestyle, and each situation must be evaluated on an individual basis. If the decision is made to recommend an alternative feeding method, then this usually means placement of a gastrostomy tube.

What is a gastrostomy tube?	A *gastrostomy tube*, or G-tube, is a tube that goes directly into the stomach through the skin, allowing the person to be fed without having to swallow. The food goes through the tube into the stomach and then is digested normally through the intestinal system. Liquids and pureed foods can be put through the tube, as can liquid medicines or crushed pills.
How is a gastrostomy tube placed?	There are four ways to place a gastrostomy tube. A *Stamm gastrostomy* involves placing a tube into the stomach either via an open operation (in which the surgeon makes an incision in the abdominal wall) or via a laparoscopic procedure (the surgeon places several thin tubes through small holes or cuts in the abdominal wall). The third method is a percutaneous endoscopic gastrostomy (PEG) and does not involve opening the abdomen. An endoscope (a long tube) is placed through the mouth and into the stomach. A needle is passed into the stomach from the skin and a tube is pulled up from the stomach onto the abdominal wall. These three procedures are done in the operating

room with anesthesia. The fourth is done by an interventional radiologist, in a special x-ray room with intravenous sedation and local anesthesia. A needle is passed into the stomach and then the tube is pushed through the opening. Once the child has recovered from the anesthesia, feeding is begun through the tube. Usually, within one to three days the child is getting all the nutrition he or she needs through the gastrostomy tube.

Which method for placing a gastrostomy tube is best?

If the child has significant gastroesophageal (GE) reflux requiring an operation called a *fundoplication* (see below), then usually a Stamm gastrostomy is placed at the same time. The fundoplication involves tightening the lower esophageal sphincter (the muscle at the end of the esophagus where it enters the stomach) by wrapping the upper part of the stomach around the lower esophagus. It can be wrapped all the way around or partially around. This may be done either by an open procedure (with an incision) or laparoscopically, depending on the preference and skills of the surgeon. If there is no significant reflux and the child only needs a gastrostomy tube for better nutrition, then a PEG may be placed. This should be done by someone who has been specifically trained to do this procedure, such as a gastroenterologist, a gastrointestinal (GI) advanced practice nurse (nurse practitioner), an interventional radiologist, or a surgeon.

Can a child with a gastrostomy tube still eat by mouth?

Having a gastrostomy tube does not prevent a person from eating by mouth. If the tube is being placed because the child was unable to eat enough—if it is being used as a *supplement* to feedings by mouth—then certainly the child can continue to eat by mouth as well. If the tube is being placed because the child was aspirating everything he or she was eating (meaning food and liquids were going into the airways or lungs, causing respiratory symptoms), then the recommendation would be not to eat by mouth, though it may be possible for the child to take occasional tastes of food.

What are the side effects of having a gastrostomy tube?

The most common side effect is irritation of the skin around the tube, causing *granulation tissue* (a fleshy projection on the surface of a wound). Infection of the skin can develop at the site where the gastrostomy tube goes into the abdomen, but this is usually a local skin infection and is easily treated with an antibiotic ointment (or antibiotics given by mouth or via the tube).

There are other, less common complications. The placement of the gastrostomy tube may worsen or cause gastroesophageal (GE) reflux in the patient who did not have severe reflux prior to having the tube placed. Also, the placement of the tube by Stamm gastrostomy can result in *adhesions*, which are bands of fibrous tissue in the abdomen. This can sometimes lead to bowel obstruction, preventing food from passing through the intestines. Such a condition would make it necessary for the child to have another operation to relieve the obstruction.

Does the gastrostomy tube have to be replaced?

Usually a gastrostomy tube is replaced every three months. This schedule lessens the likelihood that the tube will become infected. The tube may also need to be replaced if it becomes clogged, if it gets pulled out accidentally, or if it has a balloon that breaks, causing the tube to fall out. G-tubes may be replaced by physicians, nurses, or parents, who can be taught the procedure and made to feel comfortable doing this at home. If a parent does not have a spare tube at home or is unable to replace it, he or she should call the physician or go to the nearest emergency room. The tube needs to be replaced quickly to prevent the hole from closing, which can occur in a matter of hours.

Can the child with a gastrostomy tube go swimming?

Yes! The child can shower or bathe and even go swimming.

What is a gastrostomy button tube?

A button, or low-profile, tube is a gastrostomy tube that lies flat on the abdomen rather than "hanging" out from the abdomen. Many parents prefer this type of tube because it is less obvious to others that the child has a tube. A low-profile tube is also less likely to be pulled out by the child or by others or to get caught on clothing or equipment.

Gastroesophageal (GE) Reflux

What is gastroesophageal reflux?

Ordinarily, when food is swallowed it goes down a tube in the body called the *esophagus* and then into the stomach. A sphincter at the end of the esophagus acts as a one-way valve preventing food from coming back up the esophagus. In many newborn babies this muscle (known as the *lower esophageal sphincter*) is underdeveloped, resulting in what is commonly known as "spitting up." As the child grows and develops, this sphincter gets stronger and eventually stops food from coming up into the esophagus. Thus, usually by age 1 to 1½ years this "spitting up" has stopped. However, in many children with CP this problem continues, though the child may not actually vomit or have food come back up.

This condition, known as GE reflux, can cause inflammation of the esophagus, called *esophagitis*. This inflammation occurs because as the food comes up, so does acid that is normally in our stomachs. Esophagitis causes pain, sometimes to the point where the child refuses to eat. When severe, this condition can cause anemia from blood loss, as well as a *stricture*, which is a narrowing of the esophagus caused by chemical burns from stomach acid. Other complications of GE reflux include aspiration pneumonia and an inability to gain or maintain weight.

How is GE reflux diagnosed?

One test used to evaluate causes of GE reflux is a contrast study of the gastrointestinal (GI) tract, or "upper GI." In this test, the child drinks a milklike substance (barium) and, via x-ray, the radiologist watches it go down into the stomach. This x-ray looks at the anatomy of the GI tract to make sure that there are no twists or narrowings (called strictures) that might be causing the reflux. The test takes only about 15 minutes, and reflux may not be seen. If this test is normal and your physician still strongly suspects reflux, then other tests may be recommended. These could include a pH or impedance probe study and a gastric emptying scan.

What is a pH probe?	A pH probe is a thin wire coated in plastic that is passed like a nasogastric tube, through the nose and into the esophagus. It does not go all the way down to the stomach but remains a few centimeters above the lower esophageal sphincter. This probe remains in place for up to 24 hours. The child is fed as usual or with some apple juice as well, and the probe records each reflux episode and each instance of acid coming back up into the esophagus. If your child is already on an acid-reducing medication, the medication likely needs to be stopped at least five days before the pH probe study.
What is an impedance probe?	An impedance probe is very like a pH probe but is more commonly used because it can detect reflux that might be missed by a pH probe. It uses a different technique to measure reflux and can detect episodes that don't involve acid and would thus be missed by a pH probe.
What is a gastric emptying study?	A gastric emptying (GE) scan, sometimes called a "milk scan," is a study done in the nuclear medicine section of the radiology department. This test measures how well the stomach empties. The child is given a certain amount of milk or formula that contains an isotope, or dye. The scan lasts for one hour, and the radiologist calculates how fast the stomach empties and also notes any episodes of reflux. Children should empty at least half of what they drink in one hour. Less than half indicates delayed emptying of the stomach, which can make reflux worse.
How can reflux be treated?	There are several ways to help decrease reflux episodes. One conservative method is to hold the child upright for 20 to 30 minutes after feedings. Another is to avoid placing the child in an infant seat to feed, as the child is often bent forward, putting increased pressure on the stomach and making reflux worse. Thickening formula or milk with cereal or a thickening agent (like Thick-It) can help to keep food in the stomach but can also delay gastric emptying.
Are there medications that treat reflux?	There are medications that can help decrease reflux but none that stop it altogether. Two general types of medications are used: prokinetics, which help make the stomach empty faster, and medications that reduce acid or stop acid production. Examples of prokinetic medications are metoclopramide (Reglan) and low-dose erythromycin. These medications work by increasing contractions in the stomach and by acting on the vomiting center in the brain. They have potential side effects, however, including a decreased seizure threshold, drowsiness, involuntary movements, decreased urine production, abdominal cramps, and headache.

Two types of medications help reduce acid production: H_2 blockers and proton pump inhibitors. Examples of H_2 blockers are ranitidine (Zantac), famotidine (Pepcid), and cimetidine (Tagamet). These medications decrease a child's production of acid and thus decrease the amount of acid going into the esophagus with each reflux episode. Since it is the acid that causes all the complications associated with reflux, some children only need to be treated with this type of medication and do not have any further problems. They may continue to reflux or regurgitate, but without complications.

Proton pump inhibitors (PPI) inhibit the production of acid. These medications come in capsule, liquid, or granule form. The capsules can be opened up and placed in soft food or Maalox. Omeprazole (Prilosec), lansoprazole (Prevacid), and esomeprazole (Nexium) have been studied in children and have been approved by the US Food and Drug Administration (FDA) for use in children. The potential side effects include diarrhea, headache, and abdominal pain.

What kind of surgery is done to prevent reflux? The most common surgery for preventing reflux is a *Nissen fundoplication*, in which a portion of the stomach is wrapped around the lower part of the esophagus. This operation prevents food from coming back out of the stomach. It is still possible to eat after the surgery has been done, since the procedure does not totally close off the esophagus. Instead, it allows food into the stomach but prevents it from coming back up. This procedure can be done as an open procedure or laparoscopically. A gastrostomy tube is usually inserted at the time of surgery. An alternative to a fundoplication is placement of a jejunostomy tube, or J-tube.

What is a J-tube? A J-tube, or jejunostomy tube, is placed into the part of the small intestine called the *jejunum*. This procedure can be done as a temporary measure or as a more permanent one. When the procedure is a temporary measure, a radiologist passes a tube through the G-tube site, threading it down past the stomach and ending in the small intestine. This procedure must be done in the radiology department and involves radiation exposure for the child. This tube contains two ports: a gastrostomy port, to allow for venting or medication administration, and a jejunal port, to allow for feeds. This type of J-tube needs to be replaced every three months in the radiology department, and it can easily be dislodged. However, using this type of J-tube can help determine whether the child will tolerate feedings in the small intestine before placing a more permanent tube. It can also help determine whether the child needs a fundoplication. Placement of a permanent J-tube is done by a surgeon. The surgeon takes a loop of small intestine and stitches it to the skin surface. A low-profile tube may eventually be placed at this site just as at a G-tube site.

What are the possible complications of a fundoplication? The most common complication is wound infection, which may require local drainage or antibiotic treatment. Rarely, the wrap around the esophagus is too tight, making it difficult for food to get into the stomach. More often, the child may not be able to burp and release air trapped in the stomach. This can easily be treated if a gastrostomy tube is in place by letting the trapped air out through the tube. Intestinal blockage (obstruction) from adhesion formation within the abdomen can occur. These adhesive bands may require surgery to relieve the blockage. The risk of this occurring is 5 to 10 percent. Another possible complication is the dumping syndrome, in which food exits the stomach too rapidly; the causes of this phenomenon after a fundoplication are not clear. Finally, over time the wrap may become undone (especially in a child with a seizure disorder), resulting in a recurrence of the reflux. A reoperation may be necessary.

What is dumping syndrome, and how is it treated?

Dumping syndrome occurs because the shape of the stomach has changed, and it can no longer act as a reservoir to hold food. Therefore, food dumps out immediately from the stomach into the small intestine. This can result in malabsorption of feedings, sweating, increased heart rate, and a sudden increase in blood sugar followed by a sudden drop in blood sugar rather than a gradual drop. This syndrome can be treated by changing the child's formula, adding complex carbohydrates and fiber, or by offering continuous feeds rather than bolus feeds. If these measures do not work, then medications to slow gastric emptying can be used.

Is constipation a common problem in patients with CP?

Constipation is not an uncommon problem in any child, but it is even more common among children with CP, especially those who either sit most of the day or do not take sufficient liquids—or both. If the child is not taking in enough liquids, for all the reasons discussed earlier, then constipation certainly may become another problem for the child.

How is constipation treated?

Constipation is easier to prevent than to treat, and the first step in doing either one is usually to make dietary changes. In particular, an increase in fluids and fiber in the diet should help prevent or treat mild constipation. It is important to determine how constipated the child is by obtaining a careful history, taking an abdominal x-ray, and performing a rectal exam. If there is a moderate amount of retained stool, dietary changes will likely be insufficient. If the child has not had a bowel movement in a week, has had fecal soiling, or has been constipated for a long time, most likely he or she will need a "clean out" to rid the entire colon of stool before beginning a maintenance regimen. A clean out can be done "from below" with enemas, or "from above" via a tube inserted through the nose into the stomach or through an existing G-tube with an infusion of a medication called Go-Lytely. Children with CP may have decreased tone, and because the colon is a muscle, it too may have decreased tone. Therefore, the colon may be unable to effectively contract to push the stool out of the rectum. Such children may require a stimulant such as senna or bisacodyl to help make these contractions occur.

Low Bone Density/Osteopenia/Osteoporosis

Which children are likely to fracture their bones easily?

Not all children with CP are susceptible to bone fractures, but some children with CP do seem to be unusually susceptible. These susceptible children can break their bones after minimal trauma, sometimes even with no obvious trauma at all. Several factors put a person at risk for easily fracturing his or her bones. The more risk factors present, the more susceptible the child is to such fractures. Once a child has had a nontraumatic fracture, his or her risk for additional such fractures is increased considerably. The factor that seems to predict who is at risk is low bone mineral density (BMD).

What are the risk factors for low bone mineral density?

Multiple factors may affect bone density in children with severe CP. One of the most important factors associated with low energy fracture is lack of weight-bearing ambulation. Bone adapts to what is required of it: a heavier load creates stronger, thicker bones, and a lighter load yields thin, weak bones, which are more apt to break. Bones weaken after periods without minimal weight-bearing ambulation and periods of immobilization (sometimes in a cast) following fracture or orthopedic surgical procedures. Another factor affecting BMD is nutritional status. Children with compromised nutrition show poor growth and inadequate intakes or even deficiency of vitamins and minerals. Specific nutrients that are important for bone health in children with CP are calcium, vitamin D, and sometimes phosphorus. Inadequate intake of these nutrients is common in this population. Many children with CP take, or have taken, certain medications that can negatively affect BMD. These include some anticonvulsants, steroids, and hormonal birth control. Some physically impaired individuals have heat intolerance and are therefore less likely to participate in outdoor activities in the sun. Sunlight exposure contributes to higher vitamin D levels in the body. In addition, CP is often associated with prematurity, and many low birthweight premature infants have lower than normal bone mineral content when evaluated as older children (whether or not they have CP). Delayed puberty, which is not uncommon among those with CP, may also contribute to low bone density in children. Undoubtedly, the underlying pathophysiology of low BMD in children with CP is complex, but it is clear that the biggest risk factor is nonambulation. That is, children who are primarily in wheelchairs (or confined to bed), and not standing or walking, are the most likely to have low BMD.

How is bone mineral density measured?

The most commonly used method for measuring BMD is DXA, or dual energy x-ray absorptiometry. DXA is a type of imaging that uses low dose x-rays; it involves a small amount of radiation exposure. While in the adult elderly population BMD is used to predict risk of fracture, this is not the case with children. In children with CP, however, a strong association has been described between BMD and fracture history. Measuring BMD on people with neuromuscular disabilities can be challenging, since the body sites and positions typically recommended may not be attainable or valid, and use of an alternative body site, the lateral distal femur (LDF), may be required. The DXA scan should be performed at an imaging center familiar with scanning children who have physical disabilities and perhaps a center offering the LDF DXA scan. Results of the DXA study are given in measured density of the bone (grams per square centimeter) but are also reported as Z-scores. A Z-score is the number of standard deviations above or below the mean for age and gender. A Z-score of less than –2.0 (that is, more than 2 standard deviations below the mean) is considered "low BMD." There are other ways to measure BMD, including quantitative CT and MRI scans and ultrasound, but these are not as widely used as DXA.

What can be done to prevent these fractures?

Some of the risk factors mentioned above are not easily avoided. For instance, if a child needs to take seizure medications, the medications should not be stopped because the child has had broken bones. It may be possible to replace the child's anticonvulsant with one that has less potential for interfering with vitamin D metabolism. If the problem is nutritional, then it may be helpful to work with a pediatric registered dietitian nutritionist (RD/RDN) to address *what* the child is eating. If the child is eating orally, speech and occupational therapy might be helpful in addressing concerns about *how* the child is eating. Some adjustments to the diet (such as adding milk or dairy products or special formulas with extra vitamin D, phosphorus, and calcium) may be useful. It may also be necessary to provide calcium, phosphorus, and vitamin D supplements, either in liquid or tablet form, on a daily basis. Fifteen to twenty minutes of exposure to the sun without sunscreen should be safe and will help the child's body make more vitamin D. There is also some evidence to suggest that physical therapy focused on weight bearing (standing, ambulation) improves BMD in children with CP.

Currently the most promising way to treat osteoporosis (defined as a combination of low BMD and multiple long-bone fractures or vertebral fractures) in children with CP is through the administration of bisphosphonate medications, which are widely used to treat osteoporosis in elderly people. In children with quadriplegic CP, the bisphosphonate used most often is pamidronate, which is given intravenously on three consecutive days every three to four months. Pamidronate has been shown in small trials to significantly improve BMD and reduce the risk of fracture. Newer bisphosphonates and other classes of medications being used in adults are being studied in children and may become available for use in children in the coming years.

Drooling and Airway Issues

Why do children and adults with CP drool more than others?

People with CP don't make more saliva than others. Instead, the problem is lack of coordination of the muscles in the face, head, and neck, which can result in a significant amount of drooling. Just as some people with CP can't coordinate their muscles in order to swallow food, some people have such poor coordination that they can't effectively swallow their own saliva. Certain anticonvulsant medications (especially clonazepam) may contribute to drooling by increasing the amount of saliva. Of all people with CP, approximately 35 percent are said to drool significantly.

How can drooling be treated?

To some extent, drooling can be improved by modifying the person's position so that the head does not fall forward. Other measures that may help include better toothbrushing, to help eliminate dental disease; correction of orthodontic problems, which may interfere with the ability to close the mouth; and elimination of enlarged tonsils or adenoids, which may obstruct the mouth or nose.

Four primary methods have been tried to reduce drooling: (1) oral motor therapy, usually by a speech-language therapist, to improve tongue and jaw position and mouth closure; (2) behavior modification through cuing and positive reinforcement, so that the person swallows his or her saliva more often; (3) medications to decrease the amount of saliva; (4) surgery, either to decrease the amount of saliva or to divert the saliva toward the back of the throat, where it can more easily be swallowed. Neither oral motor therapy nor behavior modification works for more than a very small percentage of people. Medications and surgery can effectively decrease the amount of saliva produced, but they can have significant side effects. Because the effects of surgery cannot be reversed, most physicians will use medications first. Commonly used are anticholinergic medications by mouth or by application of a patch or botulinum toxin (Botox) injected directly into the salivary glands.

How do anticholinergic medications work, and what are their side effects?

Glycopyrrolate (Robinul) and other anticholinergic medications have been used to decrease excessive tracheal and bronchial secretions, as well as saliva. Studies of children with CP treated with glycopyrrolate have found that most showed a significant decrease in drooling (or tracheal secretions in those who have tracheostomies). Side effects included constipation, behavioral changes, dry mouth (or thick tracheal secretions), flushing, and urinary retention. A small number of those experiencing side effects were switched to an alternative anticholinergic medication and then experienced the benefit without the side effects. Such alternatives include benztropine (Cogentin), hyoscyamine (Levsin), and the scopolamine patch (Transderm Scop). The goal is not to stop all production of saliva, as moisture in the mouth is necessary for dental health and a dry mouth can be uncomfortable. Rather, the goal is to decrease the amount of saliva being made while keeping the mouth moist.

How does botulinum toxin work, and what are its side effects?

The use of botulinum toxin for muscle spasticity is discussed in Part 3. Its use in the treatment of excessive drooling is relatively new. As its name implies, Botox is a toxin that interferes with nerve function, thus blocking the action of the salivary gland when it is injected directly into the gland. Ideally, the effect lasts 4 to 6 months. As with oral medications, the goal is not to stop all saliva production. Therefore, botulinum toxin is injected only into the four salivary glands in the neck (the two parotid and two submandibular glands), not into the ones under the tongue or in the roof of the mouth, so that saliva is still produced and the mouth remains moist. In some people the parotid and submandibular glands become small (atrophic) and therefore stop working after a few injections. These people usually don't require more injections, while others may need repeat injections every 4 to 6 months to continue to control their drooling. The injections are done with ultrasound guidance by a specialist called an interventional radiologist. The main side effect is the brief pain from the injection, which can be eliminated by giving the injection with sedation.

When should drooling be treated?

The main issue with drooling is the social problems it can cause. People may not want to approach someone who is drooling because it is unattractive or because they don't want to get wet. For the child attending school, it can be helpful to diminish drooling in the daytime but not treat it once the child gets home from school. Some parents decide to give medication just for special occasions, such as a family gathering. And others have their child take it routinely several times a day, every day, so that they can be comfortably around others. Besides the social effects, drooling can cause some medical problems. Especially in the winter in colder climates, the skin around the mouth can become irritated from being constantly wet. Sometimes the child's poor swallowing of saliva doesn't lead to drooling but to aspiration of saliva into the lungs.

How can I tell when my child is aspirating saliva?

When a child has recurrent aspiration pneumonia, the physician usually looks first for aspiration of food, either from swallowing difficulties or from gastro-esophageal reflux. If these conditions have been corrected (for instance, with gastrostomy tube feedings and a fundoplication), so that there is no possibility that food is going into the lungs, and the pneumonias continue, then the physician usually begins to suspect that the child is aspirating his or her own saliva.

At this point, a test called a *salivagram* is done. This involves placing a small amount of a radioactive material called *technetium 99* on the tongue. Then a special scanning device is used to discover whether the material goes into the stomach, as it should, or into the lungs, as is suspected.

What can be done about aspiration of saliva?

Sometimes the treatments mentioned above to decrease the amount of saliva are effective in preventing aspiration. However, if use of Botox or anticholinergic medications doesn't stop aspiration, then operations such as a tracheostomy or laryngotracheal separation may need to be considered. A *tracheostomy* involves placing a breathing tube into the trachea (windpipe), at the front of the neck. This procedure is recommended when a child has a breathing obstruction in the upper part of the airway, such as in the mouth, throat, or larynx. A regular tracheostomy does not prevent aspiration and in most cases is used to treat upper airway obstruction rather than aspiration.

A laryngotracheal separation is a more absolute procedure, in that it completely separates the windpipe and lungs from the mouth. It is highly successful in preventing aspiration. The major drawback is that it is permanent. After a laryngotracheal separation, the person will never be able to speak, because air no longer passes through the vocal cords. This procedure is therefore reserved for children with severe aspiration and with significant cognitive impairment who are not expected ever to develop a significant amount of verbal speech.

What is involved in caring for a child with a tracheostomy?

Caring for the tracheostomy tube can be intimidating at first. Nurses at the hospital, where the procedure is initially done, teach parents and other caregivers how to manage the "trach" tube at home. Routine care involves suctioning the tube and periodically replacing the tube with a new one. The frequency of suctioning can range from as seldom as a few times a day, or just when the child is congested, to as often as once every 1 to 2 hours. The tracheostomy allows secretions from the lungs and the airways to be suctioned easily. The presence of a tracheostomy tube may affect the child's acceptance into schools that cannot handle the amount of nursing care required.

What equipment is needed to care for a tracheostomy?

A child with a tracheostomy usually needs a fair amount of equipment at home, including a humidifier, which provides a mist to help increase the moisture in the air, in the child's room. Many children require this only when they sleep. A child with a tracheostomy may or may not need oxygen. Many need a suction machine and suction catheters in order to help suck out the secretions in the tracheostomy tube itself and to keep it from getting plugged up. As part of tracheostomy care, parents may be taught to do chest physiotherapy, which involves pounding on the chest and draining the phlegm in the airways. The tracheostomy tube is changed at regular intervals, usually every week. Some children also may require the delivery of medications through their tracheostomy, often with a *nebulizer* (which is similar to a vaporizer in that it produces a medicated mist). These medications, such as albuterol (known as Ventolin or Proventil) and budesonide (Pulmicort) are given to children who have recurrent wheezing, either on a regular basis or just when they have symptoms.

What is a normal sleep pattern?

Sleeping habits vary widely, but most healthy people sleep 7½ to 8 hours per night, with anywhere between 4 and 10 hours considered normal. An individual's sleep needs depend on a variety of factors, including age, genetics, and activity level. Throughout the night, the brain cycles through four stages of sleep. These stages are thought to play different roles in restoration of the body, learning, and memory consolidation. The final sleep stage is called rapid eye movement (or REM) sleep; during this sleep stage dreaming occurs. As the night progresses, a person spends more time in REM sleep. Young children average seven such cycles per night.

What causes sleep problems, and how are they treated?

A regular sleep pattern is established in the first few years of life. Often, an infant or a 2- to 3-year-old child resists this pattern, wanting to stay awake. In order to help a young child establish a regular sleep pattern, parents should set a specific bedtime, using the time just before bed to help the child settle down through quiet activities such as reading.

If parents do not set a regular bedtime, or if there is a great deal of nighttime activity, the child may not develop the habit of going to bed and to sleep around the same time every night. Once a regular sleep pattern has been established, a major change, such as a hospitalization or surgery, can cause a temporary disruption. Even after the child returns home, it may take weeks to return to his normal sleep pattern.

Some children with CP never develop a sleep pattern, perhaps because of brain immaturity. In this situation, doctors sometimes prescribe a medication to help regulate sleep.

When is snoring a problem?

Snoring is very common in adults and not unusual in children. Generally it is not cause for concern. However, sometimes snoring is an indication that there is a more serious obstruction of the upper airways, especially when it is accompanied by episodes of apnea (pauses in breathing). Snoring usually results from a partial obstruction of the airways during sleep, but when the obstruction becomes more severe, *obstructive sleep apnea* occurs. If left untreated, obstructive sleep apnea can cause daytime fatigue, behavior problems, and a range of other cardiac and pulmonary complications, such as high blood pressure.

Obstructive sleep apnea is characterized by loud snoring with episodes of silence during which the child struggles unsuccessfully to breathe. After several seconds of such effort, a loud snort or gasp forces open the airways and breathing resumes. Often a child with obstructive sleep apnea will awaken partially, sometimes kicking, flailing the arms, or experiencing a total body spasm. Sometimes the child wakes up, and the regular sleep pattern is disturbed without obvious symptoms. The child may then resume sleeping only to repeat the same sequence of events again throughout the night. These problems are considered pathological based on certain criteria, including the number of times per hour the episodes occur, as well as the oxygen and carbon dioxide levels during sleep. A sleep study (polysomnogram) is an overnight test used to characterize sleep patterns and respiratory patterns during sleep and diagnose obstructive sleep apnea.

What causes this obstruction?

One or more factors may contribute to this obstruction of the upper part of the airways, which includes the mouth, throat, and larynx (where the vocal cords are located). In young children the most common cause of this obstruction is enlargement of the tonsils and adenoids. The adenoids are tissues that sit above the roof of the mouth in the back of the nose. If these tissues are enlarged, they may block the nasal passages and cause a child to breathe primarily through the mouth. If the tonsils are also enlarged, the back of the mouth becomes more crowded, and airflow through the upper airways may be reduced. In addition, children with CP may also have obstruction because of decreased muscle tone in the muscles around the upper airways. Because of decreased tone in these muscles, there can be increased collapse of the airways as well as obstruction from the tongue. Finally, a child who is overweight or obese is at increased risk for obstructive sleep apnea.

Besides snoring, are there other symptoms of obstructive apnea?

A child who hasn't slept well at night may be either hyperactive or excessively fatigued during the day. The child may have difficulties with concentration and focusing in school. Some children with obstructive apnea have a below normal body weight and have difficulties gaining weight. Another sign of obstructive sleep apnea is nighttime bedwetting in a child who has previously remained dry overnight.

How is obstructive apnea treated?

The treatment is aimed at relieving the obstruction. If obstruction is due to enlarged tonsils and adenoids, for example, these are removed. If the child is markedly obese, weight loss is recommended. Nighttime CPAP or BiPAP, which involves delivering airway pressure through a mask while the child is sleeping, is also a treatment for obstructive sleep apnea. For children whose obstruction is severe and caused by poor muscle control, or for those who don't respond to the less invasive treatments, a tracheostomy may be recommended.

What complications are possible from a tonsillectomy and adenoidectomy?

Commonly, this surgery is followed by a sore throat, which may interfere with the child's ability to eat and drink. In severe cases, a child may become dehydrated. Bleeding from the throat, although unusual, can occur even two weeks after surgery. In children with CP there are other risks, such as a decreased ability to handle oral secretions, especially when a sore throat follows surgery. Because of increased oral secretions, decreased respiratory muscle tone, and ineffective cough, children with CP may be at increased risk of respiratory complications after surgery. This operation poses a special risk for children who are very young or have complex medical needs because of increased risk of dehydration and respiratory complications. Therefore, these children will usually stay in the hospital overnight for monitoring.

Communication Issues

What makes it difficult for a child with CP to communicate?

To communicate successfully, a person must be able to receive and interpret language as well as to express it. Cerebral palsy may interfere with both receptive and expressive language skills. Poor attention span, for example, with or without intellectual impairment, can decrease the ability to process speech from other people. A hearing impairment can interfere to the point of affecting speech and language development. On the expressive side, neuromuscular disability can interfere with breath control, vocal cord movement, and lip, tongue, and palate motion—all of which can result in articulation problems and difficulty in speaking. Neuromuscular disability also can interfere with written and electronic communication, both of which are functionally and socially critical in today's world.

What can be done to help my child communicate?

Early diagnosis and identification of any factors that might be correctable (such as fluid in the ears) is the first step to ensuring good communication. If there are no factors that can be corrected—that is, if the impairment is due to the cerebral palsy itself and not to a correctable hearing problem, for instance—then the child should be referred to a speech-language therapist, who may help the CP patient improve his or her communication. For children who have normal or near normal intelligence and the ability to comprehend and express thoughts but who cannot speak because of the cerebral palsy, there are assistive devices, known as *augmentative communication devices*, that can help. These devices, ranging from a simple board with pictures for pointing to or focusing on with the eyes to very sophisticated electronic devices with synthesized speech, can help a child with cerebral palsy express himself. Such devices commonly support development of receptive and expressive language in most children who have complex communication needs associated with their cerebral palsy. As a part of an evaluation, speech-language therapists determine which of these devices are most appropriate for an individual child.

Referral to a speech-language therapist with expertise in augmentative communication as early as the second year of life can help prevent a child from falling significantly behind his peers in speech, language, and social development. (See "Augmentative Communication" in Part 3 for more details.)

Dental Issues

Oral health is being recognized as a foundation for good overall general health and wellness. The success of dental treatment and care depends on the parents and caregivers. They are important members of the oral health team. They need to become knowledgeable and competent in home oral health practice, such as toothbrushing.

At what age should a child with CP have a first dental evaluation?

Like any other child, a child with cerebral palsy should first be seen by a dentist between 6 and 12 months of age. This provides an opportunity to implement individualized preventive oral health practices and reduce the child's risk of preventable dental disease in the future. The first visit usually includes a detailed medical and dental history and a thorough examination. At about age 3, the first dental x-rays are usually taken. If the child cannot sit still, taking x-rays may require sedation. By scheduling the patient at a designated time (early in the day) and allowing sufficient time to talk with the parents or guardian and the patient before initiating any dental care, the dentist can establish an excellent relationship with the patient. The primary purpose of the first visit or visits may be to allow the dentist and patient to become acquainted. The dentist will provide a summary of the oral findings and specific treatment recommendations to the patient and the parent or caregiver. When appropriate, the patient's other care providers (physicians, nurses, social workers) might be informed of significant findings.

Do children with CP have more cavities than other children?

The incidence of cavities among children and adolescents with CP is high. Dental cavities are caused by plaque, bacteria attached firmly to the tooth. If not removed, plaque produces acids that will "dissolve" areas of enamel and eventually create a hole or cavity. Plaque can be removed only by mechanical means using, for example, a toothbrush or washcloth.

Many factors increase the likelihood of cavities. One factor is a diet high in sugar. Parents and caregivers need to be aware of medications that have sugar in them, especially liquid medicines. Another factor is decreased saliva production, so parents and caregivers need to be aware of medications that cause a dry mouth. A decrease in saliva increases the risk of cavities because there is less saliva to neutralize the acids caused by plaque. Defects in the enamel (the outer covering of the tooth) can make the tooth more susceptible to cavities. Studies show that developmental enamel defects are more common among children with CP. The risk of these enamel defects varies with the tooth type and is more common among children born prematurely. However, the major cause of cavities in children with CP is poor oral hygiene. A strong tongue thrust, as well as biting and clenching reflexes, make it difficult to get a tooth-

brush into a child's mouth. Crowded teeth can make the teeth more susceptible to cavities because cleaning these teeth is more difficult. Cavities can be
painful. Cavities should be considered as a possible reason for crying in a child
who cannot communicate.

How can cavities be prevented?

Cavities can be prevented by proper toothbrushing two times a day. The dentist or hygienist can create a customized toothbrushing technique for the parent or caregiver to use at home. Fluoride is recommended for all children. It
is a simple and cost effective means of reducing the risk of cavities. Fluoride
is often found in municipal water. If the municipal water system is not fluo-
ridated, the dentist can prescribe fluoride drops or pills to be taken daily. In
addition, many dentists apply fluoride to the child's teeth every six months.

What is gum hypertrophy?

Gum hypertrophy (also called *gingival hypertrophy*) is an enlargement of the
gums. The common causes of this condition are poor hygiene (not removing
plaque) or certain medications, such as Dilantin. Approximately 40 percent
of people taking this medication develop enlarged gums. Symptoms are more
prevalent in younger children and occur approximately 2 to 3 months after
they start taking the medication. Symptoms reach their highest level after 9
to 12 months of taking the medication. Whatever the cause, the gums can become so enlarged that they grow over the teeth. If this situation continues for
too long, the gums can become dark pink or red and bleed easily. They may
even become painful.

What is the treatment for swollen gums?

One simple way to treat swollen gums is by eliminating plaque through good
toothbrushing. If the gum tissue is swollen and toothbrushing has not helped,
the most effective treatment is to remove the extra gum tissue surgically. The
gum tissue can grow back after surgery, but the swelling will be less severe if
good toothbrushing is maintained.

Are there other dental abnormalities that are common in children with CP?

One common abnormality is *malocclusion*, meaning poor alignment of the
teeth and jaws. In malocclusion the upper and lower teeth or the upper and
lower jaws do not line up properly. Malocclusion in the child with CP involves
more than just misaligned teeth. There is also a musculoskeletal problem.
Often, the upper front teeth of a child with CP are too far forward, putting the
child at risk for breaking those teeth. Protruding upper front teeth are typically
associated with tongue thrusting. Another common malocclusion is an open
bite, which is the presence of a space between the upper and lower front teeth
when the jaws are fully closed. Ideally, the upper front teeth should come over
the lower front teeth about 1–2 mm. The inability to close the lips because of
an open bite also contributes to excessive drooling.

Muscle spasticity directly affects dental and skeletal formation. The spasticity causes pathological contraction of the muscles of the head and neck. When
the muscles of chewing are in spasm, they can remodel and reshape the bones
of the face and the upper and lower jaws. When this affects the jaw, it can re-

sult in malocclusion. Thrusting of the tongue, mouth breathing, and a poor swallow reflex can affect the shape of the jaw and contribute to malocclusion.

Can children with CP have braces on their teeth?

Braces (orthodontics) in children serve many functions. They help realign poorly positioned teeth and help the jaws come together and thus function better. When crooked teeth are made straight, the teeth are easier to clean. It should be noted that correcting malocclusion is very challenging in children with moderate or severe cerebral palsy. Orthodontic treatment may not be an option because of the risk of cavities and enamel hypoplasia seen in children with CP. The ability of the patient or the caregiver to maintain good daily oral hygiene is critical to the success of orthodontic treatment. Poor oral hygiene leads to cavities and inflamed gums. As gums become more inflamed, they can exert a pressure that can slow the movement of teeth, causing the orthodontic treatment (the braces) to take longer to straighten the teeth. However, a developmental disability like CP in and of itself should not be perceived as a barrier to orthodontic treatment. The orthodontist may elect to put the braces on over a few months instead of during a single long appointment.

What is bruxism?

Bruxism is the habitual grinding of teeth. It is common in children with CP. In extreme cases, bruxism wears down the teeth and flattens the biting surfaces of the back teeth. If this happens, the enamel can be worn away, exposing the dentin underneath. Exposed dentin can cause sensitivity to cold food and sweets. Parents often complain about the constant grinding noise their child makes while sleeping. There are several common causes of bruxism:

- Stress, such as a divorce or death in the family, a new school, changes in the child's normal routine.
- Malocclusion, which the body tries to eliminate by grinding it away.
- Habit. Back baby teeth have flat top surfaces which make it very easy to slide the teeth from side to side, especially under age 6, before the first permanent molars erupt.

Is there a treatment for tooth grinding (bruxism)?

The usual treatment is to take upper and lower impressions of the teeth and make a custom thin U-shaped plastic splint to place over the lower teeth. It is worn only at night. It is a challenge to take impressions of the teeth of most children, because they tend to gag and vomit. It is even more challenging to treat bruxism in the child with CP. First, the child's hyperactive bite reflex, greater gag reflex, and body and head movements can make it difficult to take an accurate impression, so that the splint might not fit. Second, it is possible that the splint will cause more gagging, more swallowing problems, and discomfort for the child. On the positive side, most tooth grinding that occurs in early childhood stops around age 6, when the first permanent molars come in. Unlike the baby molars, the permanent molars have long cusps. When the upper and lower jaws come together, these cusps interlock, making grinding more difficult. Some indications for treatment, regardless of age, include severe enamel wear, tooth sensitivity, and pain in the temporomandibular joint, or TMJ, the joint that connects the jaw to the skull.

Why are children with CP susceptible to dental injuries?

Children with CP have a common malocclusion in which the upper front teeth are too far forward. Seizures or an unsteady gait, which can lead to frequent falls, can result in trauma to these protruding teeth. The most common type of dental injury is fracture of the tooth's enamel and dentin. Any dental injury requires immediate attention. One severe form of dental trauma occurs when a tooth is avulsed, or "knocked out." Avulsed baby teeth should not be reimplanted. However, an avulsed permanent tooth should immediately be placed in a cup or container of milk and brought with the patient to the dentist so that the tooth can be reimplanted.

Hernias and Undescended Testicles

Are children with CP more likely to get hernias?

A hernia is a projection of a body part beyond its natural location. The most common type of hernia is an *inguinal hernia*, which occurs in the groin region. The incidence of inguinal hernias in boys with cerebral palsy appears to be higher than that in boys who do not have cerebral palsy. We know that inguinal hernias are more common in premature infants, especially those weighing less than 1,500 grams (3 lb. 5 oz.). But even among these children, the incidence is higher for those who have CP, possibly twice as great as that among premature children without CP. It's not clear why this is so. Parents and the physician of a child with CP, especially a boy born prematurely, should be on the alert for signs of an inguinal hernia, in particular swelling, either in the scrotum itself or, more usually, in the thigh area above the scrotum.

Are undescended testicles a common problem?

Normally, the testicles begin forming in the abdomen of the male fetus prior to birth and descend into the scrotum by the time of birth if the pregnancy is full term. Premature infants are more likely to have undescended testicles. However, the testicles will often descend on their own into the scrotum by the end of the first year of life. If they do not, surgical correction is recommended, because the undescended testicle can twist on itself, cutting off the blood supply and permanently injuring the testicle. An emergency operation is required if this occurs. Also, a tumor may develop in an undescended testicle later in life. It is easier to detect a testicular tumor if the testicle is in its normal position within the scrotum.

Even if the testicles are descended at birth, there can be problems later on. Studies have shown that there is an increased incidence of undescended testicles in teenage boys and young adults with cerebral palsy. According to some estimates, as many as 50 percent of males with CP have this condition. It would appear that spasticity of a muscle known as the *cremasteric muscle* causes the testis to be positioned higher as the boy with cerebral palsy grows older, thus pulling it out of the scrotal sac.

Retractile testicles are those that are not in the scrotum but can be felt in the groin and brought down into the scrotum by gently pulling with the hand. Retractile testicles do not usually become undescended and do not need surgery.

Do children with cerebral palsy have more trouble with bladder control?	Problems with bladder control are not common in children with cerebral palsy, but they do occur more often among these children than among the general population, especially in those who have constipation. These problems can include incontinence (day or nighttime wetting), difficulty starting a urinary stream, or symptoms of urgency, meaning the feeling that one has to urinate immediately, without prior warning. Some children may have subclinical voiding disorders, meaning their bladders do not work entirely normally, but they do not show any symptoms under ordinary circumstances. These children may develop symptoms, especially an inability to empty the bladder, after surgical procedures.

Issues Regarding Puberty

What physical changes should I expect when my son begins puberty?	In boys, the onset of puberty is marked by the testicles getting larger, followed by the growth of pubic hair and the penis getting larger. The onset of puberty in boys generally occurs between 9 and 14 years. It is generally believed that a boy who either starts puberty before age 9 or does not show signs of puberty by age 14 should be evaluated by a doctor for a possible medical problem. It has been found that boys with CP start puberty earlier than boys without CP, but progress through the stages is slower, and puberty ends later.
What physical changes should I expect to see when my daughter begins puberty?	Puberty in girls generally begins with breast growth, followed by pubic hair growth, followed by the start of menstrual periods. For girls without CP puberty can begin as early as age 6 but is generally around age 8. The end of puberty, considered the time when a young woman gets her first period, is at approximately 12 years. From start to finish, puberty takes about two to five years. Nutrition, body fat, racial background, medications, and underlying medical conditions affect a young woman's puberty. If there is no breast growth by age 14 or no periods by age 15, she should be evaluated by a doctor.
Will CP affect my daughter's puberty?	Although girls with CP start puberty earlier than girls without CP, they end puberty later, with periods generally beginning at age 14. In addition, in girls with CP, pubic hair tends to appear before breasts begin to grow, whereas in girls without CP breast growth is the first sign of puberty. The average age of the start of breast development in girls with CP is about 10 years, and the average age of the start of pubic hair growth is about 8 years.
How will puberty affect seizures?	In young women with CP and seizures, the onset of menstrual periods can cause seizures to worsen. The hormones that control the menstrual cycle also have an effect on the brain. Because of the monthly changes in these hormones, seizures may increase a few days before and a few days into the menstrual bleeding.
What can be done if a girl experiences increasing seizure activity during puberty?	There are several options for managing these seizures. One strategy is to give an extra dose of the prescribed antiseizure medication a few days before the expected start of the period and about two days into the bleeding. Another option is to provide hormonal therapy in the form of a contraceptive pill, patch, ring, injection, implant, or intrauterine device. A change in the dosing

of the antiseizure medications may be needed, as the way the body handles those medications changes during puberty. This should be discussed with the physician who treats your child's seizures.

What can be done about a change in behavior around the time of a girl's period?

Premenstrual syndrome (PMS) usually occurs one to two weeks before the onset of bleeding and goes away a few days after bleeding begins. Young women with PMS report a multitude of symptoms, including hot flashes, chills, difficulty concentrating, and mood changes such as irritability and depression. In women and girls with intellectual disability, PMS can cause an increase in behavior problems, seizures, aggression, tantrums, crying spells, self-abusive behavior and self-mutilation, restlessness, and agitation. Hormonal contraception, medications such as ibuprofen or naproxen, and medications used for depression can be used to treat these symptoms. Talk with your doctor about appropriate options for your daughter.

What can be done when a girl becomes agitated and seems to be in pain around the time of her period?

Pain during the time of a period is called *dysmenorrhea*. Usually it begins a few hours prior to the start of the period and lasts for one to two days. In some girls the pain starts earlier and ends later. Nausea, vomiting, diarrhea, back pain, thigh pain, and headache may also be experienced. Girls who cannot communicate may become very agitated and distressed during their periods because of these symptoms. They may thrash around or tense up. Posturing, tooth grinding, and increased irritability may occur as well. Although medications such as ibuprofen and naproxen are very effective for the treatment of dysmenorrhea, if symptoms continue, hormonal contraception may be effective.

What can be done if menstrual bleeding is difficult to manage?

Menstrual hygiene may be an issue for some teenage girls with CP. Although it is felt that with encouragement and teaching most girls with and without intellectual disability can learn to use menstrual products, some girls simply cannot change a pad or a tampon due to physical or cognitive impairment. During the first two years of starting to have periods, some girls may bleed unpredictably and heavily at times. This bleeding should be evaluated by a physician. Although most girls will outgrow it, it can be a nuisance for families and the child. In such a situation, hormonal medicines and perhaps surgery, both of which are discussed below, can be used to stop or decrease monthly bleeding.

Do females with cerebral palsy need birth control?

Teenage girls and women with cerebral palsy are capable of and interested in sexual activity in much the same way women without CP are. Studies have shown that girls with mild intellectual disability engage in sexual activity, including sexual intercourse, in proportions comparable to those in the general adolescent population. A much smaller proportion of girls with moderate or severe intellectual disability do so. Regardless of the complexity of their cerebral palsy or the level of their intellectual disability, these girls are still at risk of victimization by males in their peer group and environment. In fact, one-third of those with mild intellectual disability and one-fourth of adolescent girls with moderate intellectual disability have been reported to be victims of rape. This is the main reason why it is important to provide comprehensive sexual education to all adolescents. Important topics to discuss include safe touch, safe sex, and general changes adolescents can expect during puberty.

Parents often seek hormonal treatment for their female child with CP for hormonal contraception, hormonal control of the child's period, or control of the symptoms that accompany a period. Certain medical conditions may exclude some girls from receiving some of these hormonal treatments, but in general a therapy can be found that is safe and effective for most women.

For the aforementioned reasons, it is important to consider the necessity of birth control for all girls with CP, including those with severe or limiting disabilities. Contraceptive options include condoms and hormonal contraception. Hormonal contraception protects against pregnancy. It comes in the form of a pill to be taken daily, an injection given every three months, a patch placed on the skin and changed weekly, a ring placed in the vagina and changed monthly, or other devices that can remain in place for years. All hormonal methods can be used to decrease the frequency of menstrual flow or stop it entirely. Both the subdermal implant and intrauterine devices have the advantage of remaining in place for many (3 to 5) years and are more reliable than birth control pills, the patch, or the ring. Table 4 compares types of hormonal contraception.

Does a young woman need an "internal" exam before starting hormonal treatment?

Pelvic (or "internal") exams are no longer required prior to starting hormonal treatment. Currently young women do not need to have their first Pap smear, or cervical cancer screening, until they reach 21 years of age. Careful examination of a girl's past medical history and family history is often sufficient prior to her starting hormonal treatment. A breast or external genital exam (looking at the outside of the vagina) may be part of the physical exam prior to starting hormonal contraception.

If medications are not an option, is surgery a possibility?

Surgery may be available as a last resort for those individuals who have failed all other forms of treatments. One possible surgical procedure is a hysterectomy, removal of the uterus. However, hysterectomy raises many ethical questions (discussed in the next section). Endometrial ablation is also an option. This involves destruction of the inside lining of the uterus to decrease or stop menstrual bleeding completely. This procedure is also controversial because the lining can grow back and women can still become pregnant afterwards, with a high risk of complications associated with the pregnancy.

Can a young woman with cerebral palsy be sterilized at the request of her parents if she has severe intellectual disability?

Some parents would like to have their daughters sterilized surgically either by having a hysterectomy performed or by having the fallopian tubes tied. This is especially true of parents of women with severe intellectual disability, who would not be capable of caring for a child. Whereas years ago many women and men with intellectual disabilities were sterilized against their will, this is much more difficult today. A parent must go through the courts to obtain permission to have the procedure done, primarily because society feels that being able to bear a child is an inalienable right. Parents and legal guardians have to prove that maintaining the ability to bear a child is not in the individual's best

Table 4. Types of Hormonal Contraception

	Combined Pills	Patch	Ring	Progesterone Only Pills	Medroxyprogesterone Acetate	Hormonal IUD*	Hormonal Implant
Hormones	Estrogen and progesterone	Estrogen and progesterone	Estrogen and progesterone	Progesterone	Progesterone	Progesterone	Progesterone
Frequency	Daily	Weekly	Monthly	Daily	Every 3 months	Every 3-5 years	Every 3 years
Side effects	Nausea, bloating, breast tenderness, blood clots in legs or lungs	Nausea, bloating, skin irritation, not as effective in those weighing more than 198 pounds, blood clots in legs or lungs	Nausea, bloating, skin irritation, not as effective in those weighing more than 198 pounds, blood clots in legs or lungs	Weight gain, irregular bleeding, no menses at all	Weight gain, decreased bone density, irregular bleeding, no menses at all, delayed return to fertility, alopecia	Pain with insertion, expulsion of the device, spotting or breakthrough bleeding, uterine perforation	Not as effective in those weighing more than 130% of ideal body weight, irregular bleeding, headache, weight gain, acne
Contraindications	Certain types of migraines, blood clots in legs or lungs, clotting disorders, uncontrolled high blood pressure, liver disease	Blood clots in legs or lungs, clotting disorders	Blood clots in legs or lungs, clotting disorders	Breast cancer	Breast cancer	Uterine abnormalities	Breast cancer

*There is another type of intrauterine device that does not contain hormones but instead contains copper. This type of intrauterine device is not used for contraception.

interest. Reasons occasionally cited include profound intellectual disability and an increased risk of being victimized. Reasons that are generally not accepted are individual medical conditions in and of themselves.

Does my child need the HPV vaccine?

The American Academy of Pediatrics recommends the full human papillomavirus (HPV) vaccine series for all male and female children beginning at 9 years of age, regardless of the child's sexual activity status. The vaccine has been shown to protect against the development of cervical cancer when women reach middle age. The reason the vaccine is recommended starting at age 9 is because for those teens who will become sexually active, the vaccine is most effective prior to the start of sexual activity. Even children with CP or an intellectual disability need the vaccine series, because these children also engage in sexual activity (as discussed previously) and are also at risk for abuse of all types, including sexual abuse. In addition, even those children who might seem immature may decide to become sexually active at a later age. Finally, it is important to remember that the HPV vaccine not only protects against cervical cancer in women but it also protects against types of genital warts and head and neck cancers in both men and women.

When people with CP have children, what is the risk that their babies will have CP?

Traditionally, only 1 to 2 percent of cases of CP were found to be familial and thus to be caused by a genetic abnormality. More recent studies have shown chromosomal abnormalities associated with CP, which may or may not be the direct cause (see Chapter 1). It would be prudent for a woman with CP whose cause is not known to receive genetic counseling in order to determine whether there is a risk of passing on CP to children she might carry. The frequency of miscarriages and toxemia are no greater for women with CP than for other women. The majority of adults with disabilities have normal children, though parents with CP have more children with abnormalities of all kinds than the norm.

Pain

When my nonverbal, noncommunicative child with CP seems to be in pain, what could be the cause?

Every parent deals with this question when their children are infants and don't yet communicate verbally. Crying is a form of communication. Just as parents of infants soon learn to recognize the sound of crying because of hunger and to differentiate this from the cry caused by pain or frustration or simply being tired, parents of the nonverbal child with CP also learn to recognize the different kinds of crying.

Many of the medical problems described in this chapter need to be considered when the child with CP appears to be in pain. These could include causes of pain that are commonly seen in children with or without CP, such as constipation/impaction, esophagitis due to GE reflux, sinusitis, an ingrown toenail, or a girl's monthly menses. Conditions that are less common in the general population but occur in those with CP might be causes for the child's pain. These might include a fragility fracture due to osteoporosis, gallstones, kidney stones, or a dental abscess or cavity. Pancreatitis can be caused by some medications and is often seen after spinal fusion for scoliosis. A dislocated hip can be painful, as can a decubitus ulcer (also known as a pressure sore). If the child has a V-P shunt, this should be evaluated by the physician managing it, as a blocked shunt causing increased pressure in the brain could result in crying (or other changes in behavior, like excessive sleepiness). Spasticity itself can cause discomfort or pain; many children who awake at night due to tight muscles will go back to sleep after repositioning or a brief massage. Seizures can cause behavior changes, including crying. A new medication can cause a change in the child's behavior, including crying. Likewise, weaning a child from a medication he or she has taken for a long time, especially if it is stopped abruptly, can cause crying. And emergency abdominal problems like appendicitis or bowel obstruction can come to the parents' attention because their child is crying.

When the parent or caregiver believes that the child is experiencing pain, a full evaluation by experts in managing the child with CP should be undertaken. This evaluation should include a detailed history and physical examination, an x-ray evaluation of the hips, and possibly an abdominal ultrasound. If no source can be identified, a whole body technetium bone scan should be considered.

Poor Temperature Control

The body's temperature is usually tightly controlled. Most people have a temperature close to 98.6 degrees Fahrenheit or 37.0 degrees Centigrade. Infections of almost any kind, whether of the lungs (pneumonia) or the urinary tract or common viral infections such as influenza can cause an elevated temperature. Any temperature above 100.4°F (38.4°C) is considered a fever. Sometimes an elevated temperature is due to an inflammatory disease (juvenile arthritis or lupus are two such diseases). Environmental conditions, such as too many clothes or extreme heat, can raise the body temperature.

In all these situations, the body tries to get rid of heat by shivering and perspiring. These mechanisms are controlled by the brain. When the brain is severely damaged, as in some children with CP, these mechanisms can be damaged too. A very high or very low body temperature can result from infections or environmental temperature. Sometimes there is no obvious cause. A sudden rise or fall in body temperature needs to be investigated, as it could be caused by an infection. However, if it happens frequently and no infection is identified, it may be that the child's body temperature is sensitive to the environment and the child needs to wear fewer or more clothes. Some children with CP have a "normal" temperature when not sick that is as much as 2 to 3 degrees lower than that of the general population (meaning 95 to 96°F, or 35 to 36°C). These children may need to wear extra clothing routinely or even use a heating blanket to stay warm. When these children are outside on hot sunny days, caregivers need to keep them out of direct sun. If they stay outside for a prolonged period, their temperature should be monitored. Cooling vests are available for those who want to be outside on very hot days but cannot regulate their temperature.

Life Span

What is the expected life span of someone with cerebral palsy?

In recent years, children with cerebral palsy have survived to adulthood in much greater numbers than before. Approximately 90 percent of children with cerebral palsy will survive to age 20, compared with 99 percent of children in the general population. Among children with CP, 99 percent of those who have no severe functional disabilities survive to age 20, compared with 50 percent of those who have severe functional limitations in all three major areas (ambulation, manual dexterity, and mental ability). For all children with cerebral palsy, death is usually due to respiratory illness, often aspiration pneumonia or upper airway obstruction. A smaller number will die unexpectedly when in apparent good health, often in their sleep. This can happen especially in those who also have epilepsy along with their cerebral palsy (see "Sudden Unexpected Death in Epilepsy" in Part 3). As medical technology advances, there is a greater chance that many more children with cerebral palsy will survive into adulthood.

Despite continued medical advances, many families will still be faced with having to decide whether to let their chronically ill child die or to introduce new and more intensive treatments, such as a tracheostomy for airway obstruction. When faced with these decisions, it may be helpful to speak with a palliative care team. Palliative care is an approach that focuses on improving the quality of life of patients facing complications associated with life limiting disease. This is achieved through early identification and treatment of pain and other medical or social problems. Palliative care is often misinterpreted as hospice care. While hospice is a subset of palliative care, a child does not need to have a terminal illness to qualify for palliative care services. Many hospitals now have hospice and palliative care teams. These teams support acute or chronically ill children by helping them to manage their pain and symptom management so as to achieve the best quality of life possible. Some families will choose to provide comfort care to the child without any intensive intervention, while others will elect to do everything possible. If a family chooses to provide comfort care, the hospice and palliative care team will help with the transition to supportive care, including hospice when the time is appropriate for the child and the child's family.

It is important for both the parents and the patient to think about what life-sustaining measures they would want to take *before* a crisis arises. It can be helpful to talk this decision over with those who can provide emotional support, such as other family members, physicians with whom the family or patient has a strong relationship, or clergy. This may be a difficult conversation for parents to have with their child. If possible, the older child or adolescent, who may have his or her own thoughts about life-sustaining measures, should be involved in the decision. Of course, a patient who has reached the age at which he can make his own medical decisions might make a different choice than his parents would have done. While there is no one right answer for all patients and their families, many families have to make this decision at some point, and it is wise to discuss it in advance.

Patients may want to put their wishes into an advance directive. An advance directive is a document that specifies the patient's preferences regarding medical treatment in the event that he or she is unable to communicate those preferences to a doctor. If the patient is not of legal age to make his own medical decisions, the patient's legal guardian can complete this document for the patient. There are also documents designed specifically for children and young adults so that their wishes can also be heard.

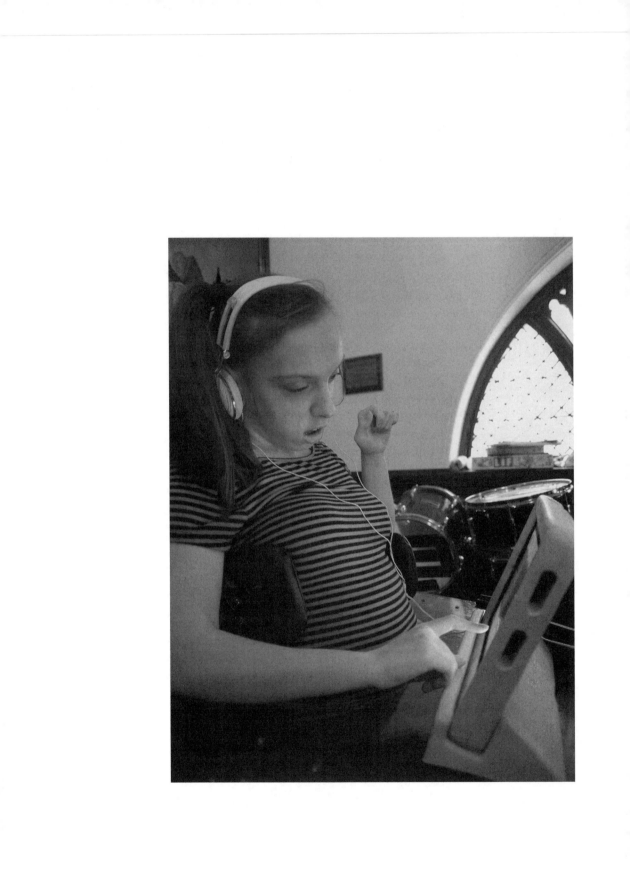

4

Intellectual, Psychological, and Social Development

THIS CHAPTER explores how cerebral palsy affects the intellectual and psychological development of the individual from infancy, toddlerhood, and childhood through adolescence and young adulthood. We focus on the emotional and social development of children with cerebral palsy, and we also look at how children develop intellectually. We explore how cerebral palsy affects psychological development differently in different children, depending upon what part of the child's body is affected and how profound the disability is. Family functioning is important to the well-being of a child with cerebral palsy, so in this chapter we pay attention to both the family and the child. In fact, since problems in the newborn can have such an impact on families, we begin the chapter with a look at how families function.

Birth to One Year

Emotional development during this period is characterized by the growing attachment between parents and their new baby. This attachment is dependent upon the interplay between the infant's characteristics (for example, his or her temperament) and the characteristics of the parents. The interplay itself influences the child's emotional development. The child's intellectual development, on the other hand, is driven by the infant's motivation to reach out and discover the world through sensorimotor actions on people and things around him or her. Cerebral palsy can affect the infant's emotional and intellectual development both directly, through the child's limitations, and indirectly, through the world's response to the child.

How might parents react when they hear that their child has cerebral palsy?

The discovery that their baby has a disability usually has a significant impact on parents and on how the family functions. Often the disability begins to have an impact before a diagnosis is made. Parents "just know" that their child is not developing or behaving as they expected. They begin to be concerned that something is wrong with the baby, even though the doctor may not yet know whether this is the case. Thus, parents sometimes experience anxiety and fear even before the doctor delivers the diagnosis. The tension and fear experienced during this period of uncertainty often lead to stress and may begin to undermine the family unit even before the diagnosis has been made.

When they hear that their baby has cerebral palsy, some parents may go into a state of shock or disbelief. Such a reaction to devastating news is understandable, especially as parents often think of the "worst-case scenario" and are not aware of the wide spectrum of this condition. But individuals who react in this way are likely to experience stress even more keenly than if they had reacted less strongly. Shock and heightened stress often make it difficult for parents to take in all the information the doctor gives them. Because of this, it's a good idea for parents to return to their doctor to go over information about their child's medical condition.

How does the initial reaction change over time?

As parents become better acquainted with their child and understand more about what cerebral palsy means, they develop different responses to their child's disability. Some parents cope by getting very involved in their infant's care. This means that they investigate the nature of their baby's disability and take an active role in the baby's care and therapy.

For other parents, the grief, pain, and uncertainty they feel about having a child with a disability is more than they can endure. To cope with these feelings, these parents may deny that their baby has a disability, or they may minimize its effects. Such denial is likely to become more apparent as the child gets older and the extent of the disability becomes clearer. Other parents, laboring under these same stresses and feelings, may feel angry about what has happened to their child and to their family.

Becoming actively involved in the infant's care and therapy is a healthy way of coping with the feelings a parent has when he or she discovers that an infant has cerebral palsy. Denial and anger, on the other hand, can have a negative effect on the child and the parents—indeed, such feelings take their toll on people and relationships throughout the family. Spouses who are persistently under stress, for example, might find that they argue more often. Sometimes the care and the long-term outlook for the child with a disability are the source of the conflict. The end result of these reactions can be that the parents emotionally distance themselves from the child. This, in turn, means that the much-needed emotional closeness between the parents and the child is diminished.

Families in this situation are vulnerable to continuing discord, which can lead to separation and divorce. Other children in the family can be affected by this persistent discord too.

What impact can cerebral palsy have on the family, including siblings?

A diagnosis of cerebral palsy impacts not only the child who has been diagnosed but the entire family. Parents feel that they must be effective advocates and caregivers for their child. To do this, they have to learn a new language made up of medical and educational terms they may never have needed before. They have to continue to provide for their family on a day-to-day basis while negotiating the ever-changing health care system, the world of insurance, and the special education system to ensure that their child receives the appropriate services.

The stress on parents is clear. However, typically developing siblings are also impacted by having a child with special needs or cerebral palsy in the family. Not only do they have to share their parents' attention with a sibling but that sibling with cerebral palsy likely requires increased amounts of adult attention and supervision due to the medical, social, emotional, and physical difficulties the child faces. Siblings may find themselves receiving less attention from their parents, who must focus their time and attention on the child with cerebral palsy. Parents may be less available for everyday activities such as helping with homework, practicing soccer, or driving back and forth to activities or playdates. They may have less time to hear about siblings' day or their friends, to help them explore new activities, or even to just "snuggle" or take part in the regular routine before bedtime.

The impact on siblings can be both positive and negative. Just as the diagnosis of the child with cerebral palsy needs to be explained in terms that the child can understand, typically developing siblings also need the information to be presented in a way they can understand. Their developmental level will dictate how much information, and in how much detail, parents should provide. And just as the child with cerebral palsy needs a "quick answer" to share with others about his diagnosis, so too will the siblings need a "quick answer" when they are asked "What's wrong with your brother?" or "Why is your sister in a wheelchair?" Parents and caregivers would benefit from meeting with a mental health professional who has experience working with families of children with disabilities to learn ways to address siblings' concerns about their brother or sister with CP and how to present the information appropriately.

There is growing recognition of the impact of having a sibling with special needs on typically developing children. Their lives are different from the lives of their peers who do not have a family member with special needs. Support groups for siblings are becoming more popular. There are also books written specifically for siblings and websites where they can go to meet other siblings of children with special needs. School counselors or psychologists may be able to help the family identify trusted resources in their area if they are not able to do so by themselves.

How does the family's emotional reaction affect the child?

If the parents deny that their child has a problem, they can't really absorb the information provided to them by doctors and other professionals involved in the care and treatment of their child. Without this information, parents may not be in a good position to make decisions about or take part in their child's treatment, or they may be unable to make proper use of the resources available.

In extreme cases, a parent's negative emotional reaction can also inhibit development of a healthy relationship with the baby. For a few parents the pain and hurt may be so crippling that they become depressed and don't interact with their baby. These parents are psychologically and emotionally unavailable to the child. The result of this is a weakened attachment that may result in the abuse or neglect of the child. In response, the baby typically becomes withdrawn and depressed.

Some parents overprotect the child in situations they view as potentially harmful or dangerous. Overprotection may stifle the child's development and inhibit the child's efforts to be more independent, which are usually seen in the second year of life.

Finally, some parents may react by overcompensating. They may ask the baby to do too much, or they may have higher expectations for the child's progress at any point in treatment than the child can realistically be expected to meet.

How can the family be helped?	Families need professional help and good support to come to terms with the fact that their baby has a disability. Ideally, counseling, therapy, support groups, and sibling groups will be made available to the family within a reasonable time after the diagnosis is made. This help could go a long way toward preventing the development of unhealthy parental coping styles. It could also prevent many of the other undesirable consequences mentioned. Furthermore, ongoing contact with a mental health professional can ensure that the family has continued support as the child with cerebral palsy ages and faces additional developmental obstacles. Adjusting to the news of having a child with cerebral palsy does not happen all at once. It will be necessary for parents to continue to change their expectations and adjust to a life that is often different from the ones many other families live. Each developmental stage the child goes through has the potential to present new adjustment issues.
How does the emotional tie between parent and child develop?	One important development in the first year of life is the establishment of a lasting tie between the baby and his or her parents in a process known as *attachment*. The strength of this tie is influenced by how the baby and the parents respond to each other. The baby's appearance, vigor, and basic way of responding to the environment (that is, his or her temperament) are important factors, as is the parents' ability to tune into the baby's feelings and "read" his or her needs. The parents' ability to adapt to the baby's temperament (especially if he or she is fussy and irritable) also plays a large role in the development of this tie. If the infant begins to develop secure attachments early in life, they will be demonstrated in many infants by a fear of strangers (which develops at around 7 to 8 months), by a sense of trust in the parents, and by a mutual love between infant and parent. The sense of trust and security, which for the young child go hand in hand, can be delayed or not fully develop if parents are not emotionally available to the baby or abuse or neglect the baby. Failure to develop this sense of trust is demonstrated when a baby fails to thrive and grow or becomes either very negative or passive and withdrawn.
How are emotions expressed?	A second major development in the infant during this first year is emotional expression, the infant's ability to signal his or her feelings through facial expression, body tone, and activity in a way that is accurately communicated to caregivers. Basic emotional expressions of joy, sadness, and anger are common by the end of this phase of life. The development of the ability to express basic emotions is important because it helps the communication between parent and baby and cements the evolving relationship between them.
What is the relationship between the child's emotions and his or her actions?	A third development that begins to appear in this period is *motivation*. Motivation is a set of feelings that makes the baby act. The important motivational factors that develop during this period are the need to relate to others, the need to learn to use the body to get around, and the need to use toys and other materials and understand how they work. The development of motivational factors during this period of life is one of the building blocks for later emotional, social, and intellectual growth.

How does cerebral palsy affect these areas of emotional growth?

The influence of cerebral palsy on emotional growth during the first year of life depends on two factors: how parents cope with having an infant with a disability, and personal characteristics of the individual infant. The role of parental coping strategies has already been discussed; the baby's role is influenced by his or her temperament and the extent of the cerebral palsy.

An infant who has an engaging style of responding to his family, regardless of how significant his disability may be, may conquer his parents' pain and fears and weave them into a tapestry of mutual love that will promote attachment and security. On the other hand, an infant who has a mild degree of disability but who nevertheless has a difficult temperament may intensify his parents' pain and fears and thereby frustrate his own emotional growth.

Much of the emotional development that takes place during the first year of life depends upon the infant's ability to signal needs and express emotions to his parents. This ability may be impeded in an infant who has either extremely low or high tone. For example, a baby who is very floppy and flaccid may not have the muscle strength to express emotions or needs in a way that will produce interaction with a parent. For an infant with very high tone (such as a child with spastic quadriplegia), the inability to control movement could inhibit or distort emotional expression. In either case, it may seem that the infant is not really responding when a parent tries to "read" the baby and interpret his needs. This can be frustrating to parents and can lead them, over time, to spend less time interacting with the baby. This in turn can jeopardize attachment and security, and it can ultimately jeopardize the infant's emotional development.

What can parents do to cope with their child's difficulty with expression?

A parent whose child either lacks expression or has distorted expression can be helped. The parent of an infant with very low tone can be taught to read the diminished or muted cues of the baby, so that a satisfying interaction takes place. The parent of an infant who has very high tone can be taught to work with the infant by anticipating the baby's schedule and providing what the infant probably needs. Likewise, parents can learn to use a variety of soothing techniques to quiet a stiff, irritable child and to arouse their infant in a way that will promote love and communication. In addition, a consultation with a qualified mental health or health professional may help parents work with these kinds of problems.

How can parents motivate the infant with cerebral palsy?

Cerebral palsy also has an impact on the baby's motivation to interact with her surroundings. Its effect is apparent in the infant's desire to master her body in order to move about and reach and grasp and to make things work or happen: to play with toys, for example. The impulse to move about and explore is thwarted by very low muscle tone. Alternatively, a child may have so much spasticity (tightness) that she can't move about or reach out, grasp, and manipulate toys and other objects. In either case, parents need to bring the world to the child. This means moving the baby to different rooms in the house or having the baby "ride along" when parents are performing common household tasks like cooking or cleaning. It also means presenting the baby with appropriate toys (like a rattle), showing the infant how the toy works (shaking the rattle to make a noise), and assisting the infant in her attempts to play with the toy.

Some babies with low tone may be less inclined to move about and manipulate toys. In such cases parents can put desirable toys just out of reach to motivate the baby to move and reach and grasp. It's especially important to teach the baby to be persistent in overcoming obstacles in order to attain a goal. The baby may have the desire to move about or to manipulate toys but may find it difficult to do this because of spasticity. Parents need to assist the baby in his efforts in a way that helps the baby reach his goal. This does not mean doing it for the baby; it means providing the minimal amount of support and assistance needed. When the child learns that he can propel himself forward on his own to get a toy or grasp and move a rattle with his hand to produce a sound, he will feel a sense of accomplishment and will be encouraged to try other things. The baby's motivation to persist and to try to master tasks should be supported in a way that allows the baby to deal with a tolerable level of frustration and yet be successful. If identifying that tolerable level of frustration is difficult for parents, they may find it helpful to consult with an appropriate professional, such as a physical or occupational therapist, for ideas and help.

How does intelligence develop?

The development of intelligence during this period of life depends to a great extent on the infant's ability to anticipate regularly occurring events (so-called contingent relationships) and to use her sensorimotor system to explore objects, to discover the permanence of objects, and to recognize the uses of some objects commonly found in her environment (like toys).

The capacity of the baby to anticipate regularly occurring events comes about when the baby learns, for example, that crying and thrashing about will bring her contentment in the form of food, a diaper change, the chance to sleep, or the experience of being comforted in her mother's or father's arms. Under these conditions the infant learns that she can have an impact on her environment. Just as importantly, this sets the stage for development of trust and security, the beginning of a sense of mastery, and the beginning of the ability to understand cause-and-effect relationships. Of course, this early line of development depends on the parents' ability to understand the baby's cues and respond to them in a sensitive and suitable manner. Consistent failure by parents to respond in this manner may interfere with this line of growth. Difficulties of this sort may be overcome by consulting a qualified mental health professional.

How does discovering the world help a child develop intelligence?

The other major intellectual development during infancy is the baby's ability to discover the world of toys and other objects, as well as people. This begins before the baby can use his hands. It starts with the baby looking at things and people and tracking them with his eyes as they move around. Indeed, by the time he is 3 or 4 months old a baby can remember familiar faces and toys. More importantly, the ability to engage in such tracking helps the baby start to develop the concept of spatial relationships and the notion that objects are "real." The idea that objects are real is constructed during this period when the baby becomes aware that objects disappear and reappear as they travel around the environment. When the baby begins to use his or her hands to reach and grasp things, the pace of development surges.

At this point, when the baby has a toy in his hands he can look at it, feel it, put it in his mouth, and listen to any noise it might make. The baby discovers that the toy makes a noise or does something else when he moves his hand. Thus the baby uses several sources of information to get an idea of what the toy is like. Thus, the baby begins to form ideas of objects that are similar (such as rattles) because they generally look and feel the same when held and they make a similar noise when the hand is waved. By the same token, the infant also begins to discover that objects are substantial or real, because he can use his hands to recover them when they fall or are dropped. Finally, the infant is further developing his sense of cause and effect, because he discovers that he can make toys do things that are interesting and fun.

How can cerebral palsy affect these experiences of discovery? Cerebral palsy can have an impact on the infant's ability to develop an awareness of shared relationships. Infants who are very tight and spastic, for example, may have disruptive feeding patterns—they may have difficulty sucking, for example. This could interfere with the baby's ability to recognize that there is a relationship between (1) his or her hunger pangs, (2) crying, and (3) being soothed by food. A child who has very high tone and has tight muscles may also be prone to fussiness and irritability and unable to appreciate his parents' efforts to soothe him at times of distress or upset. He may not be able to recognize the relationship between feelings of distress and their eventual decline.

The motor coordination involved in tracking people and objects as they move about can also be affected by cerebral palsy. The infant with either very low or very high muscle tone may not be able to engage in the kind of coordinated eye and head movement needed to do such tracking. Therefore, the beginning stages of the development of visual memory, spatial relationships, and so-called object permanence (the idea that objects are real and substantial) may be delayed or distorted.

Cerebral palsy can also disrupt the early growth of object recognition and the understanding of cause-and-effect relationships. The reason is that this early line of development normally hinges on the development of reaching and grasping. The coordination between the feel and sight of the object being grasped and whatever sound or action it produces when the hand is moved or waved is essential. Developmental delays might be expected in particular for infants whose disability affects their ability to use their hands to reach for, grasp, and manipulate toys and other objects. This would be the case when at least a moderate degree of spasticity is present in the upper trunk and upper limbs. Delays may also be seen in babies with extremely low tone, however. In any case, infants can be helped to compensate for this problem. Parents can show an interested infant how a toy like a rattle works and help the baby play with the toy. Likewise, toys adapted to the infant's needs (such as toys with special switches) can be used to foster this development. A physical therapist, an occupational therapist, or an early education specialist can suggest alternative ways to help the baby manipulate toys and interact with the environment.

Ages One to Three

At this stage, the child becomes increasingly independent. At the same time, he or she begins to master control of body functions and impulses. The child learns to use the toilet successfully and can also postpone gratification to some degree. This is also the time when the child begins to play with other children and learn the foundations of give and take.

Intellectually, this period is marked by the child's recognition that people and objects are substantial and real, by an increasingly sophisticated understanding of cause-and-effect relationships, and by the ability to imitate. There is also tremendous development in the child's imagination, and she or he begins to use language.

What are the main issues in emotional and social development at this age?

Children at this age display real evidence of emotional and social development: they strive to be independent; they test boundaries and limits; they begin to learn to control their impulses and feelings. This is primarily why children 18 to 36 months of age are described as going through the "terrible twos." This is the period when intense feelings, especially anger, are exhibited, and children throw temper tantrums as a way of expressing unhappiness and frustration.

Another hallmark of social development during this period is increased socialization with peers. The child moves from being the lone actor on the stage (except in interaction with parents) to having at least one playmate. Over the course of these two years the child comes to enjoy being with other children. He learns how to share toys and other possessions and how to deal with his own feelings and those of other children in the context of budding social relationships.

This period is marked to some extent by the struggle for independence as well as the struggle to find out where the limits are. These struggles are influenced by the child's temperament (and his or her parents' temperament) and the child's sense of emotional security. A high-strung and highly active child, for example, is generally more tempestuous and headstrong than a laid-back toddler. A more easygoing toddler may not put up as much resistance to having things done for him or having limits set on his behavior. A lack of security and trust can either intensify or stifle the striving for independence. The rearing styles and personal attributes of parents (their patience and resilience, for example) influence how both toddler and parent get through this period of development.

How might cerebral palsy affect the child's independence?

The child with cerebral palsy can have a difficult time gaining a sense of independence and learning self-control. Ordinarily children at this age develop a sense of independence by trying to do things for themselves (like using a spoon to feed themselves) and by moving about and exploring the environment. The child who does not have use of her hands or who cannot move around (such as a child with diplegia or quadriplegia) may not be able to assert her willfulness or growing sense of independence in a way that fosters both a sense of autonomy and a sense of self-control. Sometimes issues of control between parent and child are played out in an exaggerated fashion in any area where the child does have some power (such as eating).

Other factors, such as significant developmental delays, can also impede this area of development. Children who are significantly behind their peers developmentally will have a harder time learning new things, following verbal directions, and paying attention. Likewise, parents who have a hard time letting go of their child, who cannot see the child as a person in his or her own right, and who foster a great deal of dependence in the child may interfere with or distort the child's progress in this area. Finally, a child who by temperament is very passive or who perhaps has very low tone may find it hard to muster the energy to test limits or to get into things that would lead to confrontation with a parent and thus eventually promote autonomy and independence.

How might cerebral palsy affect the child's self-control?

The toddler develops the ability to master feelings (especially anger and frustration) and to control impulses by interacting socially with parents, other adults, and other children. Because a child with cerebral palsy may have restricted use of his hands and limited mobility, he may not develop these skills as readily. However, these restrictions are less likely to interfere with the child's development of self-control than with his development of independence.

Cerebral palsy *is* likely to have an impact on how the parents confront the child when he is angry or out of control or when he cannot have a desired object at the very moment he wants it. Parents who see the child as an individual, who let the child know they understand these feelings, and who nevertheless exercise appropriate disciplinary techniques will foster growth and promote the child's ability to master his feelings. On the other hand, parents who believe they need to give in to their toddler and not let him experience frustration, perhaps because of his disability, are less likely to help the child come to terms with strong feelings and impulses. This approach can delay or distort the child's development of self-control.

What is cerebral palsy's effect on socialization?

The growth of peer socialization that takes place during this time is dependent on the child's having access to other children. For a child with cerebral palsy, this access may be limited by the parents' protectiveness, the attitudes of other parents toward having their child play with a child who has a disability, and the child's own ability to keep up with other children in play activities.

About 2 years of age is an ideal time for a child with CP to play with children their age who do not have disabilities. Most children this age are very accepting of children who are different from them. They will usually adapt and adjust to the other child's limitations if helped to do so by a caring adult. (For example, the adult might model interactions or facilitate the play.) Playing with children without disabilities is easier for a child who has a mild to moderate degree of motor impairment. But it is possible to integrate a toddler with a severe disability in the extremities if this is done with careful planning. For the child without a disability, playing with a child who has one teaches tolerance, patience, and generosity. The child with a disability has an opportunity to learn that he can be accepted and to learn social skills.

It is important not to ask the child with a disability to play only with children who are much older or who are much more advanced in social and intellectual skills. (This is true for all children, whether or not they have a disability.)

What is normal intellectual development like at this age?

At this age, most babies go through tremendous changes in their intellectual development. Indeed, the 3-year-old child barely resembles the child she was at 1 year in terms of thinking and problem-solving skills. The major milestones of intellectual development during this period are the development of a sophisticated understanding of cause-and-effect relationships, the ability to imitate what has been seen and heard some time after the incident occurred, the ability to represent reality in internal thought or images and through the spoken word, and the ability to use speech as a way of communicating ideas and needs to other people.

The child continues to learn the concept of object permanence, which is necessary before she can master verbal, spatial, and mathematical concepts. It is not until the child understands that toys and other objects still exist when they are out of sight (a concept a 1-year-old cannot understand) that she can begin to lump objects together by one or more common features, to map out where things belong in the environment, and to count objects or order them according to some physical dimension (such as smallest to largest).

How does the understanding of cause and effect develop?

The appreciation of cause-and-effect relationships begins during the first year of life, such as when the baby aimlessly waves his hand to produce a sound from a rattle and then realizes that it's the hand shaking that causes the effect (the sound). Children aged 2 and 3 play with much more advanced toys (progressing from a busy box to a wind-up toy) and use more advanced methods of problem solving (for example, to get things that are out of reach). Indeed, this is when children first use tools to solve problems (standing on a chair in order to get something that is out of reach, for example). By the beginning of the third year, the child can solve a problem by thinking about it and then getting what is needed to solve the problem. At this age, solutions to problems are concrete; they are mainly carried out using motor skills and materials available in the surrounding environment. Later the child will be able to solve mental problems.

What is the role of imitation and representation?

During this period of development, imitation and representation are tied to each other. Indeed, the ability to represent internally some aspect of reality grows out of imitation. In this case, imitation means that the child can copy an act he has seen someone else perform or repeat something he has heard someone else say. As the child matures during this period, imitation becomes increasingly more sophisticated in terms of the succession of acts and phrases that can be copied and the amount of time between when the child notes the activity and when he repeats it. Thus, imitative activity changes: rather than precisely mimicking an action or spoken phrase immediately after seeing it or hearing it, the child now puts together internal thoughts or images and creates his or her own sentences or actions.

The capacity to form images stems from repeatedly imitating the same acts until, in a sense, they are committed to memory in the form of an internal picture. As the child matures, he relies less on repetitive imitation to form such images. These images are pictures or representations of aspects of the growing child's reality. It is the ability to represent reality in the mind that allows a child to engage in different forms of imaginary play, such as role-playing (pretending to be a doctor) or make-believe (having a tea party with friends). Of course, the ability to represent reality increases with age and enriches the child's play and thinking.

How does speech develop?

Speech evolves significantly during this time frame. For one thing, there is a dramatic increase in the number of words the child can string together. The child progresses from an infant who has a few words at her disposal to the 2-year-old who can combine two or three words. As a 3-year-old she can very nearly hold a conversation: stringing several words together in order to express feelings, thoughts, or needs. The child's speech evolves from one word expressing a need or describing an action to phrases or sentences that aid the child in expressing thoughts and ideas, in communicating present and future needs, and in developing her relationships with adults and peers. At the same time, the child learns to put spoken words in the correct order so that others can understand her better. The child also develops the ability to engage in the give-and-take of social conversations in a culturally acceptable manner.

How might cerebral palsy affect intellectual development with respect to these skills?

Much of the intellectual development that occurs between 1 and 3 years seems to rely on the coordination of input from the senses with movement (such as crawling or walking) and hand use. This is particularly true for the development of object permanence, cause-and-effect relationships, and representational thought. But it is also true for speech, because much of what a child knows and can talk about at this age comes from what the child learns by doing.

As already discussed, the child with cerebral palsy may meet with difficulties in this area of growth because of limitations in mobility or hand use. Development may be even further jeopardized by any reduction or distortion in the input from the senses of vision, hearing, or touch. The child who is disabled in a way that severely restricts her ability to move about could show some delays in the development of object permanence and spatial relationships. However, the child who is capable of using her hands can overcome this kind of impediment. Thus, for example, the baby who is able to search for and pick up a toy that falls behind her is getting the kind of information that will probably allow development in these areas to proceed.

Impaired hand use is often a major obstacle to development of intellectual abilities at this age. A child who has a great deal of spasticity in the upper extremities or throughout the body may be more hindered in intellectual development than if only his legs were affected. This is because ordinarily the ability to manipulate toys and objects and play with them in both familiar and novel ways is essential to intellectual development. For example, losing and finding objects stimulates the development of object permanence; making the jack-in-the-box pop up stimulates recognition of cause and effect; and giving the doll a drink is a way to learn imitation and representation. Delays in these skills can also affect speech development in the sense that because of these delays, the child may not form the ideas and concepts that most children talk about at this age. (Not to mention that speech is a highly coordinated motor activity that may be impaired due to the effect of cerebral palsy on the muscles of the mouth.)

How can a child who is severely affected by cerebral palsy be helped in these areas?

Delays in intellectual development are not always inevitable for a young child with cerebral palsy who is severely disabled in hand usage. Some young children who have severe disabilities do overcome such major obstacles and become intellectually competent. How this happens is not entirely understood, although experts believe that the child's inborn intellectual ability may have significant influence. However, it may be that the parents' bringing the outside world to such a child or allowing the child to interact with toys and people plays an important role here.

Parents who help the child play with toys or work with switches may help the child overcome the barriers posed by the disability. By the same token, parents who in a sensitive way help the child cope with the frustration of trying to reach or manipulate toys and other objects probably encourage the child's intellectual development. Parents who support efforts on the part of a child who has these kinds of limitations in hand use and mobility are most likely building the child's sense of mastery over the environment as well as helping the child learn to be persistent and diligent in the face of physical hurdles.

Finally, talking to the child and, most importantly, actively trying to understand the child's attempts to communicate can facilitate the development of ideas that might not otherwise come about in a child with a severe motor impairment. Likewise, listening to such a child in a way that allows the child to communicate, be it with language, gesture, gaze, pointing, or signing, promotes in the young child the idea that communication is an interactive and social activity. Some parents may want to wait for their child to communicate verbally rather than allow therapists to use alternative means of communication at this age (such as sign language or picture symbols). However, as discussed above, developing an effective communication system in any manner is vitally important to development at this age, as well as in all future stages of development.

Ages Four to Seven

These years are marked by an increase in the child's investment in peer relationships and forming friendships. It is also a time when the young child begins to develop a sense of identity and a sense of right and wrong. At the same time, the youngster is learning to reason concretely and solve problems, as well as to master academic subjects such as reading and mathematics.

What are the typical social and emotional developments?	The child's desire for autonomy and independence begins to manifest itself in a different way as the child begins to separate physically from his parents. Socialization includes making friends with peers, typically of the same sex. Indeed, this is an age when friendships and contacts with peers begin to play an increasingly dominant role in the child's life, starting a trend that will continue to gather strength and direction until at least the time of young adulthood. The move to peer friendships makes it more important than ever that the child learn to share, to take turns in games and other pursuits, and, most importantly, to see things through other persons' eyes.
How does a sense of identity develop?	A major development during this period is the child's increased sense of identity. The identity that begins to take shape at this age will influence the child's attitudes and aspirations for the future. Identity is often an important factor in shaping the child's idea of what it means to be male or female. Identity formation happens at this age as the child begins to identify closely with a parent or other significant adult, typically of the same sex. For example, a son may take on the personal characteristics of his father or pretend to do some of the things the father does at home and at work. This process continues throughout childhood but becomes suppressed to some extent by the onset of adolescence.
What about the child's sense of morality?	This is the time when the child develops a conscience and a sense of guilt. The development of a moral sense depends on the child's intellectual capacity, but its shape is a function of the values practiced and taught by parents and other significant adults and, to a lesser extent, by peers.
How might cerebral palsy affect these areas of development?	At this age the impact of having cerebral palsy changes. The child's sensorimotor abilities have less impact on development at this age than in earlier developmental stages. Instead, the child's access to a range of social relationships becomes increasingly important.

Specifically, children need to be around parental figures or other adults who are nurturing and caring and who will serve as role models to reinforce the child's own identity. Parents and other significant adults should work at instilling pride in the child with respect to his abilities, whatever they might be, and his physical makeup, even though the child may be different from the majority of people around him. It's important to help such a child recognize his disability and take pride in his accomplishments—it's essential to *maximize self-esteem*. One boy reflected back on his memories of his first awareness that he was different from other children and the process of coming to terms with that realization:

The first time I realized that something might be wrong with me was when I would go for therapy. At first, I thought it was a normal routine; I thought that everybody did it. Then, as I got older, I realized it wasn't something that other kids were doing. I wondered what was wrong with me. I probably should have asked, but I don't remember asking. I should have, but I think it would have been painful. I was sad. It was hard knowing that something was wrong with me. I remember thinking, "Why me? Why me?"

Another thing that I remember was when I realized that I had to have more operations than other people. That was hard. Why did I have to do this? Why did I have so much pain?

When I was very young, I also noticed that I still crawled while other kids were able to walk. I decided that it just wasn't my time yet to learn how to walk. Later I realized that I wasn't going to be able to walk. That made me sad. Getting a powered wheelchair helped. Things are much better now. I've come to accept my disability, and I will keep trying to fight on to be the best I can be.

Ultimately, helping the child understand and own his disability will help the child to cope with any ridicule or rebuff he may encounter as a result of his disability. This means describing the disability to the child in terms he can understand and helping the child come up with ways to answer questions that are asked of him. The terms used may change as the child ages and matures, but having a personal understanding of his condition, as well as a "quick answer" to give to those who are curious is important. To do other than help the child maximize self-esteem—and especially to try to make the child pass for being "typical" —is to lower the child's ability to cope with whatever emotional, social, and physical adversity he encounters while growing up with a disability. Individuals with cerebral palsy may have low self-esteem later in life. Giving them a strong foundation and maximizing their self-esteem when they are younger may help them face obstacles encountered later on.

Children with cerebral palsy also need to have the opportunity to be in social settings with children their age, such as preschools or elementary schools, in order to learn to relate to peers who do not have disabilities. The adjustments that must be made to integrate a child into such a setting is far easier at this age than later on. To some extent, moderate to severe sensory or intellectual impairments make this harder, but even a child with these impairments will profit from having some kind of access to peers without disabilities.

These arrangements also allow children without disabilities to learn to accept the kinds of differences presented by people with disabilities. Acceptance can be encouraged by providing the child who has a moderate to severe motor impairment with adaptive devices, such as computer-aided communication devices, that make it easier for the child to participate in classroom activities and to communicate with peers and teachers. Children at this age who do not have disabilities can learn to be comfortable with modifications made in classroom activities to accommodate the child with cerebral palsy. The lessons learned from these interactions as children will, it is hoped, carry over into adulthood.

How does a child's ability to think change over time?

At this age, children generally begin to think, reason, and solve problems with the help of their toys and educational materials. For example, preschoolers learn to count and to sort and group objects by use (such as things that bounce), by name (such as cars), and by physical attributes like size and color.

Children at this age are able to think about what they are doing with their toys and other objects and sometimes invent new ways of using them. They are also able to think about their friends, recognize that their friends and playmates have feelings of their own, and take these feelings into account in their peer relationships.

In general, this is a period when thinking becomes more abstract, but the child still must rely on objects to support her thinking. The development of such thinking skills is essential to the child's early academics (counting and letter recognition, for example) and to her later ability to think more abstractly.

What is the role of speech?

The speech of 4- to 7-year-olds resembles adult forms of speech in terms of grammar, since the child's grammar at this age is nearly as sophisticated as an adult's. By this time most children have acquired an extensive vocabulary corresponding to the world around them, although the child does not yet have the vocabulary of an adult. Finally, it is at this point that the child becomes aware of the speaker-listener relationship and begins to learn the rules of conversation, so that he can effectively communicate with others. Development of language skills—grammar, vocabulary, and rules of conversation—is of course important for the child's ability to communicate, but it also plays a significant role in his ability to learn how to read and write.

What kind of impact can cerebral palsy have on these developmental issues?

During this period, intellectual development usually progresses through play and schooling. Cerebral palsy may interfere with development in this area because it may interfere with integration of the child's motor and sensory skills. A child who has severe to moderate impairment (such as spasticity) involving the upper extremities may have difficulty engaging in the kind of play that ordinarily results in the ability to think about how different things relate to one another. Other factors such as native intelligence can work in such a child's favor. That is, the brighter the child, the more likely he is to learn these thinking skills, even without the usual play activities.

The child's efforts to learn from play should be promoted by parents and others who can support the attempt to manipulate educational materials. Professional therapists who work with the child can provide some of this encouragement. Toys and equipment can be adapted to fit the needs of a particular child. The child can also be encouraged to experience play vicariously, by watching other children. The overall goal is to help children with an impairment experience this level of play in some way so that the impediments to intellectual growth posed by their disability are diminished.

Unlike intellectual development, the development of communication skills is very closely tied to social interaction. To develop communication skills, a child with cerebral palsy—especially one with moderate to severe motor impairment—must have the chance to relate to people in a way that encourages communication and teaches the child the rules of conversation. But speaking is only one way of communicating. The child with cerebral palsy may have to rely on gesture, signing, or a communication device to "talk" to others. All efforts to communicate, whatever form they take, should be encouraged at this age. If language skills and relationships with friends who are not disabled aren't fostered until later on, the child with limited ability to communicate may find that his peers have less patience with his limitations. He may also be less motivated to communicate if prior efforts at earlier ages were not reinforced.

Ages Eight to Twelve

During these years the young child is working on peer relationships and refining her sense of right and wrong. It is also a time when the child becomes more independent of her parents in terms of activities and relationships. Finally, it is a time when a great deal of energy is devoted to schooling and to learning the basic academic skills involved in reading, writing, and mathematics.

What are the social and emotional milestones of this age span?

Personality, peer relationships, and the development of a sense of morality take on more importance. In the early years of this period, the family still has a major influence on the child's personality and moral development. Values embraced and expressed by peers also contribute to the child's emotional and social development. Indeed, by age 12 a good deal of a child's personality and moral sense has usually been formed. The child's own inherent makeup also influences this development.

Especially toward the end of this period, the child develops relationships and friendships, particularly with children of the same sex, that last for a long time, sometimes for a lifetime. The child's social world begins to be dominated by friends rather than by his parents. The child's friends begin to serve as important models in terms of gender roles and in terms of determining, in some part, the child's interests, social mores, and value systems. Since choice in friends is to some extent influenced by values already established by the family, this wider social network and its influence is typically consistent with the child's family background.

What about increasing freedom at this age?

This is also a period during which the child gains greater freedom from the home and becomes less reliant on parents for entertainment. The child begins to learn how to get around the neighborhood and the community by himself. He may travel to school independently of his parents, and in a few years he may go shopping or participate in social or sports functions without always having one or both parents present.

How does cerebral palsy affect these developments?

Cerebral palsy can influence social and emotional development since it sometimes has an impact on peer relationships. A child with a motor impairment, especially if it is moderate to severe, may be impeded in her ability to get around with her nondisabled peer group. Also, the kind of activities that bind children together at this age involve the ability to converse freely with one another and often involve the use of both the legs and the hands (in sports activities, for example). Thus, a child who lacks the motor ability to talk or whose movement is impaired even to a mild extent, may have less access to peers and peer socialization.

Another reason cerebral palsy may affect social and emotional development is that the child begins to stand out as being different from most children his age. Marked physical and cognitive differences sometimes result in the child's being rejected by children who don't have disabilities. Even the child with a very mild degree of cerebral palsy may be socially isolated.

What qualities enable the child to cope best with these stresses?

There's no question that the child with cerebral palsy must have a lot of courage and determination to deal with the possible rebuffs, cruelty, and rejection she may encounter. The child must reach out to people in spite of rejection and must continue to want to achieve in school and other settings. In order to do this the child must already have a very strong, positive self-image. In fact, a positive self-image is probably what keeps the child moving ahead during this and the next phase of life (adolescence).

What can parents do?

To achieve this kind of positive self-image, the child needs to have—and to continue to have—parents or other significant adults who nurture and care about him and who see him as a person in his own right. Parents should promote interactions between their child and adults and other children by introducing him into settings where peer interaction is more likely to be successful. While their child may not be able to physically keep up with peers in activities like soccer or baseball, there may be other ways or other activities in which the child can participate with peers. The child may need to use adaptive devices to achieve better communication, mobility, and hand usage. Parents must begin early in their child's life to encourage and reward him for mastering a variety of social and play situations and for all the special talents the child may possess. Rewarding efforts and attempts, not just complete success, is vital for all children, but particularly for children who have disabilities.

During this period, the child with cerebral palsy needs his parents to be available to listen when he is wounded by peer rebuff or cruelty. Given proper support and encouragement, the child can effectively communicate and vent his feelings. The parent can help the child understand why other children behave this way. More importantly, they can interpret such incidents in a way that does not undermine the child's self-esteem and self-image.

Finally, parents must continue to be effective advocates for their child. In the area of social and emotional growth, this means allowing the child access to peers who are likely to be accepting. It may mean fighting hard to prevent the child's segregation into a special school or a restrictive classroom setting. The child who is in a regular classroom benefits from having relationships and friendships with children without disabilities who are at his social and intellectual level. It may also mean that parents and other significant adults have to challenge the child at times to behave in ways that will foster such relationships. Parents may need to seek the help of a skilled counselor to guide them and their child through what can sometimes be a turbulent period of life.

What are the major intellectual tasks at this age?

The major intellectual tasks for children during this age occur at school, where they learn to read, to express themselves in written language, and to perform fundamental mathematical calculations. Additionally, this is the time when the child learns to accept the structure and rules of the classroom and to obey the teacher.

How can this stage of development be affected by cerebral palsy?

Cerebral palsy can affect schooling and classroom learning in a number of ways. The level of the child's intelligence and thus the child's ability to learn are scrutinized at this time, especially if the child has a severe disability. It is difficult to evaluate the intellectual ability of the child with restricted hand use and limited speech, and it is not uncommon for such children to be judged as intellectually less proficient than they are. Inaccurate assessment frequently results in inappropriate classroom placement.

Many of these children have disabilities that make it difficult to assess what they know and what they have learned. Indeed, it is important to distinguish between learning and performance. It is likely that many children with cerebral palsy with moderate to severe impairment can learn, sometimes on a par with their peers. The problem is that the child cannot communicate this to others by writing or speaking.

Children with cerebral palsy may have other subtle impairments that interfere with learning and performance in the classroom. Some children have a learning disability such as dyslexia (normal vision but an inability to interpret written language), which is tied to their central nervous system disorder. Some children may also, for the same reason, have a short attention span or an inability to store or retain knowledge. For other children, anxiety or worry may interfere with their ability to concentrate or focus on tasks being presented. Finally, the child with cerebral palsy may have a limited ability to accept adult authority and classroom rules and structure, depending on how much past opportunity the child has had for this kind of interaction.

A child who has already learned to share with peers and to accept rules when playing with other children will have an easier time. By the same token, the child who has learned to accept the authority of his parents and to take responsibility for his own acts will find it much easier to be an active and appreciated participant in the classroom.

How can teachers and parents help?

Educators first must identify children who cannot demonstrate their level of learning. Then they must provide the child with the means to get over this barrier. This can be accomplished by providing her with suitable alternatives for expressing or demonstrating what she is learning. The child might do very well working at a computer, for example, or using computer-assisted communication devices. Sometimes a tutorial or one-on-one session between a teacher and the child is the best way to unblock communication. Also, parents need to be aware of possible problems with reading, and teachers should be on the lookout for telltale signs of such problems and be available for extra help. When teachers and parents are insensitive to a child's individual learning capabilities, they may condemn the child unnecessarily to academic failure. This may lower the child's self-esteem and decrease the child's motivation to learn.

Ages Thirteen to Eighteen

More often than not, these years are marked by emotional turbulence. During this period the adolescent struggles with self-identity, with increased physical and emotional independence from parents and family, with sexual impulses, and with the growing influence of his or her peer group. Likewise, the adolescent's thinking, problem-solving, and reasoning skills often move from the concrete to a more abstract and mature level. Finally, during this time youngsters begin to make career or vocational choices that may carry into adulthood.

What are the primary areas of social and emotional development?

Sooner or later, almost every adolescent goes through a stormy period. The major issues of the turbulent teens include striving for independence and autonomy, the increasing importance of peer relationships, and most of all, managing the surge of sexual feelings and impulses.

It is during this period that many young people gain a conclusive sense of their own identity and autonomy. It is also the time when young people gain mobility, as they are increasingly able to come and go from their homes and other places in the community without continual adult supervision. They learn to drive and find other ways to get to and from activities without adult assistance. Social activities at this age often do not include parents or other family members.

Most young people at this age form long-term friendships with peers that sometimes last a lifetime. Indeed, the young person typically develops a social circle of peers who help define her interests and recreational activities and to some extent dictate who and what is socially acceptable and unacceptable. Being part of a peer group often leads young persons to rebel against family and cultural traditions and expectations.

During this period, sexual feelings and impulses develop, and adolescents begin to recognize and express them. Sexual expression often develops against the backdrop of family, religious, cultural, and peer group value systems—which are frequently at odds with one another. The young adolescent also begins to recognize his sexual identity and orientation and to come to terms with it in some fashion. Adolescents begin to develop relationships that have sexual overtones, typically involving members of the opposite sex. This ushers in a period of dating, of expressing sexuality with someone else (including often deciding if and when one should become sexually active), and of moving into short- and long-term relationships with a partner.

Although most adolescents will make it through this period of development intact and doing well, there are times when social and emotional development do not go "as planned" and difficulties emerge. For example, late adolescence and early adulthood are times when mental disorders or emotional difficulties can begin. Mental health disorders are identified by significant changes to the teen's or adult's baseline level of functioning. Anxiety disorders can appear at this time. The symptoms of these disorders include clinically significant levels of worrying and anxiety that interfere with the individual's functioning on a daily basis. Symptoms of bipolar disorder include fluctuations in mood, activity, and energy levels. For example, the individual may appear sad or "down," lose interest in activities he used to enjoy, and experience changes in the amount of sleep he needs and in appetite (either increases or decreases). They may also demonstrate an atypically elevated mood, confusion, or "reckless" behavior or speak more quickly than usual. It is important to remember that most, if not all, adolescents and adults will demonstrate some of these symptoms at one point or another. We all have days when our mood is down, or we feel more energetic, or we are excited and speak quickly. When diagnosing bipolar and/or mood disorder it is important to consider whether these symptoms have lasted beyond a specified time and whether they represent a significant change from the individual's baseline level of functioning. A mental health professional such as a licensed counselor or psychologist will be able to help determine whether the symptoms exhibited meet criteria for a psychiatric diagnosis.

Another mental health issue that emerges in the late teens and early adulthood years is schizophrenia. This disorder is characterized by symptoms including delusions and hallucinations as well as flat affect and lack of motivation to complete activities. These symptoms can be difficult to detect and differentiate from those of other disorders. Therefore, it is strongly recommended that parents pursue an evaluation with a qualified mental health professional if they are concerned for their adolescent teenager or young adult.

In what ways can cerebral palsy affect social and emotional development during adolescence?

As previously mentioned, motor impairment that interferes with mobility and communication can restrict autonomy as well as access to peers and members of the opposite sex and the expression of sexual feelings and impulses. Likewise, severe or profound intellectual disabilities can diminish interest in sex and the expression of sexual impulses. But often the impediments to full development in these areas are more emotional and social than physical. The young adult with cerebral palsy may already have encountered so much rebuff and ridicule from peers that he or she is afraid of rejection or failure and therefore is unwilling to take a chance on dating or intimacy. Thus the experiences that normally lead to a mature expression of sexual feelings are often avoided or put off until sometime later. While it may be thought that adolescents who have a diagnosis of mild cerebral palsy do not experience the fear of rejection or failure as much as those who have more significant motor difficulties, this is not always the case. Adolescents who have been diagnosed with mild cerebral palsy may still have difficulties with their self-image and self-confidence because they have had problems keeping up physically with peers despite their "almost typical" appearance. In some cases, it can be easier for a teen diagnosed with spastic quadriplegia to explain why he cannot play an informal game of soccer after school than for the teenager who has a very mild hemiplegia. Some teens may feel a need to "hide" their diagnosis from their classmates for fear of being ridiculed or otherwise singled out. In a time when most of their peers are trying to figure out ways to "fit in," standing out is not always rewarded or celebrated. For adolescents and young adults diagnosed with mild cerebral palsy who choose not to share this information with their friends and peers, this can be a difficult secret to keep.

Growth may also be hindered by lack of social access. For some adolescents, social isolation (due, for example, to the adolescent's need to attend a separate school) may be the reason there is not much opportunity for interaction with peers, and especially with potential sexual partners. But lack of opportunity for interaction may also be due to the fact that young people with cerebral palsy, regardless of the type or severity of their disability, are often viewed as "different" by able-bodied peers and thus rejected. Sometimes such a young person is accepted only in a very limited sense. He or she may be seen as a great pal, for example, but not as a prospective dating partner. This is particularly true in early adolescence.

Most young adults with cerebral palsy have the same sexual feelings and impulses as their able-bodied peers. Denying this—which happens frequently—robs young people with cerebral palsy of their dignity and their right to experience the fullness of life. It is therefore essential that parents and other significant individuals give these young adults the opportunity, over time, to explore and express their sexual nature within the context of the family's value system. Professional advice and counsel can be invaluable here.

Regarding the emotional difficulties or mental health issues that tend to emerge in the late teenage to early adult years, individuals with cerebral palsy are believed to be at the same risk as individuals in the general population. The diagnosis of cerebral palsy is not known to be associated with specific symptoms of mental health issues; however, this does not mean that these disorders cannot develop in an individual with cerebral palsy. Depending on the level of motor impairment and cognitive difficulties, it may be more difficult to diagnose mental health conditions accurately in these individuals. The assistance of a well-qualified mental health professional who has experience working with individuals with disabilities like cerebral palsy can be very helpful in identifying whether the symptoms being seen meet criteria for a specific psychiatric or psychological disorder.

What are the major characteristics of intellectual development at this age? In this period the young person develops the ability to think abstractly. This means that ideas, words, and other abstract symbols dominate when the individual is trying to solve a problem. The ability to think abstractly is seen in the young person's schoolwork (when doing algebra problems, for example) as well as in social relationships, in which more abstract moral and ethical considerations color how young people relate to one another.

Whether an individual can reach this stage of thinking depends in part on her or his cognitive abilities. However, every individual needs a certain amount of social and intellectual experience, as well as schooling, in order to reach this stage of thinking. Individuals who are delayed in their intellectual development, and particularly those who meet criteria for a diagnosis of intellectual disability, either will be delayed in reaching this stage of thinking or will never reach it.

Another significant milestone that occurs during this period is that young people begin to make and sometimes finalize their vocational and career choices. Adolescents, especially by the time they get to high school, typically start making choices that will lead them into a trade or profession. A young person's choices are often dictated by his or her interests and talents, but these factors may be circumscribed by family background and tradition, perceived gender roles, and ethnic and socioeconomic considerations. Encouragement and nurturing from parents, other significant adults, other family members, and friends may also influence a young person's career aspirations.

How might cerebral palsy affect this development?

Cerebral palsy may or may not affect the young person's capacity to engage in abstract thinking and problem solving. For example, the young person who has a disability that has produced moderate to severe intellectual deficits most likely will not attain this level of thinking. Associated visual, hearing, or learning handicaps may also delay or inhibit such development. However, many people with cerebral palsy, even those with significant physical impairment, have typical intellectual abilities and can achieve a great deal, as this letter from one child with CP testifies:

My name is. . . . These are my thoughts on obtaining membership in the Order of the Arrow and the rank of Eagle Scout.

When I was sworn into Scout Troop 652 on . . . , I didn't really know what to expect. I wanted to explore things for a bit. At that time I remember one of my friends was going to get his Eagle rank. I was, of course, happy for him, but I didn't know what it entailed. I went to his ceremony. When I saw all they gave him and did to honor him, for the first time in my life I wanted that—badly. I knew that I would have to try my best to get it. I knew that you couldn't get Eagle after you turned 18, and I was 14. I only had a few years to work on this. After one camping trip, I remember coming home and saying to my father, "Dad, I want to be an Eagle." And so we went to work. Dad agreed to help me. I attacked this like I never worked on anything before. I realized this was something I could do. I can't play football or any other sports, but I knew I could do this.

Now, it is 3½ years later and I am waiting for my ceremony. My badges are complete—25 of them. I worked on three projects for the three highest ranks. For Star projects, I raised $6,500 to have a hydraulic lift installed on the Scout bus. Before that my Scoutmasters would have to lift us, our wheelchairs, and all the gear for the camping trip into the bus. For Life project I painted, with lots of helpers, an auditorium in the church where our troop meets. For Eagle project I realized the need to have badge books put on cassette tapes. This is how I did all my merit badges, because of my vision problems. My father recorded the ones we did at home, and I used those plus several more that Scout friends recorded for me.

On September 18 I passed the Eagle Board of Review, which is the final test before the National Council scrutinizes the folder with the application, the summary of projects, and letters of recommendation. I feel that I have achieved a lifelong dream. It makes me feel fulfilled and proud. This is the one thing that I tried and came out successful. I can say to any other disabled kids who are thinking about doing something and are not sure they can, "Try your best. Don't give up. If you do it, great! If you don't make it, at least you know you tried your darndest."

Many factors influence the young adult's ability to attain the capacity for abstract thought. Previous stimulation and social experience can either aid or stunt such development. Access to appropriate schooling can also promote or arrest the child's progress toward attaining this kind of thinking ability.

The impact of cerebral palsy on vocational and career decisions has many facets. Significant impairment in intellectual, learning, visual, or hearing capacity may ultimately restrict the kind of education and training the child receives, limiting the young person's vocational choices. But even the choices of the less involved child or the child who is bright but quite physically disabled may be unnecessarily limited. In this case, it is vital to recognize the child's potential early on and assist him (with therapy and educational assistance) to overcome these barriers so that he can more fully develop his abilities.

What can be done to help children overcome these problems? Children with cerebral palsy must be able to obtain an education that will put them in a position to exercise their choices to the fullest extent possible. Parents and other significant adults must, on the one hand, advocate for the child's appropriate educational needs and, on the other hand, provide the child with the assistive devices, aids, and tutors that may be necessary in order for him to learn and express what he knows. The child needs to be stimulated and challenged educationally. At the same time, people who matter to the child must consistently motivate him or her to persist in the face of whatever odds are stacked against short- and long-term success.

It's important not to undersell or oversell the child. Thus, good counseling and assessment are important in the decision-making process. Likewise, every attempt must be made to ensure that as he grows toward adolescence the child is exposed to the social world in a way that enables him to interact appropriately with people in a variety of situations. Good social skills are a significant determinant of the young person's access to employment. Finally, it's important to know and understand the laws with regard to the right to an appropriate education and to employment without discrimination for individuals with disabilities. If the parents and their child understand their rights in this regard, the young person with cerebral palsy will have a better chance of attaining his or her ultimate career or vocation.

Adulthood

The major issues of adulthood revolve around the formation of long-term relationships such as marriage, the direct expression of love and sexuality, the raising of children, and finding a job or career that will firmly establish independence.

Most adults who are able to express sexual feelings and impulses are interested in settling into a suitable relationship. This involves finding a partner, making a commitment, and, often, working toward making it a long-term relationship. Such relationships are dependent on communication; only through communication can the needs of the involved individuals be met. And relationships involve practical issues as well as emotional ones. Decisions about bearing and rearing children, household responsibilities, and finances must be made and carried through.

How might cerebral palsy affect adult developmental issues?

For adults with cerebral palsy who have adequate intellectual skills, quality of life and adjustment are influenced more than anything else by the attitudes they hold about themselves and by the attitudes of able-bodied people toward them. It is true that moderate to severe motor impairment of any kind, particularly if it extends to all areas of functioning, can be a stumbling block in working out a long-term relationship, having sex, and rearing children. However, the willingness of each partner to explore these limitations and to seek out the appropriate professionals (such as physicians, therapists, and psychologists) who can help the couple confront the physical barriers to a meaningful relationship can go a long way toward overcoming such problems.

What is crucial, then, is that the adult have a sense of self-esteem and self-worth. For many, if not most, adults with cerebral palsy, it takes a good deal of strength, persistence, and courage to socialize with adults without disabilities and to reach out to try to form relationships that are deep and lasting. For it is likely that at some time in their lives most individuals with cerebral palsy will have encountered some degree of rejection and even cruelty when trying to form friendships.

The physical disability of the adult with cerebral palsy may create some obstacles to employment. The more the impairment limits mobility, hand use, or communication, the greater these obstacles will be. Nevertheless, assistive devices like computers can be used to integrate the adult with cerebral palsy into the workplace. Again, it is important that individuals become familiar with federal and state laws governing employment of individuals with disabilities so that they can act to make certain that their opportunities are not being unfairly—and unlawfully—limited.

What tools are most important to the adult with cerebral palsy?

The adult needs the kind of self-esteem and strength that allows her to weather rebuff and rejection while continuing to risk finding friends and partners. The sources of self-esteem and persistence have been discussed throughout this chapter: these attitudes come from being loved and held in high esteem by family members and friends, and from being seen as a person with talent, value, and skills that can be put to use in the everyday world. An infant, child, adolescent, or young adult who has support from parents, friends, and perhaps an encouraging counselor is better prepared to handle problems.

The attitudes of able-bodied people toward the adult with cerebral palsy also play a role. It is likely that some adults with cerebral palsy only find a limited number of people who are available for friendships, and perhaps even fewer who are open to sexual or long-term relationships. High self-esteem, courage, and persistence are important assets for the adult with cerebral palsy.

Likewise, such adults benefit from having had experiences with peers in late childhood and in adolescence that taught them appropriate social skills.

Finally, it is important for parents, relatives, and other significant adults in the individual's life to recognize that this person is going to experience the same need for a sexual outlet and a loving relationship as anyone else. Disability should not automatically exclude young adults from experiencing the fullest measure of life possible. Parents, relatives, and friends must encourage and pave the way for such experiences rather than prevent them.

In addition to job-related training, the adult needs good work skills and the ability to get along with others in the workplace, both of which are known to be highly related to success and stability on the job. The experiences the child has all through the growing-up years influence his or her ability to succeed as an adult.

In this chapter we have described how cerebral palsy affects intellectual and psychological development. We have seen clearly that the life pattern for the person with cerebral palsy is set early. In the end, parents and the person with cerebral palsy walk a fine line throughout life in terms of expectations. It is easy to set expectations either too high or too low. There is no easy way to manage this tightrope act. Seeking appropriate counsel from physicians, therapists, and other professionals along the way is often helpful, but in the final analysis, parents and children need to know when to forge ahead and when to pull back in the face of stresses and barriers. The real goal is to help children with cerebral palsy grow into adults who feel good about themselves and their abilities, adults who are fulfilled because they are able to experience the joys and disappointments that life has to offer.

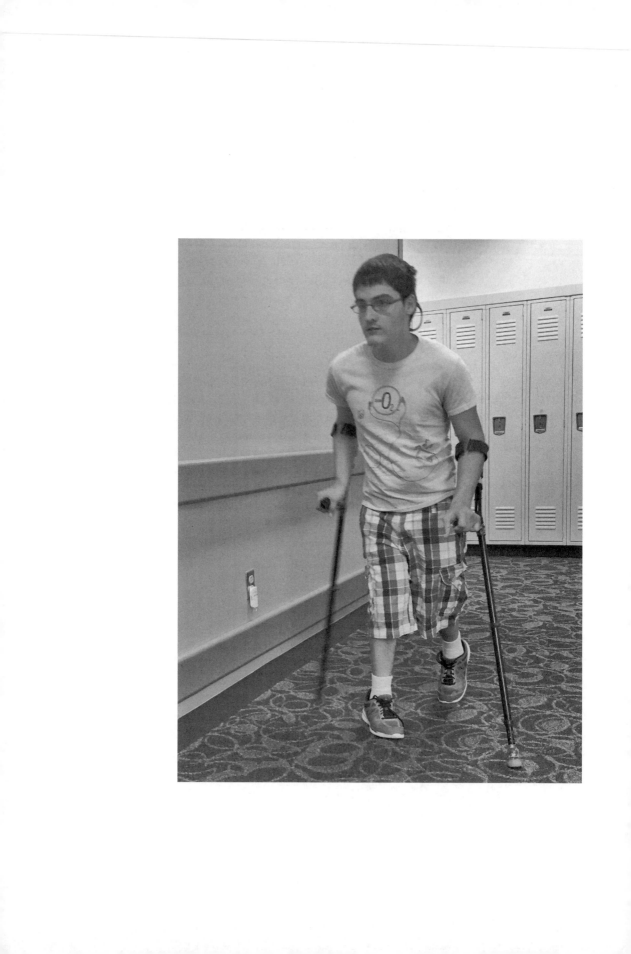

5

Hemiplegia

HEMIPLEGIA is a form of cerebral palsy in which one arm and one leg on the same side of the body are affected. Another term for this form of cerebral palsy, one that is gaining popularity, is *unilateral involvement*, meaning only one side has an impairment. The majority of children with hemiplegia have normal intelligence, go to regular, age-appropriate schools, can expect to have relatively normal function as adults, and have few problems beyond the physical difficulties of the arm and leg involved.

The term *hemiplegia* is sometimes more broadly used to describe children with mild involvement of one limb (also called *monoplegia*). A child whose primary motor dysfunction involves both legs and one arm may also be diagnosed with hemiplegia, although this pattern is more properly called *triplegia*. *Double hemiplegia* is a sometimes confusing term that is used to describe cerebral palsy that affects all four limbs but with asymmetry between the right and left sides. Children with this diagnosis have very different physical problems from the problems of children whose CP involves only one side of the body and more closely resemble those with diplegia or quadriplegia.

If your child's CP involves one arm more than it involves the legs, then this chapter addresses most of your concerns. However, Chapter 6, on diplegia, better addresses issues concerning a child whose more severe involvement is in the legs and a child with double hemiplegia who can walk. Chapter 7, on quadriplegia, is most relevant if your child cannot walk.

What does hemiplegia usually look like?

For most children with hemiplegia, the arm is usually more affected than the leg, and the problems are usually worse at the end of the limb. The child with hemiplegia has a harder time with hand and wrist movements than with shoulder function, and problems with the elbow fall somewhere in between. Similarly, the child's foot and ankle present more difficulties than his knee. Hips are seldom significantly involved. The child's most significant problems are usually related to spastic muscles and decreased growth of these spastic muscles. This growth abnormality causes the muscles to be short and the joints to be stiff, so that as the child grows, he has progressively less range of movement in the affected limbs.

Birth to One Year

What physical abilities can the newborn's parents expect to see? At first the typical infant's hands and legs function only immaturely, and the infant has poor trunk control. As the first year of life progresses, however, the infant rapidly develops many new abilities, though of course different infants develop these abilities at different ages and in different ways. This is an exciting time for parents. Because of the natural variation in development and the rapid changes that are taking place, mild abnormalities often go unnoticed by parents and physicians alike.

Can hemiplegia be diagnosed at this age?

The diagnosis of hemiplegic cerebral palsy is very seldom made in the first year of life, primarily because it is virtually impossible to determine conclusively that a child has this condition at this young age. A child's first year is a difficult time for parents if they suspect that their child has a problem. Because it is often easier to deal with bad news than it is to handle an unknown diagnosis and the waiting required before the outcome can be determined, many parents push for an early diagnosis. But the only reliable way to determine the outcome of a child who has a brain injury is to wait and see. During this wait-and-see period, therapy interventions can begin. Such intervention shows parents how to facilitate their child's emerging development. If it turns out that the child is typical and does not have CP, this intervention does no harm.

A prediction of the future outcome for the child who has been diagnosed with a birth abnormality that is not specifically related to a syndrome or a more specific diagnosis is only slightly more reliable than an educated guess. When a syndrome is identified or a specific diagnosis is made (such as Rett syndrome, Tay-Sachs disease, or trisomy 18), much more accurate predictions can be made, because these syndromes tend to follow a more predictable course. Cerebral palsy is not predictable in this way, because it is not a disease, nor is it due to a specific chromosomal abnormality. The symptoms depend on where the brain damage is and how the brain compensates for this damage during growth. These details cannot always be seen even using the most sophisticated brain-imaging techniques, like MRI. Although imaging has been improving, providing better detail, it is still not clear how this improvement will impact predictions of outcome in the young child.

Some parents may have been prepared for a diagnosis of severe cerebral palsy, particularly when their newborn was premature or had intracerebral bleeding, only to find that at age 4 the child has mild hemiplegia. In contrast, some parents who have been told their child will be normal, or at most mildly affected, discover when the child is older that the child is more severely impaired. In cases such as these, the conclusion must be that the initial diagnosis involved an incorrect prediction, not that the initial brain injury has changed in any way. When a child is diagnosed at a later age, and with reliable criteria, predictions about abilities will be more accurate; parents should not be anxious that the prognosis will become worse over time.

As a parent, what early signs can I watch for?

If your child has very mild hemiplegia, there are usually no noticeable signs or symptoms, with the exception of early hand dominance. Preference for the left or the right hand usually is not well established until 18 to 24 months of age in a typically developing child. Therefore, if your 5-month-old always reaches out with the same hand for toys or food, you should talk to your child's pediatrician. The normal hand is the one your child is using; the affected hand may be held in a fist most of the time, or you may notice that one arm or leg seems stronger or stiffer than the other. The fisted hand or the tightly held thumb is usually flexible and can be gently pulled out, but this is evidence of early spasticity in the affected limb, which gradually increases as the child grows. The position is sometimes referred to as a *contracture* even though it is flexible.

If the arm appears weak or does not move normally, this may be a sign that the nerves in the infant's shoulder were stretched during birth. If your child has this condition (called Erb's palsy), you'll notice that he usually moves his fingers well but does not move his arm from the shoulder normally. Diagnosis of Erb's palsy requires a neurological evaluation. This condition should not be confused with cerebral palsy.

The child of 4 or 5 months who shows an unwillingness to use one hand or who consistently holds a fisted hand should be evaluated. However, a full-scale evaluation, which includes the appropriate scans, might not show a definable abnormality even though the child clearly appears not to function normally. Scans taken at this early age do sometimes reveal cysts or other deformities in the brain, but these findings may not correlate with the pattern of the cerebral palsy or how severe it will be.

Between the ages of 5 and 8 months, children typically start sitting. Children with hemiplegia have a tendency to fall to the side. They may realize that they are falling, but they may have trouble reaching out with their involved hand to stop themselves. As their balance improves, however, these children are able to sit very well. In the more severely involved child with hemiplegia, the ability to sit well may be delayed until 16 to 18 months. However, all children with classic hemiplegia eventually become good sitters.

As the child starts crawling "commando style," the involved side is often held in more rigidly at the hip, knee, and elbow. It look as if the child is holding the affected side more closely to his body. It may even look as if the child is dragging this side.

Children with mild hemiplegia may walk by 11 to 14 months of age. Many children with hemiplegia walk late, however, and many of them start walking on tiptoe. Walking late and continuously walking on his toes are two strong indications your child has CP. As he develops balance and confidence in walking, he may very well outgrow toe walking.

Are there treatments available for children who show these signs?

A child with these early symptoms should undergo a thorough medical evaluation by the child's pediatrician or by a specialist such as a pediatric neurologist or developmental pediatrician. If the diagnosis of CP is made, then referral to a therapist is indicated. The primary treatment for the 5-month-old who shows an unwillingness to use a hand is to present the child with toys directed at the affected hand or with toys too large to hold with only one hand, such as a large ball. Finger foods can be presented in the same way. Some extra care may be necessary in opening and cleaning the fisted hand. Occupational therapists will direct therapy for the child with an affected hand.

For the most part, however, your child should be treated like a normal child.

One exception is a child with an extremely tightly fisted hand. In a child at this young age an extremely tightly fisted hand occasionally requires a splint. Only in a child with severe CP do hand contractures occur at such a young age.

If your child is having problems crawling, this is a good time to start seeing a physical therapist. Advice from a physical therapist can provide you with both direction and reassurance. Special braces or shoes are not needed at this age unless the child is trying to walk and is a persistent toe walker.

Is a walker recommended?

Some parents enjoy seeing their child move about on her own in a sling-seat walker, but parents need to supervise the child very closely to prevent accidents. One safety guideline is to tie the walker to a post or piece of furniture in order to limit the distance the child can travel. It is essential that a child in a walker stay away from stairs, as this is where most accidents occur. Also, the walker must be one that is engineered to be stable. Many physical therapists discourage the use of walkers because they are concerned that bad movement patterns will be reinforced. Many pediatricians discourage the use of such walkers for all children. They fear that the child's increased ability to get around in the walker will increase the likelihood that he will fall off porches or down stairs, resulting in severe injuries.

The use of a sling-seat walker will not teach the child to walk sooner and can create dangerous situations. There is no evidence that the use of walkers does any long-term harm, however. The walker will not prevent a child from learning to fall, cause foot or hip problems, or delay the time when the child is able to walk independently.

Ages One to Three

During this period most children with mild hemiplegia are diagnosed, usually because they are toe walking and have not started to walk by age 15–18 months or because it is clearer that they are not using one of their arms normally. If it hasn't been done before now, a full neurological evaluation is necessary, although it may not reveal any definable problem in the brain. The main reason for this type of evaluation is not to find a cause of the cerebral palsy but to be certain that no other condition is causing the child's symptoms. If there is a condition other than cerebral palsy, then it needs to be treated properly. An evaluation at this age is also useful for parents who are considering having another child and want more information about the cause of their toddler's problems.

In many ways, caring for the child with hemiplegia at this age is not very different from caring for the child without a disability, except that it may be a little harder to determine the proper level of expectation. But parents can work with health care professionals to develop a level of expectation that is consistent with the individual child's ability. This is usually established by consulting with occupational and physical therapists, who often offer valuable counseling.

For example, it's not reasonable to expect any 6-month-old to eat with a spoon. Most parents know this from talking to other parents, consulting their child's pediatrician, or reading books. It is just as unreasonable to expect the child with severe hemiplegia to hold a cup in the midline (at the middle of the body) if the child is physically unable to hold a cup and bring it there, even at age 16 months. Parents need help from professional therapists to learn what to expect from their individual child at each stage of development, such as when the child might be expected to bring the cup to midline.

How should the affected hand be treated?

During this period it is important to present your child with toys that re-quire two-handed manipulation and that stimulate your child to use the in-volved hand, even if only to assist the good hand. Give your child toys such as large stuffed animals or large balls and dolls too big to hold with one hand. Encourage her to hold a bottle or cup with both hands if she is able. Don't try to force your child to do anything that she is physically unable to do, however. If your child can't open her affected hand to hold a large bottle, then it is better for her continued development to get a bottle that she can hold with one hand, such as those that have an open split in the middle. A physical or occupational therapist can make equipment recommendations.

At this age the development of fine motor skills can be encouraged by play-ing with your child in stacking blocks and putting pegs in holes. It's difficult to get your child to do these activities with the involved body part, especially if she is not motivated. It's best to encourage her in these activities but not to push her to the point of frustration. If your child refuses, the refusal is prob-ably due to her impairment; it's not possible for her to do this task at this time. As your child continues to grow, she may suddenly begin to perform activities such as these with the involved hand, though much later than she did with the normal hand.

Because each child is an individual and there are no tests that can define expectations for a specific child with CP, it's important to work with a therapist and a physician to help define these abilities. They may also be depended upon to make suggestions about hand braces.

When and how are braces used for the hand?

Generally, the fisted posture in which many children with hemiplegia hold the hand starts changing as they reach 2 to 3 years of age. This is also the time when muscles start tightening up, and it is the right time to consider bracing. The brace is used to prevent the muscles from becoming tighter.

There are a number of different types of braces for the hand. The two most frequently used types are those designed to keep the thumb out of the palm and those designed to keep the fingers and wrist extended. The specific de-sign used depends on the experience and philosophy of the therapist and the physician, as well as on the needs of the specific child. Generally, hand braces are very well tolerated by children in this age group, but they usually do not improve the hand's functioning.

One drawback of the brace is that it reduces the feeling in the hand, which can make a child ignore the hand even more. At this age your child is develop-ing use patterns, so it is not a good idea to keep the hand covered by a brace all the time, as this encourages the child to ignore the hand during play. Also at this age, muscles generally don't become tight quickly, and function often improves nicely if the child is encouraged to use the hand. For these reasons, the brace should be worn only at night or for short periods during the day.

Is there any harm in not bracing?

The use of hand braces varies greatly, and the benefits and risks are not very well defined. Therefore, it is generally best to continue with whatever seems to provide the most benefit to your child and to stop doing those things that don't seem to work. For example, if your child refuses to wear a brace and continually removes it, he does so because it hurts him or because it is in his way. This should be a sign to stop using the brace, or at least to try another one. The focus of treatment should be to encourage the use of the hand for functional activity, which in this age group means during play time. It is important not to try to force your child to do something that he physically is not able to do or that he does only with great difficulty.

What about my child's normal hand?

In the past, it was often recommended that the normal hand be restricted to encourage use of the affected hand. This philosophy was later abandoned in recognition of the stress this placed on the child. Until recently parents were urged never to impair the normal hand. Restricting the use of the normal hand has been shown sometimes to cause significant psychological distress, which can have long-term consequences. However, recent studies have demonstrated positive outcomes from a program of restricting normal hand use for a limited amount of time. This program, "enforced use therapy" or "constrained use therapy," is not well accepted at this age. It is addressed below, when discussing the 3- to 6-year-old child.

We recommend encouraging use of the impaired hand at 1 to 3 years, but not by restricting the normal hand, except for short periods during active therapy.

What about walking?

A child who has not yet attained the developmental ability to walk cannot be made to walk. Consider this: no matter how hard a parent or therapist may try, it is impossible to make a 5-month-old normal infant walk by himself. Many moderate to severely involved children with hemiplegia at 15 months old are like a 5-month-old normal child in that they do not have the developmental ability to walk. Therefore, parents should not insist on their child walking. Rather, they should focus on the things that the child *is* doing (such as crawling), expecting that in some months the child *will* walk.

Involvement of the leg becomes more noticeable at this age and is a significant factor in the delay in walking. But children with a typical hemiplegic pattern of cerebral palsy become good walkers if there are no other underlying problems. The child with mild hemiplegia typically walks within the same age range as a child without a disability. Children with moderate involvement are often delayed, however, beginning to walk between 18 and 24 months. The child with more severe involvement may not walk until between 24 and 30 months of age. Assistance from a physical therapist can be very helpful, especially for a child with significant developmental delay.

Each child has his individual schedule based on his development and level of involvement. Encouraging your child to stand and to take steps is fine as long as it is approached with a healthy attitude—similar to the approach you would take with a normal child who is learning to walk. Always be sure your coaching is in line with what your child is physically capable of doing.

Does a child have to crawl before walking?

Several therapy theories suggest that all children have to crawl in a specific way before they go on to walk in order to develop a normal gait pattern. However, there are no empirical data to justify these theories. There are children who never learn to crawl but just stand up and walk, and there is no harm in this.

Children's crawling styles vary greatly. Most children with hemiplegia learn early on to do an asymmetrical "commando crawl" (similar to the low-to-the-ground crawl of the soldier under fire). Some can progress to a four-point crawl, on hands and knees, as a normal 8-month-old baby would, but others cannot. The crawling pattern that works for the child should be encouraged, and there should not be too much emphasis placed on perfecting a particular type of crawl if the child does not seem comfortable with change. If a therapist insists on a specific crawling pattern, parents should consider switching therapists.

What problems do the feet present?

Foot problems in the child with hemiplegia are primarily due to a tight Achilles tendon. The muscle that runs to this tendon, the *gastrocnemius*, seems to be the slowest of the muscles in the leg to grow. It is the dominant muscle below the knee and the largest, and it is usually the most spastic. Problems with this muscle and this tendon are seen in the persistent toe walker.

Often when children begin walking they walk on tiptoe. This may in fact be normal in a child up to the age of 2 or 2½, but a child should be walking flat-footed six months after he begins to walk. Children with hemiplegia toe walk for a prolonged period, often for several years, and they toe walk on both feet, resulting in tightness on both the uninvolved and the involved sides.

The child with hemiplegia may also have a problem with his foot turning in, as do many normal children at this age. Although the foot may be flat, the whole foot appears to turn in. This pattern, which is due to a twist in the bones of the leg, often corrects itself as the child grows and develops better muscle control. Because the condition self-corrects, surgery, exercises, and braces are rarely necessary. If parents are very concerned, activities that require pointing the foot forward can be encouraged. These include roller-skating, ice-skating, and ballet—activities that are often preferable to physical therapy or home exercises because they involve the child in normal activities.

Can stretching or other exercises help?

Opinions vary widely on the usefulness of physical stretching as therapy. The child with spasticity is no different from anyone else in that she will benefit from stretching after being in one position for a long time: it feels good to get up and stretch after lengthy sitting. The child with spasticity needs help to stretch out the affected muscles. But the tightness that develops from the spasticity will not be overcome by physically stretching the child. It would actually require 8 to 12 hours of relaxed stretching each day to make a muscle grow. Clearly, devoting several hours a day to stretching a child is impractical.

It's good practice to stretch for short periods of time (5 to 10 minutes) twice a day. This can be a regular part of your child's daily routine, like bathing and toothbrushing. Your child's spasticity will not go away; however, it will change over time. This spasticity, or tightness in the muscle, has been shown to worsen until about age 4 or 5 and then slowly decrease until adolescence. Although no exercise program has ever been shown to make a long-term difference in a child's disability, exercises prescribed by a therapist or physician should be considered. However, your role is that of parent, not therapist. It's important to consider the rest of the family, job obligations, and educational goals, as well as how the involved child is responding to other demands.

Exercise for the child with hemiplegia should be approached in the same way that physical exercise is approached for the nondisabled individual. The purpose is to keep the child fit so that he or she feels and functions better. There is room for flexibility, and no great harm is done by skipping a day or taking vacation time off. As with other exercise programs, the benefits are ultimately lost when the exercises are discontinued.

When are foot braces suggested?

The AFO (ankle-foot orthosis) or MAFO (molded ankle-foot orthosis) is a commonly used brace worn for the purpose of stretching the Achilles tendon. An AFO can be helpful to children with hemiplegic involvement who are walking on tiptoe, usually more so on the side affected by the spasticity. The brace is applied if the foot can be brought to a neutral position. If the foot cannot be brought to a neutral position, then surgery or another kind of treatment needs to be considered (see below).

Although there is no commonly accepted routine for using an AFO, it's generally true that children who need to use the brace should wear it during the day in the same way that they wear shoes. There is no harm in the child's walking barefoot for periods of time in the evenings or after a bath. If the muscle is very tight, there may be some benefit to wearing the brace at night for an additional stretch.

A child will need time to get used to a new AFO, just as most of us need time to break in a stiff new pair of shoes. The AFO must be adjusted if areas of skin become red or if the foot does not stay down in its correct position. The AFO will feel very restrictive to the child, so even though the child looks better walking and standing, the AFO will not feel natural or comfortable to her. Once the child is used to the AFO, often several months later, it should feel very comfortable. Even then it is preferable for her to spend some time out of the brace. If a child is braced continuously, the foot may become hypersensitive and feel much like a limb feels after being in a cast for several months. Also, the muscle will get weaker and weaker.

If the child continues to complain about the AFO, it should be carefully checked. To check an AFO, look for wrinkles in socks (a telltale sign that something is wrong); determine whether the foot has been positioned correctly; and find out whether the toes are curled up inside the shoes. Also, make sure the AFOs have been placed on the correct feet. If the AFO is applied by many different people (parents, siblings, daycare teachers, and so on), it is especially important to make sure that the AFOs are clearly marked as right or left. Applying the wrong AFO to a foot is a common error.

The type of AFO used depends on what is locally available. For the child who is running around, the best brace is a thin, light plastic, custom-molded brace, sometimes with a hinge at the ankle to prevent the child from toe walking. It is imperative that the brace not restrict the calf area too much. As the child grows, braces are reevaluated for size, and new braces must be made. Generally braces are replaced yearly because of the child's growth. However, during rapid growth spurts it may be necessary to replace them more often. Some orthotists make AFOs whose length can be extended, but this feature adds very little to the length of time the brace will fit. Adjusting only the length of the AFO might be compared to attempting to make a pair of pants last a child for five years by making the legs longer each year.

Another problem with the hemiplegic foot involves a spastic *tibialis posterior muscle*, which is located on the inside of the ankle and pulls the foot so that the toes point toward each other. This can cause the child to walk on the inside border of the foot. An AFO is a recommended treatment for this problem in a young child.

Are there any options other than surgery when braces don't work out?

If the child's spasticity is the primary reason he cannot tolerate the brace and stretching has reached its limit, Botox injections may be used. Used appropriately, this medication can delay surgery for the very young child. Botox (botulinum toxin) is a chemical that significantly weakens a muscle when it is injected directly into that muscle. It is injected with a small needle, much like those used for immunizations. Most children tolerate the injection well in the outpatient setting, although the injection may be administered after sedating the child or after numbing the skin with a local anesthetic. The chemical stays in the muscle where it is injected, and its use is safe, but there are potential side effects, such as spreading weakness and muscle scarring. Unfortunately, the beneficial effect is temporary, lasting only 3–6 months. Additionally, although Botox can be injected multiple times, in most children each injection is less effective than the preceding one. This is because the body manufactures antibodies to the Botox, recognizing it as a foreign substance. For many children, after three to four injections over a period of 9–18 months, one sees little or no effect. But it is useful in delaying surgery for that amount of time. Unless the parent or therapist see a clear change after the Botox injection, further injection should not be given.

If the child is not able to tolerate a brace because the tendon is contracted and spasticity is *not* a major component, Botox is unlikely to help. Botox can also be used in the hamstrings and adductor muscles, as well as in the spastic upper extremity muscles.

Another possible option is serial casting. Serial casting, which involves placing the leg in casts that are changed every two weeks, is a method for lengthening the tendon that was popular in the past but now is seldom used. In cerebral palsy, this is almost always a temporary measure; the foot returns to its former position within several months of removing the cast. Once in a while a child who has a very mild tightness and is not tolerating an AFO may benefit from serial casting for six to eight weeks. If serial casting fails, proceeding to surgical intervention allows the family to get back to normal functioning with fewer disruptions than repeated cast changes and long-term cast wear involves.

When is surgery for the foot advisable?

When the foot can't be brought to a neutral, or normal, position despite the use of braces and/or Botox, then surgery to lengthen the Achilles tendon is indicated. Surgery is usually the best lengthening method. The younger the child is when the Achilles tendon is lengthened, however, the more likely he will need to have the procedure repeated as he grows. Ideally, a single carefully planned surgery for lengthening suffices. Surgical correction is also possible for the foot that is turned in severely, but it is preferable to put this procedure off until a child is at least 8 years of age so as to permit growth in the tendon.

Formal gait analysis has become an integral part of the evaluation of children who walk. It is a complex procedure that takes approximately 3 hours. The child is first examined by a physical therapist, who records measurements of each of the muscles. The therapist then places sensors on the major muscles, and the child is asked to ambulate on a specific walkway while computers register the changes occurring at the various muscle sites. These computer data are analyzed at a later date by a team made up of an orthopedic surgeon and therapists. Their analysis could include recommendations for bracing, orthotics, therapy, and/or surgery when any of these modalities are indicated. Typically, the gait analysis is ordered when surgery is being considered. In that case it is usually covered by insurance.

What other muscle spasticity problems can children with hemiplegia have at this age?

Some moderate to severely involved children with hemiplegia may have tight hamstring muscles. Usually all that's needed at this age is exercise and stretching. Braces fitted to above the knee aren't helpful. The severely involved child may have some spasticity about the hip, although this is less common. Should it occur, it would be handled in the same way that spastic hip disease is treated in the child with diplegia (see Chapter 6).

Ages Four to Six

The problems of the child with hemiplegia in this age group are similar to those of the younger child. It is uncommon for children at this age to be self-conscious about bracing, and they seldom object to wearing a brace as long as it is comfortable and not too restrictive.

Therapy benefits the child most if she enjoys it. Most children resist therapy that consists in long periods of passive stretching or in being urged to pull the foot or wrist up. It is not advisable to force a child to participate in an activity that she dislikes. At this age reluctance can also be due to the child's repeated failure or fear of failing. If a child is reluctant, parents may help to motivate the child by focusing on the result of the activity rather than on the activity itself. However, choosing an alternate form of therapy is often the better solution.

What forms of therapy are most helpful at this age?

Therapy should now be focused on activities of daily living, such as learning to put on and take off shoes, use eating utensils, and ride a bicycle. The child can get stimulation from playing with large balls requiring two-handed play and from reaching for and holding on to playground equipment such as jungle gyms. Bike riding, swimming, and ballet are activities that stimulate the development of coordination—and they're also fun. A basketball hoop placed at the appropriate height allows a child to play while shooting and dribbling the ball, both of which are beneficial activities.

Should I be concerned with hand function at this age?

A child with severe spasticity can develop significant tightness at this age. It's very helpful for the child to wear a brace that lifts the wrist, extends the fingers, pulls the thumb out of the palm, and turns the palm upward. If your child is using his hand, it is crucial not to cover his palm, since this decreases sensation and will decrease function. Occupational therapy is usually best aimed at this age group, since this is the age for learning skills such as dressing, bathing, and using eating utensils. In addition, fine motor skills such as writing and coloring can be addressed more intensely. Hand surgery is only recommended for a small number of children, and then not until after age 6.

What is enforced use therapy, also called "constrained use therapy"?

Enforced use therapy is a structured program currently in use that has had encouraging short-term results. However, there aren't a lot of long-term data. Currently there is very little evidence that it improves function 1, 5, or 10 years after the therapy is discontinued. It also has few side effects, except causing frustration in some children. It is applicable to children with hemiplegia who have a potentially functional affected hand and arm but tend to totally ignore it. They appear to not be aware that the extremity "works." These children are ideal candidates for this therapeutic treatment because they actually have the ability to use the extremity.

The treatment involves a short period of casting the "normal" arm and hand (usually 4 weeks), forcing the use of the affected limb. A therapist is an essential part of the treatment. The therapist works intensively with the child during this period, guiding her to use the "ignored" limb by restricting the more functional limb. The goal is for the child to continue using the arm and hand after the cast is removed. In programs that have employed this therapy, benefits have been reported 3 to 6 months after cast removal. These benefits have included improved motor skills and increased unprompted use of the arm. However, it seems most of the benefits are slowly lost over time, although this outcome has not been well documented. It is, however, extremely important to only use this therapy with children who understand the purpose and who have agreed to the therapy. Restricting the "normal" extremity of a child without cooperation can produce significant distress and is not recommended.

How does spasticity affect my child at this age?

Problems relating to the arm and leg often become more noticeable as the child of this age begins to adopt an adult pattern of running. A normal running gait involves high lifting of the feet and reciprocating arm movements. When children with hemiplegia try to run, they tend to flex the affected elbow and wrist and turn the palm down. The arm tends to move away from the body. This arm pattern is typical and usually quite noticeable. It tends to be worse at this age of 4, 5, or 6 years and then gradually approaches normal during walking in most children. As the child's running gait matures, this arm posturing slowly improves, though usually not completely. At this age a child is not generally very concerned with appearance, and parents should avoid focusing on appearance as well.

As the child runs, the lower extremities also experience spasticity. The knee tends to be held in a stiffened position, which makes the affected leg swing out. The affected foot, if it is not braced or surgically corrected, tends to cause the child to trip. The foot may drag or turn in or out. Occasionally a severe flat foot develops.

What roles do casts, alcohol or phenol blocks, Botox, and surgery play?

Casting at this age has the same limited use as it does at younger ages. Casting is helpful only for spasticity that is not severe enough to need surgical treatment and yet interferes with the fitting of an AFO.

Alcohol and phenol blocks, used extensively in the past, are injections of these medications into the spastic muscles. These injections must be administered under general anesthesia, since they are very painful and cause severe muscle scarring. The decrease in spasticity that is achieved is temporary, lasting five to six months, leaving a stiff, scarred muscle that does not work well. Phenol and alcohol injections in the calf and hamstring muscles should be avoided. Botox has replaced these blocks for children in cases where temporary relief of spasticity is desired.

Surgical lengthening of the Achilles tendon must also be done under general anesthesia. This procedure, if it is done at an appropriate age, can benefit the child for as long as five years. In many cases surgery can even result in permanent correction.

What is the role of the AFO at this age?

The AFO helps keep the Achilles tendon from becoming too tight and the foot from becoming flat. It can also help to keep the foot from rolling in. Heel cups and arch supports are usually less effective. This is an appropriate time in a child's life to prepare him to enter school with as normal a gait as possible, without the need for bracing, and it may be the appropriate age to consider surgery on the Achilles tendon.

What kind of surgery is usually recommended at this age?

The most common surgically correctable problem is a tight Achilles tendon, which that prevents the child from placing his foot flat on the ground. Lengthening this tendon involves a relatively simple procedure with few risks. Sometimes the procedure needs to be repeated as the child continues to grow, but often one lengthening is sufficient. If the child is tolerating an AFO, it is best to delay this surgery until 7 or 8 years of age.

A foot that has a tendency to pull in while the child walks on the outside edge can be corrected at the same time by a split transfer of the *posterior tibialis tendon*. Severe flat feet that roll in may need to be surgically corrected with a fusion (in which several bones are made to grow together). This procedure can often be postponed until the child is fully grown, however. An AFO will usually take care of the problem in the meantime.

Tight hamstrings cause the child to walk with a crouched gait. This condition can be greatly improved by a lengthening as well. Occasionally a child walks with his entire leg turning in. In this case the leg can be surgically derotated and realigned correctly. Seldom would one of these surgeries be done in a child with hemiplegia under age 7.

Shortness of the involved leg generally becomes noticeable at this age. Interestingly enough, this shortness can be helpful for a time, as it prevents the child with a tight Achilles tendon from catching his toes when walking or running. A shoe lift on the involved side can actually cause the child to trip more often. For some children, however—those who have a severe disparity in leg length (more than ¾ inch) just prior to or during the adolescent growth spurt—this difference in leg length needs to be addressed. Special x-rays called *scanograms* accurately determine the difference in length between the two legs, and surgical options are available to equalize the leg lengths permanently.

The age of 6 to 7 years is an excellent time to consider surgical correction for a number of reasons. First, the child is old enough to understand most of what is involved, and this lessens anxiety considerably. Procedures should be scheduled so that the child will not have to miss valuable school time. This means that procedures, together with the necessary recovery, should take place before the child enters school or during school holidays. Additionally, improvements attained through surgery will most often be maintained for five or more years, as the child undergoes a slow, steady growth until the adolescent growth spurt.

Surgeries should be coordinated to minimize disruption to the family's life. It is beneficial to the development of a child to keep his hospitalizations to a minimum rather than have him undergo various minor surgical procedures every year or so. A team of physicians familiar with the multiple problems of children with cerebral palsy can predict what a child might need and then effectively limit the number of surgeries and hospitalizations. This approach allows for more than one corrective procedure to be performed while the child is under anesthesia. In this way the child spends less time in the hospital and has less exposure to anesthesia risks. We want to stress the importance of consulting a surgeon who is experienced with cerebral palsy so that a practical, coordinated plan for all surgery can be formulated.

Ages Seven to Twelve

At this age children are developing a self-concept and becoming more aware of how they are different from their peers. To diminish those differences, it helps to direct therapies toward specific goals. In addition, it is preferable to use school vacation time for treatment or intensive therapy so that time is not taken away from academic efforts. For example, if a child with moderate to severe hemiplegia is experiencing difficulty in self-dressing (handling buttons or tying shoes), the summer break can be the best time to work on improving this skill.

Almost all children with hemiplegia function well in normal age-appropriate classrooms. Teachers can easily be made aware of the child's special needs, and they can be called upon to help design and implement classroom adjustments. The teacher can also play a significant role in helping the other children in the class understand and be supportive of the child with the disability.

The goal at this age should be to place the child in the best situation for learning. A physical therapy program that detracts from this goal is not good for the long-term well-being of the child. After-school activities such as ballet, gymnastics, or karate provide the benefit of stretching along with the opportunity to function and interact with children without disabilities. Teachers who love to work with children to help them grow and enjoy sports without training them to become world-class athletes often welcome the opportunity to work with a child with a disability. Thus, the child can concentrate on academics in school and work out physically during extracurricular activities.

How are the hand and arm best treated at this age?

This is the age at which children begin to object to using arm splints or braces because wearing these devices makes them look different. If your child feels self-conscious and does not want to wear a brace, it is best not to force the issue, especially since arm braces provide little functional benefit at this age.

Mild arm involvement refers to the limb that is used almost normally but has a tendency to flex at the elbow when the person is excited or running. This pattern continues throughout adulthood and is primarily a cosmetic concern. It is frequently handled by acquiring habits that control or conceal the movement in socially acceptable ways. For example, females may learn to carry a purse (and males a book bag), even purposely weighted, on the affected arm. Or they learn to place the hand in their pants pocket. When preadolescent children first become self-conscious about the arm, they often hold the affected hand with the unaffected hand to cover up and control the deformity.

The moderately involved arm is one that is always flexed and pronated at the wrist and elbow to some degree. *Pronation* refers to the rotation of the forearm and hand such that the palm of the hand is always turned away from the person's face. The hand may also have abnormal sensation, and the moderately involved arm is quite noticeable cosmetically. Although the arm can be used well as an assist, its pronated position prevents the child from being able to fully see what he is trying to pick up because he can only see the top of his fingers and hand.

This kind of involvement usually responds very well to surgical correction. The amount of *functional* improvement achieved varies depending on the pre-surgical status, but the *cosmetic* result is invariably excellent. If the child has been using the arm readily in most activities of daily living and also has fairly intact sensation, the surgery will allow for easier use and the child will naturally use the arm more. The child is often more aware of the cosmetic result, while the parents notice improved function.

The severely involved arm is one that is used only to perform an activity that is impossible to execute with one hand. This hand usually has poor sensation as well as poor muscle control. Surgical treatment for this type of involvement is indicated purely for cosmetic improvement, because function is rarely improved, even though the hand may be better positioned. Poor brain control and poor sensation preclude significant functional improvement. Sometimes, if this is not well understood by parents prior to surgery, conflicts arise. Because the arm *looks* so much more normal, parents and teachers may expect more functional ability. They may even attempt to force a child to use an arm that he simply is incapable of using.

Age 7 to 12 is the best time to correct the arm surgically, if indicated. Children are now old enough to understand a great deal about the procedure and the recovery. They are also capable of fully participating in the rehabilitation process. Children at this age generally do not have well-formed or unrealistic expectations, which is an added benefit, since they are invariably pleased with the surgical result.

Delaying surgery until after age 12 can present some problems. As children go through the adolescent stage of development, they may become unrealistic in their expectations and are often self-deprecating. Many adolescents may in fact breeze through this period as easily as they did childhood. Those who are more upset over perceived as well as real deficiencies tend to be affected in two ways. First, they are more concerned about their appearance and are unhappy with braces or splints. Second, they have unrealistically high expectations about the outcome of corrective surgery and frequently are disappointed with the results. Choosing the right time for surgery is essential. And the importance of making certain that the adolescent is fully prepared—that he has as complete an understanding as possible of various outcomes—cannot be overemphasized.

What are the specific surgical procedures?   The specific surgery is dependent on the level of involvement as well as on how well the involved muscles function. Surgery might be approached one way if there is a possibility of increasing function and another way if there is no such possibility, but in practice, function and cosmetics are generally approached similarly. A strict rule of medical treatment, of course, is to avoid doing harm. In this case, surgery must be designed and carried out in a way that doesn't *decrease* function (with a few exceptions, as described below).

Before performing surgery, the surgeon will obtain a detailed history of the patterns of use and will give the child a careful physical examination. In some institutions, an electromyography, or EMG (a diagnostic procedure to evaluate coordination between nerves and muscles), is performed before surgery in order to assess the level of muscle function in upper extremities. This is not standard practice at the present time, however, since EMGs are used more in the area of research than in therapeutics. A tool that has become more useful for determining the specific surgery required and problems of the involved hand is the SHUEE (Shriners Hospital Upper Extremity Evaluation). In the SHUEE, the child attempts to perform a series of tasks, such as getting money out of a wallet, while the hand is video-recorded for later careful review. Combined with a detailed physical examination, the SHUEE can be very helpful in understanding the deformities that limit specific functions.

Most surgery involves transferring muscle tendons, in order to achieve balance, or lengthening tendons, in order to relieve tightness. The flexed wrist is the most noticeable problem. It is usually addressed by transferring to the top of the hand the tendon end of the *flexor carpi ulnaris* muscle, which then pulls the hand and wrist into the extended position. In this new position it is attached to a wrist extensor muscle tendon or to the finger extensor muscle tendons. If the fingers do not extend, the finger muscle tendons need to be lengthened. If the thumb is pulled into the palm, this is corrected by releasing the *adductor pollicis* muscle tendon in the palm or by moving a muscle tendon to help the thumb extend, or both.

Frequently, the forearm is in a pronated position, palm down. This can be addressed by transferring or releasing the *pronator teres* muscle tendon in the mid-forearm. Occasionally the forearm is flexed at the elbow and contracted. In this case the *biceps* muscle tendon is lengthened. Infrequently a thumb joint fusion is indicated, and rarely a wrist fusion is performed. Wrist fusions were popular in the past, but today they are only performed on a child who has a severely contracted hand or whose hand is completely without function. A fusion of this type should almost never be done at this young age, because although the cosmetic result is good, the procedure almost always reduces functional ability.

One guiding principle in this type of surgery should be to attempt to address as many problems as possible at the same time, taking advantage of *one* anesthesia exposure and *one* hospitalization. If they have any concerns about specific recommendations, parents should seek a second opinion, preferably from an orthopedist who is experienced in treating people with cerebral palsy. By taking these precautions a parent can hope to avoid subjecting the child to surgery again.

What is the usual postoperative course?

If surgery involves the hand and wrist, the arm is placed in a cast extending from the fingers to the elbow. If the elbow has been surgically addressed during the same surgery, then the cast extends to the shoulder. The arm remains in the cast for four to six weeks. Analgesics (pain medication) may be necessary in the immediate postoperative period, but patients are generally quite comfortable in the supportive cast.

When the cast is removed, a short course of intense occupational therapy (1 to 3 times weekly for 1 to 3 months) is very beneficial and helps the child achieve the maximum benefit from the surgery. In addition, resting splints are often used full time for 6 to 12 weeks and often for a longer period at night in order to maintain correction.

Generally, continued use of the night splint is most important for the growing child. There is little rationale for a child who has finished growing to use a night splint for more than 12 months, since by this time the situation is unlikely to change, with or without splinting.

What is the role of bracing for the lower extremity?

The issues and problems of the lower extremities in this age group are much like those of younger children. The use of the AFO to help control the foot is often well tolerated. This is especially true if the child notices that the brace makes it easier to walk and run. In addition, the brace is fairly easy to hide with clothing, and peers may not even be aware that the child is wearing a brace. A good compromise for brace wear is to have the child wear the brace all day during school but allow him to remove it in the evening and on weekends. However, when an activity involves a great deal of walking, an exception needs to be made to include the brace.

During the summer, children generally go without their braces much of the time, especially if they swim a great deal. There is really no need for a child to wear braces in the water. One of the disadvantages of constant brace wear during childhood is the development of very small, thin calf muscles. A significant cause of the small calf is that spastic muscles don't develop normally, and using braces constantly or using braces that are too small serves to keep the muscle smaller. (Repeated surgical lengthenings of the Achilles tendon also cause thin calf muscles.) Allowing the child to go without his brace, as well as taking care to see that outgrown braces are replaced, can help minimize this problem. The muscle only grows bigger and stronger if it is used actively in activities such as walking, running, and jumping. Bracing and casting are the most effective ways we have of making a muscle weaker and thinner. Therefore, a delicate balance must be found between using the AFO to improve walking and going without the brace to stimulate the muscle to make them stronger.

What surgery is suggested for the lower extremity?

For most children of this age with hemiplegia, the goal should be to release them from the necessity of bracing. Doing so may include a weaning period as well as surgery. Early adolescence, when a child has begun the adolescent growth spurt but is not fully into puberty, is a good time for surgical corrections to be made. Surgery on the lower extremities can frequently be combined with surgery on the upper extremities.

The most commonly performed surgery on the lower extremity is the lengthening of the Achilles tendon, which is appropriate for almost any child who is walking on her toes. If this procedure was previously done when the child was 3 to 4 years old, then age 7 to 12 is often when it needs to be redone. This also is the age to correct a foot that turns in. If the entire foot is turning in, this is corrected by externally rotating either the *tibia*, in the lower leg, or the *femur*, in the upper leg. This is accomplished by an osteotomy, which involves surgically breaking the bone and realigning it in an appropriate position. If the foot tends to roll in as the child walks, causing her to walk on the outside edge, a split *posterior tibialis* muscle tendon transfer, which involves moving half of the tendon to the outside of the foot so the muscle will provide a balanced pull to the foot, may be indicated.

A severe flat-foot deformity is best treated at this age with either a limited fusion procedure or *calcaneal osteotomy*, in which the bones of the foot are realigned to create an arch. This procedure might also be indicated for a very stiff foot that is turning in.

Additionally, leg length discrepancies should be closely assessed, and decisions concerning equalization should be made during this period. If the length discrepancy between the two legs is 1 centimeter or less, this actually represents an advantage, because the child will trip less often. Even if the discrepancy is 2 centimeters (approximately ¾ inch), there may not be a significant problem. A larger difference is very easily treated surgically by stopping the growth in the longer leg. This procedure, called an *epiphysiodesis*, is timed to make the most of total growth while correcting length differences between the two legs.

What is the usual postoperative course?

The child who has had an Achilles tendon lengthening and split tibialis transfer procedures will go home with a leg cast, most commonly one that stops below the knee. This is usually a walking cast that will be worn for four to six weeks, followed by bracing for a short period in order to maintain correction. A child who has had an osteotomy (to correct a foot that points in) that involves the tibia is placed in either a short or a long leg cast for four to six weeks. An osteotomy that involves the femur may include metal fixation, which means that a plate is inserted during the surgery.

A child who has had a foot procedure will be in a cast (usually short leg) for four to eight weeks after the surgery. The first month after surgery he or she may be placed in a nonwalking cast, especially if the bone is thought to be weaker than normal. If two months of cast use are needed, weight-bearing exercise is encouraged during the second month, as it will help bone healing and prevent more bone weakness from developing.

After an epiphysiodesis procedure the knee is immobilized in a brace for approximately three to four weeks.

Ages Thirteen to Eighteen

This may be an extremely difficult time for the adolescent with a disability, or it may present few problems. The degree of physical disability does not appear to have much bearing on the child's experience. Rather, the child's personality and temperament, his family's and peers' acceptance of his disability, as well as the child's and family's goals, seem to have the most impact. Some of our most difficult adolescent crises have involved children with the mildest physical disabilities, because they are insistent on passing in public as being completely typical, and they focus huge energy on trying to hide their disabilities.

Children this age who have disabilities generally no longer enjoy participating in organized sports. They have usually accepted the fact that their success in this area will be limited, and they prefer to eliminate the stress of competing with their nondisabled peers. The adolescent who redirects his energies to areas in which he is likely to have more success, such as music or academics, is often happier.

What is the role of physical therapy and exercise at this age?

Adolescence is the period in which children actively work at separating from their parents as they move toward adulthood and independence. Children with a hemiplegic disability usually enter into this process just as children without disabilities do. For this reason exercise programs orchestrated by parents tend to be met with various forms of opposition. Rather than imposing an exercise program on the adolescent, parents should encourage their child to exercise to maintain his flexibility in the same manner that they encourage him to accept responsibility for his personal hygiene and appearance. Parents may have to allow the maturing adolescent to suffer the consequences of not having taken responsibility, but this often proves to be the best learning experience, a far more lasting and effective experience than parental harassment.

There is no reason for ongoing, or "chronic," therapy, which only tends to foster dependence and magnify the significance of the disability. Occupational therapy and physical therapy should be limited to short-term intervention either to help the child accomplish a specific activity or to provide postoperative rehabilitation. Whenever possible, everyone around the child should avoid connecting the concept of chronic illness with the disability.

What are the surgical considerations at this age?

While some surgical procedures may have been done at an earlier age, parents should not preclude the possibility of making improvements, and the teenage years are certainly a time when the physical disability should be reevaluated. One patient who was a schoolteacher with a mild right hemiplegia had spent her entire teaching career being limited by significant walking difficulties because she could not place her foot flat on the floor. When she retired she hoped to travel, and she decided to find out whether something could be done for this problem. After a simple operation, her foot was flat and she could walk as much as she wanted to!

The positive aspect of surgery in the teenage years is that whatever corrections are made are permanent—they will not be outgrown. However, this is a somewhat tumultuous period for teenagers who have unreasonable expectations. A child or a teenager who has psychological or behavioral problems should not have surgery until he or she becomes more stable and more mature.

The specific problems and possible surgical corrections for the affected arm are almost the same as for younger children. In some adolescents with severe involvement, there may be a great deal of stiffness. For some of these young people a wrist fusion is suggested, but the consensus among surgeons who treat individuals with cerebral palsy is that wrist fusion should be avoided unless there is no other way to deal with the problem.

Surgery on the affected leg and foot includes all the procedures outlined for ages 7 to 12 for all the same problems. If there has been no prior surgical treatment of the foot, the foot may be very stiff. In this situation, tendon transfers are not possible and an arthrodesis (bone fusion) may be indicated. An Achilles tendon lengthening procedure is often necessary because of the increased growth at this age.

The correction of leg length discrepancies should be made with careful attention to keeping the affected leg slightly shorter to prevent the individual from catching his toes and tripping. In adults, generally a 2-centimeter (¾ inch) difference is well tolerated. If the problem must be addressed, the best approach is to shorten the longer leg surgically, either by arresting its growth or by removing a piece of bone. The first procedure is simpler but somewhat less predictable, since it involves estimating future growth. When a piece of bone is removed, it is usually taken from the hip or from the middle of the femur. The bone is then fixed with a plate or rod.

Another option is wearing a shoe lift. The shoe lift will be fixed to every pair of shoes worn by the individual during her entire life. In view of the simplicity and excellent outcome of surgical correction, surgery is usually the preferred option.

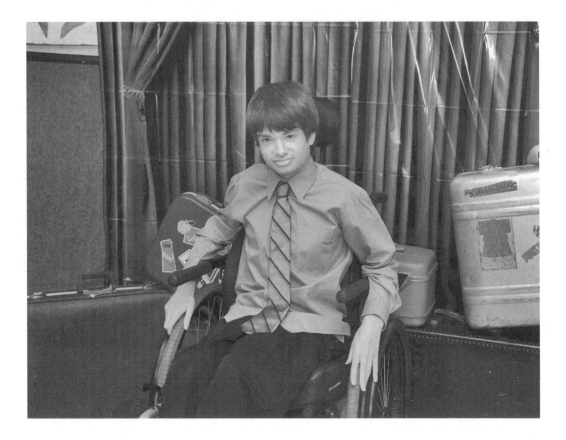

৳ 6

Diplegia

DIPLEGIA is a form of cerebral palsy primarily affecting the legs. Most children with CP have some problems with their upper extremities, but for a child with diplegia the upper extremities are clearly much less involved than the lower extremities. Almost all children with diplegia have spasticity, but they also have difficulty with balance and coordination. There is a good deal of variation among children with respect to involvement and severity of involvement. *Bilateral cerebral palsy* is another term used to describe diplegia. This term does not differentiate between those with diplegia and those with more severe arm involvement, more typically called quadriplegia.

If your child has as much involvement in his upper extremities as in his lower, then the chapter dealing with quadriplegia will probably be more appropriate for you to read, especially if your child has an athetoid component. If your child has asymmetrical involvement, with one side of the body clearly more affected than the other, almost normal side, then the chapter on hemiplegia will be more relevant. A child whose primary motor dysfunction involves both legs and one arm is termed *triplegic*, and this child's challenges are addressed in this chapter.

What does diplegia look like?

The child with diplegia generally has nearly symmetrical involvement of both legs with only mild clumsiness in the arms. Spastic muscles and delayed growth of these muscles cause leg muscles to be short, and as a result the joints become stiff and the range of motion decreases as the child grows. For most children with diplegic involvement, the foot and ankle present more of a problem than the knee, and the hips may become dislocated (for this reason, the child's hips must be closely monitored).

Many children with diplegia were born prematurely and had respiratory problems. Many children with diplegia have normal or near-normal learning ability. Mild eye problems, such as crossing, are common. For the majority of children with diplegia, growth and development are not a problem. Children with diplegia are eventually able to walk, although most of them begin walking late, and they generally attend regular schools and become independently functioning adults.

Does diplegia have degrees of severity?

Diplegia is generally classified as mild, moderate, or severe. A child with mild diplegia is an excellent walker, walking without aids such as crutches. Such a child has a normal tolerance for walking and can keep up with nondisabled children of similar age in activities requiring walking. Children with mild diplegia are classified as GMFCS I on the CP severity scale. With moderate involvement, a child is able to walk for most daily activities but may sometimes use aids such as crutches or a walker. They would usually be classified as GMFCS II on the severity scale. A child with moderate involvement needs to use a wheelchair for activities involving extended walking, such as going to a shopping mall or an amusement park.

The child with severe diplegia requires an aid, such as a walker or crutches, for managing even small distances within a room and walks only in level, uncrowded areas. To get around in public the child uses a wheelchair. These children are classified as GMFCS III. Usually, even the most severely involved children are ambulatory enough to lift themselves into their wheelchairs independently and to move about their own rooms. A child who is not able to do this minimal amount of maneuvering should be diagnosed as quadriplegic even if the upper extremities are not significantly involved.

Birth to One Year

Many infants who are born prematurely spend the first year trying to catch up with their age-matched peers. This first year sees the development of many milestones, such as head control, reaching out for a toy, sitting, starting to vocalize sounds, and finger feeding. Even though every infant has her own schedule and special circumstances, parents are often concerned about the rate at which these developments are taking place. There is a fairly wide range of normal development, and rates of catching up for premature infants vary. These circumstances make it very difficult to predict whether the infant who was born prematurely will eventually catch up or will have CP or some other developmental problem.

Can diplegia be diagnosed this early?

Diagnosing CP is difficult early on, although as a parent you may have been advised of the possibility because of your child's problems at birth. If your baby was born prematurely and had significant medical problems, such as bleeding in the brain or breathing difficulties, he is at risk for developing diplegia. However, in order to know for certain whether your child has or will have cerebral palsy, you must wait for the child to grow and develop. Once her development starts to lag behind or is obviously abnormal, there is still very little anyone can say with certainty about how your child will eventually function. Based on the child's age and function some general predictions can be made. There are no specific tests or scans that can definitely prove that your child does or doesn't have CP, though several patterns of abnormality are often seen on CT or MRI scans of children with CP (such as periventricular leukomalacia, PVL) (see Chapter 1). There are certainly no tests that will demonstrate how he or she will function at maturity.

Are there some warning signs?

The severity of involvement, even if diplegia is suspected, is extremely difficult to predict on the basis of any examination in the first year of life. Most commonly a child with a diplegic pattern has stiff lower extremities, with comparatively less than normal movement, and relatively normal upper extremities. Initially the child may appear to be exceedingly strong, but often this is a manifestation of spasticity.

Floppiness is also frequently seen at this young age. Some children are very floppy from birth and may appear to have no spasticity. They may eventually develop the same appearance of stiffness as the child who is initially stiff, however. Some children with diplegia appear completely normal, particularly in the first six months. Even examination by neurologists may not uncover an abnormality.

If your child was born prematurely, then normal development for him is counted from the day the child would have been born had he been born "on time" (at "term," which is 40 weeks' gestation). This means that if he was born at 36 weeks' gestation (4 weeks early), we expect that his social smile should develop by 10 weeks of age rather than the 6 weeks we usually expect. This "correction" for prematurity continues for the first 18 to 24 months.

By 6 months of age (corrected for prematurity if necessary) your child should roll over, start to develop a sitting balance, and move his legs in a fairly normal fashion. If this occurs, your child most certainly will not have severe involvement. At this age, children who have severe involvement will show significantly decreased movement, stiffness, or severe floppiness in the legs. If your child is sitting independently by 9 or 10 months and is pulling himself up to a standing position, he is likely ultimately to have mild or at most moderate involvement. Even children who are not doing these things at this age may end up having mild involvement. It is simply too early to make an accurate prediction. Few children with even mild diplegia walk independently by 12 months of age.

What treatments are recommended at this age?

Although it is rare for a child younger than age 1 to have leg problems (and tightness or spasticity almost never require bracing, special shoes, or surgery at this age), exercise, especially gentle stretching, is good for the child who is not moving his legs on his own. It is best to incorporate this stretching into activities of daily living, such as diapering and bathing. The stretching should never be done so vigorously that it makes the child cry.

Infants generally respond well to infant stimulation programs. These programs also put parents in touch with professionals who are comfortable with their infant and can tell parents about activities that will help stimulate the infant in a way that is appropriate for his level of development. These programs also reassure the parents that their efforts are helping the child and that their child is developing at his maximum ability. Generally, taking part in a group program with other parents once a week or every other week is sufficient.

Is a walker recommended?

Many parents enjoy seeing their child move about on her own in a sling-seat walker, but parents need to supervise the child very closely to prevent accidents. One safety guideline is to tie the walker to a post or piece of furniture to limit the distance the child can travel. It is essential that a child in a walker stay away from stairs, as this is where most accidents occur. Also, the walker must be one that is engineered to be stable. Many physical therapists don't recommend walkers, because they are concerned that bad movement patterns will result. The use of a sling-seat walker will not teach the child to walk sooner and can create dangerous situations. There is no evidence that the use of walkers does any long-term harm, however.

Ages One to Three

This is the age at which the characteristics of diplegia become more noticeable, mainly because unlike other children at this age, the child with diplegia is not walking. This major developmental milestone becomes the focus for many parents. While the delay in walking is certainly important, it is much more important that at the age of 14 months the child be fairly healthy, eating well, growing normally, gaining weight, and developing hand function and speech.

By the age of 3 years, it is usually helpful for the child with diplegic CP to be involved in a specialized school environment, such as a cerebral palsy center, which as a site of therapy is preferred by many medical professionals over the home. In a peer environment, focus can be placed on physical and occupational therapies, with emphasis on the child's disability. For children without brothers or sisters, the group environment is also helpful in developing interactive social skills.

What can I do to help my child walk?

A child cannot be made to walk before she is developmentally able to do so, and a child does not need to crawl in order to be able to walk. As a parent, you may work at offering the best possible environmental stimulation, within the scope of your personal schedule and the therapist's judgment. But you should never *force* your child to walk or make her feel inadequate for not being able to do so. Providing a loving, supportive environment is the best gift you can give her.

How can I tell if and when my child will walk?

Normal children start walking sometime between the ages of 8 and 18 months. Most children with diplegia are delayed in walking and do not walk until between 2 and 4 years of age. Children with mild involvement are usually learning to walk at age 2 to 2½. At this age they pull up along furniture and cruise just as normally developing 10- and 11-month-old infants do. Some children with diplegia don't start walking until as late as age 8. Therefore, there are a good many years when it's possible that the child will begin walking. Once a child starts walking, she almost always continues to make progress in her gait. In general, by age 8 to 10 years the child has developed the pattern of mobility she will have for life.

Are there special positions my child should avoid?

This is an area that sometimes generates conflict between therapists and physicians. Between 1 and 3 years of age, children with diplegia have a tendency to sit in a W position, with their legs bent backward at the knee. This provides a very stable sitting posture and frees up the child's hands for play. It is also a very comfortable sitting position due to the rotational alignment of their legs.

Although there is no scientific evidence that this position is damaging or dangerous, there are those who think that this position causes hip and gait problems. In fact, however, children who sit in this position walk with their feet turned in only because the alignment of their legs, which allows them to sit this way comfortably, also causes them to walk toeing in. Most professionals recommend that parents allow children to sit in a comfortable position, particularly if they function well. Therapists may try to improve the child's sitting posture and utilize long sitting (sitting with the legs extended in front) and tailor-style positions. Size-appropriate chairs are important as well, as they can help the child develop a good sitting posture.

As your child starts to move on the floor, she will probably use a commando type of crawl, dragging herself with her arms, her legs following. Allow your child to move and explore with whatever pattern of crawling works for her, bearing in mind that therapists will probably work to establish a four-point crawl, on hands and knees, like that of a typical 8-month-old baby. Although you may certainly work on the crawl at home, you should never prevent your child from using a crawl that works well for her.

What walking aids should my child use?

While children without diplegia start cruising at 9 months, children with mild involvement usually start to cruise at approximately age 2. The best walking aids are push toys such as small shopping carts and baby buggies, which work best when weighted down with sandbags because otherwise they tend to be very light. Children at this age seldom need walkers or crutches and usually do not like to use them.

If your child has moderate involvement and is just starting to pull himself up to a standing position at age 2½, he will most likely be cruising at age 3. He will probably enjoy using a walker because of the freedom of movement it offers. Try letting your child use the walkers that push in front as well as the rear walkers. Experimentation allows the child, with the help of therapists, to determine which kind works best for him. Even at age 3 he will often enjoy pushing toys.

If your child has severe involvement, he will most likely be standing with support by age 3. If by age 2½ your child is not pulling himself up to stand, a standing program should be initiated. Therapists usually recommend the use of ankle-foot braces (AFOs) to help with foot control and a stander, usually the prone type. We also recommend one to two hours a day of standing if your child tolerates it. The use of a stander helps give children a sense of being upright, encourages head and trunk control and balance, and stimulates the normal development of bones and joints in the legs. Remember that most children with diplegia *will* be pulling up and standing early enough that a standing program will not be necessary.

As children with diplegia start to stand, they usually go up on their toes. If they have good balance, they may walk around like little ballet dancers, but if balance is a problem, they frequently have difficulty walking. Ankle-foot braces, particularly molded ones, can help stabilize the child's feet and ankles. At this age, the goal of using these braces is to help the child get his feet flat and stable, eliminating the need for concentrating on controlling movement at the foot and ankle. Another condition that responds well to the brace is that of the very flat foot that tends to roll in; for this we recommend the use of a rigid brace, without hinges. It should extend to the tips of the toes so that the child does not curl his toes over the end of the brace in a gripping fashion. It is more difficult to fit shoes over these longer braces, but generally a style of sneaker that opens far toward the front fits very well.

In the past, orthopedic shoes with attached braces were commonly used. While they may provide a benefit to a small number of children who react allergically to plastic, the vast majority of children are happier in plastic braces, concealed by clothes and worn with regular shoes. The cost, when one considers shoe wear, is comparable. There is almost never a need to use long leg braces or braces above the knee for children with cerebral palsy. Although children with disabilities such as spina bifida, polio, and spinal cord injuries benefit from using these braces, they tend to make walking more difficult. At this age, continuing to work with therapeutic exercises has the best effect. Surgery is seldom recommended at this age.

Is a wheelchair or a special stroller needed?

Between the ages of 1 and 3 most children with diplegia have good trunk control and sitting balance. Regular child or infant strollers are usually adequate for mobility. Special adaptive strollers or wheelchairs are not needed at this stage unless your child doesn't have good trunk control and needs additional support.

What are the concerns regarding the hips?

By the time a child with diplegia reaches the age of 2, there is a need to begin close and regular examination of the hips for possible spastic hip disease. The spasticity in the muscles around the hip joint puts the child at significant risk for hip dislocation. Hip dislocation occurs very slowly and gradually. The head of the femur (which is round like a ball) moves out of the socket of the hip joint. The most serious consequence occurs when the hip becomes completely dislocated, eventually causing early arthritis and pain as the child grows. Pain sometimes occurs as the hip is dislocating too. This process of gradual dislocation is called *subluxation of the hip*. Spastic hip disease can be detected by close observation and appropriate *x-rays*; a hip examination is necessary every six months, and x-rays need to be done every year if the child is not walking without a walker or crutches. At this young age, muscle release surgery can usually prevent the hips from becoming completely dislocated if the hips begin to sublux.

What problems do the feet present?

As we pointed out earlier, at this age it is very common for children to be walking up on their toes or, alternatively, to be noticeably rolling their feet in. Both of these problems are best controlled with foot braces (AFOs) and very rarely need surgical correction at this young age. These braces must be replaced as the child grows. A few children have a lot of spasticity and find the braces uncomfortable. Injections of botulinum toxin (Botox) usually will make the orthotic wear more comfortable. Typically this will only work for three or four injections spread 4 to 6 months apart. After that, surgery may need to be considered, but seldom before the child is 5 or 6 years old.

Some children will have excessive turning in from the foot or leg, causing them to trip a good deal. Heavy braces to try to correct this should be avoided. Rather, the child should work with therapeutic exercises. If necessary, the problem can be dealt with at an older age with surgery.

Ages Four to Six

Between 4 and 6 years the child with diplegia makes the most significant physical improvement in motor function. By the time your child reaches age 6, he or she should be ready to devote time and energy to school. Once the child reaches kindergarten or first grade, the focus should be on cognitive issues. If at all possible, therapy should now be deemphasized, even discontinued, and children who are able to should be in a regular school setting.

How much therapy, and what kind, might my child need at this age?

The frequency and specific type of therapy is dependent on the severity of your child's involvement, the child's response to therapy, the availability of services, and the parents' ability to provide services. The child who is more severely involved will probably benefit most from therapy because he is less able to stimulate himself. The child with mild involvement moves about and plays fairly readily, thus providing a good deal of his own therapy.

There is agreement, professionally, that the period from age 4 to the time when a child is entering kindergarten or first grade is the best time to focus on therapy. However, there is no absolute agreement on the ideal number of sessions. Most children at this age will not tolerate more than five half-hour sessions a week. Some children will tolerate considerably fewer. If your child is resisting, back off and give him time to explore on his own. If you are involved in the therapy, it should be a pleasant experience for both parent and child. Your role is not that of physical therapist but that of parent, a role that includes many things more important than exercises. Community-based physical activity is better than not doing any exercise, but you should not feel guilty if other necessary activities at home prevent supervising your child's exercising.

There is very little evidence that physical or occupational therapy is directly related to a child's long-term functioning. Therapy *does* provide benefits to the child, and the therapist can provide significant help to the parents in the form of direction and suggestions. The benefit of therapy is somewhat similar to that of reading to a child of this age. Most children enjoy being read to, and it appears to stimulate a later interest in reading and possibly in school. It is hard to prove, however, that reading to a child two hours a day is better than reading two hours a week or two hours a month.

What types of walking aids are now appropriate?

There are no hard-and-fast answers to this question, as each child will choose the walking aid that best suits her needs and her social situation. It helps to keep in mind, however, that this is the age for assessing and working out the child's mobility status. The goal is for the child to be as mobile as her peers by the time she begins school. The focus should be on mobility, and not just on walking. A child who can walk very fast with a walker in almost every situation and on any terrain but is quite slow with crutches should not use crutches for school. The crutches should be used at home and in the context of therapy, allowing her time to become more proficient with their use, with school use as a goal.

For the more severely involved child, whether he will *ever* walk may still be unknown. This is impossible to know until the child is in fact walking or has reached the age of 7 or 8. Even at that point, walking is not an all-or-none issue. Many children are able to walk short distances around the house but never walk long distances independently outside. The question then becomes one of which means of mobility works best for the child. In home situations he may hold on to walls and furniture; in school he may use a walker or crutches; for an all-day excursion to an amusement park he may choose a wheelchair. In this he is comparable to the individual without a disability who walks at home, rides a bike to go short distances, takes a car for longer rides, and gets on an airplane for great distances.

Could my child need a wheelchair? What type of stroller or wheelchair is best?

Most children at this age who still need to be pushed in a stroller have outgrown standard-size strollers. Families need to evaluate what kind of replacement they need based on how it will be used, where it will be used, whether the child will be able to manipulate it, and how it will be transported in the car. Large strollers are generally quite light and appear less medical than wheelchairs, in addition to being easy to fold up and transport. Their wheels are small, however, and this makes them difficult to push on rough ground. The child can't push herself in a stroller, and she may be concerned about its appearance because it resembles a baby stroller.

The standard wheelchair is certainly more costly, as well as clearly medical in appearance. However, children often prefer it because they don't want to look like a baby in a stroller. They can also help choose the color. Most children with diplegia can independently manipulate a chair (power wheelchairs are discussed in Chapter 7 and in Part 2). Clearly, the family's environment, as well as the individual child's needs, must be considered when choosing a chair.

My child isn't walking at all. Can I do anything to encourage her?

Problems with balance, muscle coordination, spasticity, and leg alignment are the main general causes of *delayed* walking. Any of these problems may also *prevent* a child from walking. Some children may have only one of these areas, while others may have problems in several. Generally at this age it's possible to begin to identify and address the specific problems preventing the child from walking.

Difficulty with balance (*ataxia*) is a common problem that prevents a child from being able to walk. Even children who walk well with a walker may not be able to progress to crutches because of balance problems. Typically these are children who cannot stand without holding on to furniture or another person. The balancing mechanism, located in the brain, continues to develop and mature until a child reaches 8 to 10 years of age.

Physical therapy can be very helpful in maximizing your child's balance. Therapists help children exercise and practice falling in much the same way that gymnasts and dancers learn to perfect maneuvers with good balance.

Many children between the ages of 4 and 6 develop a protective fear of falling. It is important during this stage not to force them to use crutches. It is better to work in a therapeutic environment in which falls will be cushioned by mats, allowing the child to develop a sense of safety. Some therapists suggest heavy shoes to help with balance. Braces usually are not helpful, and there is no surgical treatment that will improve a child's balance.

Lack of muscle coordination makes it difficult for the child to place his feet in the proper position for walking. At an early age, this phenomenon shows up as the inability to initiate steps. The process of taking steps involves the co-contraction of two muscles successfully working in harmony. If muscles are working against each other, the child cannot take any steps. Again, therapy can be helpful in working with the child to develop strategies to control his muscles. Usually by age 8 to 10 the combination of maturity and therapy yields significant improvement with respect to this problem.

Surgery can be helpful in improving the balance between different muscles. This is accomplished by transferring the overpowering muscle in a way that increases the ability of the weaker muscle. Sometimes the knee is prevented from bending because of muscles pulling excessively in the front; this is improved when part of the muscle is transferred to the back of the knee. Sometimes a child's foot rolls in or out excessively. This imbalance can often be corrected in a brace, but if it is severe, it can also be addressed surgically with transfers or lengthenings of muscles about the ankle.

Spasticity is another problem that contributes to a child's difficulty in walking. Spasticity causes the stretched muscle to pull back and other muscles to become tight as the child attempts to move. Spasticity varies with the child's activity, state of health, growth, and mood, as well as with the time of day. Stretching the muscle and putting it through its range of motion helps to keep it loose but has no effect on the underlying spasticity. Spasticity also prevents muscles from growing normally. As children grow, the very spastic muscle becomes shortened, resulting in a joint that cannot move normally.

A number of oral medications help reduce spasticity (see table 5). However, for most children the side effects and complications of these medications outweigh the benefits. The decrease in spasticity is often short-lived, and withdrawal of the medication typically leads to a temporary increase in spasticity. Botulinum toxins A and B are available for off-label use (the medication is approved by the US Food and Drug Administration, but not for this purpose) to control spasticity in some tight muscles. Botulinum toxin is best used when there are specific muscles (six or fewer) that are spastic. It is a relatively safe drug without known systemic effects if it is not injected into the bloodstream. It acts locally within the injected muscle to block the release of some of the nerve signals to the muscle. There are rare side effects, the most common being some temporary soreness within the injected muscle. The FDA has required that the drug company include a black box warning stating that injected toxin can spread to muscles beyond the injection site, resulting in breathing and swallowing problems. Deaths have been reported, though the data are not clear about whether it was the botulinum toxin that caused the

Table 5. Medications for Spasticity

Name (Generic/Trade)	How Given	Possible Side Effects*
Diazepam/Valium	By mouth; via G- or J-tube; rectally	Sedation; fatigue; weakness; memory disturbance; ataxia; respiratory depression
Dantrolene/Dantrium	By mouth; via G- or J-tube	Weakness; drowsiness; lethargy; dizziness; nausea; diarrhea; liver damage
Tizanidine/Zanaflex	By mouth; via G- or J-tube†	Sedation; decreased blood pressure; liver injury
Baclofen/Lioresal	By mouth; via G- or J-tube	Sedation; weakness; fatigue; abrupt withdrawal can cause hallucinations
	Intrathecally (injected into spinal fluid in back via a pump)	Dizziness; lightheadedness; drowsiness; nausea; vomiting; decreased blood pressure; respiratory depression
Botulinum toxin A/Botox	Injected into spastic muscle	Localized pain; generalized fatigue; transient weakness

*One or more of these side effects may occur.
† Simultaneous use of tizanidine with fluvoxamine or ciprofloxacin is contraindicated

deaths. However, it is generally believed that children with severe CP are those at most risk for severe complications from very high doses. Therefore, most physicians now limit the dose to 10–12 units of botulinum per kilogram of body weight and inject it into no more than four large muscles. If the muscles are small, as in the hand or forearm, then more muscles can be injected.

Additionally, two surgical procedures involving the brain or spinal cord are in use today to treat spasticity. The *selective dorsal rhizotomy* (SDR) involves cutting the nerves coming from the spinal cord (see Part 3 for details). The second procedure involves placing a pump under the skin of the abdomen that feeds an antispasticity medication, baclofen, via a catheter to the fluid surrounding the spinal cord. The physician can adjust the level of medication as needed. This procedure is reversible, and little postsurgical rehabilitation is necessary. No studies have been published regarding the long-term outcome of either procedure.

The best results from rhizotomies seem to be in young children who have excellent balance and few muscle coordination problems and are walking fairly well despite severe spasticity. Children between the ages of 3 and 7 have the best results. A child who is making good progress in walking would not be a candidate for surgery until he has reached a point where he cannot progress because of the spasticity. Also, problems with balance can actually increase with a dorsal rhizotomy. There is very little long-term experience with baclofen pumps or rhizotomies in ambulatory children with diplegia, although these approaches may have a more defined role in years to come.

Any child who might be considered for selective dorsal rhizotomy might also be considered for pump implantation for intrathecal baclofen. Parents may perceive advantages and disadvantages to each approach. SDR involves a single operation, whereas intrathecal baclofen requires operations to replace the pump when its battery is exhausted, pump refills in the doctor's office every few months, and unpredictable additional operations to repair problems with the spinal catheter. Wound complications are more common after pump implantation than after SDR. Intrathecal baclofen therapy carries risks of drug overdose and drug withdrawal, although these problems can be avoided by careful attention to pump refill procedures. Intrathecal baclofen requires implantation under the skin of a device the size of a hockey puck, but there are no implants with SDR. On the other hand, the effects of SDR are immediate and permanent, which means that if the loss of tone makes the child less functional (which can happen if the child's tone helped him stand and walk), it cannot be undone. Also, SDR requires a period of intensive rehabilitation immediately after surgery. The effects of intrathecal baclofen can be adjusted slowly and are entirely reversible, and if the patient or the family becomes dissatisfied, the pump can be removed.

Bone and muscle malalignment is another problem that interferes with walking. Most frequently children have difficulty with their feet turning too far in, causing them to trip as they walk. Feet that are rolling in or out and mild toe walking can usually be corrected with an AFO. A hinged AFO should be worn if possible. If the turning in is coming from the hip, thigh, or lower leg, no brace or cable can be applied that will result in better function for the child, although the cosmetic appearance may improve. Children without spasticity often show improved alignment as they grow. However, children with spasticity may improve less as they grow, and surgical correction of the problem may be necessary, usually before the child begins first grade. After 5 to 6 years of age, the spasticity tends to slowly decrease. Timing the procedure to prepare the child to enter grade school in the best possible condition is a reasonable goal.

Bone malalignment is corrected by surgically cutting the bone (called an *osteotomy*) and resetting it in a corrected position. Muscle lengthenings involve cutting the tendon. The entire muscle system must be evaluated so that lengthening one muscle does not create an imbalance. Typically, a child who needs his Achilles tendon lengthened has tight hip and knee muscles as well. If only the Achilles tendon were lengthened in a child who is toe walking and has tight hamstrings, the child would walk flatfooted but with a crouched gait. Thus, the timing of muscle lengthenings is crucial, because as a child grows the muscles retighten.

I've heard about surgery to help children walk better. When is the best time for this?

A highly individualized, often subjective evaluation is necessary to determine when to perform surgery to make a child walk better. On the one hand, a child's progress should not be impeded by putting off necessary corrective surgery. On the other hand, surgeries should be timed so that a child has a minimum number of operations in his lifetime. The younger a child is when muscle lengthenings are done, the more likely it is that the child will need to undergo additional lengthenings as he or she grows. But delaying necessary surgery will often impede a child's progress in walking.

Minimizing the number of surgeries a child has helps keep the child from seeing himself as "sick." Operating on a child at an age when he can understand some of his experience and cooperate with postoperative therapy is also beneficial to the child. Generally, just before a child enters first grade is an appropriate time for the first surgery. Most children with diplegia can be treated surgically at this age, with the final adjustment made at the end of adolescence.

With good planning, including grouping procedures, the majority of children will undergo only two orthopedic surgeries in the preadult years. This ought to be the goal, and it certainly is the ideal situation. Even if this goal can't be met, there is no reason for a child with diplegia to have an operation every year for four or five years, as was typical in the past.

To avoid repeated surgeries and recoveries, it's essential for the child to be evaluated by an orthopedist who is experienced with cerebral palsy and who can perform several necessary procedures while the child is under one dose of anesthesia. The orthopedist must be highly skilled and able to predict the impact of one procedure on another.

Should I be worried that my child might have a hip dislocation at this age?

Hip subluxation and dislocation are certainly significant concerns. Your child must be examined at least every six months and x-rayed every year if he is walking without a walker or crutches. The risk of developing hip problems is related to the severity of involvement. Children with very mild involvement are at low risk for developing hip problems, but as many as 50 to 75 percent of children with severe diplegia develop hip abnormalities that require surgical intervention. Releasing the muscles in the groin that are applying abnormal forces to the hip—the adductors—is the simplest surgical procedure. It should be done as soon as recommended because of its simplicity and generally excellent outcome.

Should I be concerned about my child's back?

Although back problems are a concern, the back does not need to be monitored as closely as other areas at this age. There may be the appearance of a *scoliosis* (curvature to the side) or *kyphosis* (round shoulders), but these are almost always flexible deformities. X-rays and treatment generally are not considered at this age because the deformity is not fixed. However, these conditions do require periodic evaluations by a physician.

Are there any upper extremity problems?

The child with typical diplegia by definition has no significant problem with her upper extremities. However, children with diplegia do frequently have difficulty with fine motor coordination, such as that required for coloring and writing. Some children do have a significant problem with one arm or hand even though they have a diplegic pattern. Refer to the discussion of the upper extremities in Chapter 5 if your child has such a problem.

Ages Seven to Twelve

The early school years usually bring significant changes for children, including children with a disability. By the time a child reaches this age, the rate of physical improvement has leveled off in areas such as balance and coordination, and it's a good idea to refocus the child's attention away from additional physical improvement and toward intellectual learning. Children without a disability are also being encouraged to concentrate more on academics and less on play at this age, but for the child with a disability these years usually involve coming to terms with a decreased level of physical function.

What school environment is best for my child?

The choice of school environment is often difficult. In some districts parents are not given reasonable options, which of course complicates the process of placing a child with special needs. The current trend is for inclusion of most children with diplegia, meaning that they are placed in regular classes. This tends to work well for the mildly affected child, as the child can be integrated into most normal activities. Children who have more significant cognitive disabilities are sometimes included only for classes such as music and art, allowing for some interaction with peers. Children with a significant physical disability need to attend school in buildings that are accessible to wheelchairs, walkers, or crutches. An appropriate and accessible toileting facility must also be available.

It is important to consider many factors when choosing a learning environment for your child. Children need to be in an environment where they can feel successful while learning, without constantly being frustrated. Children with learning disabilities clearly benefit from interacting with children who don't have disabilities, but they need to be placed in an appropriate learning environment as well. Make certain that properly trained staff are available to meet the needs of your child and to manage interactions with the other children. It is often uncomfortable for the child to be identified as different from the other children, so it's important for you to strike a balance when choosing the appropriate school environment.

What is the role of adaptive physical education?

Many children with mild to moderate diplegia can enjoy normal activities of physical education (PE) until they are approximately 10 or 11 years old, when sports tend to become more competitive and the child cannot compete effectively. Alternative PE) activities, such as adaptive PE, are beneficial. Adaptive PE can be structured by a physical education teacher, providing good physical activity while enhancing the child's self-esteem. If it is desirable and available, informal physical and occupational therapy may be provided for the child with cerebral palsy while children without disabilities are engaged in routine PE.

How much therapy is necessary now?

For the child with mild diplegia, the start of first grade is a good time to discontinue formal physical and occupational therapy. These therapies should be replaced by physical activities such as swimming, dance classes, karate, or horseback-riding lessons. Children are often involved in these activities at an even younger age, usually because the parent has identified an interest and located a capable teacher.

Formal therapy at this age has less long-term impact and is similar to an athlete's daily training routine, in that when the training is discontinued, the athlete's ability starts to regress. Because a child cannot be expected to continue physical therapy indefinitely, cultivating her interest and ability in an activity that she can continue throughout her lifetime is a healthier option. Additionally, formal therapy takes time away from the child's schooling, study time, and possible interaction with other children. An exception should be made for therapy that focuses on teaching specific activities of daily living, such as dressing, and postoperative rehabilitation therapy. These types of therapy are recommended as needed.

The child with severe diplegia may not be able to participate in extracurricular physical activities. Again, it is extremely important to make sure that therapy, especially for children with normal learning abilities, doesn't interfere with academic learning. Academic subjects and knowledge are most beneficial for the child in the long term. Certainly, a routine home exercise program has many benefits, and parents can stress the importance of such a program just as they do the importance of daily hygiene.

Will my child's walking continue to improve?

A child reaches his maximum physical ability to walk by 8 to 10 years of age. The child who has limitations in terms of endurance and distance when he is 8 to 10 almost certainly will not do better when he is 16. In fact, the adolescent growth spurt typically adds 12 inches and 50 to 75 pounds to the child's frame. Because his muscle control and coordination do not improve, this extra height and weight make walking more difficult. This period of adjusting to new body dimensions, often referred to as the clumsy period, is experienced by adolescents without disabilities as well.

The 8-year-old with diplegia who is using all his ability to walk is not going to walk as well when he ages and has extra height and weight. This does not mean that a child who walks well at age 8 will need a wheelchair at age 16. It is likely, however, that a child who is worn out from a shopping trip at age 10 will need crutches for a shopping trip at age 16. The child with severe involvement who has to struggle with a walker at age 8 will probably be a full-time wheelchair user except possibly in his own home. In short, parents should not expect major regression, but they can anticipate that their child's walking skills will plateau, with some mild decreases in function.

For both child and parent, frustration can easily result if these changes are not anticipated or haven't been planned for. Up until the age of 8, continuous gains are being made and it is easy, though incorrect, to anticipate that these gains will continue. Frequently, the parents or the child will want to increase the amount of physical therapy, under the false assumption that even more therapy will result in greater gains. As mentioned previously, a far more rewarding approach is to increase the focus on academics.

At this time, both parents and child should be working to accept the reality of the child's level of function. Often this is easier for the child than for the parent. Clearly, the child will be at a distinct disadvantage if her parents have not been able to deal with their expectations, particularly as the child enters the difficult period of puberty.

What is the best type of walking aid?

The specific aid will most likely vary with the walking environment. A child may hold on to walls in his home, use crutches at school, and prefer a wheelchair for the amusement park. What the child finds works best for him is what he should be allowed to use. Generally children want to use the least obtrusive assistive device that they are comfortable with. Therefore, a child who wants to use crutches usually needs them; the child who does not want to use them is probably stable without them. Parents and therapists should help the child find what works best for him and not force their preferences on the child.

Some children need an assistive device but are unable to understand the need because of a moderate to severe cognitive disability. Some children who have not developed a healthy fear of falling don't understand this either and may need to wear a helmet to avoid injury.

Children with severe involvement are at risk for becoming less interested in walking as they get bigger and walking becomes harder. A similar phenomenon occurs in children without disabilities; as they gain weight, they watch more TV, eat more food, and get less exercise. Because obesity poses a significant problem for children with diplegia, parents and others need to work with these children to help them avoid obesity. As a parent you should establish firm guidelines requiring your child to get some exercise appropriate to her ability. Your child needs to learn that exercise and good eating habits are the cornerstones of good health and that it is especially important for her to work on these areas.

What braces are indicated at this age? The use of braces is usually limited to molded foot braces (MAFOs) or, occasionally, smaller shoe inserts for children who may need them. Usually foot deformities can be corrected with surgery. However, delay of surgery for optimum effect may make it necessary for the child to wear a brace for one to two years. Most children will not object to wearing braces when they are young, but any objections can be dealt with by adjusting the brace or clothing so that the brace is covered up. When the child's reluctance to wear the brace involves other children's reactions, the teacher may find that explaining the use of the brace provides both an excellent lesson for other children and a solution for the wearer.

What shoes should my child wear? Usually the best choice for the child with diplegia is an athletic shoe, with or without a MAFO. Today, athletic shoes are well constructed and well accepted in almost any social setting. Since the MAFO provides almost all of the foot support, it is not necessary to purchase an expensive shoe. There is no harm in a child wearing more formal dress shoes on special occasions, with or without braces. Even if a child does not walk as well without braces, occasionally wearing dress shoes can provide a psychological boost without causing any long-term physical damage.

Will surgery improve walking at this age? At this stage of development, improvement in walking has reached a plateau. If a child is walking without difficulty but has some mild problems, it is best to address these after puberty. On the other hand, if a child has significant problems that can be improved with surgery but were not dealt with before the child started school, they should be addressed now. There is almost no doubt that existing difficulties will increase in severity with the adolescent growth spurt in puberty. Not confronting significant problems also puts the child at risk for additional psychological stress.

My child walks with her knees bent. What can be done?

Walking with bent knees is referred to as a crouched gait. It is the most common gait problem in children with diplegia in this age group. If the crouched gait is severe, it should be treated, since it can prevent a child from getting around. Once a child has become wheelchair bound due to this problem, it is extremely difficult for her to return to her prior level of walking ability.

The crouching is caused by tight muscles, specifically the hamstrings and *iliopsoas* muscles. It can be treated by surgical lengthenings and occasionally by using a MAFO to help the child stand straighter. There are some other, less common causes for the crouching, such as overlengthened Achilles tendons or severe flat feet, and these have their own treatments. The child who has increased crouching will tire more easily and want to walk shorter distances. During rapid growth spurts crouching usually gets worse, because the muscles aren't growing as fast as the bone.

The causes of the crouched walking pattern are often complex. The primary problem is increased contracture of the hamstring, but there are usually significant secondary problems, such as feet that turn out or are severely flat. A gait analysis is often required to determine all the causes of crouched walking and to plan a correction of these various components of the problem. After surgery, intense physical therapy is recommended to improve the gait pattern, and the child will need to wear special AFOs that help to support the knee when the child is standing. Usually some crouching persists, but this outcome is preferable to a gait pattern in which the knee snaps back into hyperextension (also known as back-kneeing). This complex problem should usually be addressed by an orthopedist who has experience with children who have gait problems secondary to cerebral palsy.

What is the treatment for severe flat feet?

Wearing an AFO is the preferred treatment for severe flat feet at this age if the position of the child's foot can be adequately corrected this way. There are surgical procedures that stabilize the foot; for example, the deformity can be permanently corrected with an arthrodesis, which involves fusing together the bones around the heelbone (*calcaneus*). But it's best to delay this surgery until the child's growth is almost completed, since the procedure will stop some of the growth in the foot. As always, to minimize disruptions the child should undergo the fewest possible surgical procedures. If the child cannot function well, of course, then surgery must be considered.

Is there any treatment for spasticity?

As mentioned earlier in this chapter, a number of oral medications are helpful in reducing spasticity (see table 5). For most children, however, the side effects and complications of these medications outweigh the benefits. The decrease in spasticity is often short-lived, and withdrawal of the medication typically leads to a temporary increase in spasticity. Spasticity may be treated at this age with a selective dorsal rhizotomy, which involves cutting nerves close to the spinal cord (see Part 3 for details).

As mentioned above, botulinum toxins A and B are available for off-label use to control spasticity in some tight muscles. Botulinum toxin is best used when six or fewer muscles are spastic. It is a relatively safe drug without known systemic effects if it is not injected into the bloodstream. It acts locally within the injected muscle to block the release of some of the nerve signals to the muscle (see pages 149 and 171–72).

Intrathecal baclofen pumps are being used for some children with this level of disability, and while short-term results appear favorable, the long-term outcome is still largely unclear. Muscle releases and lengthenings are well-established procedures that predictably work well, though they do not directly decrease spasticity.

Should I still have concerns about hip subluxation and dislocation?

Hip subluxation does continue to be a concern, although the child with diplegia who walks well and has had no hip problems by this age is unlikely to develop problems later. Children whose hips show mild to moderate subluxation must continue to be watched closely, with x-rays every one or two years through the teenage years. By this age, any child with severely subluxed or dislocated hips should have been treated. If a child with severe hip problems has not been treated, then the child should have bone surgery, usually involving additional reconstruction of the hip socket.

Are there back problems that I need to monitor?

As a child approaches puberty, she needs to be watched more closely for scoliosis, since the adolescent growth spurt can produce a larger curve and eventually a stiffer curve. Back curvature can be monitored by physical examination, and with x-rays when necessary. The severity and pattern of increase of the curve will dictate how often x-rays are needed. The risk of developing scoliosis caused by cerebral palsy is fairly low for children who are walking. If scoliosis does develop and become severe, however, professionals usually recommend surgical correction.

Ages Thirteen to Eighteen

During this period of a child's development, a major issue is separating from the family. Adolescents with mild to moderate diplegia and normal intelligence often cope with this issue similarly to the way children without disabilities do. It's not uncommon for young people to feel as if their parents are trying to control their lives. It is, in fact, often difficult for parents to allow a child who has a disability to be independent and to separate from them. This is especially true for children with more significant disabilities—children whom parents feel a need to protect.

What can I do to help my child develop independence?

As they enter the adult world, a world in which they will interact mostly with individuals who don't have disabilities, teenagers with CP will of course experience failures and disappointments. But these experiences will help them develop a sense of self, something that all children need to do.

It is important to allow the teenager to make reasonable decisions and to give him choices in the decisions being made for him. Adolescents often resist having anything to do with outward signs of disability, for example. They may not want to see doctors or therapists, and they may be opposed to wearing braces or exercising. As they mature, teenagers must be allowed to make decisions about such things for themselves whenever possible, even when the outcome of those decisions is likely not to be as good as the outcome would be if the teenager followed parental advice (see the next question, below).

The teen with moderate to severe involvement who is handicapped will probably experience more difficulty separating from his parents and developing independence. A person who needs assistance in the activities of daily living, such as dressing, will of course have a more difficult time. Such teens should be offered as many choices as possible and should be allowed the freedom and distance from their parents that will allow them to interact with other caregivers. Children who aren't able to get out of a wheelchair by themselves can develop a sense of independence by being permitted to give instruction to the people who assist them.

Using service dogs to help persons with disabilities is a relatively new concept, similar to the use of guide dogs to help people who are visually impaired. These dogs can be very helpful in fostering independent living. They are taught to retrieve needed items and to help with such tasks as opening doors, and they can be trained to assist the individual who has specialized needs. It goes almost without saying that "man's best friend" can be a wonderful companion.

My child refuses medical care. What should I do?

Although the adolescent should continue to have yearly general medical checkups and orthopedic evaluations every six months to two years, the severity of the diplegia will dictate the frequency of medical visits. If the teenager resists this type of routine medical care, parents should first attempt to address any objections: might the teen be more comfortable with a different doctor, for example? Clearly, if a teen who needs care is not able to respond reasonably to a parent's attempt to help, then parents must assume more responsibility for seeing that he or she receives proper medical attention.

Suppose that the young person recognizes that wearing a brace improves the function of his limb but resists wearing it anyway because self-image and peer acceptance are more important to him than limb function. A flexible approach by the parents would be best. In this case, they can recognize that doing without the brace at this age will not have a long-term negative effect. On the other hand, a significant advantage of MAFOs is that they are easy to conceal under clothes, so a compromise with a resistant teen may still be a possibility.

What can I do to help my teenager deal with diplegia?

Adolescents frequently have a difficult time as they go through puberty and attempt to develop a personal value system. The teen with diplegia is certainly no exception. What's interesting is that there does not seem to be a significant correlation between the severity of a teen's involvement and her response to the involvement. In fact, it is not uncommon to find a teen with a very mild disability having more trouble accepting the disability than a child who has a severe involvement.

Much of an individual's coping style is derived from the individual's personality. The teen with very mild involvement may have difficulty because she is "almost normal," while a teen who has severe limitations and knows that she will never be in a situation that is physically similar to that of individuals without disabilities may have less difficulty.

Many adolescents with moderate diplegia go through puberty and develop a healthy self-concept with more ease than a child who has no health problems at all. Other children need extra help in accepting their disability. This help can be obtained from licensed, trained counselors. There are psychologists, social workers, and psychiatrists who specialize in helping children deal with disabilities, and the child who is having significant behavioral difficulties should be referred to one of them for professional counseling.

My teenager walked better a few years ago. What happened?

There is no further improvement in walking after a child reaches the age of 8, 9, or 10 unless he undergoes surgery for a correctable deformity. Adolescent growth leads to a decrease in endurance and coordination that is related to adjusting to the increase in body size. This is rarely a serious problem unless it is not anticipated or understood. At times a parent assumes his or her child is getting lazy or is less motivated, and this often fosters conflict. Parents must balance the need to encourage a teenager to stay active with the need to allow her to accept a comfortable level of mobility, as determined by her disability.

There is a normal decrease in mobility as individuals mature. The 16-year-old certainly spends less time running around than the 6-year-old. For the individual with a disability, the frequent side effect of less activity—weight gain—can make walking more difficult, which in turn can mean more weight gain as a result of less walking. This cycle can be a lifelong concern for some individuals.

Why is my daughter starting to walk with her knees bent again?

The most common recurrent problem for the adolescent with diplegia who has had previous surgery is the crouched gait and flat feet. The crouch is most likely a result of hamstrings that have not been able to accommodate to the increase in height. The crouched gait can be a significant problem if left untreated. If it becomes severe, it is harder to treat and puts the teen at significant risk for no longer being able to walk, so it should be addressed immediately. A moderate degree of crouching that does not seem to be getting worse is best dealt with when the teen stops growing. Then there can be a final surgical correction.

The fact is that for a number of reasons surgery to correct a crouched gait frequently does not result in a 100 percent correction. Because teenagers often have unrealistic expectations concerning surgery—even after the surgeon has provided a thorough explanation of the anticipated outcome—it's often beneficial to the whole family for the teen to be involved in making decisions about surgery. The physician or surgeon should allow ample time to explain the procedures and answer questions. Taking these steps preoperatively often leads to better cooperation by the teen in the postoperative therapy program.

The teen needs to understand that while no surgery can completely take care of the problem, he has some influence over the outcome.

After surgery to lengthen the appropriate muscles, short-term intensive physical therapy is usually necessary. Once the teen has good correction, it is important for her to keep active doing things to maintain the correction. A therapist can suggest appropriate activities.

What can be done to treat increasing flatfoot deformity?

As a child gains weight, the feet become increasingly flat and pronate more. MAFOs, which are usually effective when a child weighs 50 pounds, generally can't be used when the adolescent reaches 150 pounds. Then there is simply too much weight, causing painful skin pressure as the MAFO holds the foot in position. Surgical correction may involve fusions of the small joints in the foot or different kinds of osteotomies (bone cuts) to correct the flat foot. The degree of severity and the surgeon's experience will determine the specific procedure that is likely to be recommended.

Often it is not easy to decide when feet need to be surgically corrected, though a general rule is that the foot that is causing problems for a person as an adolescent will most likely cause problems for him as an adult. When foot pain is not relieved by adjustments in shoes and inserts, there is definitely a need for treatment. Problems with foot position and shoe wear provide less clear guidelines. Keep in mind that this surgery can easily be done at any time from age 10 to age 40 with little difference in outcome. Of course, delaying surgery may also mean delaying relief of symptoms.

What about toe problems that cause pain and calluses?

During adolescence the toes often begin causing problems. The big toe may develop a painful bunion (a large bump on the side of the toe that rubs on the inside of the shoe). The toe with the bunion may begin to bend toward the second toe and even overlap it, causing more discomfort. The easiest solution is to wear soft shoes that are not tight.

Surgical correction is recommended if the pain continues in the foot with the bunion. There are many different bunion operations for individuals who don't have cerebral palsy, but most of these will not work well for individuals with CP. Again, it is important to consult a physician who has expertise in treating cerebral palsy before having surgery.

Other toe deformities, such as hammer or claw toes, can cause calluses and be very uncomfortable. They often make walking more difficult, and they may make it difficult to wear shoes. These problems are easily treated with surgery.

Are there other leg and foot problems that can be corrected at this age?

In most cases leg and foot alignment has been corrected by this age, but adolescence is certainly an excellent time to make a correction, particularly after the growth spurt is completed. Bone procedures can be combined with muscle lengthening, making it necessary to expose the child to anesthesia only once.

These alignment corrections range from the straightforward to the complex. Most professionals recommend that a gait analysis be performed to help make decisions about proper treatment. Such analyses are conducted in a laboratory specializing in analyzing the gait problems of children with cerebral palsy. This evaluation can provide excellent information prior to surgery.

Should I be concerned about hip development?

For some individuals, hip subluxation needs to be monitored through adolescence. If the teen has a mild to moderate involvement and his hips have been normal up to this age, it is very unlikely that any problems will develop. X-rays generally are not needed in this group of teens.

Children who have had hip problems or subluxation need to be followed closely by physical examination and x-rays through the adolescent growth spurt and into the teen years. Any change in the hips during the adolescent growth spurt usually needs to be treated with surgery, with both bone procedures and muscle lengthenings. Also, it is often necessary to address the hip socket surgically at this age.

Continued monitoring and treatment as necessary will help the child reach adolescence and adulthood with hips that are as near to normal as possible. This is the child's best hope of avoiding the early development of arthritis, which can cause significant walking problems and pain.

What about scoliosis?

Scoliosis, or side-bending curvature of the spine, as a result of cerebral palsy is not a common problem in children with a mild to moderate pattern of diplegia. However, when it does occur, it becomes severe during the adolescent growth spurt. It must be carefully monitored with physical exams, and x-rays should be taken when the physical examination shows signs of scoliosis. This type of scoliosis should not be confused with *idiopathic scoliosis* (spinal curvature), which can occur in adolescents, usually girls, who are otherwise normal.

The spinal curve in the teen with cerebral palsy is usually not helped by wearing a brace. Doctors often suggest surgery if the curve progresses to 45 to 50 degrees. A spinal fusion prevents any further progression and corrects a significant portion of the curve. (Scoliosis is discussed in more detail in Chapter 7.)

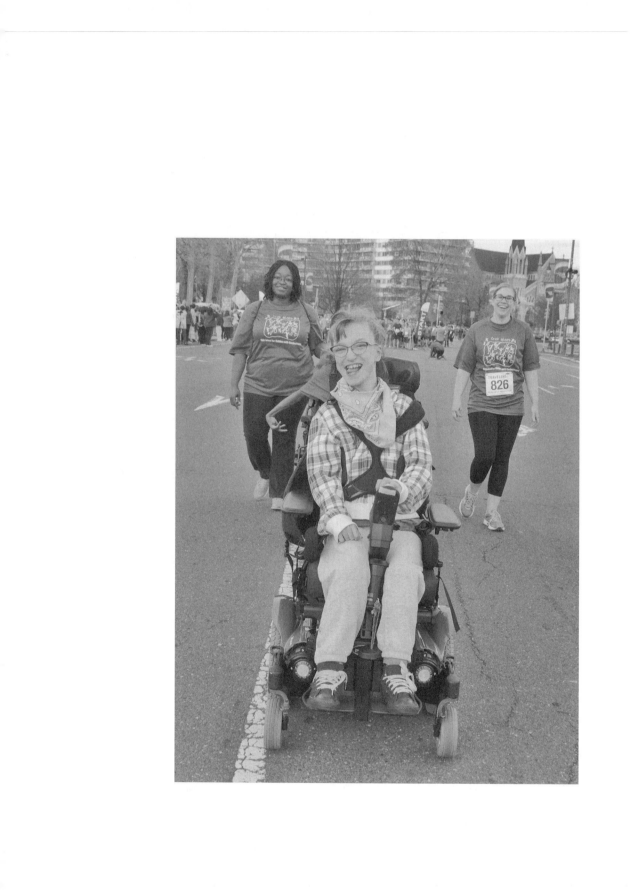

Quadriplegia

QUADRIPLEGIA, also known as *bilateral cerebral palsy*, is a form of cerebral palsy in which both arms and both legs are affected. Severe diplegia can be mistaken for mild quadriplegia, primarily because almost everyone who has diplegia has some involvement of their arms as well as their legs. For people with diplegia and for those with mild quadriplegia, there is mild dysfunction of the arms, but it is not a significant disability. The terminology used to describe the degree of involvement can vary greatly, even among specialists, because it is so difficult to fit a great number of individuals with differing functional factors into a specific category. There are always overlaps, and opinions vary regarding the proper diagnosis.

There are many people whose degree of cerebral palsy is not properly described by a broad term like *quadriplegia*. For this reason, several different kinds of quadriplegia have been identified. This chapter focuses on the orthopedic issues of quadriplegia. The medical problems often associated with this condition are covered in Chapter 3.

What do the different kinds of quadriplegia look like?

The child with *moderate spastic quadriplegia* (GMFCS IV) sits quite well, can lift himself into a wheelchair independently or with assistance, may be able to do very limited walking with a walker, and has enough hand function to feed himself. (Someone who primarily has spasticity and can walk well has diplegia. The needs of such a person are addressed in Chapter 6.) A child with *severe spastic quadriplegia* (GMFCS V) can't walk even with assistive devices, is not able to move to and from a wheelchair independently, usually isn't able to feed herself, and has difficulty sitting.

Athetosis (making large, uncontrollable movements) usually affects the upper extremities more than the lower. Most individuals with athetosis have a quadriplegic pattern, although the degree of involvement varies widely. Children with *moderate athetosis* are able to walk and can use their extremities well enough to perform most activities of daily living on their own. Children with *severe athetosis* are not able to walk independently and often are not able to transfer (move into and out of a wheelchair) by themselves. Some children with severe athetosis are unable to feed themselves and have speech problems as well. Many children with severe athetosis have difficulty sitting and need special seating support.

Other terms that are often confused with the terms described above are *pentaplegia*, *tetraplegia*, and *triplegia*. *Pentaplegia* refers to poor head control and four-limb involvement. *Tetraplegia* is essentially another term for quadriplegia. *Triplegia* refers to involvement of three limbs: both legs and one arm. Children with poor head control and quadriplegia are discussed in this chapter, in the context of severe spastic quadriplegia or severe athetoid quadriplegia. Parents whose children have triplegia, are mildly affected, and can walk will find the most relevant information in Chapter 5, on hemiplegia. Parents whose children have moderate leg involvement but walk with assistive devices will find the most relevant information in Chapter 6, on diplegia. The child with triplegia who can't walk is considered in this chapter, in the context of moderate spastic quadriplegia.

Birth to One Year

The first year of life is one of rapid changes. The infant learns to control the movement of her head, reach for a toy, roll over, and sit by herself without support. A delay in the development of these abilities is often the first sign of a problem in children who have quadriplegic pattern involvement. Experienced parents or grandparents will often notice that the infant does not "feel normal" when they hold him in their arms. They may say that the infant doesn't move normally or is either stiffer or more floppy than expected. But such signs of problems may be subtle and hard to put a finger on.

Can quadriplegia be diagnosed at this age? The early diagnosis of quadriplegia is difficult, as is the early diagnosis of diplegia and hemiplegia. However, children who had certain kinds of medical problems at an early age are at higher risk of later being diagnosed with spastic quadriplegia. Certain complications in the early development of the infant are associated with quadriplegia. These complications include extreme prematurity (less than 28 weeks' gestation), very low birthweight (less than 1,500 grams), bleeding in the brain, severe asphyxia (lack of oxygen), bacterial meningitis, and shaken baby syndrome (see Chapter 1). Children who survive these complications may have mild, moderate, or severe involvement, or they may be normal. As mentioned in Chapter 1, other disorders can look like CP, especially quadriplegia. Particular suspicion should be raised in the infant without any risk factors for CP. These infants should have appropriate testing done for other neurological diagnoses.

Although many children with traumatic beginnings grow and develop normally, parents' and physicians' suspicion and concern is raised when children have a history of early significant problems. A definitive diagnosis is rare during infancy, but parents are often given an idea of what might be ahead for them and their child. However, it is important to remember how tentative these predictions are.

What can be done for the high-risk infant during the first year of life? For the infant who is considered high risk because of medical problems in infancy or because of early signs of developmental delay, an infant stimulation (also known as early intervention) program is often recommended (this is addressed further below). In addition, any ongoing medical issues need to be addressed, and the infant's growth and development should be optimized.

Nutrition is one of the most important issues during the first year of life. A child who is not growing either is not getting adequate nourishment or is having severe medical problems that are inhibiting growth. The brain needs energy to grow and develop, and it uses the same energy as the muscles and bones. Therefore, if the muscles and bones are not growing, it's likely that the brain is not growing either. Medical problems can drain a lot of energy from a child or can be part of the reason a child does not want to eat.

Children with quadriplegia may have hydrocephalus, a condition that makes it necessary to place a shunt, a surgically implanted device that prevents fluid from building up, in the brain. Shunts must be checked periodically, and a child who has frequent infections should be checked carefully and often. Infection around a shunt—or any other infection—must be treated aggressively, and attempts must be made to prevent such infections by treating their cause. (See Chapter 3 for more discussion of shunts.)

Do children with quadriplegia often have seizures?

Seizures are frequently associated with quadriplegic cerebral palsy. Because seizures can have a significant effect on the growing child, careful attention to seizures, and treatment to achieve maximum control of them, is strongly advised. (Seizures are discussed in Chapter 3.)

What kind of feeding problems might a child with quadriplegia have?

Feeding problems caused by oral motor dysfunction are commonly associated with quadriplegia. This dysfunction of the muscles of the tongue and mouth can make chewing and swallowing difficult. Feeding problems can affect the child's nutrition and can also lead to chronic aspiration and pneumonia.

Gastric reflux, in which food comes back up the esophagus, can cause spitting up or vomiting. Sometimes the child coughs when this happens, and then food particles are introduced into the lungs, causing bronchitis and pneumonia. Some children have a poor gag reflex, and they too are susceptible to respiratory infections. It is often helpful to sit the child up after feeding him or her. Several medications may be used to help control these problems. In the most severe situations, surgical options ranging from placement of a gastrostomy tube to a fundoplication may be recommended. (See Chapter 3 for a full discussion of feeding problems and their treatment.)

Should I start my child in therapy at such a young age?

Although no absolute proof exists that early therapy changes the functional outcome of the child, most children benefit from early developmental stimulation therapy provided by physical and occupational therapists. Early exposure to a therapist is often an invaluable resource and support for parents. Therapy should be delayed until the baby is medically stable, however, and until it can be handled without putting too much stress on the heart and lungs. Premature babies usually need to gain at least enough weight to be at approximately normal newborn weight. After a severe brain trauma, such as a near drowning, therapy should not be started until the blood pressure and heart rate are stabilized and do not change when the child is handled. The therapy, when initiated, must be administered gently so that the child isn't agitated, as agitation can cause the blood pressure to rise.

Ages One to Three

Abnormal development in a child becomes easier to clearly recognize and define as the child approaches his first birthday. Most children at this age are rolling over, sitting, pulling to a standing position, starting to say words, and even walking independently. Of all these developmental milestones, walking is usually of greatest concern to parents of a child with a developmental delay. Parents naturally become concerned about the long-term prognosis if their child has not achieved head control when other children his age are walking. Often it is at this time that a diagnosis of quadriplegia is made.

Some parents adopt the mistaken notion that more therapy or use of a special brace or a walker will make it possible for their child to walk. This notion is often fostered by a combination of factors, most importantly by a lack of understanding of the child's problem or difficulty accepting how severe the problems are. Physicians need to spend time with parents in order to help them understand the complex problems facing them and their child. Parents should be encouraged to focus on the developmental skills that can be addressed now and to set aside, for the time being, their concern about developments that will only become clear with the passage of time.

What are the most important health issues at this age?

The most important health issue at this age is whether the child is thriving, gaining weight, and growing in height and head circumference. The long-term best outcome for any child requires that he get adequate nourishment in order to grow and develop. The child's actual weight is less important than whether the child is gaining, staying the same, or losing weight over time. The child who is not getting enough nourishment and not growing is also not going to develop optimally. The child's overall nutrition and health are much more important than any therapy, brace, or other device. Good nutrition is essential to normal growth and maximum development.

Another health issue at this age is constipation. The child who cannot get around on her own may become constipated and uncomfortable and may express this discomfort by becoming irritable. An appropriately designed bowel program can be a great help in this area (see Part 2 for a description of such a program).

Are physical and occupational therapy beneficial?

Physical and occupational therapy are important for the child's stimulation and to help the family develop realistic expectations. The therapist is a great resource for the parents. Therapists can provide parents with information about future equipment needs and serve as a "doorway" to the medical community. They can also teach parents how to touch and hold their child. However, it is important to understand that there is a limit to what the therapist can do. A physical therapist, no matter how experienced and knowledgeable, can't *make* a child walk. He or she can work to keep the child's joint range of motion at its maximum and provide valuable strategies for helping with balance so that the child has the best possible chance of walking if she is capable of doing so. The actual ability to walk and to balance are functions of the brain. At present, no one knows how to overcome the damage the brain has suffered and get it to function normally.

Similarly, occupational therapists can help enormously with activities of daily living such as self-feeding, but they can't make a child who has quadriplegia have normally functioning hands and fingers. The goal of any of the therapies should be to help the child achieve those skills they can achieve within the limitations resulting from their cerebral palsy. Therapy itself should not be the goal. Therefore, therapy should not consume the child's life. Nor should anyone suggest or believe that therapy will satisfy unrealistic expectations. The child can receive therapy in various ways, some of them of benefit to both the child and the parent; for example, there are infant stimulation day care centers where the child can be placed for both day care and therapy.

Parents need to maintain contact with the therapist. The therapist can answer many of the parents' questions as well as provide suggestions for home activities that would help the child and family. Many of these suggestions will be practical, while others will be fun and stimulating.

In terms of when therapy ought to begin, the situation is somewhat different for the child who sustains a brain injury between 2 and 5 years of age. After an injury, a child may very quickly develop severe muscle tightness and contractures. Parents may believe that this possibility should have been addressed earlier by therapy, but the safe time for starting therapy varies with each child. Just after an injury the brain swells. Everything possible must be done to reduce this swelling and prevent additional swelling, including avoiding agitating the child and raising his or her blood pressure. At some point, from several days to a month after the injury, the swelling diminishes and the brain begins to heal. This is the time to start therapy.

How many doctors does my child need? Generally, by age 1 or a year after brain injury, a child can be followed by a family pediatrician. Specialists can then be consulted as the need arises, thereby limiting the time the child and parent spend in doctors' offices. Not only is this helpful in a practical sense but it is also psychologically beneficial. Most children with cerebral palsy need to be seen by specialists at times—a pediatrician can't provide for *all* the child's needs. What the pediatrician can do is refer the child for dental, orthopedic, neurological, and other consultations when necessary.

Do many children with quadriplegia have cognitive impairment? Children with quadriplegia may have cognitive impairments, but many who are thought to have cognitive limitations in fact are only very limited in their ability to communicate. Having a child tested by appropriately trained individuals is essential in order to evaluate his or her potential. (Cognitive impairment is further discussed in Chapter 3.)

What about self-injurious behavior? Self-injurious behavior, or SIB, often begins at this time. It is usually seen in children with spastic or hypotonic quadriplegia who have some degree of cognitive impairment. It is very rarely seen in children with athetosis. (During the adolescent period, athetoid movements can become strong enough to cause injury accidentally. The treatment for this problem is different from the treatment for voluntary self-abuse.)

The most common self-abusive behaviors are hand biting, hand hitting, head banging, and eye scratching. The behavior generally is worse when the child is left alone or is not involved in some activity. Treatment should focus on finding ways to keep the child occupied and distracted. Other methods, such as rewarding desired behaviors, may be tried but may not be successful because of the child's cognitive limitations.

Occasionally, restraints such as elbow extension splints, helmets, and face guards are used, but they may only frustrate the child and make matters worse when the restraints are not in place. Clearly, if the self-abusive behavior is causing significant bodily harm, such as risking blindness or the loss of fingers, the child must be protected from himself. (See Chapter 3 for a more complete discussion of self-injurious behavior.)

What type of seating is best?

Most children with quadriplegia are not sitting well by age 1, although many of them eventually develop the ability to sit. At this age parents should concentrate on supporting the child's upper body, encouraging head control and providing head control as needed. This is especially important to improve the child's feeding, communication, and interaction with the environment. Between the ages of 1 and 2, the child should be fed while seated in a seat facing the person feeding him. The seat may be a chair with special trunk (upper torso) supports or with a special contour (plastic contoured seats such as the Tumble Forms chair are one alternative). For best results, the child's needs should be assessed frequently by an occupational therapist, who can recommend the best seat for the individual child. (See "Choosing Appropriate Seating" in Part 2).

In choosing a seat it's important to consider whether only a feeding chair is desired or whether a combined stroller and feeding seat would be more useful. These combination devices are popular, and there are a number of them on the market. Generally, they have a nice appearance and resemble a standard baby stroller rather than a medical wheelchair. The chair should be ordered with a lap tray. Toys can be placed on the tray in front of the child, and the chair can be used as a desk as well.

There are also a large variety of positioning and play chairs available, which the child may use in school or therapy. If one of these seems especially well suited to the individual child, the parents may want to order one or make one for use at home. These chairs include corner chairs, saddle chairs, benches, cylinders, and swing chairs.

Is a walker recommended?

The use of a child walker is controversial. Some therapists believe that walkers are detrimental to development, and others see them as useful. Many parents prefer to use them because children seem to enjoy the increased freedom of movement, though sometimes the movements consist in stiffening or flailing rather than being purposeful. The walker will not prevent a child from walking independently if he is capable of doing so. Nor will the walker make a child who cannot walk do so.

There is no scientific evidence that a short period of time spent in a walker is either harmful or beneficial, but the walker may represent an emotional issue for parents. Children without disabilities use this type of seated walker, and when a child with cerebral palsy uses a walker he may appear more like a normal child. This is in contrast to the child's use of a stander, which a child without disabilities would not use. Our position, simply stated, is that using a walker is not going to harm the child as long as safety precautions are taken with regard to staircases and objects that can tip the device over. This is crucially important, because many children have been seriously injured when left unattended in a walker.

Is standing important? There are many benefits to standing, among them improved bone health, less constipation, and better endurance. Many therapists and doctors believe that standing also helps the development of balance, head control, and spatial conceptualization. Thus the child who may later be able to use a power chair gains a better sense of the three-dimensional space in which he will eventually move around. These beliefs of doctors are difficult to prove, but we do know that children without disabilities develop these concepts in just this way. It seems logical that children with cerebral palsy need the same stimulation to develop their abilities to the greatest extent possible.

How can I tell whether a stander would be helpful for my child? Between 18 and 24 months of age is usually a practical time to start considering a stander. By this time the child's acute medical issues are mostly resolved and parents and doctors have a good sense of the rate of gain in development. Also by this time, many children with quadriplegia are able to move by crawling or rolling on the floor. Some are able to scoot in the sitting position, and some are able to pull to a standing position. If a child is able to pull himself up to a standing position by 24 months, she can bear her weight and most likely will progress with time to a walker. If a child has not reached this milestone at 24 months, she should be started in a standing program with a stander.

There are four types of standers: prone, supine, sit-to-stand, and parapodium. The parapodium, or freedom, stander is most useful for children with spina bifida who have a normal upper body. It has almost no usefulness for children with cerebral palsy, because most children with CP have poor upper body control and will end up falling forward in this type of stander. Those children with CP who have very little upper body involvement usually are able to pull themselves to a standing or are able to use a walker.

Children with poor or no head control should be started in a supine stander. The disadvantage of this type of stander is that the child leans backward and therefore his field of vision is limited to the ceiling. This can be compensated for by hanging interesting objects above the child's head to provide stimulation or by positioning a mirror to reflect the activity that's going on in the room.

For children with some head control, the prone stander is better because it stimulates them to hold up their heads. In addition, a lap tray placed in front of them can allow them to play while they are standing. The tilt of both the supine and the prone stander can be adjusted so that the child is as upright as possible and yet comfortable. (See "Choosing a Stander" in Part 2 for a more complete discussion of standers.)

How much time should my child spend in the stander?

It is usually best to start off by having the child spend just a short period of time, typically 10 to 15 minutes, in the stander. As the child becomes accustomed to the stander, a parent should try to work the child up to a one-hour stretch twice a day if the child tolerates it. Standing should not be a period of great difficulty for the child, however. By working with different positions and involving the child in activities, the parent can make time spent in the stander more enjoyable for the child. Physical therapists can help parents design a successful program for their child.

If the child develops a severe aversion to the stander, it may be better to stop working with it for several months and come back to it with a new approach. For the child who is not walking, the goal should be to stay with a standing program into and through adolescence. There are many adults who still find the stander useful.

Are motorized wheelchairs appropriate at this age?

No, they are not. Motorized wheelchairs are often very appealing because they are "state of the art." For many parents, they may represent the best they can provide for their child with a disability. However, a motorized chair for a child with cerebral palsy should not be considered until the child is approximately 6 years old.

A child with CP who is able to drive a motorized chair at age 3 is most likely capable of cruising (walking around by holding on to furniture) and will be a very functional walker within a year or two. An expensive motorized wheelchair will provide little benefit to such a child. On the other hand, the child who will eventually need a chair is unlikely to be able to drive a motorized chair at age 2 or 3, because of other impairments (such as visual difficulties, attention deficits, fine motor dysfunction, or cognitive impairments). There are a few exceptions, mainly children with various conditions that have no intellectual impairment associated with them. These children might appropriately and effectively use a motorized chair at this young age.

Are there other pieces of equipment that might be helpful?

For the child who is not able to sit independently, a bathing chair can be very helpful. Several different types are available commercially, or they can be constructed using PVC pipes and cloth or netting. Purchasing these devices puts a financial strain on some parents. It's usually easier to obtain funding for seats and wheelchairs than for standers and bathing chairs. Sending letters of medical necessity (provided by the physician's office; see Part 2) and being persistent are often the best ways for parents to approach insurance carriers. Community service organizations may also provide financial assistance for such purchases.

What are the predomi-
nant bone and joint
problems at this age?

Until a child reaches the age of 1 there are almost no cerebral palsy–related problems with the bones and joints that need to be addressed by anything other than evaluation and observation. Starting at 1 year of age, however, close follow-up is important. The most severe problems, which often start to become evident at this age, are hip subluxation and hip dislocation.

The hip is a ball-and-socket joint. *Subluxation* refers to the condition in which the ball slowly pulls partially out of its appropriate position in the socket. *Dislocation* is the condition in which the ball has come completely out of the socket. Both conditions are called *spastic hip disease* and are caused by tight or spastic muscles about the hip. Spastic hip disease is a common problem for children with quadriplegia; as many as 80 percent of children with severe involvement are affected. Pain is sometimes associated with spastic hip disease and can cause a child to be irritable.

With proper monitoring, follow-up, and treatment by an orthopedist familiar with spastic hip disease, hip dislocation can be avoided. Monitoring begins with a physical examination. If the examination reveals a limitation of motion in the hip such that the legs cannot be spread apart to a total of 90 degrees, an x-ray needs to be taken and repeated every six months. The x-ray indicates whether the hip is properly located within the socket. If the hip starts to move out of the joint, the tight muscles need to be treated. Nonsurgical treatment has proven unsuccessful in preventing hip subluxation. Braces, casts, and exercises have been used extensively without much success, so these approaches have been almost completely abandoned by most orthopedists treating children with cerebral palsy. To date, there is no proof that botulinum toxin prevents hip subluxation.

The medical community agrees that spastic hip muscles need to be treated surgically. However, opinions vary a good deal regarding exactly which muscles should be released and how the child should be treated after surgery. Some surgeons prefer the use of casts or braces postoperatively to maintain correction, while others prefer to use only therapy or exercises. Because of the variety of treatment possibilities, finding a surgeon who is thoroughly familiar with spastic hip disease becomes crucial.

If muscle release surgery is not successful, a *varus osteotomy* of the femur bone may be needed at an older age. In addition, an *acetabular osteotomy* (reshaping the socket) is sometimes also necessary. Both surgeries are very successful if done at a young age. Occasionally with severe spastic hip disease, a muscle release that initially was successful ends up needing to be followed by a varus osteotomy. The key to the successful treatment of spastic hip disease is close observation and early treatment. The greatest problems arise from late recognition of the problem. Bones in a hip that has been out of place for a period of time undergo changes in shape, making the best treatment outcome far more difficult to achieve for even the most highly skilled surgeon. All children with quadriplegia should be evaluated every six months by a physician who understands these issues.

Scoliosis, which is side bending of the spine, and *kyphosis*, which is bending forward, are also common problems. At this age, these are only symptoms of the child's poor upper body control, and they should be observed over time by the physician. The child must be provided with adequate support in seats and standers. This curvature is not related to the structural spinal curves that develop later, frequently at adolescence.

Feet can also present problems. Because of poor muscle control, they are often very flat, or if there is spasticity, they may point down, so that the child only bears weight on her toes. As the child is started in the stander, small braces on the feet are often needed either for support or for position. These AFOs (ankle-foot orthoses) may be made by a therapist or an orthotist. At this age they are used mostly when the child is standing. Some children will have less spasticity or will be able to move more easily when sitting in a chair wearing braces. The braces inhibit spasticity and may be worn most of the day for comfort. If the child has severe spasticity and the foot cannot be positioned properly in a brace, botulinum toxin injection of the gastrocnemius muscle (calf muscle) may be helpful in controlling foot placement within the brace. Surgery for foot problems is rarely recommended at this age.

The use of hand and upper extremity bracing at this age may or may not be recommended. It is most useful for the child who is developing severe *contractures*, in which the fingers or limbs assume a fixed position. Braces are usually made by an occupational therapist and are worn by the child for anywhere from one to six hours a day in an attempt to keep the muscle stretched. If a child tolerates the braces well, they may be left on during the night. Splints made from a neoprene material allow for more functional hand mobility during daytime use. Rigid braces are less functional but have the advantage of controlling more severe contractures. Children who are using their hands for reaching or manipulating objects should not have the hand covered for prolonged periods of time. This is extremely important, because the brace will decrease sensation in the hand and may discourage children from using their hands.

Ages Four to Six

Children in this age group continue to develop rapidly both mentally and physically, and patterns and potential abilities become much more clearly defined. By the time the child reaches the age of 6, his or her basic pattern of involvement and abilities can be determined, although neurological development will continue at a significant rate for at least several more years. The child who is not able to sit independently by age 5 will almost certainly never walk independently but will continue to improve in head and upper body control. The cognitive abilities of the child can also be much better defined at this age and will progress as he or she gets older.

The primary goal for children in this age group is to prepare for school. By this age children with disabilities should already be in a program with other children and therefore should be somewhat accustomed to separating from their parents and interacting with peers in a structured setting. A major concern should be that the child continue to grow physically, because the brain can only develop if it has enough nourishment. The best indication of adequate nutrition is good overall growth in the child.

What role does physical and occupational therapy play at this age?

As the child approaches school age, education should be the predominant concern, and therapy that contributes to this goal should be stressed. Occupational and speech-language therapy, as well as communication efforts that make the most of the child's learning potential, are most important. Therapy that is focused on physical gains can be incorporated into the school program or even accomplished through play. An appropriate balance prevents the child from regressing physically while making it possible for him to grow intellectually.

What is necessary in terms of vision and hearing screening?

It is vitally important to evaluate your child's vision and hearing as part of preparing him for school. If your child was tested at an earlier age, then a simple checkup is appropriate. A child who has never been fully evaluated, however, should be examined within the limits of his or her functioning level. That is, the examining physician, audiologist, or optometrist must know whether the child is unable to respond to questions because of deficits in her sight or hearing or whether the problem is due to cognitive impairment or inability to speak or communicate due to motor problems. In the latter case, the child may see and hear perfectly but may not perform well on a vision or hearing test because of cognitive or motor limitations.

An accurate assessment of the child's visual and auditory capacity will help to place her in the appropriate school or classroom and to develop a communication system for her to use. Eyeglasses and hearing aids, if indicated, may have a significant impact on the child's interest in her environment, as well as on her ability to learn.

My child has communication problems. What can be done for him?

This is a good age to begin teaching simple nonverbal communication skills to children who aren't able to talk. If your child can use his hands, he may begin on his own to develop a sign language that works for him and his caregivers. Around age 3, many children can begin to learn formal sign language, although the ability to learn formal sign language, like the ability to learn any language, depends on the child's cognitive level. For children who have limited hand function, eye signing and facial expressions make communication possible.

At this age, communication allows the child to understand that she can influence and to some extent control her environment. Another way for the child to learn this is by playing with toys, a computer laptop, and TVs that she can control by using electrical switches or joysticks. A proficiency in manipulating these devices will be valuable later, when the child uses computers, communication systems, and motorized mobility devices. Many electric toys can be very easily adapted for the child with a disability. Sometimes all that is needed is an on-off switch that the child can control by touching it. (Communication systems are discussed more fully later in this chapter.)

What decisions need to be made about seating?

Appropriate seating continues to be important for feeding, transportation, and positioning for maximum hand use. All these functions can often be accomplished with one wheelchair that is fitted with a lap tray, good chest supports, and, if needed, a headrest. Hip guides and hip abductors are sometimes necessary for proper lower extremity alignment. Some parents prefer to use one chair for feeding, a stroller for mobility, and a separate seat with a lap tray for play activities. One reason parents like this arrangement is that it seems less medical and makes the child appear less disabled.

As the child grows older and begins riding the bus to school, multiple seating arrangements become more difficult to manage. The problems arise not only in terms of providing all these different seating arrangements in different settings (at home, at school, and elsewhere) but also in maintaining two, three, or four seats with proper adjustments for support. If the family goes to a restaurant, for example, all the child's needs—transportation, the freedom of mobility, and the assurance of a proper feeding position—can be met with just one chair, a properly fitted wheelchair adapted for feeding.

Strollers have the advantage of not looking like a medical device and of being more easily transportable, but they have the disadvantage of providing poor trunk support for the child. The older child may object to the appearance of the stroller because she associates it with babies. And it's impossible for a child who is sitting in a stroller to propel the stroller herself. For these reasons, a wheelchair can be a significant symbol of growing up and independence. A child with some limited ability to use her arms may be able to push a regular wheelchair quite well if it fits her properly. Wheelchairs come in a variety of colors, and most children enjoy having a say in choosing the color.

Is this the right age to introduce a motorized wheelchair?

It's often difficult to decide whether to provide a child with a motorized chair. The decision is usually complicated by the fact that not everyone involved in the decision agrees. There has been much debate about fitting power chairs to 2- or 3-year-olds, for example, but this is almost always appropriate only for children with *osteogenesis imperfecta* (very brittle bones) and *arthrogryposis* (very stiff joints). Children with these conditions are cognitively normal and have normal balance and motor control. If they aren't walking by the age of 2, they aren't likely to become fully functional walkers and will be dependent on the chair for long-term use.

Children with cerebral palsy, however, are very different, in that most of the children who would be capable of using a motorized chair at age 3 are already cruising and will be very functional walkers within the next year or two. Getting a motorized wheelchair for such a child would be counterproductive. Conversely, most of the children who will eventually need a chair are not able to handle the controls at a younger age, so a motorized wheelchair would be of no use to them. Thus, it seldom makes sense to introduce a young child to a motorized wheelchair.

The most appropriate age at which to introduce a power chair is around 6 years. As with other things, this is an average, and some children who will be able to handle a chair later, after they have grown and developed, will not be ready for a power chair at age 6. Some children get around pretty well with a walker from the age of 6 through age 8 or 9, while they are small and in the lower grades. However, as time passes, the child's need for motorized transportation will probably have to be reevaluated. For one thing, as children move into the upper grades the schools get larger, and managing the long hallways with a walker may be tiring. Another consideration is the child's increasing weight, which may also make it difficult for her to use a walker.

There are two areas of controversy regarding motorized chairs. Some parents want their child to have a power chair even though it would not be appropriate for her. These parents are often motivated by a desire to provide everything possible for their child, and in their eagerness to provide for her, they sometimes do not consider her functioning level and her safety awareness.

At the other extreme are parents whose child does some walking but is too slow and unsteady to be a functional walker in a busy school environment. These parents sometimes worry that the child will stop walking and regress if he has a motorized chair. This fear is unfounded. The situation is similar to that of a 16-year-old who gets his first car. Initially, certainly, he wants to drive everywhere, and he does walk less often. But he doesn't forget how to walk, run, or ride his bicycle. It soon becomes apparent to the 16-year-old that it is easier to walk to his friend's house down the street than to open the garage door, back the car out, and drive 100 yards. In the same way, the child with some walking ability soon learns that it is easier to walk around the house than to try to maneuver the wheelchair in close spaces.

Just as the teenaged driver must demonstrate competence before she can get a driver's license, the child with a disability must demonstrate competence before being allowed to operate a power chair. She must be able to understand that pushing forward on a stick causes her to move forward (playing with a video joystick is good practice for this). She must also understand about danger areas so that she doesn't drive over curbs or down stairs. If she should drive into a corner, she must be able to back up and turn around to get herself out. She must be able to see in order to drive a chair, but she doesn't have to be able to use her hand or fingers to control the chair. There are joystick controllers for power chairs (like the ones used in video games), as well as head, mouth, leg, and foot controllers. The sensitivity of the controller and the speed of the chair must be adjusted according to the child's age and abilities.

When children with cerebral palsy start to use power chairs, they may have trouble with spatial perception at first. For many children, this is because they have never moved around on the floor independently and thus lack experience. Some children have vision problems as well, or their balance may be poor, and this can further limit their ability to move appropriately in space. The bottom line is that any child who is using a power chair for the first time needs training and guidance.

It is usually best to work with the child in a confined space, such as a room in which objects are arranged closely together. This type of close maneuvering is usually easiest for the child to learn, because he or she has more experience manipulating objects in a small environment. The best way to provide training for the child is to walk in front of him, providing a focus of attention. It may take some children months or even several years to learn to drive in a relatively open area and to stay on a sidewalk.

Parents should choose their child's chair and controller, as well as seating support systems, only after getting advice from school therapists and their child's doctor. The home environment and transportation systems must be taken into account, and parents should be prepared to describe any limitations posed by either or both of these. For children who are easy to fit, selecting a chair can often be done within the school system, where the child may even be able to take several different kinds of chairs for a test drive. For other children, it may be best to make these decisions based on a short-term admission to a hospital's rehabilitation unit, where the child can be evaluated on several systems and the parent's home and the available transportation system, as well as the school environment, are carefully considered.

It is usually not a good idea to select a chair in the salesroom of a wheelchair dealer. Typically, the dealer will carry only one or two brands and may be motivated to encourage you to choose one of them. It's possible that the salesperson won't even be well trained in satisfying the mobility needs of a child with a disability. Our recommendation is to choose a chair in a setting that provides both an unbiased opportunity for choice and the help of trained personnel, as described in the preceding paragraph, and then purchase the chair through a dealer with a reputation for good service.

For more information about different styles of chairs, you might consult the section on wheelchairs in Part 2 of this book. Another good source of information is other owners of motorized chairs, who can provide valuable advice about the reliability of local sales people and repair shops. Motorized chairs generally require more repair and service than cars, so before you buy a chair, it's essential to know how and where you are going to get good service. Some hospitals have wheelchair clinics staffed with persons who can service the chairs.

What about walking?

You may have ongoing concerns about how or if your child will walk. As your child grows older, predictions become more reliable, so by this age things are certainly becoming clearer. Again, it's important to remember that a child must have head control before he can sit independently, and he must be able to sit before he can walk.

Can standers, braces, and walkers help?

By this age, almost all children should be in a standing program for weight bearing to help with bone development, body control, coordination, and balance. Children who have difficulty controlling their ankles, either because they go up on tiptoe or because their foot turns or rolls into a flatfooted position, should have plastic ankle-foot braces made to help them stand. Only children with the most severely affected feet need ankle surgery, and even then it is usually only a minor lengthening of the Achilles tendon or transfer of half of the tibialis posterior tendon. Either of these procedures will allow the foot to fit properly into a brace. (Surgery for flat feet is discussed in the next section.) Braces above the knee have no benefit. Children who can't control their knees need to be placed in a stander that provides knee control.

Commercial infant walkers in which the child sits continue to be controversial. Some therapists believe that the child's posture and movements in the gait trainer impede the development of balance and upper body control. However, we know of no scientific evidence to support this. Positioning devices (e.g., ankle prompts) can be added or subtracted from the device to assist with controlling the position of the upper extremities, the trunk, and the lower extremities. The biggest concern with walkers is safety. It is our opinion that if the child enjoys being in the walker, his parents want the child in a walker, and there is someone who can watch the child very closely to keep him safe while he's in it, then there is probably no harm in using a walker for short periods of time, about one hour daily.

What hip problems can occur at this age?

Spastic hip disease, or hip subluxation or dislocation, continues to be a big problem at this age. Children with severe quadriplegia have an 80 percent chance of developing hip subluxation, while children with moderate quadriplegia and those with athetosis have a slightly lower but still very high risk for this problem.

Hip dislocation, the end result of subluxation, can only be avoided if it is detected and dealt with early. The surgical release of the tight, spastic hip muscles is a relatively simple procedure and can often prevent dislocation. Many children with severe cerebral palsy need bone surgery to place the hip in a more stable position, however. If the dislocated hip remains untreated, the surgical procedures for correcting the problem become much more complex, placing the child at an increased risk for complications. To avoid extensive surgery and the possibility of complications, it is essential to continue close monitoring, with a physical examination every six months and x-rays once a year or more frequently as needed.

Should I be concerned about my child's spine?

At this age, spinal deformities are generally less of a problem than spastic hip disease. Many parents are concerned about scoliosis, although at this age it is still mostly due to poor upper body control and is best managed by good seating support and by a standing program. Kyphosis (forward slumping), which is also due to poor upper body control, may be more difficult to manage than scoliosis. A harness or a reclining, tilting seat can be helpful. For some children a body brace is useful for postural control, although this can create feeding and breathing problems. Only rarely does kyphosis become stiff and permanent. Your child's spine should be routinely examined as part of his scheduled medical care.

What about my child's upper body?

Some children with severe athetosis may dislocate a shoulder because their posture is abnormal. For example, they may keep their arms above their head and behind them. Lifting the child by the arms may also result in a dislocated shoulder. The best treatment for dislocation is to avoid the activity that caused the dislocation in the first place, which may mean using a splint that keeps the arm at the child's side. This is especially helpful at night.

Elbow tightness may make dressing and bathing difficult, but the elbow is usually flexible at this age. Short-term splinting is helpful. Splinting may also be suggested as treatment for wrist flexion and to keep the thumb out of the palm. The advantage of a splint is that it keeps the tight wrist, elbow, or thumb stretched out. The disadvantage is that the splint can decrease hand function. While it may be true that the contracted upper extremity becomes useless, it is also true that a continuously splinted upper extremity doesn't have a chance of learning to function. For this reason, we only recommend short-term splinting—usually just at night. Botulinum toxin injection into spastic muscles can often be helpful whether or not it is combined with splinting.

Could my child have knee problems?

The child with very tight hamstrings will not be able to extend his leg at the knee. At this age tight hamstrings, though a common problem, are not likely to be as troublesome as they may become in adolescence. Physical therapy stretching exercises are generally sufficient, and splinting is only occasionally used. The child may get stiff knees, but usually due to spasticity; again, stretching exercises are usually sufficient treatment. Botulinum toxin injections into the hamstring or quadriceps muscles for tightness may be helpful if a contracture of the tendon has not occurred.

Do the feet pose specific problems at this age?

The most common concern for parents is a tight Achilles tendon. This often can be managed with stretching exercises, Botox, and the use of a molded ankle-foot brace. A severe tightness that cannot be modified by these methods may need to be lengthened surgically. If your child cannot be fitted with any type of acceptable footwear, or if the position of his or her feet causes difficulty with standing, surgery is recommended.

Flat feet or feet that tend to roll out are also problems. They are most easily noticed when the child is standing. Using an AFO or a shoe insert, such as a heel cup, is a good idea if it helps your child stand, but some braces try to create an ideal arch and may cause your child discomfort. If the brace causes pain, it must be repaired or removed permanently.

There is no scientific evidence that these braces permanently change the shape of the foot. In particular, there is no evidence that they shape an arch. Sometimes the feet get better as the child grows and muscle control improves, and sometimes they get worse. The braces probably don't have any effect on the developing foot position. Comfortable braces often do make it easier for the child to stand, however, and in this case they are helpful.

At this age, surgery should only be considered in cases of the most severe flatfootedness, when bracing has proven to be completely unsuccessful. Those who do have surgery have a fairly high recurrence rate and may need to have repeat surgery at an older age. There continues to be a wide range of opinions about flat feet in children with cerebral palsy, and there aren't many scientific studies to back up any one opinion. The best thing to do, generally, is to weigh all other options before turning to surgery for this problem at this age.

What about my child's toes?

For the child with overlapping and cocked toes caused by spasticity, it is usually difficult to wear shoes. At this age, the best treatment is to provide your child with soft, roomy shoes. Soft silicone toe spacers that can be placed between the toes may help prevent callouses. If the toe condition worsens, simple surgical treatment is available and often provides good correction

Ages Seven to Twelve

During these years a child's physical and cognitive potential can usually be determined. By ages 8 to 10, a child's ability to sit, walk, and use his arms has fully developed. Children may still learn to function more effectively, but unlike in earlier years, significant new abilities do not emerge.

As a parent, you may find this to be an especially hard time as you continue to work hard with your child and hope for gains while seeing less progress. In addition, you may be receiving a good deal of input from your child's teachers and therapists, as well as medical personnel. Your child has now been in the school system long enough, and therapists have worked with your child often enough, that your child's abilities can be defined with a fair degree of accuracy.

Certainly, your child will continue to learn and will improve in some physical abilities, as all growing children do. However, the pattern will now be clearly established. This means that if your child is not walking by age 10, he or she will never be an independent walker. If your child has not learned to recognize any words by age 10, he or she clearly has a cognitive impairment and will never learn to be a functional reader (unless the cause of the reading problem is an untreated visual problem).

You can prepare yourself for this stage of development by accepting the difference between the rapid developmental gains of the period from birth to age 6 and the much slower rate of gain after age 6 and understanding that this contrast in development exists in normal children too. Your child's slowed development after age 6 may, however, affect you psychologically and emotionally more than their child's slowed development affects the parents of a child without disabilities. This is to be expected.

What kind of therapy is most important?

When adults with cerebral palsy are asked this question, their response is speech or communication therapy. These skills are especially important for children who have a high cognitive level. If their oral speech is too difficult for strangers to understand or the child's ability to speak is very limited, augmentative communication should be provided.

What is augmentative communication?

Augmentative communication refers to methods of communication other than speech. Signing, a method of communicating with hand signals used by people who are hearing impaired, may be useful, although children with quadriplegic cerebral palsy have too much upper extremity involvement to sign efficiently, except for a few basic signs. The simplest augmentative communication device is a communication board that displays pictures or words appropriate to the child's functioning level and current situation. More advanced technology systems may use smart devices or tablets to develop alternative communication skills for these children. These devices can be hooked up to computers with speech synthesizers. Speech-language therapists who work with children who have disabilities should be able to help you evaluate what would work best for your child. (See "Augmentative Communication" in Part 3 for more information on this topic.)

For the child who is severely involved physically and who has difficulty using his hands, the use of eye signs is a good, simple way to communicate. This form of communication is slow, however, because it essentially limits responses to either a yes or a no answer. Head pointing sticks with computer attachments are another option.

Developing an efficient communication system should be a major part of your child's early education. Hospital centers with augmentative communication clinics can use a number of different systems to evaluate your child. But you need to keep in mind that this process is much like buying a wheelchair, in that there are many different options and prices, and it's not wise to go to a dealer, who may be influenced by what he sells.

Parents may find that paying for these devices is difficult, since Medicaid coverage varies from state to state and insurance coverage may vary as well. In regard to insurance, it is important not to accept an initial rejection but to continue to resubmit until you have exhausted the appeals process. Organizations such as local variety clubs, the Easter Seal Society, and churches may provide assistance with funding. (See Chapter 10 for more information about finding sources of funding.)

Is speech-language therapy helpful for the child whose cognitive abilities are severely affected?

Yes. Most speech-language therapy for children with quadriplegia and severe cognitive disability, in which communication is not a goal, focuses on teaching swallowing and feeding techniques. The therapist will evaluate swallowing function if this has not already been done and provide pointers to parents for preparing food and feeding their child (see Chapter 3 for more details).

What is the role of an occupational therapist?

An occupational therapist works with your child to develop functional skills involving his or her hands. At this age, the focus should be on becoming independent in activities of daily living. For children who can write, improving handwriting is a goal. For those who may have more upper extremity involvement, an occupational therapist helps the child develop skill in using a keyboard. The occupational therapist also focuses on improving function in the tasks of daily living, as well as finding positions in seating and hand use that allow for optimum function. This becomes increasingly important as children grow. At this age, the therapy should be much more function oriented; focusing on stretching and exercising at this age is inappropriate. If stretching is needed, passive stretching through the use of nighttime splints is more time efficient and cost effective.

The amount of time the therapist spends may vary from three times a week with the child who is working on learning a specific new task to a monthly evaluation for the child who seems to be functioning well. If your child is doing well in the classroom and functions well during play, it's best not to take time away from those things for therapy.

How much physical therapy is needed?

This depends a good deal on the individual child's needs and on the availability of therapy. Like occupational therapy, physical therapy should be balanced with school and play time. The child who is doing well academically should not be removed from the classroom for therapy unless there is a specific short-term goal he or she is trying to achieve. In general, though, therapy gradually takes on the role of *maintaining* function rather than stimulating *new* function.

For the child who is moderately affected by CP and who is cognitively normal, therapy should be functionally oriented, offering as little interference as possible in the child's education. Such a child will be able to become a contributing adult member of society by virtue of her cognitive abilities, and her physical limitations will not be significantly changed by hours of therapy in late childhood. She needs to learn early on that her time and energy are more effectively used in developing her intellectual abilities, and she should be encouraged to succeed in this area.

As parents, you need to ensure that therapy time is spent on functional skills and not on hours of preventive stretching exercises. These exercises may temporarily prevent some stiffness, but they take valuable time from the child's educational development or from opportunity for socializing with peers in play. Parents need to strive for a balance, keeping in mind that correcting a little knee stiffness is much less important than the development of a child's intellectual potential.

Children who are wheelchair dependent should not remain isolated in a seated position all day. They need to have an opportunity for some exercise, ideally by taking part in an enjoyable activity, preferably one that they can participate in for a lifetime. Swimming and adapted horseback riding are excellent options. Engaging children in sports with team play, such as bocce or adaptive sporting events, encourages socialization, which is very important for the child's sense of friendship, joy, and overall well-being.

The child with severe physical involvement may find it difficult to get exercise. He may need continued therapy provided by a physical therapist or an exercise program prearranged by a physical therapist and executed by school personnel. Children with severe cognitive and physical involvement should have routines worked out for positioning changes, adequate seating with support, and a regularly scheduled standing program. The therapist may also help the self-abusive child by describing methods of prevention and protection so the child does not injure himself or caregivers.

How much physical therapy is appropriate for a given child depends upon many variables. At this age, the child who is doing well in school and is not having specific new problems may touch base with his therapist once a month or every six months if he is in a program designed by the therapist and carried out by school personnel. By contrast, the child who has a specific problem that the therapist is currently working on with him may need to be seen three times a week.

What kinds of problems are there with therapy in school?

There are two basic conflicts here. The first is an issue of cost versus gain in terms of the child's development. Not every child with cerebral palsy, even those with moderate to severe quadriplegia, needs therapy. In fact, taking some children out of the classroom for therapy might actually be harmful in terms of intellectual growth. Second, in many schools therapists' time is quite limited, so that choices must be made about which children will benefit most from the available services. The Individualized Education Program (IEP) process provides the opportunity to evaluate the child in terms of his best interests, but the parent who does not feel comfortable with the outcome of that process may have to pursue the issue further.

Sometimes the child's doctor prescribes therapy. If the child has had surgery and postsurgical therapy is indicated, it is not necessarily the responsibility of the school to provide this kind of therapy. Postsurgical therapy is medically indicated and most likely is covered by medical insurance.

Separating therapy as part of education from therapy as a medical treatment can be difficult and may be complicated by the fact that schools often don't have enough therapists to meet their students' needs. In addition, there are no absolute criteria for deciding which children need therapy in school. The parent or caregiver is usually the child's strongest advocate, but the parent also needs to weigh carefully the classroom time lost for the purpose of therapy. If the school's lack of therapists poses a significant problem, parents may consider forming parent groups and becoming active at school board meetings to insist that the number of therapists in the school system be increased.

Should my child be placed in a special school, or would he benefit from "inclusion"?

The answer to this complex question depends on what's available within the educational system in your particular geographical area, as well as on the cognitive, physical, and psychological needs of the individual child. The purpose of the IEP is to evaluate the child in terms of his or her educational best interests. But if parents or caregivers do not agree with the recommendation of the IEP, they should be willing to take on an advocacy role and try to get the recommendation changed. (See Chapter 11 for more on dealing with the educational system.)

What can I do about my child's drooling?

At this age excessive drooling can cause significant physical problems, such as wetting books, papers, and computer keyboards. Occasionally if drooling is severe, skin irritation can develop around the mouth and face. It is also cosmetically unappealing, of course, and has the potential of being emotionally disturbing to the cognitively aware child. There are several options for treatment, including therapy (with a speech-language therapist), medication, and surgery. (Drooling is covered in more depth in Chapter 3.)

What about feeding problems?

Feeding problems encountered when your child was younger may continue at this age. (Problems related to swallowing, reflux, regurgitation, and constipation are all addressed in depth in Chapter 3.) It is of tremendous importance to involve experienced physicians in managing feeding intolerance and nutritional status, because conditions such as weak bones leading to fragility fractures may occur as a result of poor nutritional intake alone or in combination with some medications and lack of weight bearing (see Chapter 3 for more details on the evaluation and treatment of low bone density).

Should my child be in a wheelchair?

Concerns about wheelchair use are essentially the same as those encountered in the previous age group. However, there are several issues that now become more important and need to be addressed for the 7- to 12-year-old. The child of school age usually has started to become concerned about appearance. By age 6 or 7, strollers should not be used, especially for children who want to start feeling grown up. An adult-type wheelchair, particularly in a color that the child has chosen, is usually far more appealing.

Children who are dressed neatly and are seated in a good-looking chair are attractive. Often people who come into contact with them will react more positively toward them than toward a child whose physical appearance has been neglected. This is especially true in public areas and in schools. For the child who is aware, an attractive appearance also instills self-esteem. But even when the child is not aware, parents will feel better if the child looks comfortable and well cared for. Discussion about the use of a power wheelchair ought to be ongoing, especially for the child who is not quite able to keep up pushing a manual chair and for the child who is making cognitive progress and is able to use power responsibly.

Is my child likely to break bones?

Osteoporosis (weak bones) occurs most commonly in the quadriplegic child over 9 years of age who is unable to bear weight. The causes of this problem appear to be multiple. These include lack of weight-bearing exercise, poor nutritional intake, and the use of some seizure medications. Poor bone strength may predispose the child to fractures of the long bones. The most common fractures are seen in the lower extremities, especially above or below the knee. Most broken bones occur from very minor trauma, such as when a child is being moved or during a physical therapy session. Many such fractures may go unrecognized at first, with the child having unexplained pain and crying for several days before the diagnosis is made. Initial x-rays may even appear normal if the fracture is nondisplaced. In such cases a special imaging study called a bone scan is helpful. Nonambulatory children who are at risk for weak bones or who have had more than one broken bone should be monitored with a bone density test (DXA) and evaluated by experienced pediatricians for possible medication intervention. The diet of a child with low bone density measurements should be assessed for mineral and vitamin content and be supplemented if some or all of these nutrients are deficient compared with the recommended dietary intake (RDI). More severe cases may require treatment with a medication (called a bisphosphonate) that helps to improve bone strength. Treatment of a fracture is usually nonsurgical and involves a very well padded cast. Surgical treatment is only necessary in some severely displaced fractures. (See Chapter 3 for more on the evaluation and treatment of low bone density.)

What ankle and foot problems might my child encounter?

This is the age when the severe flat foot causes problems with standing. If the foot cannot be held in a good position with a molded AFO, then surgical intervention is recommended. A lengthening of the heelbone (calcaneal lengthening) or realignment of the heel (calcaneal osteotomy) can be performed in some patients with the proper indications. These procedures avoid fusion of the joints. Surgical treatment for severe foot deformities usually requires *subtalar fusion*, the fusing together of two bones in the heel. The *triple arthrodesis*, in which four bones are fused, yields a more predictably permanent result. A lengthening of the Achilles tendon may also be recommended at this age and rarely needs to be redone at a later age.

Ankle deformities in children at this age usually make it difficult for the child to wear shoes or to stand properly. Addressing these problems is usually deferred until the child is older. There are some minor toe problems at this age that will become more prominent in adolescence. (On addressing these problems in adolescence, see below.)

What about my child's knees?

Tight hamstrings cause difficulties in standing and possibly also in sitting or lying down. When the child with tight hamstrings sits down, the pelvis tends to roll back, causing the child to sit bent forward. As before, physical therapy stretching is usually adequate. However, when the problem interferes with activities of daily living such as standing and sitting, surgical release or lengthening is recommended. Tight rectus muscles cause the knee to be held straight all the time and make sitting difficult. If this is a significant problem, then surgical release of the rectus muscles can be very helpful.

Will my child's hips still cause problems?

Yes, the hips still need to be watched, especially if they are borderline normal or have been surgically treated for dislocation. This is especially true as the child approaches the adolescent growth spurt, when the hips may again start dislocating after being stable for a number of years. Hips that are changing must be x-rayed every six months until they are treated or are again stable for two years. As the child gets older, simple muscle releases are less reliable as treatment and usually need to be accompanied by varus osteotomy of the femur and often a pelvic osteotomy as well. These surgeries correct the problem. With close follow-up and most importantly appropriate treatment, a child will not end up with a hip dislocation.

Sometimes longstanding, neglected hip dislocations become very painful. The first step in addressing this difficult situation is to decrease the activity to the hip, stop physical therapy exercises, and start anti-inflammatory medications like naproxen (Naprosyn or Aleve) or ibuprofen (Advil). If this doesn't work, then reducing the hip surgically may help, or the hip may be totally replaced with an artificial joint. Excision of the femur (castle or girdlestone operation) is almost always ineffective at this age because the child will continue to grow and the hips will become painful again.

Are there any problems with the arms? During childhood the function of the arms becomes fully developed and contractures also start to develop. Occupational therapists will work to help the child use his or her arms as much as possible, especially for activities such as self-feeding, manipulating switches, and using joysticks and keyboards.

Some children with severe functional motor involvement develop contractures that make dressing and bathing difficult. Surgical release of arm contractures may be considered, but surgery is usually not performed until early adolescence. Splinting should continue as long as it does not interfere with the child's functioning.

Is spinal curvature a problem now? As the child gets older and taller, especially as puberty begins, scoliosis often starts to worsen, and the child may bend more and get stiffer. The best way of dealing with spinal curvature at this age is to make sure that the wheelchair has good lateral chest supports. A brace is one way of helping the child sit better, but usually the problems caused by the brace outweigh the benefits. Also, the brace does not have any impact on the eventual outcome of the scoliosis. (For a full discussion of scoliosis, see below.)

Kyphosis, or forward bending of the spine, is usually at its worst at this age. Even positioning a child in a chair may prove difficult because the child will tend to roll forward into a ball. Using a soft plastic body brace can help correct this problem and make seating easier. Many children outgrow this deformity. The few who don't, particularly those with poor head control and movement disorders, may need to undergo a spinal fusion, usually in early adolescence.

Ages Thirteen to Eighteen

At this age independence is the primary goal, but how it is achieved varies greatly depending upon the child's physical involvement and cognitive ability. Normally during adolescence, children start to separate from their parents and make plans for the future. The process of achieving independence, though necessarily modified, should be encouraged in the child with cerebral palsy. The level of CP involvement clearly must be considered, but the disability should not be considered to be inconsistent with independent living. From a psychological perspective, it's crucial to communicate this conviction to the adolescent.

Some adolescent personalities develop rather abruptly, whereas others undergo a long period of maturation. Either way, adolescence is often a stressful time, whether or not the child has a disability. It may be difficult for parents of a child with cerebral palsy to separate the normal turmoil of adolescence from the problems related to the disability. It is important to keep in mind that the growth spurt and hormonal changes of adolescence can affect seizure patterns and otherwise affect behavior in a child with CP.

After addressing some specific questions about problems that develop or become more severe in the adolescent years, the remainder of this chapter discusses issues of independence. In this discussion, we group individuals according to their predominant disability. Although categorizing children this way is not simple and far from ideal, it does make it easier to take differences into account. (Chapter 4 discusses many of these issues from a developmental perspective.)

At this age, what problems occur in the upper extremities?

Adolescents with an athetoid pattern may develop shoulder dislocation that produces some discomfort, though the shoulder rarely remains out of the joint. The best treatment is for the teen to learn to avoid the positions that cause the dislocation. Sometimes this means avoiding holding the arm in a certain position while sleeping (using a splint at night to keep the arm positioned at the side may solve this problem). Shoulder dislocation can be surgically addressed with soft tissue repair. However, it may recur. Shoulder fusion can be used to treat recurrent dislocations. Fortunately, surgery is rarely necessary.

People with severe spasticity sometimes develop elbow contractures that make it difficult to clean in the elbow crease, which can make dressing difficult too. To address this problem, the biceps and brachialis muscles in the elbow may be lengthened or released; the surgeon will be careful to retain enough muscle to keep the arm flexible. In a similar fashion, the thumb can become contracted (fixed to the palm), making it difficult to clean the hand. This too is best addressed with surgery, which fixes the thumb in a straight position, permanently allowing easier dressing and cleansing.

Contracture is also common in the wrist, with severe flexion to the palm side. A minor surgical procedure in which a tendon is transferred in order to keep the wrist extended can be very helpful. Small joint fusions in the hand are sometimes helpful, but these should only be performed by surgeons experienced in the particular problems associated with cerebral palsy.

Some people gain significant functional improvement, along with improved cosmetic appearance, following upper extremity muscle release or tendon surgery. Improved hygiene and cosmetic appearance are the most likely results, with improved function a pleasing but uncommon result of surgery. The hand of the individual with athetosis is problematic. Surgery in these children is frequently complicated by a return of the hand to its former position. For this reason, surgery is best avoided in the child with athetosis.

What treatment is available for scoliosis?

Scoliosis, or side bending of the spine, occurs in children with hemiplegia and diplegia, but it occurs most commonly in children with quadriplegia. Scoliosis is caused by poor muscle control. There is no known method of prevention nor any form of nonsurgical treatment.

This scoliosis is very different from the scoliosis that nondisabled children, most often girls, develop, which can be treated with braces. Unfortunately, there continues to be a great deal of confusion among physicians and therapists who are unaware of the intrinsic difference between the scoliosis related to CP and the scoliosis of normal teenagers. The treatments that are somewhat effective for normal individuals have no effect on the individuals with cerebral palsy because their scoliosis is directly related to the CP.

Braces may be temporarily helpful for the child with cerebral palsy for position, particularly sitting, but it is often easier to use wheelchair modifications to help the child sit upright because these don't have to be applied to the child. However, neither wheelchair modifications nor wearing a brace will have any effect on the development of scoliosis. In other words, by age 20 the spine will be just as curved if a brace has been worn full time for 10 years as it would have been if a brace had never been worn.

Braces give some children gastrointestinal and/or respiratory problems and need to be remade as the child grows. Rigid braces can cause pressure sores. When a brace is used, we prefer a soft brace made from a more flexible synthetic material. This type of brace is better tolerated by the child. One advantage of the brace, however, is that it is worn under clothing and therefore does not interfere with wheelchair support positioning as seasons change and bulky coats are added and removed. Another advantage of the brace is that it gives better support because it fits more securely. There is no harm in using both wheelchair modifications and a body brace.

In deciding whether to modify a wheelchair or apply a brace, the possible risks and complications must be considered, with the overriding understanding that neither will have any impact on the continued development of the spinal deformity. Some doctors think that the scoliosis may be slowed, but there really is no evidence for this, and the consensus among orthopedic surgeons who care for children with CP is that neither modifying a wheelchair nor applying a brace has any impact.

For the child who has severe spastic quadriplegia (GMFCS IV and V), there is a 75 to 90 percent risk of developing scoliosis, and the only effective treatment is a spinal fusion. This surgery involves straightening the spine, placing steel rods along the spine, and implanting bone graft so that the spine and the rods heal together as one bone. There have been great advances in this area of surgery. Even children with severe curves can be adequately straightened to sit in a straight-backed chair.

Spinal fusion is a major operation, usually lasting three or four hours, and must be performed by a surgeon who has experience with surgery for scoliosis associated with cerebral palsy. The surgery for this scoliosis is different, and uses different rods, from the surgery for scoliosis in normal adolescents. Most children recover rapidly and are sitting up in a chair three or four days after surgery, without the need for casting or bracing. And most of them are ready to go home 10 to 14 days after surgery.

For children with very severe and stiff curves, it is sometimes necessary to perform an additional, smaller surgical procedure (called an anterior release) before approaching the back. In an anterior release, some of the deformed and stiff discs between the vertebrae are removed. Although this adds approximately one week to the average hospital stay, it allows the surgeon to achieve a far better result in the correction of the curvature.

Once the spinal fusion is complete, growth is no longer possible in the spine, although the legs and arms continue to grow. Therefore, the ideal situation is for the child to grow as much as possible before the surgery without the curvature becoming stiff and fixed. This usually means delaying surgery until the child is between 12 and 16 years old, but then only one surgical procedure is necessary and usually provides excellent correction.

Sometimes a curve has become so severe by the time the child reaches age 8 or 9 that surgery must take place, sacrificing some growth. This is a rare occurrence and is most likely in a child who begins to develop scoliosis between 2 and 5 years of age.

What other spinal deformities might occur?

Kyphosis is a curvature of the spine in which the child bends forward and has a posture similar to that of an elderly individual. While kyphosis is very common in young children with CP, most will outgrow this condition as they achieve better upper body control. A few children develop stiffness and become fixed in this position, however, which may make sitting very difficult. For these children, surgery can correct the deformity by fusing the spine using bone graft and metal rods, similar to the procedure described above for scoliosis.

Lordosis, the least common spinal problem in persons with CP, refers to the curve in the spine that makes the arch in the lower back. This can become severely exaggerated in some children with cerebral palsy, causing problems with sitting and often back pain. The only treatment is the surgery described above.

Spinal surgery sounds frightening. What complications can occur?

No surgery is without risk of possible complications. The parent and surgeon should spend time together discussing the risks and benefits of surgery. Clear and realistic goals and expectations must also be discussed. If the child is medically involved, the parent must be prepared for a higher risk of complications after spinal surgery. The most frequent complications include gastrointestinal problems, respiratory problems, and wound infection. The child's surgery should be performed at a hospital with an experienced pediatric intensive care and medical staff, as all these complications are treatable. In addition, intraoperative bleeding that requires blood transfusion should be expected. An experienced pediatric anesthesia staff is critical during the surgery to help manage this potential problem. It is important to keep in mind that although complications can occur, the long-term benefits of spinal deformity surgery and keeping a child in a well-balanced upright position outweigh the risks in the majority of children with CP. The decision to proceed with surgery is ultimately up to the parent, and the benefits should be carefully weighed against the potential risks.

Do adolescents generally have hip problems?

Children who have had problems with subluxating hips earlier in life need to continue to be watched, but not quite as closely as when they were younger. Now x-rays only need to be done every one to two years, and if the hips are normal, only a physical examination may be necessary. Sometimes the hips start to sublux again at the same time that the scoliosis is developing. If the hips are dislocating at this age, surgery involving the bone rather than just muscle usually needs to be done. Often, a pelvic osteotomy is also needed to reshape the acetabulum, or cup of the hip.

All efforts should be made to prevent the hips from dislocating, because dislocated hips often become painful later, and then they can be very hard to manage. Orthopedic surgeons experienced in dealing with CP are able to keep the hip in the socket and, with good treatment, to keep the hips almost normal. It's essential for the child to be checked regularly by a surgeon who is experienced in the treatment of spastic hip disease.

This is the age at which the problems associated with the neglected dislocated hip become most painful. The first course of treatment involves avoiding activity that irritates the hip and using arthritis medications like naproxen (Naprosyn, Aleve) or ibuprofen (Advil, Motrin) to decrease the inflammation. Acetaminophen (Tylenol) is effective for the relief of pain, but it is not effective for the treatment of inflammation, which is thought to be a major source of pain in a condition such as this. If taking medications and avoiding certain activities does not effectively manage the pain, then surgery is the next option. There are a number of available procedures, but unfortunately none has a high rate of success.

Putting the hip back into the joint is the first step if the arthritis is not too severe. This procedure has the best long-term results, although sometimes persistent stiffness or pain makes a second surgical procedure necessary. The real advantage to this surgery is that there are good second choices. Total hip replacement is another choice, but it is often technically difficult and potentially problematic. When it is successful, however, it gives an excellent result. *Proximal femoral excision* is yet another alternative. This surgery involves removing the top portion of the femur (upper leg bone). Although this surgery is used fairly frequently, it can often result in a hip almost as painful and occasionally as stiff. It is important to keep the child in traction for six weeks following a proximal femoral excision to allow a scar to form.

Unfortunately, the high failure rate of the proximal femoral excision leaves only the alternative of removing more bone. Each successive removal of bone makes seating more difficult, as the legs become shorter. This operation is the procedure of last resort. Another option may be to fuse the hip joint, but this makes the child completely stiff. *By far the best course of action in terms of hip dislocation is prevention.* For children who have had dislocated hips for several years without pain, we would recommend leaving the hip dislocated. A surgical attempt to put the hip back in place would certainly cause the child pain.

As teenagers grow and hip muscles become tighter, diapering and perineal care can become difficult, particularly for menstruating females. When the condition has reached the point where one person must hold the child's knees apart while another washes the child or changes the diaper, then some surgical muscle releases should be considered. Osteotomy of the bones at the hip or relocating recently dislocated hips with little associated arthritis is a possibility. Without surgery, this difficulty with personal care will only become worse as the child gets older, stiffer, and stronger.

Another common hip problem is so-called windblown hips. This occurs when one hip is contracted inward (adducted) and the opposite hip is contracted outward (abducted). The primary problem is with positioning the child in a sitting and lying position. The adducted hip may be dislocated, requiring both muscle release (adductor release) and bone reconstruction (varus osteotomy and acetabular osteotomy), whereas the abducted hip usually requires varus osteotomy only. The goal of the surgery is to realign the legs to point them straight ahead as well as to treat the dislocated side (if a dislocation is present).

What if my child has both scoliosis and a dislocated hip? Should one be treated before the other?

It is not uncommon for scoliosis and hip dislocation to occur together. If both are equally severe, the spine is usually treated first, followed six months later by treatment of the hips. Some children with severe hip pain and mild to moderate scoliosis should have their dislocated hip treated first, to alleviate hip pain, before the scoliosis is treated.

What are some common knee problems at this age?

Tight muscles behind the knees (the hamstrings) that prevent the knees from straightening out are the most common problem in children who don't stand. These muscles sometimes become so tight that the child has a problem settling her feet comfortably on the footrest of the wheelchair. It may also be difficult for the child to lie down if she can't straighten out her knees. Children with this problem often position themselves so that one leg is turned out and the other in, or they lie and sit with both knees spread far apart. This makes sitting difficult and is also not cosmetically appealing, especially for females.

If the child is able to stand and these muscles become tight, they should be surgically lengthened in a procedure that will allow the child to stand as straight as possible. Occasionally, though rarely, the hamstring contractures are so severe that they can't be released sufficiently to correct the problem. When this occurs, a distal femoral osteotomy, in which the femur bone is cut and extended just above the knee joint, often produces good results.

In contrast to hamstring tightness, in which the knee is fixed in a flexed position, there is a condition in which the knee is unable to bend. This is usually caused by spasticity or contracture in the rectus muscle, which is located in the front of the thigh. This situation makes it very difficult for the child to sit in a wheelchair. Sometimes the muscle is so tight that the child's feet become sore from being kept forcibly secured to the wheelchair.

Mild cases of rectus tightness can be treated with stretching exercises that are done when the child is being dressed or transferred. The surgical release of the rectus muscle is a fairly simple procedure that should be considered if seating is a problem. Knee problems that are more of an impediment to walking or standing are covered more fully in Chapter 6.

Could my child have problems with his feet?

Two common types of foot problems occur in older children: equinovarus foot, in which the feet point down, and equinovalgus or planovalgus foot, in which the feet point down and out. A good foot position is necessary to allow for proper standing and shoe wear. Treatment options include (1) accepting the deformity and accommodating the deformed foot with soft comfortable shoes; (2) controlling the foot deformity with bracing; and (3) correcting the deformity with surgery.

Although standing is recommended, there are children who do not stand. If these children have foot position problems, it is preferable not to force their feet into shoes or braces. Rather, their feet can be kept protected and warm with slipper socks, slippers, or soft moccasins. There are many readily available options that are both inexpensive and comfortable. Most children who do not stand do very well in soft shoes and do not require surgery.

In the case of a weight-bearing child who has a less severe (flexible) foot deformity, the foot can usually be held in a brace in a good position. It must be remembered, however, that bracing has not been shown to prevent or permanently change any foot problems. When a child's foot deformity is severe, causing difficulty with standing in a child who weight bears, or the child's skin is breaking down because of rubbing against shoes or braces, the problem needs to be addressed surgically. Equinovarus foot deformity may be due to spasticity or contractures. Releasing or lengthening the Achilles tendon and lengthening or transferring part of the *posterior tibial tendon* are helpful procedures when there is minimal bone deformity in the foot. Equinovarus deformity with deformity in the bone and most severe equinovalgus deformities do well with a triple arthrodesis or subtalar fusion, in which the joints that are causing the problem are fused.

What about the toes? A common toe problem is the severely cocked up, or flexed, big toe. This occurs most commonly in adolescents with athetosis. Wearing shoes is often difficult and painful, because sores develop. Two options are available: the child can wear very large, soft shoes with a large toe box or the deformity can be corrected surgically, by fusing the big toe joint. The first option offers the easiest solution, although the surgical procedure is relatively simple and usually gives an excellent result that lasts the rest of the child's life.

Cocked-up toes or overlapping toes may be a problem in the small toes and may also cause sores when the toes rub against a shoe. They can be dealt with surgically by a minor procedure in which a small joint is excised and the toes are fused straight, or the adolescent can wear large shoes to prevent the formation of sores. None of these toe problems should be seen as an emergency. The surgeries can be done with the same success at age 10 or age 80.

Similar problems may be caused by severe bunions, and these too are best treated with correction and fusion. A person with cerebral palsy has a different kind of bunion from the bunion deformities that other people get, and this bunion should not be treated in the same way that those other deformities are treated. If the person with CP has a standard bunion operation, the bunion will recur. It is generally best not to have the same surgeon who did a good job on grandmother's bunions operate on the adolescent with CP unless that surgeon is familiar with the essential differences between these deformities.

Ingrown toenails can also be a problem. They usually result from trimming the nail back too far at the edges or by the nail's rubbing against the shoe, causing the shoe to dig into the flesh of the toe. If the toe becomes inflamed, it can be treated initially with warm water soaks twice daily. Continued irritation from wearing shoes should be avoided. For severe inflammation, antibiotics may be needed, and some people develop an abscess that needs to be drained. Nails should be trimmed frequently and straight across, not rounded. Recurrent ingrown toenails may require partial toenail excision.

What methods can be used to control my child's spasticity?

Increased muscle tone, or spasticity, may cause difficulty with positioning, problems with proper hygiene, or sometimes pain. The role of muscle surgery in treating tight muscles has already been discussed. Other methods used to help control high muscle tone include oral medications, medication that can be injected directly into the tight muscle, and surgical implantation of a pump to reduce muscle tone.

The usefulness of oral medications in helping control muscle tone is usually limited. That these drugs are noninvasive is a misconception. These drugs all act at numerous sites in the brain and the spinal cord and therefore can alter or depress many functions of the brain, including alertness, mood, cognition, and personality. The physician prescribing these medications should carefully monitor for these side effects. Two commonly used drugs are Valium and oral baclofen. Valium is best used for a short time, such as to help control post-surgical muscle spasm. Long-term use frequently results in tolerance, so that the drug becoming less effective. Drowsiness is another common problem. Oral baclofen has been shown to have better efficacy in head and spinal cord injuries to children with spasticity. Its use in the child with CP is limited. It may cause difficulty with seizure control in some children with seizures. And children must be weaned from it gradually.

Botulinum toxins A and B are available for off-label use (the medication is approved by the FDA, but not for this purpose) to control spasticity in some tight muscles. Botulinum toxin is best used when specific muscles (six or fewer) are spastic. It is a relatively safe drug without known systemic effects if it is not injected into the bloodstream. It acts locally within the injected muscle to block the release of some of the nerve signals to the muscle. There are rare side effects, the most common being some temporary soreness within the injected muscle. The FDA has required that the drug company include a black box warning stating that injected toxin can spread to muscles beyond the injection site, resulting in breathing and swallowing problems. Deaths have been reported, though whether it was the botulinum toxin that caused the deaths is not clear from the data. However, it is generally believed that children with severe CP taking very high doses are at the highest risk of severe complications. Therefore, most physicians now limit the dose to 10–12 units of botulinum per kilogram of body weight and inject it into no more than four large muscles. If the muscles are small, as in the hand or forearm, then more muscles can be injected.

In children with generalized spasticity (increased muscle tone involving arms, legs, and the trunk muscles), baclofen can be delivered directly into the spinal canal by means of a small pump surgically implanted under the skin. Called intrathecal baclofen therapy, this method allows the baclofen to be given in much smaller doses than the oral medication because it is acting directly on the nerves in the spinal cord to control the high muscle tone. The pump is about the size of a hockey puck and is surgically placed under the skin in the lower abdomen. A small plastic catheter is tunneled under the skin around to the back and then inserted into the spinal canal, where it infuses a very small but constant dosage of baclofen. It can help to relax high muscle tone in the legs, trunk, and arms. Parents must be willing to bring the child in to the physician who manages the pump every 3 to 6 months to refill the medication in the pump. This is done by inserting a small needle stick through the skin into a port in the pump. Intrathecal baclofen has been extremely helpful in managing high muscle tone in the quadriplegic patient. The pump is best placed and managed at a medical center that is set up to do a preoperative assessment and trial to test the effects of the medication on the child before the pump is actually surgically implanted, as well as follow-up care after implantation.

Another option is an operation called selective dorsal rhizotomy (SDR). SDR is usually recommended for children with diplegia who are walking. Less commonly SDR may be considered for more severely affected children who need lower limb tone reduction to facilitate care such as bathing and diapering. Pump implantation for intrathecal baclofen is the standard recommendation for such patients, but if practical obstacles (such as living too far away from a center to get the pump refilled) or aversion to an implanted device makes this option unattractive, SDR may be considered.

What are the issues of independence for adolescents with various degrees of involvement?

Adolescents who are cognitively normal and mildly involved physically. For adolescents who have normal intellectual function and are able to walk with assistive devices, the issues are essentially the same as for normal teenagers—allowing for a great deal of variation with respect to individual response. All teenagers want to be "normal," but their idea of normal is often based not on reality but on perceptions acquired from the media and on their personal fantasies. They may form unrealistic goals about their weight, their skin, and their muscle strength. Ultimately, most children in this group will be incorporated into society and will have jobs and families.

Some children with disabilities focus so intently and exclusively on overcoming the disability that they require psychological counseling to help them gain perspective. Some children in this age group have unrealistic expectations about the outcome of surgical procedures too, and they may perceive surgery as unsuccessful. This is primarily due to the child's unrealistic hope for a cure. That expectation may persist even when the treating physician gives the child a detailed explanation of the procedure and its expected outcome. The focus should be on realistic goals that will improve the daily life of the child.

Adolescents who are cognitively normal and moderately involved physically. Children with more severe involvement, and especially those with speech and movement disorders, often find adolescent socialization, including dating, difficult. Most teens are initially awkward with members of the opposite sex. As a coping mechanism, they often strive for conformity in dress and values. The adolescent with a physical disability clearly has more to deal with in terms of socialization. It is therefore not unusual for teens with disabilities to have limited sexual and socialization experience.

Adolescents who are not able to walk and need some assistance with activities of daily living, such as bathing or dressing, can be fairly independent most of the time and usually have adequate communication skills. Their problems are very similar to those of the previous group, but they have obvious limitations and they need help in areas where normal children have outgrown the need for help. Since teenagers typically become secretive and self-conscious about their bodies at this age, a teen who requires assistance with bathing or dressing is likely to experience some conflict. It is important for the teen to learn how to address these feelings so he can become his own person and eventually learn how to teach someone to be his or her caregiver. This will allow the teen to prepare for going away to college and moving toward a more independent life.

During the teenage years it may become apparent to the child that total independence is not a realistic goal. If a child has not achieved physical independence in self-care and other activities of daily living by the age of 16, it's unrealistic to expect that he will be capable of complete independent self-care in the future. Accepting his limitations may take considerable psychological work. Parents and therapists should focus on helping the adolescent learn how to direct his own care, providing both realistic goals and a sense of control.

One way to foster maximum independence is through independent living training, which is often available in rehabilitation facilities. The goal is for the child to learn to do all he can for himself, as well as to learn how to direct untrained individuals to help him do the things he cannot do. The best age for the adolescent to work on this training is between 12 and 16 years.

Independent living training in a rehabilitation facility is also an excellent method of working on separation issues. The training usually takes place over a period of weeks at a residential facility. It may be the first time the parent and child have been separated for an extended time. This may actually be as hard for the parent as for the child, if not harder. However, it is an essential part of growth and maturity, and the child should be provided the opportunity and freedom to develop his independence. Parents need to let go, understanding that they will not always be around to provide for their child. Additionally, the important planning for the possibility of college or work cannot be effectively accomplished if the issue of separation has not been addressed.

It is important to respect the maturing child's right to privacy, though this may be somewhat difficult for a teen who needs help with toileting. Closing doors and respecting the teen's requests for privacy whenever possible is essential. Adolescents in this group often have little opportunity to work on issues of sexual socialization, primarily because they are still working on issues of separation. These teens need to be offered opportunities to be involved with their peer group within the community.

Adolescents who are cognitively normal and severely involved physically. All the issues that apply to adolescents with moderate physical involvement also apply to adolescents with severe involvement. But the adolescent with a severe disability also needs help with all activities of daily living and usually requires an alternative means of communicating. Difficulties in the areas of daily living and communication can be very frustrating and energy consuming. It is understandably upsetting for the adolescent when people don't take the time to try to understand her and assume that she is cognitively impaired. Every effort should be made to plan for the future; adolescents in this group eventually need to become self-sufficient with the help of a full-time trained aide.

A child who is severely involved is usually not able to direct an untrained individual in her own care. Plans should be in place to ensure that trained caregivers with whom the child is comfortable are always available. This is especially important in the event the child needs to spend time in a hospital or be cared for by a caregiver other than the one to whom she is accustomed. For a child who is unable to communicate orally, it's imperative to seek medical treatment at a facility whose staff are familiar with the needs of individuals with severe disabilities or to make certain that knowledgeable, trained caregivers are present to be sure that the child receives adequate care.

For a child in this group, there is almost never an opportunity for sexual socialization as a teenager, and there are only occasional opportunities as an adult. He or she has sexual feelings and desires, though they may be difficult to address. (This aspect of development is discussed further in Chapter 4.) The teen's difficulty in communicating, as well as the attempt to cope with normal maturation issues, often leads to withdrawal and depression, which may not be recognized or addressed properly because of the communication difficulties. Providing communication systems for these adolescents is probably the single most important service that the medical care system can provide. (See "Augmentative Communication" in Part 3 for information about communication systems.)

Adolescents with mild cognitive and physical involvement. Adolescents with mild cognitive impairment who are able to walk, with or without the use of assistive devices, face issues that are very similar to the issues facing children without disabilities. However, they need additional structure and guidance concerning schooling, training, and, ultimately, job opportunities. They also need to be given the same opportunities to fail that parents give to normal teenagers, although achieving a balance of help, guidance, and letting go is never easy.

Adolescents in this group may have significant difficulty dealing with social interactions. This difficulty may show up as depression or anger. Parents should make it possible for these teens to discuss their feelings with a professional counselor before the feelings become overwhelming. With proper guidance and within the appropriate environment, most of these youngsters can become fully self-sufficient members of society.

Adolescents with moderate cognitive and physical involvement. Although many of them are able to walk with assistive devices, these adolescents need to be in a structured and supervised living and working environment because of their cognitive limitations. If the adolescent is presently cared for at home, the main issue of concern for the family is to plan for the time when the current primary caregiver will be unable to care for the child. These plans should be recorded in writing, and they should be described to the teen's next of kin.

If institutional care is likely to be needed in the future, facilities should be investigated in advance. One of the very attractive alternatives to institutionalized living is the structured group home, which makes it possible for the person to move away from home but still live in the same community and go home on weekends and holidays. This arrangement closely parallels the situation of the child who leaves home when he finds a job but continues to be involved with his family in the same community.

Adolescents with severe cognitive and physical impairment. Adolescents in this group need full-time trained custodial care. They don't have all the psychological problems that beset adolescents with milder involvement, however. The main issue for this group is the need for good planning for the future. If the parent is the sole full-time care provider, then plans must be made for alternative caregivers. The parents of severely involved children often have the misconception that their child has a short life expectancy. However, the majority of individuals who reach their teenage years will probably outlive their parents. Thus, long-range planning really is a necessity. Additionally, unexpected events such as an accident or illness sometimes make it impossible for the primary caregiver to continue to provide care.

If no alternative plans have been made, the state social service agency will assume responsibility for the child, who will be placed in whatever facility is available, often without regard to what the parents may have wanted. Rather than let this happen, it is far better to make arrangements with a facility or with other individuals willing to provide the necessary care before something interferes with the present arrangements. Ideally, an alternative caregiver will previously have provided some care, perhaps as respite care, and will be familiar with the teenager and his needs. Having some familiarity beforehand with the new caregivers also provides the child with comfort and security in a new environment if a move becomes necessary.

Parents must allow themselves the opportunity to ask how much longer they can continue to care for their child. This is a difficult issue and one that can lead to conflict between parents. Unfortunately, divorce is a fairly common result of the strains and conflicts that prevail in the family of a child with a severe disorder. Some parents are poorly equipped to handle the extra stress, and some are not willing to give up a previously pursued career in order to care for the child full time. Once a parent has psychologically come to terms with the extent of care that he or she is personally willing to provide, there are various alternatives to consider.

After taking into account many factors—such as the home environment, schools, siblings, availability of respite care, and financial resources—parents may decide that it's better for the child to be in another environment. They may choose to relinquish parental rights and never see the child again, or they may place the child in a group home or chronic care facility and visit the child there or bring the child home for weekend and holiday visits.

Another option is foster care, in which the child is placed with another family for care. In this arrangement, the parents retain their rights and have the opportunity to take the child on weekends, special occasions, or whenever they want to spend time with the child. There are some caregivers, mostly women, whose occupation as foster parents is to care for children with disabilities. Many of these persons provide excellent care, although their services are in great demand and they are hard to find. Some individuals providing foster care, however, lack either the appropriate skills or other options for work; they may be motivated by selfish needs, which do not always lead to the best care for the individual. Thus foster care may provide the child with the best of care or with very poor care, primarily because there is little supervision over the care provided. Parents need to thoroughly investigate any situation they are considering for their child.

There should also be some discussion about the level of medical care parents want to provide in life-threatening situations. This is an emotionally charged subject in which religious, ethical, and practical factors are intricately interwoven. Parents need to reach an understanding in advance about their wishes for their child's care and then put this into writing. That way they won't suddenly be faced with a difficult decision for which they are unprepared. Parents should also make sure that any doctor treating their child is well aware in advance of their wishes regarding medical treatment in a life-threatening situation. Discussing these decisions allows the parents and the physicians to become comfortable with them. Many parents decide to provide all the care necessary to ensure the child's comfort (such as correcting scoliosis) but not to take heroic measures to prolong life (such as permanently putting the child on a ventilator). This includes doing everything possible to improve the ability of caregivers to care for the child.

Often there are difficult decisions to make, and it seems as if a fine line is being drawn between providing medical care to improve the child's quality of life and providing care to prolong life. If, for example, a child's kidneys fail, a plan to transplant a kidney in order to prolong the child's life might well be rejected fairly readily. A decision regarding gastric surgery for a child who experiences frequent pneumonias related to reflux and aspiration may be more difficult to make, particularly if the pneumonias respond well to antibiotic treatment.

The decision to operate on a severely involved child can be very difficult. Scoliosis is usually treated with surgery because even though it is major surgery, the result allows for better seating and more comfort. But if a child develops a severe bowel obstruction, the parents may elect not to have surgery because a bowel obstruction usually quickly leads to death without much pain, whereas the surgery for bowel obstruction may involve a very long recovery period with a great deal of discomfort.

Clearly, such decisions must be made on an individual basis. They are easier if parents and physicians have established a compatible working relationship before an acute situation arises. Then parents can be more comfortable with their decisions and confident that the physician is prepared to abide by those decisions, which are made with the child's best interests in mind and in accordance with the parents' wishes and values. (For more on end-of-life issues, see "Life Span" in Chapter 3.)

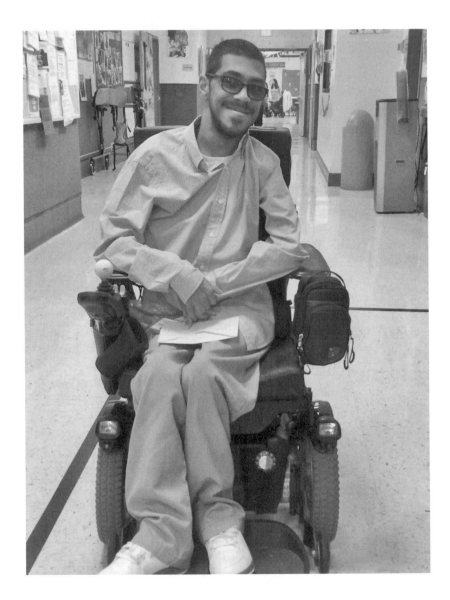

❧ 8
The Adult with Cerebral Palsy

AS CARE continues to improve with medical advances, many children with cerebral palsy become young adults, middle-aged adults, and older adults. The adult with cerebral palsy faces many of the same issues that all people experience as they age but also has unique experiences. The purpose of this chapter is to provide some understanding of how the adult with cerebral palsy grows while aging mentally, physically, and socially.

Aging can be considered similar to growth and development in a child, with the principal difference being that aging takes place over a longer time and with variation from one person to another. Concerns usually center on independence, intimate relationships, and employment. As he attempts to meet the challenges of adulthood, the individual with a disability has to deal with issues not faced by the person without disabilities. There may be significant psychological concerns for the adult with cerebral palsy, who may find it more difficult to obtain independence, social acceptance, work opportunities, and medical care because of his or her unique needs.

The degree of difficulty a person encounters in establishing independence depends on the individual, the severity of the individual's disability, and the individual's family and support systems. The transition to adulthood can be much harder for adults who have more intense support needs. Generally, children who have functioned well in a typical school environment can be expected to meet the challenges of the transition to adulthood and independence in much the same way that their classmates or siblings who do not have disabilities do. For some teenagers or young adults, however, having a disability makes it psychologically more difficult to establish a positive and healthy self-image. For those who have previously functioned well in a typical school setting, this is most likely an adjustment reaction to the transition process. This experience is very similar to the struggle the child without a disability has in adapting when moving on from high school to college or adjusting after breaking up with a boyfriend or girlfriend. Throughout the transition process, however, variability in support systems becomes the norm. Whenever problems such as unhappiness, depression, or behavioral changes emerge, they should be taken seriously, and guidance, often including psychological evaluation or counseling, should be obtained.

The Transition from Childhood to Adulthood

From birth, the human experience is the result of multiple transitions. As children with cerebral palsy grow and mature, they also move through different phases of life. The transition can be explained in a couple of ways.

One approach divides the transition into three stages. In the early stage children become aware of growing up. Becoming an adult comes with responsibilities, including maintaining one's own self-worth and happiness, addressing one's medical conditions and associated problems, along with healthy living, including engaging in physical activities. The middle stage focuses on the development of goals, starting with school and educational interests, leading to a career through employment or as a volunteer, and progressing to living independently or in a community setting. This middle stage also includes understanding the importance of routine medical visits and knowing what to do when a medical problem occurs. In the last stage, one makes decisions on his or her own regarding education, health, socialization, and living, reaching out for advice as needed but maintaining autonomy.

Another approach also divides the transition to adulthood into three stages, but in this case the process involves more reliance on others. In the first stage the child is completely dependent on the guidance and care of the parent or guardian. For children with CP, the duration of this stage can vary greatly based upon age as well as functional abilities. In the second stage the child experiments with increasing independence, with parents and other support systems present to coach and assist as needed. This is also the time when the parents learn that the child has to be given more opportunities to make independent choices about his or her life in order to move to the final stage. The third stage is independent living as appropriate for the individual. Some individuals can live alone and care for themselves, while others must have supports and direct caregivers to perform certain activities of daily living. Having a conceptual understanding of the transitional process can help both the child with CP and the family adjust as the child becomes a more independent member of adult society.

What are the important relationship and socialization concerns for the person with cerebral palsy during the transition to adulthood?

The adolescent moves toward adulthood by gaining independence in relationships, health care, employment, and residential living. Relationships and socialization are often regarded as the highest priority for the typical adolescent. The important skills learned at this stage focus on the development of not only friendships but also intimate relationships. Dating and trying to gain acceptance from peers can be very traumatic for any young adult, but the additional effort required of people with CP can be overwhelming. Much more energy is devoted to just keeping up with their peers. As they move into the adult environment, with more competition and without the protected environment of school and/or a supportive home environment, simply trying to keep up may wear them down. Individuals with CP often experience fatigue, both from the increased psychological stress of dealing with a less receptive environment and from the physical stress of a college or work environment.

Many young adults are concerned about their appearance. The stresses generated by the cultural focus on physical appearance are often magnified for the person with cerebral palsy. Fortunately, as young people mature, they learn that there is more to a person than physical appearance. It becomes clear that a relationship is much more dependent on communication, understanding, and mutual concern. This lesson can be fostered in group environments, which allow individuals with disabilities to learn socialization and intimacy skills and to meet other self-advocates, future colleagues, and potentially suitable partners. Many group environments are organized around special interests, social activities, and spiritual interests. This type of socialization certainly has advantages. Meeting people under traditional dating circumstances can be especially hard for people with a disability because of the physical and psychological barriers present between themselves and the nondisabled population. People living in areas where they have difficulty meeting others for friendships or romantic relationships might consider using an online dating service, a means of meeting people that is popular among adults with or without disabilities.

Another source of stress that may not be fully encountered until the person leaves school and tries to enter the job market is prejudice against people with a disability or handicap. It is important for the person with a disability who is dealing with prejudice to understand the rights of individuals with disabilities, form alliances with others, and become a self-advocate willing to speak up against inequalities.

Adults with Impairments

Adults with impairments due to cerebral palsy are typically people who can manage all activities of daily living without needing to expend significantly more effort than the typical population. This includes most people with hemiplegia and many with diplegia who have typical cognitive function. By definition, an impairment is an abnormality of body structure or function, such as spasticity or contractures, that does not prevent one from performing one's usual activities.

What are the usual living arrangements for adults with impairments?

Adults with impairments generally enjoy a lifestyle very similar to that of the general population, often including marriage and children.

Howard is a 39-year-old man with mild to moderate right side hemiplegia who currently works as a computer program systems analyst. Howard is generally healthy and has not had any medical problems since a foot operation at age 17. He can't fully straighten his right arm, and he has a slight limp. These impairments are so well integrated into Howard's movements that very few of his coworkers even know he has cerebral palsy. He golfs, swims, water-skis, snow-skis, and goes sailing. He does not have a special exercise program, but when he notices some tightness or stiffness, he knows he should increase his physical activity. He does sometimes worry about developing a neurological or orthopedic problem that would significantly alter his activity or functional level.

Howard started as a physical therapy major in college, but in his third year he switched to nursing. After graduation he trained as a rehabilitation nurse specialist and worked for 10 years, until he felt a need for a change. By working evenings, he earned a degree in business administration and changed his career from nursing to computer systems analysis.

Howard has been married for 10 years and has three healthy, active boys aged 2, 5, and 8. Howard and his wife, Joan, have always had open communication concerning his cerebral palsy. The only problem CP caused him in terms of parenting was in learning to carry and care for his newborn infants. Due to his affected right arm and hand, Howard was afraid that he might drop them, but this was easily solved with a little practice.

Having children made Howard think about how he would approach raising a child with a disability and, more importantly, how he would teach the child to live with a disability. He wanted to be sure his children knew the value of finding one's own way and creating a path to achieve one's goals. While his children knew that their father did things differently—typing with only one hand, for example—they also knew he was able to accomplish his goals. And they saw that he was confident and sought out assistance when he needed it.

What are some of the challenges the person with an impairment due to cerebral palsy faces in gaining employment?

The medical problems related to CP faced by adults with impairments are usually minor in comparison with the problems they face in relation to occupational choices. Howard has experienced some discrimination. When he wanted to enlist in the Air Force Reserves to earn extra income as a rehabilitation nurse, he was told that he could not apply because he had CP. This was especially frustrating because he was not properly evaluated to determine whether and how much his impairment would affect his performance. And once when he went to renew his driver's license, he was asked if he had a physical disability. When he said yes, he had to repeat the entire driving test, even though he had been driving for six years with no change in his condition. This almost resulted in his having to pay higher insurance premiums. He learned quickly that using the right terminology is important in many situations, and he began to understand the differences between those who have impairments and those who have disabilities.

The Americans with Disabilities Act (ADA), passed in 1990, makes employment discrimination illegal. Individuals who suspect that they are being discriminated against should check with legal counsel to advocate for their rights. Job discrimination against individuals with impairments still goes on, although with the extension of equal opportunity rights to people with disabilities, the incidence of discrimination should decrease. While there are still disparities in access to health, disability, and life insurance, the health insurance system is changing rapidly, and there is increasing public recognition of the need to reduce the disparities. Educating lawmakers about the needs of people with disabilities has had a very positive impact. You can participate by contacting your representatives and expressing your concerns.

Adults with Functional Limitations

Adults with functional limitations are primarily those who have moderate to severe diplegia or mild to moderate quadriplegia. Adults with functional limitations are able to live independently, but their condition significantly restricts their ability to perform certain activities of daily living. Their occupational choices and relationships may be influenced by their limitations. Most people in this category have typical cognitive abilities, although some people with mild intellectual disability could also fit into this group. People with primarily physical impairments face different challenges from those faced by adults who also have cognitive difficulties. The discussion in this section focuses on the issues faced by people who have only physical limitations.

Sam is 46 years old and works as a mechanical engineer in the research division of a major company. He has athetoid patterned cerebral palsy with a moderate degree of involvement in his hands and arms. He is able to walk without using any aids, but he has speech difficulty, especially when communicating with people who do not know him. He grew up in a very supportive family. In his view, his mother was overprotective and his father pushed him with appropriate expectations. Because he loved to build things, his father encouraged him to pursue his interests, never pressuring him to try to do things more quickly. His father's patience fostered an early interest in engineering. In grade school he was thought by several teachers to be slow or delayed because of his speech difficulty, especially during his initial encounters with people who did not have the patience to listen and learn to understand him. Because of this difficulty, and at the insistence of his father, he was placed in a special education class, where the teachers took the needed time and interest in his abilities. In the special education classes he excelled academically.

After Sam graduated from high school, his vocational rehabilitation adviser, who thought Sam's interest in going to college was a waste of time and money, discouraged him from applying to schools. Sam feels that this was in part due to the fact that the state vocational rehabilitation system was always short of money and tried to find the least expensive approach for clients, sometimes without thoroughly considering their interests and abilities. Initially, too, he was told that he could not pursue a major in engineering because he could not draw. By devising his own mechanical aids for drawing, he managed to draw so well that his instructors told him he had the best mechanical drawings they had seen in a master's degree thesis.

Ellen and Sam met through personal advertisements placed with a dating service for people with disabilities. Ellen is 44 years old with a moderate to severe spastic quadriplegic pattern involvement of cerebral palsy. She has normal speech (no impairment) but is not able to walk. She uses a wheelchair, which she can push for short distances. She can perform most activities of daily living by herself. Ellen also grew up in a very supportive family. Both her parents encouraged her to be all she could be within the scope of her physical limitations. She entered a traditional kindergarten class and remained in mainstream classes through high school. She completed four years of college and works as a travel agent. Ellen remembers a more positive educational experience than does Sam because she was not labeled "slow" or "learning disabled," largely because her speech was not affected.

What are the usual living arrangements for adults with functional limitations?

Most adults with functional limitations live either independently or in close proximity to their families or other support systems. Many young adults with functional limitations have adult relationships or get married, although often later than adults without such limitations. However, compared with the nondisabled population, fewer adults with disabilities marry.

Lack of mobility can be an obstacle to achieving independence. Having access to appropriate, reliable public transportation or obtaining personally adapted transportation, such as a van equipped with a chair lift can solve this problem. Customized vehicles are financially out of reach for many people, and external support is often limited or frequently requires innovative approaches to fundraising. A number of community agencies, such as United Cerebral Palsy and the Easter Seal Society, are interested in helping people with disabilities access what it takes to remain a functional contributing citizen in the community. Even if they cannot provide funds themselves, these agencies can provide pathways to appropriate resources. Obtaining a driver's license and a personal motor vehicle is a measure of independence.

Sam and Ellen were able to purchase a modest house, but the house required modifications, including a ramp for Ellen's wheelchair and wheelchair accessibility in the bathrooms; the laundry area had to be moved upstairs as well. All of these changes added significant expenses for which limited financial assistance was available. If Sam and Ellen had not been working, the county welfare agency would have provided wheelchair-accessible transportation. However, because they were earning money, this assistance was not available. Their income did not allow them to purchase a hand-controlled, wheelchair-accessible van, which Ellen needs for transportation. Modifications to the house may also be tax deductible if the modifications are needed because of a person's disability. A tax adviser can help determine which of these expenses can legally be claimed for tax purposes.

What are the prospects for employment?

In the 1980s, studies showed that only a small percentage (12 to 17 percent) of adults with CP were employed. More recently, published reports have shown far more adults with CP (as high as 50 percent) achieving competitive employment and independent living. People with milder physical and cognitive impairments, good family support, and proper medical treatment had the highest rate of employment. People whose speech impairment was a major part of their disability had lower rates of employment.

A common misperception in the general population about people with functional limitations is that they are also cognitively impaired. This misperception should be confronted immediately with a discussion of the person's abilities. As an example, if the person with a functional limitation is seeing a physician who ignores the person and only talks to the sponsor, the person being examined should openly say, "I know that I'm occasionally hard to understand when I speak, but I understand what you're talking about very well." It may be helpful to have a card that says, "It takes me a little longer to speak. Please be patient. I have thoughts and opinions to share." The person with CP can address the communication barrier head on by presenting this card to his new provider immediately.

Sam and Ellen were married 16 years ago, and both have continued to work. During their adult years they have experienced discrimination due to their functional limitations. While there may be challenges with real or perceived prejudice in obtaining a job, federal protections through the Americans with

Disabilities Act should alleviate some of the challenges Sam and Ellen experienced.

How can the person with a disability overcome barriers to employment?

Although current laws are designed to protect individuals with disabilities from discrimination, in reality there are both physical and psychological barriers to overcome. In the past, many employers made their workplaces physically accessible only when economically motivated to do so. However, providing physical access in the workplace is now legally required by the Americans with Disability Act.

Typically, people with disabilities are better accepted in the educational community (as students as well as teachers) and in the health care community. Certainly, individuals who have attained a college education, and particularly those with a graduate degree, have less difficulty finding a job than those without degrees.

The first step in dealing with barriers to employment is understanding that they exist and anticipating them. Networking with known contacts often yields better results than trying to enter the open market. This style of job hunting is the most fruitful for everyone, regardless of education, skills, or other capabilities: if you have access to a network in the area in which you would like to work, use it.

Adults with Disabilities

Adults with disabilities vary greatly in their cognitive and physical function and needs. By definition, a disability is a limitation severe enough to interfere with one's ability to participate in a typical societal role.

John was cared for from birth by a foster mother, Mary, who had five older children in school. Mary was a secondary school teacher and writer who felt called to adopt a child with special needs.

John started walking at age 5 with poor balance. He is considered to have moderate spastic quadriplegic CP with moderate speech impairment and a moderate degree of intellectual disability. John has an outgoing personality, is always in good spirits, and possesses an obsessive will. His intellectual disability affects his judgment, impairs his perceptions, and causes perseveration (persistent repetition of a word, gesture, or act). He is happy in his family, his closely knit local community, and his church, and he is never moody or persistently angry. In general, he has unquenchable optimism and a positive outlook on life.

Throughout his life, John has continued to need supervision for daily living activities, as well as direction to maintain appropriate behavior. When John turned 18, Mary became his legal guardian. This means that Mary was given full rights to make all decisions for John, and he was determined to be legally incompetent to make any decisions for himself.

By the time John was 26 years old, Mary had retired and was in her seventies. She started to plan for John's future care with the support of the entire family to ensure that John's wants and needs would be met. The decision was made that when Mary was unable to care for John, or in the event of her passing, John would be cared for by Hal, her oldest son, who had four children of his own in grade school. Subsequently, there was a local discussion about building several group homes for adults with disabilities in the community. The family felt this might be an even better option for John, who could live in the community with his peers and still have family and his church community close. Two homes were built, one for men and one for women. An application was made, but the family was concerned that John would not be chosen because other families seemed to have a much greater need for custodial care.

The group directing this effort felt the start-up would be easier if they began with adults who were well known in the community and who had a limited number of medical and other issues that would require management. Because of John's good nature and community ties, he was chosen as an initial resident. During the transition John stayed at his new home and returned to his family's home every other weekend. Since the new home was only several blocks from his old one, it was easy for John to come home for special occasions. John quickly adapted to his new environment and was happy.

Mary's adjustment to the changes was more difficult. Her friends would typically greet her with statements like, "How wonderful that you're free now, with John in the group home." Many did not notice her sadness. Although John's father seemed to welcome the new freedom, Mary continued to struggle and grieve. For the first time since the birth of her oldest son 46 years earlier, she awoke without anyone to care for. Mary had enjoyed caring for John and had not seen him as a burden, but instead appreciated his humor and lively engagement as a conversational partner. With John gone and her husband focusing more on his hobbies, Mary became depressed. After several sessions with a psychologist, Mary came to understand that the sadness she had experienced when John moved was a natural consequence of change and loss. It was also a reasonable cause for grieving, even if others around her could not appreciate it. With time, Mary found peace in her new life.

What are the usual living arrangements for adults with disabilities?

Personal care and housing arrangements for adults with disabilities vary from one community to another. Many adults with severe disabilities remain in the care of their parents. As parents age and people with severe disabilities outlive their parents, the caregiver role is often assumed by siblings or other family members. Care in the home is often supplemented with home health aides and/or nurses, depending on the adult's needs. A small group home with full-time support staff is a good option for many, although it may not be available in all communities. Some adults with disabilities require a significant amount of medical care and are fully dependent on others for all activities of daily living. Larger group homes with staff rotating by shifts can accommodate more complex care needs and still allow the adult to live in a community setting. Adult foster homes are another possibility. Options that many parents and adults with disabilities find less desirable are nursing homes or state hospitals. Although these are not ideal environments, there may be no other alternative for some adults requiring very intensive or skilled care. These facilities are falling out of favor nationally and are becoming harder and harder to locate.

Parents of adults with disabilities should find out what options are available in their community long before a person is expected to transition out of the home. Many of the resources available in the community have long waiting lists. If adequate facilities are not available, parents may want to consider forming a church or community group to establish a group home. This is how many group homes are developed. In many ways the transition from parental home care to outside care for the adult with a disability should follow a pattern similar to that of any child who eventually leaves the parental home to live independently. Many adults with disabilities continue to live with their families until circumstances necessitate a change in living arrangements. Planning for the time when a change may become necessary is extremely important for the adult with a disability as well as for the family and can make the transition much easier for everyone. While there are options available for emergency situations, such as when the principal caregiver becomes seriously ill or dies, a well thought out process for transition to living in the community can result in a positive experience and better accommodations for the adult and their families.

What are the prospects for employment? Individuals with severe physical limitations but normal cognitive function may find getting a job in the private sector extremely difficult. These individuals should push state agencies to help set up or find jobs. Employment is an important aspect of an adult's psychological health. Volunteer organizations can help with special circumstances, especially when being employed prevents the person from getting assistance from government agencies.

Special Medical Problems in Adults with CP

Children with CP usually have access to comprehensive medical care. However, the same specialists may not be available in adult centered care. While growing children undergo many changes and thus need close medical monitoring, adults with special health care needs need primary care physicians and specialists available for periodic evaluation. Unfortunately, many adults with disabilities endure physical problems that are preventable and treatable, but they lack medical or surgical providers with expertise to treat their unique medical needs. Finding a general physician who is knowledgeable about cerebral palsy is critical to good health. Sometimes a family physician or internal medicine–pediatrics physician is able to treat the individual from childhood into adulthood. More commonly a patient will need to transition from a pediatric provider to an internal medicine or other adult care provider. Lastly, some patients have found a medical home in the pediatric specialist's care and need to transition to a primary care doctor in the adult world.

A number of issues are more common to people with impairments, functional limitations, and disabilities, although the issues are generally the same as those faced by the general population. Many adults with CP get good care for acute problems but do not receive adequate *preventive care*, such as periodic general health evaluations and screenings (blood pressure and cholesterol monitoring, Pap smears, cancer screening). It is best to research and interview potential new physicians before there is a need for change, such as when the person is approaching adulthood or is considering moving. Establishing care and a relationship before an urgent need arises is best; it may be difficult to do at an initial emergency meeting.

Fairly common among people who have cerebral palsy are disabilities including *hearing and vision impairments, epilepsy,* and *gastroesophageal reflux.* These problems (discussed in Chapter 3) may worsen in the adult even if they were adequately dealt with in childhood. *Dental care* is also a problem for many adults with CP. Many individuals have poor dental hygiene, and finding a dentist who has the skills and is willing to devote the time necessary to treat more complex patients may be difficult. Many people with CP also have problems with drooling, which may be treatable with medication or surgery (see Chapter 3).

Adults with functional limitations are also vulnerable to chronic *dehydration* as a result of reducing their fluid intake to avoid difficulties in public toileting. Limiting fluid intake can also contribute to *constipation.* Constipation is a common problem for aging adults as well as for people who have functional limitations. This problem can be addressed by changing the diet and using stool softeners as needed, with the goal of having bowel movements on a regular schedule. Regularity can be achieved with improved toilet accessibility in the workplace and, sometimes, attendant help. Adequate water intake is essential.

The young adult with a disability is also prone to some special medical problems. One set of problems is *urinary tract infections and incontinence.* Infections are often associated with poor perineal hygiene and/or the use of a urinary collecting device or Foley catheter. Bladder incontinence is a particular problem among those who spend most of the day in a wheelchair or bed and can be improved by following a regular toileting schedule. Incontinence often occurs late in the day after the person has not voided all day, as well as during transfer activities. As noted previously, deliberate restriction of fluids to avoid this problem often leads to constipation as well.

Finding physicians has been difficult for Ellen and Sam. Ellen has had an especially difficult time finding a gynecologist who will take the time to deal with her spasticity, which is always a problem. On one occasion, she tried to tell a new gynecologist which positioning and speculum size would work best and found that he was offended. Sam has had similar problems finding a dentist because of his difficulty in controlling his mouth movements. He suggested a clamp to hold his mouth open, but several dentists ignored his suggestions.

As adults neither Sam nor Ellen has had serious medical problems, although both have to deal with chronic constipation. Sam has also had some problems with arthritis in his neck, although so far he has been able to deal with it with rest, therapy, and medication. Sam and Ellen do both worry about maintaining their current level of functioning and remaining independent.

Adults with *spasticity* must get adequate exercise to avoid stiffness. This need often conflicts with increasingly busy lifestyles, just as a full schedule interferes with the nondisabled person's ability to exercise. The same discipline is required to set up a routine that allows the person to exercise and stretch. A person is likely to stick with an activity he enjoys, such as swimming. Many adults with CP give up walking by age 25 because of fatigue and inefficiency of walking and because wheelchairs provide greater mobility and independence.

Musculoskeletal problems become common as young adults get older. Cervical neck pain (especially in those with athetosis), back pain, and pain in the weight-bearing joints (hips, knees, and ankles) is experienced by a high percentage of adults with CP, especially after age 40. Of those who are still walking at age 40, many decide to use ambulatory supports such as walkers or wheelchairs to minimize pain. Contractures of the lower extremities are also common, especially among those who have stopped walking. Carpal tunnel syndrome is a source of pain that develops because of chronic, repetitive, and atypical use of muscles or joints. It is often experienced by people who work at a computer keyboard many hours a day or by those who use crutches or push manual wheelchairs over many years. Shoulder pain may also affect those who spend a significant amount of time using ambulatory aids (crutches, walkers) or a wheelchair. The additional repetitive strain and weight bearing through the arms and shoulders can lead to overuse injuries or arthritis.

Dislocated hips, scoliosis, or foot deformities may continue to be a source of pain in the adult if they have not been fully corrected in childhood. Postural back pain is often associated with inadequate wheelchair fitting and maintenance. Crutches, canes, braces, and wheelchairs need to be reevaluated periodically to make sure they are still appropriate for the individual and continue to fit his or her needs. Some adults with CP struggle with correctable foot deformities until finally deciding at retirement to see if something can be done about them. With the help of an informed and interested orthopedist or physiatrist who is familiar with his issues, an adult with CP can remain at his optimal level of function and comfort longer. Many individuals with disabilities get used to putting up with pain and discomfort and in fact are counseled to "just to live with" their problems. Certainly, there is a limit to what modern medicine can do, but many issues can be improved or alleviated. Medications, therapies, and other nonpharmacological approaches can be implemented to minimize the impact of pain on the lives of people who have CP. The psychological impact of chronic pain should also be assessed on a regular basis. New discoveries are being made all the time, and every effort, within reason, should be made to relieve any discomfort.

As discussed in Chapter 3, *osteopenia* (low bone density) and *osteoporosis* can have a significant impact on many adolescents with CP. This problem gradually worsens into adulthood, especially if the person engages in fewer activities that involve weight bearing, such as walking or other exercise, or stops them altogether. Fractures may occur after minimal trauma, or after a fall in those who are ambulatory. A person who has had one such fracture is at an even greater risk for recurrence. Osteoporosis is a concern for the elderly population at large, especially postmenopausal women. In the disabled population, this problem is present among both men and women, and at much younger ages than in the rest of the population. Consideration needs to be given to early evaluation of bone density (usually with a DXA scan) and to possible treatment with medications (such as vitamin D and/or bisphosphonates).

The Young Adult with Cerebral Palsy

Some of the problems people with cerebral palsy have are specifically related to the person's age. One common problem that develops in this group is loss of motivation and a desire to pursue goals once the person is no longer in the school system. Some mentally high-functioning but severely physically involved individuals become disheartened when they are unable to go to college or struggle to find employment. For those who have been able to attend college, facing unemployment related to their disability is profoundly disturbing and can seriously affect their motivation.

What can be done for the person who is no longer motivated?

When an adult is no longer motivated, it is important to determine whether he or she is clinically depressed. The person who loses interest in his normal activities, is not interested in interpersonal relationships, and becomes withdrawn should not be ignored. Depression is just as likely to affect a young adult as it is to affect anyone else and should be treated with psychological counseling and, when appropriate, medication. Early intervention with referrals to a clinical social worker, psychologist, or psychiatrist can have more positive outcomes. Families and caregivers also need to be assessed and supported during difficult times.

What problems are encountered by people with disabilities who have never functioned independently?

People with cerebral palsy should be encouraged to function as independently as they are able to. There are people with disabilities who have never functioned independently; some of them have severe physical disabilities with adequate cognitive function. It is important for them to be able to articulate their life goals and direct implementation of those goals. For these people, a major obstacle to gaining maximum independence is their need for attendant care to help them in activities of daily living. Parents and/or caregivers need to be careful not to impose their desires unilaterally just because the person can't physically live independently.

Other adults with disabilities who have never functioned independently require total care in all activities of daily living as well as in making decisions. Advanced care planning is essential for the families of these adults to ensure that their quality of life and care plans are articulated. Most of these children will outlive their parents. The most beneficial contribution a parent or caregiver can make is to formulate a good long-term plan that includes residential considerations and financial estate planning (see Chapter 10).

What sexual issues need to be addressed in young adulthood?

Sexuality and sexual health should be discussed with all adolescents and young adults regardless of the degree of their disability. Often, even cognitively typical but physically involved men and women have a limited understanding of sexual health and reproductive issues, primarily because they have less opportunity to learn. The general population contributes to this lack of opportunity because of the erroneous belief that the individual with a disability lacks interest in sexual activity. This bias may even be seen within the medical profession. The adult with a disability should not be embarrassed to raise this issue with caregivers or with his or her doctor.

An example of this problem is illustrated by the comment of a young adult man who was asked how he had managed to deal psychologically with the need for therapy and bracing to deal with his difficulty in walking. He replied that as a teenager he had spent much more time thinking about sex than about how he was walking, but the doctors and therapists had only wanted to talk about his walking. People with intellectual and physical disabilities need to be educated about and given protection against pregnancy and STIs (sexually transmitted infections). They need access to preventive sexual health services, as they are able to have intimate relationships and unfortunately are at high risk for abuse.

What specific problems might the young adult female have?

Access to physically accessible preventive women's health care can be a challenge. Women need to seek care in facilities that provide Pap smears and mammograms. Young women should strongly consider the HPV vaccine, since routine screening for cervical cancer may be more difficult to obtain. Parents need to consider the potential for unintended sexual contact and the need for close personal care, as well as the potential that their daughter will eventually desire sexual activity. Young women who are interested in childbearing also need education about the impact their disability may have during a pregnancy. There are generally no medical reasons why a woman with cerebral palsy should not bear children. Individuals with seizures or other medical conditions must discuss the additional risks associated with those conditions and the medications that they are taking, as well as the effects these medications might have on conception or development of the fetus. Most women, even those with significant spasticity, can have a vaginal delivery, although a cesarean delivery may be necessary for a woman with significant hip deformities or spasticity. Even a completely paralyzed woman may have a vaginal delivery, although her blood pressure needs to be closely monitored to avoid stroke, which can occur if the blood pressure rises extremely rapidly to high levels.

What are the stresses of parenting for the parent with cerebral palsy?

The anxiety that all new parents feel may be magnified for the parent with CP, but this usually subsides as the parent finds special ways to adapt baby care to fit his or her abilities. Being a parent is a great equalizer. One man whose disability required him to use a wheelchair said that caring for his infant son made him feel like a full person because his son did not care that it was difficult for him to get out of bed in the middle of the night. When the baby was hungry, he cried until he was fed.

The Person with Cerebral Palsy at Midlife

For most of the population, the most significant aspect of midlife is experiencing and coming to terms with the physical problems associated with aging. For the person with cerebral palsy, the effects of aging are noticeable at a younger age. Adults in their twenties and thirties start to notice that they are getting stiffer and weaker, particularly if they have not stayed active and maintained an exercise routine. Many adults with CP also commonly report significant physical fatigue associated with bodily pain, deterioration of functional skills, and reduced life satisfaction. Although the normal process of aging tends to come on prematurely for the person with CP, in other respects it is no different from the process for individuals without CP. Aging does not directly change the level or degree of spasticity; however, the slowly increasing stiffness and weakness contribute to decreased function.

Adults in the general population must make an ongoing effort to counteract the effects of aging, but again, this is substantially the same effort that individuals with cerebral palsy must make, though beginning at a younger age. Good exercise habits should be learned early, but it is never too late to start. Water activities such as swimming or stretching in warm water are often the easiest and best-tolerated exercises for people with spasticity. Strength training for adolescents and young adults with CP has been shown to improve muscle strength and walking ability without increasing spasticity. Participants in such programs also report psychological benefits, such as a feeling of increased well-being. Since insurances typically will not pay for routine maintenance therapy services for adults, a home routine for exercising and stretching is something to consider.

Do people get weaker as they age?

To some extent getting weaker is a normal part of aging, but it happens at a different rate and level for the person with CP. For adults with a disability, who often push their bodies to the maximum to accomplish the activities of daily living, the muscles may wear out prematurely from overuse. This doesn't mean that the muscles stops working; rather, there may be increasing weakness as the muscles are continually stressed. The main treatment consists in modifying one's activity, for example, by using a power wheelchair for long distances, such as when shopping at the mall. As noted above, strength training, especially for the lower limbs, may increase strength and walking ability without increasing spasticity.

What are overuse syndromes?

Overuse syndromes are conditions in which pain or disability results from repetitive activity. The most common problem of this kind in the general population is carpal tunnel syndrome, in which there is irritation of a nerve in the wrist caused by repeated wrist activity such as typing. People who use crutches or push manual wheelchairs are at high risk for developing carpal tunnel syndrome. The symptoms include numbness in the thumb and in the index and long fingers. The sensation can cause individuals to awaken from sleep and often is relieved by hanging the hand over the edge of the bed.

The initial treatment for carpal tunnel syndrome is the use of an anti-inflammatory medication such as salicylic acid (aspirin) or ibuprofen (Advil) and wearing a splint at night. If this does not give relief, a very simple operation to relieve the pressure on the nerve is usually done under local anesthesia, often on an outpatient basis. The results are usually quite satisfactory.

Tendinitis of the wrist is another condition that commonly results from using crutches and pushing manual wheelchairs. It is usually treated with anti-inflammatory medication and splinting. If this treatment does not provide relief, a minor surgical release may be necessary.

Are individuals with cerebral palsy more likely to have arthritis?

Two conditions related to cerebral palsy place individuals at a significantly higher risk for developing arthritis: athetosis and a subluxated or dislocated hip. The person with athetoid cerebral palsy has frequent movements of the neck, causing increased wear and early arthritis. Despite this, many adults with athetosis do not develop neck problems.

Arthritis most commonly begins in a person's thirties, forties, or fifties, but people in their twenties or even younger may have arthritis. Usually it begins as neck pain, but it can also be associated with arm or shoulder pain. The primary treatment for arthritis in the neck caused by athetosis is wearing a soft neck collar to try to decrease the movement slightly. Muscle relaxants (such as Valium) are sometimes helpful in decreasing movement, but most muscle relaxants can cause drowsiness, which may interfere with an individual's lifestyle.

Taking anti-inflammatory medications is helpful in decreasing the soreness caused by arthritis. Such physical therapy approaches as traction, heat, massage, ultrasound, and electrical stimulation may also help. Often, over a period of several weeks to two months this discomfort settles down and the pain goes away. Rarely does the arthritis become severe enough to necessitate a cervical spinal fusion.

The other cause of early arthritis and pain is hip dislocation or subluxation. This problem can now be completely prevented by proper treatment in childhood. Many adults were not properly treated for this problem in childhood, however, because they grew up at a time when there was not a good understanding of how to treat or prevent it. If the affected hips become painful, decreasing activity and using anti-inflammatory medications is the first line of treatment, but painful hips usually require surgery. For the alert and walking patient, a total hip replacement usually gives the best result, although this operation may not completely alleviate the pain. Removing the arthritic ball of the hip joint is another option, but often this does not completely remove the pain, and it typically significantly shortens the limb, so that sitting may be difficult.

The Older Person with CP

The age-associated problems of stiffness and arthritis tend to continue as a person gets older. This typically is a time when it also becomes increasingly difficult to continue certain activities, especially walking. The older adult should be encouraged to reassess and make necessary adaptations. A change in lifestyle may give rise to depression, which, if it continues, may call for professional counseling.

Friends and relatives may make comments such as "Don't give up," "Keep fighting," or "If you don't keep going, you'll never walk again," which, although well intended, demonstrate insensitivity and do little to boost one's spirits.

Whenever possible, the person with CP should address these types of comments directly by explaining that while slowing down is a known characteristic of aging in any person, it is magnified in the person with CP. Society doesn't expect the 20-year-old, the 40-year-old, and the 80-year-old without CP to have the same endurance and ambulating abilities; the same expectations should apply to the maturing person with cerebral palsy.

A person needs to find a balance between too much and too little activity. The person with the disability is the best judge of what level of activity is best for him. He must learn to tell other people gently that he is managing the problem with medical supervision.

A Final Thought in Planning for the Future

Day by day life goes on, and for better or worse, events occur over which we have no control. In order to prepare for such events, one can make a list that includes important people and their contact information, as well as other helpful information and documents. These may include confidants to whom health information may be disclosed; health providers for routine and special problems, such as primary doctor, rehabilitation and/or orthopedic specialist, dentist, orthotics and equipment specialists; living, housing, and financial support; and important legal documents such as powers of attorney or guardianship.

Continuing to maintain an active lifestyle and taking part in recreation, worship, volunteering, and social interaction can be sources of self-worth, communal accomplishment, and joyous times. Difficulties and growing pains at any time of life don't have to destroy us. They can help us realize our potential and perhaps serve as models for those who follow us.

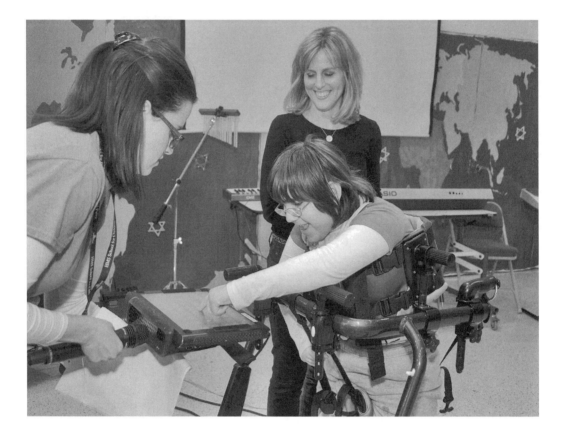

§ 9

How the Health Care System Works

WHEN PARENTS seek professional help in caring for their child with significant long-term disabilities secondary to cerebral palsy, they will encounter several different systems. One of these, the health care system, exists to provide for the physical and psychological needs of the child with CP and to address problems, whether these problems are acute (happening suddenly and/or lasting for a short time) or ongoing. Dental care, nutritional support, immunizations, and surgical procedures to maximize function are all provided by the health care system.

The other professional systems for supporting the child with significant long-term disabilities are the educational system, the legal system, and the community/social service system. The function of the educational system is to teach the child to use his cognitive abilities as fully as possible. The legal and community/social service systems help families to manage the day-to-day financial and emotional needs of the child and the rest of the family. These systems, which interact with one another and with the health care system, are discussed in Chapters 11 and 12. Financial aspects of health care, such as insurance, are discussed in Chapter 10.

In this chapter, we describe the various components of the health care system and how they work.

How many and what kinds of doctors does my child need to see?

Many families with children who have multiple disabilities find it difficult to determine how much and what kind of health care is right for their child. As it turns out, some children receive insufficient health care, while other families are burdened with excessive or redundant care for their child. In the latter case, taking the child to see specialists and trying to keep up with all their recommendations can become a full-time job. For example, one 2-year-old child over time developed ongoing relationships and had appointments with 24 health care providers. This is clearly excessive, and yet for a parent it is sometimes difficult to know which health care services provide exactly what they need.

What kind of doctor is best for my child?

First and foremost the child needs a primary care provider (PCP). This provider, who may be a physician (generally a pediatrician or a family practitioner), nurse practitioner, or a physician assistant, will direct the family's use of other health care specialists whose services are needed by the child. For children with complicated medical problems, a pediatrician is the preferred health care coordinator or director, since the pediatrician is likely to have had specialized training as well as experience in managing these problems. It is this PCP who will provide a "medical home" to the disabled child.

What is a medical home?

The medical home is an approach to providing care that is accessible, continuous, comprehensive, family centered, compassionate, culturally effective, and coordinated. There are many advantages to having a medical home. Children with a medical home are less likely to experience delayed or forgone care, less likely to have unmet health care needs, and less likely to have unmet needs for family support than children without a medical home. In families with a medical home parents miss significantly fewer days of work and children have significantly fewer hospitalizations.

In addition to coordinating chronic and acute medical needs, the PCP provides preventive care, including immunizations. Having a regular source of care was found to be the most important factor associated with receiving preventive care services. (For more on the medical home, see Chapter 3.)

What if my PCP is unfamiliar with CP?

Not all PCPs are familiar with the health care needs of the child with cerebral palsy. They may be slow to make referrals to appropriate specialists, for example. When this occurs, it may be difficult for the family to know how to proceed. One point to remember is that parents are a child's best advocates. Never fail to make your observations and recommendations known to the physician. If you believe that a more timely referral to a specialist is in order, tell your child's physician. You and the physician must forge a collaborative relationship on your child's behalf, and open, direct communication is important to successful health care management.

How can I improve communications among my child's health care providers?

When you begin a new relationship with a physician, take to the first appointment the names and addresses of the other specialists involved in your child's care. At each visit, ask that copies of all relevant dictations be sent to the specialists you designate.

According to the Health Insurance Portability and Accountability Act (HIPAA) of 1996, such requests must be put in writing and signed by you. In your request, include the following information: your child's name, birth date, and address; parents' names and address(es); a statement indicating that you want information from that day's visit to be sent to someone else, with the name(s) and address(es) of the person(s). Most facilities have their own forms for authorizing the release of information for your use. Bringing with you the names and addresses of the appropriate physicians and others who should receive this information will make filling out these forms easier.

You also have a right to obtain a copy of the records for yourself. You will, however, need to put that request in writing; add your name to the list of people you want to receive records. Be aware that there may be fees attached to these requests. Bring copies of all recent records in your possession each time you visit a specialist. The specialist needs to know what's going on, and by sharing these records, you will help to enhance communication.

If your doctors use an electronic health record (EHR), much of this record sharing will be done electronically. You still have to give written permission, but the exchange of information will be easier and quicker. Such coordination will help avoid duplication of x-rays or lab tests and should enhance the care your child receives. Also, most EHRs can make it possible for patients, parents, and guardians to see their own medical records, including lab tests and x-ray results. Be sure to ask your doctors if this is possible for you. Also, be aware that when your child turns 18 you will no longer have access to his or her medical records without permission from either the child or the courts via a durable power of attorney or guardianship.

How can I make the best use of information from my child's doctors?

Some children with CP have a relationship with a different medical specialist for each body system, as well as relationships with a variety of other professionals such as physical therapists, occupational therapists, nurses, and social workers. For a child to benefit from the evaluations of these various health care professionals, all the information they generate must be coordinated. This serves the dual purpose of keeping all the child's medical caregivers informed about the child's condition and progress and preventing redundancy in care (for example, the unknowing repetition of expensive and sometimes painful diagnostic tests).

As noted above, the parent must make certain that information from each visit with a specialist is sent to the PCP and to other specialists by way of the medical records. The PCP will help the parent understand the findings of the other specialists, and these specialists' reports will assist the PCP in managing the child's care.

Another helpful professional is a case manager, who may be employed by an insurance company or a state agency. Case managers can help coordinate your access to care, help you understand the recommendations of various specialists, and help provide direction for the care of your child.

What is a patient case manager?

Because so many health professionals are involved in the care of children with complex medical problems, the role of a patient case manager (also called a patient care manager) has evolved. Most case managers are nurses or social workers who provide excellent support to the family and assist in coordinating the child's many health care providers. The case manager may make recommendations regarding specific health care specialists.

Government agencies or specialty clinics may assign a child a case manager. This person will generally have the family's and the patient's best interests as his or her goal. But insurance companies have also begun to employ patient case managers. The primary goal of these case managers is to avoid duplication and the redundant use of resources. In dealing with case managers hired by insurance companies, parents will need to be especially strong advocates for their child (see Chapter 12, as well as "Managing the System" in Part 2).

What if I do not receive
public assistance, do
not have access to a
case manager, and do
not meet eligibility cri-
teria for various public
support programs?

If you are living just above the poverty level, you may be ineligible for many social service programs. If you have no medical insurance for your child, you may have difficulty finding a doctor to see your child for regular care. Contact your local Department of Public Health, as many states operate primary care health clinics for just such families. In addition, many states have a program known as CHIP (Children's Health Insurance Program) or SCHIP (State Children's Health Insurance Program), which provides medical insurance coverage for children who are not eligible for Medicaid and are uninsured.

An alternative is to sign up for medical insurance through the Federal Insurance Exchange (healthcare.gov), made possible by the Affordable Care Act (also known as Obamacare) of 2010. By having medical insurance, your child will be able to get care from a variety of needed specialists. Many parents will qualify for a subsidy to help pay the insurance premiums if their income is low. (See Chapter 10 for more details.)

Parents who are in a difficult financial situation often take their acutely ill child to an emergency department (ED). Each time a child goes to the ED, she may be seen by a different physician, who most likely will be unaware of the child's specific health issues and therefore may not be able to provide the best care for the child. A series of visits to the ED is not a good way to provide medical care for any child, in part because it makes it impossible to coordinate care. Instead of relying on the ED, parents should find out where the local public health clinics are located.

State and local agencies such as the public health, social services, and health and social services departments can provide this information. Call the public health clinic to find out who manages the clinic and whether you would be required to pay for any service (there may or may not be fees associated with the service). It's very possible that you and your child could receive primary health care through a clinic program.

What can I expect my child's PCP to do?

The PCP may be a doctor, a physician assistant, or a nurse practitioner. The PCP should get to know your child and your family so that he or she will be able to integrate the child's care with the family's needs. The PCP should specifically be interested in observing the growth and development of your child and making certain that routine physicals are performed and immunizations are up to date. Usual childhood illnesses such as viral illnesses, ear infections, and rashes should all be treated by the PCP. Questions about specific problems should also be addressed first to the PCP. If your child has an illness that is very rare or very complex, the PCP may choose to consult with other specialists.

It is important not to try to diagnose your child. That is the job of the PCP. The Internet is a good tool for gathering information, but it should not be used as a source of medical advice. Many websites provide medical information, but it is hard to know which ones have information from experts. It is always best to talk with your PCP or specialist about any medical concerns you have and allow them to help you determine the correct diagnosis or path forward.

What should I do
if my child's PCP is
uncomfortable with my
child's condition?

Children with multiple or complex medical problems can be a challenge for a PCP, who is often under stress because he sees many patients and may have very limited time. Providing health care for your child should be a cooperative effort, in which both the family and the PCP share what they have learned about the child and the PCP continues to support the family and help them sort out complex and confusing issues. If the PCP is not willing to take the time to help the child or appears intimidated in dealing with the child who has a disability, it may be necessary to find another provider with whom you and your child can develop a good rapport.

Who should be my
child's PCP—a pediatri-
cian, a family physician,
a physician assistant, or
a nurse practitioner?

Family physicians have medical training that includes health care for children and adults, though usually their experience with children, especially children with disabilities, is limited. The advantage of having the family physician as your child's PCP is that he or she will have a broader view, one that includes all the members of the family. In this way, a family doctor may be more helpful to parents, because he or she can incorporate and deal with general family dynamics and monitor the effect of the disability on the different members of the family, especially the parents. In addition, the family physician will be able to continue as the PCP for the disabled child as he or she grows to adulthood, whereas many pediatricians stop seeing patients after a certain age (often, but not always, at age 21).

The advantage the pediatrician brings is more specialized training and experience in the problems of children, especially more training and experience in the problems of children with disabilities. If the family develops a comfortable relationship with the pediatrician, one that allows for a free and comprehensive exchange of information, then this is the person who ought to provide primary care for your child.

There are also physicians trained and certified in both pediatrics and internal medicine (called Med-Peds training). These physicians combine the advantages of the pediatrician and those of the family physician. Their training in pediatrics is far more extensive than that of the family physician, and they have an advantage over the pediatrician in that they can treat the entire family and continue to treat the disabled child into adulthood.

There are also nurse practitioners and physician assistants (PAs) who may work with any one of these physicians as part of their practice and can function as the PCP for your child. These nurses and PAs may also specialize in the care of children, and they often have a bit more time than the physician to answer questions and help provide training in procedures or specific care techniques.

In the end, parents have to find the physician or practice that best meets their needs. They must balance the medical knowledge and skills that the nurse or doctor brings with the willingness of the doctor or nurse or PA to spend the extra time needed in providing care to the disabled child and answering the family's questions.

How often does my child
need to see the PCP?

This depends on the problems and the nature of the child's disability. As a minimum, your child should be seen by his or her PCP at least as often as the schedule recommended by the American Academy of Pediatrics for well child care (at ages 2, 4, 6, 9, 12, 15, 18, 24, 30, and 36 months, then yearly thereafter). It is very important for children with disabilities to have a complete routine physical examination periodically and not to ignore check-up visits. Immunizations are often delayed and common childhood problems such as hernias and undescended testicles may be missed in children who visit the physician's office for acute problems but never undergo a full physical examination.

Which specialists does my newborn need?

If your child had significant medical problems at birth, he or she may have been admitted to a newborn intensive care unit (NICU), which is usually managed by a neonatologist, who is a pediatrician specializing in the care of ill newborn children. These specialists generally care for the infant with special needs until the infant leaves the intensive care nursery and goes home. They are the primary attending physicians during this period and consult other specialists as needed.

When the infant is discharged, the neonatologist generally transfers care to a PCP of the parent's choice in the community, although the neonatologist may also see the infant after discharge to follow up on any outstanding medical problems. Neonatologists are generally not involved in the child's care after the child reaches the age of 1 or 2.

When my child is first discharged from the hospital, what physician does he or she need to see?

After your child is discharged, you should follow up with your PCP. If specific problems were identified and evaluated in the intensive care nursery, such as breathing problems as a result of prematurity, your child may need to be followed up by other physicians as well. As your child grows and his or her needs change, referrals to other health care specialists may be needed. As noted earlier, the PCP and the family need to work together in making decisions about calling in specialists.

Who should check my child's eyes, and how often?

If the child was in intensive care as a newborn and exposed to oxygen, as many premature babies are, an ophthalmologist should check the child's eyes before he or she is sent home. For the infant who has no such history, assessing a child's vision is part of a routine physical examination performed by the primary physician. It may be difficult to get young children to cooperate during an eye examination, especially children who have spasticity or a variety of disabilities. If the extent of the child's visual abilities cannot be conclusively determined by the physical exam, then your child may need to visit an ophthalmologist or a neurological specialist to determine whether more sophisticated vision tests would be helpful.

Depending on what the examination or specialized tests reveal about the child's visual function, follow-up eye visits may be necessary. If the child is found to have normal eye function, then visual screening at school age is the usual next step. If significant disability is present, then follow-up as indicated by the specialist is appropriate. Ask your PCP about making a referral to an eye specialist if you are concerned that your child cannot see properly.

When should my child's hearing be tested?	The newborn's hearing is now routinely screened in nearly all newborn nurseries in the United States. As with vision, the child's hearing should be assessed as part of routine health visits to the PCP. If there is any question about the child's hearing, various tests can be done to clarify the level of function. Audiometric tests can be performed by an audiologist, for example, often in coordination with an ear, nose, and throat surgeon. If this isn't helpful, then a brainstem auditory evoked response (BAER) can be done. This is a special test that can be used even for a very young child. Discuss your concerns and questions with your PCP or case manager.
Who should I see concerning my child's difficulty with her arms, legs, or back?	The problems related to the bones and muscles are addressed by pediatric orthopedists. The pediatric orthopedist generally addresses deformities and problems with the functioning of the hands, arms, legs, and feet, as well as deformities of the spine such as scoliosis and kyphosis. This health care specialist attempts to improve alignments to make the child function better and works to *prevent* deformities as far as possible.

After a consultation or treatment with a pediatric orthopedist, it is generally best to schedule routine follow-up examinations, because a child's deformities change as the child grows. Follow-up with an orthopedist every six to twelve months is usually indicated, and it is preferable to follow up with a pediatric orthopedist who is interested in the child with CP (see table 6).

Table 6. Recommended Evaluations of Musculoskeletal Function in Children with Cerebral Palsy

Age 1–9 months. Newborn hip examination: Check for hypotonia, hypertonicity. Use ultrasound for any questionable abnormalities; refer to an orthopedist if there is any abnormality on the ultrasound.

Age 1–2 years. Hip abduction: Check with hip and knee extended. If the hip abduction is less than 45°, the hip should be x-rayed. If the child is not sitting independently, he or she needs to be fitted with adaptive seating for feeding and play. Refer the child for seating to a physical therapist, an occupational therapist, or a seating clinic.

Age 2–3 years. All children should now be standing. If the child is nonambulatory, he or she should be referred for a stander evaluation. Referral for orthotic assessment should be made by an orthopedist or a physiatrist. If the child is not walking without a device, a hip x-ray is needed.

Age 3–5 years. If the child is not walking without a device, the child should have a hip exam and x-ray every 12 months and an orthotic check every 6 months. Gait problems requiring assistive devices or orthotics should also be evaluated every 6 months by an orthopedist or a physiatrist.

Age 5–9 years. Orthopedic surgery, a baclofen pump, or a dorsal rhizotomy may be considered to improve gait. A power wheelchair prescription is usually considered first for a nonambulatory child. A child not walking without a device needs a hip x-ray each year.

Age 9–13 years. A hip x-ray should be given every two years if the hip x-ray remains normal; otherwise, an x-ray is needed every year or orthopedic intervention is needed. The child should be examined for scoliosis; x-ray if any spinal deformity is present.

Age 13–18 years. If the child is nonambulatory, progressive scoliosis requires fusion. If the child is ambulatory, final surgical gait correction is needed. In either case, the child should be seen yearly by an orthopedist or physiatrist.

Who will tell me what kind of bracing my child needs?	Recommendations for bracing vary, depending on the child's problems and on the specialist making the recommendation. A physical therapist may assess a child for the possible benefits of bracing the legs, and an occupational therapist evaluates and makes braces for the child's hands and arms. The orthopedist or physiatrist (physical medicine specialist) usually evaluates the child and writes the prescriptions for bracing. In some communities, pediatric physiatrists routinely follow children with CP and prescribe braces. In other communities, pediatric orthopedists routinely follow patients and provide brace prescriptions.

If the child is followed only by a physiatrist, the physiatrist must be a pediatric physiatrist who is familiar with all types of deformities and who will actively monitor the child for the development of problems that will need an orthopedic surgeon, such as hip dislocation and scoliosis. If the child is followed by a pediatric orthopedist, then the pediatric orthopedist should pay attention to the child's bracing and seating needs. In some circumstances, therapists recommend braces and PCPs write the orders. This situation is less than ideal, because few PCPs fully understand the appropriateness of the brace. |
Who should evaluate my child's seating and recommend an appropriate chair?	Seating is much like bracing, in that it involves the disciplines of physical therapy, occupational therapy, orthopedics, and physiatry. In ordering a chair it is important to take into consideration the family's needs as well as the child's. (On the appropriateness of wheelchairs, see Chapters 6 and 7, as well as "Choosing Appropriate Seating" and "About Wheelchair Maintenance" in Part 2.)
Which specialist should treat seizures in a child?	Some PCPs are comfortable testing and treating children who have seizures, but most will want to refer your child to a specialist. Children with a first-time seizure would be referred to a pediatric neurologist, a physician who specializes in treating illnesses of the nervous system in children. Seizures that are easy to control and for which no specific cause has been found might continue to be treated and followed up by the child's PCP. Seizures caused by fevers (called febrile seizures) are limited to one or a few episodes and do not need treatment. These can be evaluated and followed up by your PCP. (For more information about seizures, see Chapter 3.)
Does my child need to see a specialist to follow up on a cerebral shunt?	The surgery to place a shunt in the brain to drain excess fluid from the ventricles of the brain is performed by a neurosurgeon (see the section "Hydrocephalus" in Chapter 3). There are pediatric neurosurgeons who specialize in treating children, but many neurosurgeons treat both adults and children. The child with a shunt may be followed by a pediatric neurologist or a pediatrician, and if there are no problems a neurosurgical evaluation every one to two years is a good course of treatment. If the shunt functions well, more frequent follow-up is not necessary.

My child has problems with swallowing and poor weight gain. What kind of doctor do we need?

The PCP should be the first to evaluate this type of problem. He or she may make a referral to a specialist—a developmental pediatrician, for example, who specializes in the evaluation of these problems—to help evaluate swallowing function and poor weight gain. The developmental pediatrician often works with a team, who participate in the evaluation. The team may include a dietitian, who can evaluate how much nourishment your child is actually getting and how much he needs; a speech pathologist or an occupational therapist, who is trained to evaluate swallowing; the staff of an x-ray department, who can perform special tests, such as x-ray swallowing tests; and a pediatric gastroenterologist, who can evaluate your child's gastrointestinal system. Swallowing and weight gain problems can be very complicated to treat, but treatment is exceedingly important to the child's growth, and therefore it is important to make use of a full team of specialists. (See Chapter 3 for more details of this problem.)

Who should my child see if he vomits frequently?

This is another situation that should first be brought to the attention of your child's PCP. If referral is needed, the PCP will probably recommend that your child see a gastroenterologist. Chronic or recurrent vomiting is best evaluated by a pediatric gastroenterologist, who specializes in caring for the gastrointestinal system and may utilize tests such as endoscopy (looking into the stomach) and a pH probe. If a problem such as gastrointestinal reflux is identified and medicine can't control it, then a pediatric general surgeon may be called in to perform a surgical procedure to correct it. Pediatric radiology specialists are also called upon to perform sophisticated x-ray tests and to evaluate the function of the stomach and intestines (see Chapter 3 for more details).

Who should clean my child's teeth and how often?

The first dental visit should occur no more than 6 months after the first tooth erupts or no later than age 12 months. After that, the visits should be every 6 months. This schedule is important for the child with CP because of issues with chewing, normal saliva flow, and swallowing. The professional cleaning and evaluation for any cavities or gum problems that the child receives at a regular dental visit are also important. If your family dentist is not comfortable treating a child with a disability, then your child should be referred to a pediatric dentist, called a *pedodontist*. These dentists specialize in the dental care of children, including children with disabilities. If your child has gum overgrowth, he or she may be referred to a specialist who can treat the condition.

Who can help me with my child's severe constipation?

Severe constipation can be a difficult problem. It is a problem seen frequently in children with CP. It is important to bring this problem to the attention of your PCP so he or she can monitor and treat your child. If your PCP is not comfortable treating this problem in children with CP, your child should be referred to a developmental pediatrician specializing in the care of such children or to a pediatric gastroenterologist, who will be able to set up a program to help with this problem.

Who can help with
toilet training?

Often, special education teachers and school nurses and therapists can suggest a routine that can be used in toilet training children with disabilities. They can describe a routine for you or provide a written explanation of what's involved. You can also request information from your PCP or a developmental pediatrician. (See also "Toilet Training Your Child" in Part 2.)

If your child resists behavioral attempts at toilet training for urine and is believed to be cognitively able, then an evaluation by a pediatric urologist may be suggested. He or she can test your child's bladder function and abilities to make certain that a physical problem is not causing problems with incontinence in your child.

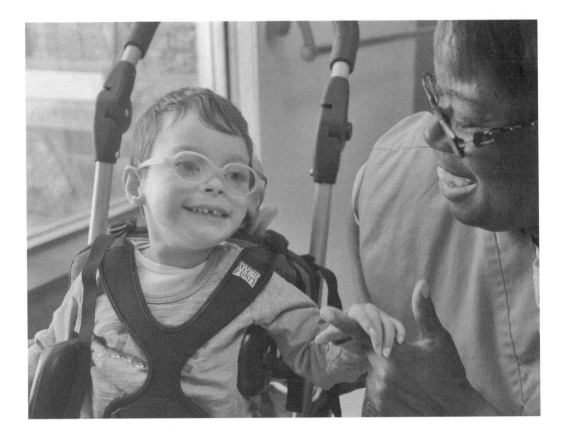

Financing Care for the Child with Cerebral Palsy

IN THE PAST, the cost of caring for a person with a chronic condition was extraordinary compared with the cost of caring for a person who did not have a chronic condition. Typically families bore the brunt of the costs in the form of high deductibles, premiums, and caps. In the age of health care reform and the Affordable Care Act (ACA), much has changed. This chapter is a starting point for families and individuals seeking information about how to afford health care for a loved one who has a chronic condition.

How is health care financed?

Health care is paid for in a variety of ways. Most often individuals are provided coverage through private health insurance (commercial employer-sponsored or self-employed), government-sponsored programs (Medicaid or Medicare), out-of-pocket funds, or charitable or philanthropic organizations.

How much of the cost does the family cover?

It depends on what type of insurance you have. With private insurance, when you choose a plan, you agree to the cost of premiums (the amount you pay each pay period) and deductibles (the amount you will pay before the insurance picks up any of the cost) that will best fit your family's anticipated needs. Families who do not frequently need health care may choose a low-premium, high-deductible plan. Families who need more extensive services may choose a high-premium, low-deductible plan. It is up to you to decide what is best for your family's needs. Government-funded programs like Medicaid and Medicare tend to absorb more of the costs and may charge the patient nothing, or just a nominal co-pay. Commercial plans may not cover any care that is considered custodial and that does not warrant a certain level of medical need. Government programs may cover some or all of custodial or medically necessary care.

What is private health insurance?

Private health insurance is insurance provided for by private individual or group funds (such as from an employer), as opposed to insurance offered by public funding through a government unit or agency (Medicare, for example). For the most part, private health insurance that covers a dependent child's medical expenses is group coverage that is part of the parent's work benefits package. Group coverage private insurance of this type can be a fee-for-service plan that pays for the service after the service is provided or a managed care type of insurance. Typically, a group insurance program obtained through employment is more generous with benefits, but this must be evaluated by the family. The Affordable Care Act eliminated a company's ability to deny a person insurance based on a preexisting condition. The ACA extended the age of coverage to 26 years old. This means that a child can remain covered under his parent's insurance until he is 26 even if he is married, working, or not in school.

Managed care came into existence to deal with rising health care costs. Its primary purpose is to contain costs (this is known as *cost containment*). Currently, many policies are administered through a primary care physician, who makes necessary referrals to other health care professionals. Many policies include specific physicians within the "network" of the plan, and patient-subscribers are fully covered only if they are treated by those physicians. Some policies allow for treatment by physicians who are considered "out of the network," or privately chosen, but the patient bears an additional expense for consulting these physicians. Sometimes private insurance companies have a *disabled child clause*, which allows the adult child with CP to remain covered indefinitely as long as the parent keeps the same insurance. Be sure to confirm this with your employer and your insurance company. If an employer is changing group insurance companies, it would be wise to check on continued dependent coverage prior to the plan change. If a person with CP is a full-time employee of a company providing group benefits, she cannot be discriminated against and must be offered *all* of the programs (medical, dental, pensions, and short- and long-term disability) that are available to other employees.

The scope of coverage and the benefits available in private health insurance vary significantly from policy to policy and from group to group and can often be confusing. It is critically important for parents to check policy provisions. Parents seeking employment should carefully check on the benefits offered. Employers who self-insure can make their own plan provisions.

What services are covered under private insurance, and what are the limitations?

Each policy must be read carefully and judged separately. No assumptions can be made about the extent of coverage. The family must investigate their own coverage and become knowledgeable about their benefits before they incur large costs. The employee should consult with the personnel office or the office that oversees administration of the health insurance plan for assistance in understanding benefits and gaining access to them. Commonly covered expenses include such things as a hospital room, surgeons' and physicians' services provided in a hospital, and outpatient diagnostic tests, such as x-rays.

Private health insurance may be adequate when a child's needs are limited to basic physicians' services and basic hospital services. When the child with a disability has multiple needs that include both community and home service and care, however, private insurance may not provide enough financial protection. States may offer a disabled child a medical assistance program if the out-of-pocket costs of commercial insurance are too high for your family.

What do I need to know about any health insurance policy I'm considering?

Deductible clauses, co-insurance, maximum benefit levels, and limits on out-of-pocket liability are the four parts of any health insurance policy that require close scrutiny. You want to understand how much you may have to pay in any given year if your child is healthy or if your child requires a lot of medical attention and services. A deductible is the amount of money a family must pay before the insurance company will pay anything. When considering an insurance policy, evaluate what the deductible will mean to you in terms of out-of-pocket costs. Co-insurance is the portion of charges that must be paid by the family after the deductible portion has been met. It is not uncommon for the family to bear 20 percent of hospital, physician, and related fees even after the deductibles have been met. The ACA eliminated the ability for an insurance plan to limit the maximum amount it would pay in a year or a lifetime for any covered member, for ten essential benefits. A few insurance plans have been grandfathered in, so they can still have maximum limits. You should check to make sure that your plan has no such maximum limit.

The limit on out-of-pocket liability, as provided in a *stop-loss clause*, is the limit the insurance company imposes on the family's out-of-pocket expenses for a given calendar year before the insurance company pays 100 percent of further covered charges. Covered charges vary from policy to policy, and the family must not assume that a specific treatment is subject to this limit without first verifying this with the insurance company.

If my insurance will not cover all my expenses, can I purchase more insurance?

Yes, but insurance policies covering a broad range of catastrophic problems are very expensive. You can also go to healthcare.gov to shop around for better insurance plans or to add coverage if you feel it is necessary.

Are there limitations for services in commercial plans?

The Affordable Care Act requires that insurances cover *essential benefits*. These include outpatient services; emergency services; hospitalizations; pregnancy, maternity, and newborn care; mental health and substance abuse services; prescription drugs; rehabilitation services and devices; laboratory services; preventative and wellness services and chronic disease management; and pediatric services. Oral and dental care must be covered until age 18, so check your plan to see if it extends beyond age 18.

What limitations can the insurance company impose on care or treatment?

The insurance company may recommend that you seek treatment from one of its preferred providers, usually within its network, who agree to provide service at a predetermined cost. If you agree to use a preferred provider, the insurance company pays the physician a higher percentage of covered charges—approximately 90 percent instead of 80 percent.

Insurance companies often require a second surgical opinion. In certain types of surgical cases, a second opinion must be obtained or the insurance company will not pay the full benefit. Often, the second opinion must come from one of the company's preferred providers.

What do HMOs provide?

Health maintenance organizations (HMOs) are a form of managed care. They can be both insurers and providers of care; they offer prepaid health plans. Employers may provide HMOs as part of their benefits package, in which case a monthly premium is paid by the employer, with the employee usually contributing a specific dollar amount to the premium as well. HMOs usually provide preventive services as a benefit, while most fee-for-service programs do not. Families select a primary care physician within the plan, who then authorizes required care from other physicians or hospitals within the plan or network. The idea is to keep all needed services within the network in order to keep costs under control. If a referral is made to a physician outside of the plan or network, there is no way of controlling charges, because the plan does not have a contract with that physician.

What government assistance is available?

Medicaid, also known as Medical Assistance, is a program of federal grants to states that pays for certain health services for eligible people. Known by different names in different states (such as TennCare in Tennessee and Equality-Care in Wyoming), Medicaid is run by the states; a percentage of the costs is funded by the federal government. The eligibility criteria, which are specific to each state, are based on financial need. Each state may add services over and above those required by the federal law. Medicaid eligibility also differs in the pediatric and adult systems. When the child is under age 18, his or her parent's income and/or assets may prevent the child from qualifying for Medicaid. Some states have special disabled children's Medicaid, which is based on the severity of the child's condition and does not consider the parent's income and assets. When a child with CP reaches age 18, the income and assets of the child (not of parents) become the critical factor in determining eligibility.

What kinds of services are covered by Medicaid?

Generally, inpatient hospital care, physicians' and other outpatient services, skilled nursing services, and lab tests are covered by Medicaid. Coverage of things such as medications, home health care, eyeglasses, and dental care are determined by the individual state. Investigate the limits of Medicaid coverage in your state. Medicaid regulations change from time to time because of budgetary constraints and use of resources, and Congress continues to reform laws with respect to eligibility, reimbursement, and benefits.

For children highly dependent on technology who might otherwise remain in the hospital to receive skilled nursing care, Medicaid has a program for those seeking greater independence that is aimed at reducing the costs of hospitalization and decreasing unnecessary hospital stays. Referred to as the Medicaid Home and Community Based Waiver, the program pays for the needed care, but the care is given in the home or in a community setting certified to provide such services, such as a group home. Because eligibility requirements vary from state to state, you'll need to call your Medicaid office or social services department for assistance in determining whether your child can benefit from this program.

Medicaid also covers long-term care. Benefits vary among the states, and in order for an individual to be eligible, his or her assets must be below $2,000. Some people try to rid themselves of (or spend down) their assets to qualify. This "spend down" can be avoided by creating a *special needs trust* and transferring the person's assets to this trust. Some states now require a person to be eligible for Medicaid in order to receive intellectual/developmental disabilities (I/DD) services. Therefore, if your child has more than $2,000 in assets in his name and you anticipate that he might need long-term care services or Medicaid in the future, consider creating a special needs trust now. (For more about special needs trusts and estate planning, see "Life Planning Process" in Part 2.)

Medicaid eligibility is required to access some services. Many families have indicated that the services offered do not meet their child's unique needs, and therefore many states have waivers. Waivers allow services in addition to those Medicaid routinely offers, effectively "waiving" traditional services and electing other services. States can have multiple waivers, so it is important to ask your child's case manager about the waiver options and eligibility so you can decide how best to meet your child's and your family's needs.

What is nursing home insurance?

This is insurance that would cover basic care in a nursing home or other long-term care (LTC) environment. Some policies may include coverage for long-term skilled care, but the operating word is *skilled*. *Skilled care* means that the individual requires nursing care under the policy definition of nursing. The cost of long-term care for individuals who require custodial care rather than nursing care will not be covered. Custodial care is rarely covered by insurance policies. LTC is getting more expensive as elderly citizens continue to live longer. This coverage is far more affordable if parents have the foresight to purchase this type of policy prior to age 65. In addition, it is important that those buying LTC are willing to go to a nursing home. Anyone who is unwilling to live in a nursing home would be wasting his money. An alternative is an *at home care policy*. These policies typically are less expensive. Many provide for both professional services and services provided by a family member or friend.

Are there other programs for children with special needs?

Yes. Under Title V of the Social Security Act, every state has a program for children with special health care needs. These programs are included under the Maternal and Child Health (MCH) Block Grant Program and provide case management and other health services such as nursing, social work, and physical and other therapies to eligible children with chronic illness. Each state sets its own eligibility criteria and its own list of services covered. Information on programs for children with special health care needs may be found at the local office of the state health department.

What is SSI?

Supplemental Security Income (SSI) is an income support program for aged, blind, and disabled adults and for children with disabilities. Eligible children live in low-income households (with less than $2,000 in assets and less than $2,100 per month in income) and must meet the SSI disability criteria. If a child is eligible to receive SSI, health care services are received through Medicaid. Contact the local office of the Social Security Administration (SSA) to determine eligibility. The SSA requires documentation regarding your assets, income, and age and the child's age. The adult with a disability is reviewed independently of the family. Adults with CP who have limited assets and are unemployed or underemployed may qualify for SSI funding.

SSI eligibility for children under 18 is based on the parents' income and assets as well as the child's. After age 18 it is based solely on the income, assets, and medical eligibility requirements of the adult with CP. Parents face the problem of how to keep their child eligible throughout his lifetime. Certified special needs planners should be consulted for assistance. Most financial planners, insurance agents, and attorneys are not familiar with or qualified to advise on the proper way to protect assets for a person with a developmental disability. Through proper special needs planning, parents will be able to pass on assets for their child's care and have these assets protected from being used to reimburse the government for Medicaid services received by the child. Without proper planning, it is possible that the child will become ineligible for Medicaid when receiving assets from family members. In addition, if a proper will has not been prepared by parents, at their death the state of residence for the person with CP will appoint his or her guardian and trustees and decide who gets the parents' assets. Medicaid could immediately take assets received by the person with special needs for reimbursement. Grandparents also need to be part of this planning, because their will can negate a properly prepared plan by parents. (To learn more about special needs trusts and estate planning, see "Life Planning Process" in Part 2.)

What is CHIP?

The Balanced Budget Act of 1997 established the Children's Health Insurance Program (CHIP), which gives grants to states to provide health insurance coverage to uninsured children living in families whose income is at or below 200 percent of the federal poverty level. States may provide this coverage by expanding Medicaid or by expanding or creating a state children's health insurance program. The legislation sets eligibility criteria. States can decide to cover all of those children or to target a narrower group of children. The eligibility criteria are to cover uninsured children who are

- not eligible for Medicaid;
- under age 19; and
- at or below 200 percent of the federal poverty level.

Where can I get information on these and other programs?

For the most part, it is up to you to pursue support that may be available to your child. Some people who may be helpful include your child's PCP, community and public health nurses and social workers, teachers, members of voluntary organizations, and members of your local Developmental Disabilities Council. You can also contact the various departments listed in the appropriate chapters of this book, as well as the organizations listed in the Resources section at the end of the book. "Managing the System" in Part 2 may also provide useful information.

Who can help me find resources to help my child?

You will find that other parents are a phenomenal source of knowledge, wisdom, and support. Every state has a chapter of Family Voices, a grass-roots organization run by parents who have children with special health care needs. Call on Family Voices for information on state programs and eligibility, insurance questions, advocacy support, and general information. Because the members of Family Voices are all parents, they understand the maze you are faced with and know the importance of timely, accurate information.

Professionals who work with children and adults with disabilities can be very helpful. If they do not have an answer for you, they can usually refer you to someone who does. Search the Internet for keywords such as *cerebral palsy*, *developmental disability, intellectual disability, support, services, family*, and the name of your state. Every state has a federally mandated Developmental Disabilities Council. You can check out their website or call them for resources. As you'll soon discover, there are many ways to gather information on resources and programs, services, and agencies, but it is mostly up to you to do the investigating. There is no "one-stop shopping." Every state also has education advocates for students with disabilities. You can search the Internet for your state's Parent Training and Information (PTI) Center, which specializes in education law, IEPs (Individualized Education Programs), 504 plans, accommodations, and parent support.

Many associations can provide a list of resources available for people with cerebral palsy. One of these, United Cerebral Palsy (UCP), is listed in the phone book and on the web under "United Cerebral Palsy." Each region has a chapter that can provide information on local resources. One thing to remember is that community agencies usually are knowledgeable only about the services offered in their community. If you require broader information, you will have to contact federal agencies or the national headquarters of UCP.

It is often helpful to contact the offices of your state senator, assemblyperson, federal congressperson, and other politicians for assistance in locating the governmental office that can help you gain access to services. It's a good idea to keep a log of all contacts. Record the names, phone numbers, addresses, and days and times called. Indicate whether the office was helpful and what your conversations were about. You may not need the agency at the present time, but you should tuck the information away for future reference.

Group activities and support groups are valuable for a number of reasons. For one thing, the people who attend can share resource information with you. While getting out of the house one night a week to attend a support group may not seem like the most exciting use of your time, it is a good way to find out from other parents what kind of help they are getting and how they are getting it. Additionally, the emotional support, both given and received, can be of great value. Many agencies offer parent and/or family support or respite opportunities. If you can't attend all the meetings, at least try to attend a few. Get to know other parents. You may learn a lot from them. Your local children's hospital may also have a list of family support opportunities.

What organizations in the private sector provide help for families?

Many agencies provide a multitude of services and supports based on age or other criteria. You can find a list of these provider agencies through your state Office of Intellectual/Developmental Disabilities, a division of your state Department of Health and Human Services. Additionally, look at diagnosis-specific groups, such as United Cerebral Palsy, the Brain Injury Association, and similar organizations, to find additional options. Private agencies offer a wide range of services and assistance, such as residential day programs, recreation services, home case management, and respite services. Call these agencies to find out about the scope of services they offer and whether you would benefit from them.

From time to time as you look for services, you may come across a fund available for specific purposes. This may be a scholarship fund or a fund for vacations for people with special needs, for example. Finding these opportunities requires persistence. When conducting an online search, try to list as many characteristics of your child and his or her situation as you can. This will help you uncover less common scholarships, grants, and funding sources.

You may also want to consider fundraising on your own. If you are interested in fundraising, the sky seems to be the limit in terms of what people will do for you and offer to you. Parents and friends of children with cerebral palsy have organized all sorts of community activities, from car washes, school dances, and marathons to direct solicitation of donations in containers at local convenience stores. Parents have mailed out letters to every organization imaginable in an attempt to obtain donations for equipment, health care, special schooling, and communication devices not covered by their insurance plans. An effort of this magnitude requires a good deal of work and persistence. It is common today for families to try online fundraising too. Furthermore, it is critical for individual fundraisers to work only within the legal guidelines established by the federal and state governments. You needn't be dissuaded by these guidelines; you only need to be aware of them and follow them.

Are there social service agencies I can call for assistance?

Your state Office of Intellectual/Developmental Disabilities is a good starting point. The office often lists its providers for residential, vocational, respite care, and family supports. Many agencies provide a variety of services. Some services are provided by more than one agency, while others aren't provided by any agency. Your state or local department of social services can offer a great deal of guidance about how to proceed on a variety of issues. Many but not all states have a book listing available services and agency offices that is available to the public for a price. It gives an excellent accounting of all the human service agencies involved in the care of individuals in a particular state or region.

Contact the Developmental Disabilities Council in your area for information. To locate the one nearest you, contact the National Association of Developmental Disabilities Councils. Groups like United Cerebral Palsy, Easter Seals, and the March of Dimes can direct you to appropriate local services. All social service agencies are community specific, meaning that the organization and administration of the services and the channeling of funds are unique to each region. Contact your local agencies for help.

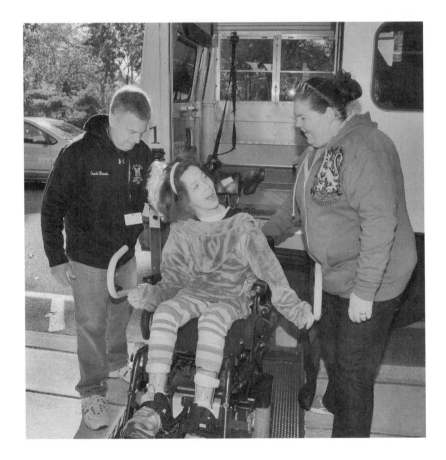

Navigating the Educational System

THIS CHAPTER discusses issues related to the education of children with disabilities. Much of the material in this chapter comes from federal public laws and regulations, which can be accessed from a number of sources, some of which are identified at the end of this chapter and in the Resources section at the end of this book. Among the most helpful to parents is the Center for Parent Information and Resources (CPIR), which houses many of the resources previously maintained by the National Dissemination Center for Children with Disabilities (NICHCY), a federally funded project that ceased operation in September 2014. Other resources may be found at a regional Parent Technical Assistance Center (six nationally), at the state Parent Training and Information Center or Community Parent Resource Center (find your state center at http://www.parentcenterhub.org/find-your-center), or at UCP, with centers throughout the country. These organizations provide information to parents, often in both English and Spanish, which will help them help their child.

The inclusion of children with disabilities in public schools or the opportunity to participate in publicly supported education, currently assured under the Individuals with Disabilities Education Act (IDEA), is now a decades-old phenomenon. Federal laws requiring public schools to provide "free and appropriate public education" to children with disabilities originated in 1970 with the passage of the Education of the Handicapped Act (EHA). This act established minimum requirements with which states had to comply to receive federal financial assistance. The amendment of the EHA in 1975 as the Education of All Handicapped Children Act (EAHCA, Public Law 94-142) marked a watershed in providing many important legal protections that remain intact today. These protections have been carried into its subsequent revisions and renaming as the Individuals with Disabilities Education Act first in 1990, then again in 1997, and most recently in 2004 as the Individuals with Disabilities Education Improvement Act.

Core principles of Public Law 94-142 that survive through IDEA and its reauthorizations ensure that students who are determined eligible for special education are provided an appropriate educational program and have access to the same educational opportunities as students who do not have a disability in the "least restrictive environment" possible for them to achieve academic success. It also ensures that parents participate in the decision making about their child's education with full due process guarantees, including written notices in an understandable language, requirements for informed consent, access to educational records, "stay put" rights during dispute resolution, and ultimately access to civil action if due process is not satisfactory. Over the years, and with the last reauthorization in 2004, goals have focused on strengthening the role of parents in working in partnership with educational professionals, ensuring access to the general education curriculum with the participation of students with disabilities in statewide assessments (to align with the No Child Left Behind Act of 2001), encouraging use of mediation to settle disagreements between parents and educators, increasing the focus on effectiveness of teaching and learning, and reducing paperwork requirements.

Important highlights of the reauthorization of IDEA in 2004 included emphasis on the importance of positive behavioral supports and the use of behavioral reinforcement as a component in a student's individualized plan. It also provides funds for teacher training in this area. The bill for the first time includes consequences for schools that fail to comply with IDEA, with the possible loss of some federal funding for schools found to be in noncompliance with the law for more than two years. Another provision prohibits school officials from forcing parents to medicate their children as a condition for attending school. Eligibility for special education services must be based on many components of a student's life, not just test scores

States are required to have policies that guarantee certain procedural safeguards. These ensure that parents are provided with the information they need to make decisions regarding which services their child will need and in which setting he will be educated and that procedures are in place to resolve disagreements between parties. Congress recognized that families should have "meaningful opportunities to participate in the education of their children at school and at home."

Features of IDEA include the following:

- Free and appropriate public education is to be provided to *all* children with disabilities, regardless of the severity of the disability.
- As much as possible, children with disabilities must be educated in settings with children who do not have disabilities.
- Age limits are established for children to receive educational services.
- Services the child will receive must be defined and periodically reviewed at least annually.
- Mechanisms by which this program must be carried out are stipulated.
- Mechanisms for conflict resolution between parent and professional are in place.

The term *special education* in the context of the law and entitlement to services means specially designed instruction, at no cost to parents, to meet the unique needs of the child with a disability. This can include (1) instruction conducted in the classroom, in special schools, in the home, in hospitals, and in other settings; and (2) instruction in physical education. In all cases, eligibility for special education services centers on whether the child can succeed in the general education program with supplementary aids and supports. If the answer is no, then the terms of this law apply.

Children who are eligible for special education services have the right to a clearly written Individualized Education Program (IEP). The IEP is the keystone of the process that assures an appropriate education for each child. It is the document that responds to the strengths and needs identified in the child's evaluation. It reports the student's current level of function and progress, describes the child's needs for specially designed instruction (which might include curriculum modification, specialized equipment, and individualized techniques), annual goals, and how progress toward those goals will be measured and reported to parents. Also included in the IEP document are related services and supports that will be provided; transportation; the extent of participation in programs for students without disabilities; what, if any, modifications will be necessary in the administration of statewide assessment of student achievement; and, beginning at age 14, the inclusion of transition planning as a part of the process. Additional related services may include speech-language pathology and audiology services; psychological services; physical and occupational therapy; recreation, including therapeutic recreation; social work services; counseling services, including rehabilitation counseling; orientation and mobility services; and medical services (for diagnostic and evaluation purposes only) in order for the child to benefit from the education program.

The IEP is developed jointly by parents and school personnel at a meeting convened at a mutually convenient time. Parents have the right to be included and to approve the educational plans for their child, or if there is not agreement, they also have the right, through a due process procedure, to appeal any decisions made about identification, evaluation, and placement of their child.

Specific health-related services may be included as a school district obligation under IDEA, according to the findings of two US Supreme Court cases. In 1984, *Irving Independent School District v. Tatro* established that the medical service exclusion of IDEA did not apply when "clean intermittent catheterization" was necessary for the student to benefit from the special education program and could be performed by a nurse or other qualified person, not necessarily a physician. More recently, in 1999, the Court determined in *Cedar Rapids Community School District v. Garret F.* (Garret F. was a special education student and also ventilator-dependent) that the school district was responsible for providing full-time nursing services at school, citing justifications similar to those in the Tatro case. Specifically, because someone other than a physician could administer the services needed by this young man, he was entitled to receive them as related services that were not subject to the medical exclusion of IDEA.

IDEA requires that states provide public education for children with disabilities aged 3 to 21 no matter how severe the disabilities. Preschool services for children with disabilities or developmental delay are available with the same requirements, protections, and rights that are assured to school-aged students under IDEA, with services available through the public education system.

Early intervention services for infants and toddlers birth to age three and their families are administered at the state level under part C of IDEA. Assistance is provided when an infant or toddler is experiencing delays in the areas of cognitive, physical, communication, social, emotional, or adaptive development or when an infant or toddler has been diagnosed with a physical or intellectual disability that has a high probability of resulting in developmental delay (being "at risk"). Specific eligibility for services is set by each state and often differs from eligibility for special education under Part B of IDEA, affecting children aged 3 to 21. Moreover, services are not necessarily free. They will make use of public and private insurance and community services and can include an adjusted fee for services. In addition, services must be provided in "natural environments," which include home and community settings in which children without disabilities participate.

Individualized plans for infants and toddlers as well as for their families are determined at a meeting that is similar to the IEP meeting for school-aged students. An important difference is that the Individualized Family Service Plan (IFSP) is also intended to assist the family in meeting their child's developmental needs.

The process of determining whether a child is eligible to receive special education services begins with a full, individual, and appropriate evaluation that may be the result of a parent's or the school's request. If the school makes the request, parents must be asked for their written approval to evaluate their child, and they must be given notice of their right to object. Similarly, if a parent requests the evaluation, the school may deny the evaluation, but it must assure the parents of their due process rights to continue to pursue evaluation and possible eligibility for special education services. In certain circumstances, an additional evaluation by an independent evaluator may be warranted, in which case there may be no charge to parents. The purpose of this evaluation for students already in the education system is to gather information related to the child's progress in the general education curriculum, to determine the educational needs of the child, and to determine whether the child needs special education and related services. One of the purposes of reevaluation is to review and evaluate the need for continuing special education services. Some students require special education supports for only a short time.

Students who have significant and/or complex disabilities should be evaluated and identified for early intervention before they are school aged. The evaluation and appropriate evaluators are determined by the needs of the child. If the child appears to have only cognitive delays, a certified school psychologist may be the only evaluator. If the child has motor delays, a physical and/or occupational therapist may need to be part of the evaluation, together with a speech-language therapist if there are communication and/or feeding needs.

What is the definition in these laws of a child with a disability?

IDEA defines a "child with a disability" as a child

(i) with mental retardation [cognitive impairment], hearing impairments (including deafness), speech or language impairments, visual impairments (including blindness), serious emotional disturbance (referred to in this title as 'emotional disturbance'), orthopedic impairments, autism, traumatic brain injury, other health impairments, or specific learning disabilities; and

(ii) who, by reason thereof, needs special education and related services.

What are the confidentiality protections that must be provided to my child and family?

The Buckley Amendment (Public Law 93-380), also known as the Family Educational Rights and Privacy Act (FERPA), gives parents of students under age of 18 and students 18 and older access to the student's educational record. This law also gives parents and students the right to review the record and to receive a copy of it. They have the right to a full explanation of the contents of the record. If they believe the record is inaccurate or misleading, they can ask that it be changed. School personnel may not destroy any part of the record if there is a pending request to review its contents. If there is a disagreement about the record, then the parents must be advised of their rights to a due process hearing. This might happen if the parents requested that the record be changed and the school objected to changing it, in which case the school must tell the parents that they have the right to a due process hearing.

The schools have the right to release part of the record to certain other education and social service agencies without parental permission. A record of all requests and a listing of the parts of the record that were released are included in the student's record. The schools are obligated by law to communicate with parents and students in their primary language even if that language is not English.

Certain school activities involving a special education student's health information are required to be carried out in ways that protect confidentiality and comply with the Health Insurance Portability and Accountability Act (HIPAA) of 1996. The extension of HIPAA to students requires schools to ensure that safeguards are in place for the disclosure and electronic transmission of "protected health information." However, a student's health information that is considered part of the official education record of that student and covered by FERPA is not "covered" by HIPAA. The US Supreme Court decision in *Falvo v. Owasso Independent. School District* (2001) provides further guidance by narrowing the definition of educational records to those maintained by the school district or other school entity, extending FERPA protections only to those records. The confidentiality rules will vary based on whether or not the records are "educational."

What other education laws apply to children with CP?

One other such law is the Carl D. Perkins Vocational and Technical Education Act of 1998, which provides funding for secondary and postsecondary vocational training while the students are still in school. Its purpose is to develop more fully the academic, vocational, and technical skills of secondary and postsecondary students.

In accordance with this law, vocational education programs and activities must be organized in the least restrictive environment, and these activities must be part of the IEP. This law gives disabled students equal access to a full range of programs available to nondisabled students, including apprenticeship programs, career guidance and counseling, cooperative education programs, and occupationally oriented courses of study.

What are the provisions for early intervention?

Early intervention services are designed to address the developmental needs of eligible infants and toddlers, birth through age 2, who have an identified disability, experience delays, or are at risk of becoming developmentally delayed. Importantly, assistance to the families of eligible infants and toddlers is also integral to this program. IDEA was initially enacted in 1986, then updated in 2004 and 2011. Early intervention is authorized by Part C of IDEA and specifically addresses the significant brain development that occurs during a child's first three years of life; and enhancing the capacity of state and local agencies and service providers to identify, evaluate, and meet the needs of all children, particularly minority, low-income, inner city, and rural children and infants and toddlers in foster care. The services may be offered in the home, or they may be center-based. The child should have access to the same related services that are provided by IDEA: occupational therapy, physical therapy, speech-language therapy, school health services, social work, and so on.

Check with your state department of education to learn about the programs available in your state. It may also be useful to contact other relevant departments (public instruction, education, health, and social services) in your state to find out which agency is primarily responsible for implementing the law.

What does the "Lawyer's Fees" Bill of 1986 provide?

In 1986 Congress addressed the issue of parents' recovery of attorney's fees for successful special education claims made under IDEA. The "Lawyer's Fees" Bill of the Handicapped Children's Protection Act provides that in a legal dispute brought by the parents over special education placement, if the parents win the suit, the courts may order the school district or the state to pay the parents' legal fees.

What about the Rehabilitation Act of 1973 (section 504) and the Americans with Disabilities Act of 1990?

These two compatible federal laws exist to prohibit discrimination against individuals with disabilities in employment programs or services if that individual is otherwise qualified to participate. Section 504 provides that "no . . . qualified individual [with a disability] . . . shall, solely by reason of his [disability], be excluded from participation in, be denied the benefits of, or be subjected to discrimination under any program or activity receiving . . . federal financial assistance." Under both acts, a person with a disability is defined as any person with a physical or mental impairment that substantially limits one or more major life activities. Discrimination against such a person is prohibited by any group or activities receiving federal funds. These include programs and activities that provide vocational training or education, public and private colleges, public and private day care centers, preschool programs, public and private elementary schools, and public and private adult programs. Employers and service providers must make an effort to make their services, facilities, and programs accessible to individuals with disabilities.

The Americans with Disabilities Act guarantees individuals with disabilities equal access to transportation, public accommodations, state and local government services, employment, and telecommunications. Employers must provide reasonable accommodations to individuals with disabilities, such as restructuring or modifying jobs or equipment, as long as those accommodations do not impose undue hardship on the company. Public transportation must be accessible to people with disabilities. Special transportation services must be made available to those who cannot use fixed route bus transit unless this poses an undue burden on public transportation.

Private establishments like restaurants, stores, and hotels cannot discriminate. Physical barriers to access must be removed, or another means of access must be arranged. (This means that these establishments must install ramps for wheelchairs, doors wide enough to accommodate wheelchairs, bathrooms that can accommodate wheelchairs, elevators with buttons in Braille, and so on, unless to do so imposes an unusual economic hardship.) All new construction must be accessible.

What are the implications of the No Child Left Behind Act for children in special education?

Although not specifically designed for special education, the federal No Child Left Behind Act (NCLB) of 2001 contains several items that are relevant to children with cerebral palsy who are in need of adapted or specialized instruction. No Child Left Behind represents comprehensive national education legislation that intends to improve school accountability for achievement and safety and to provide school performance information and some increased control to parents. It directs states to create grade-level standards for what students should know and requires testing of that progress annually in grades 3 to 8 and again in grade 10. Consistent with requirements of IDEA as reauthorized in 2004, states are required to include students with disabilities in regular assessments. Students unable to take part in a state's regular assessment with accommodations are to be provided alternative assessments. NCLB builds on IDEA and requires that the assessment scores of students with disabilities, including some of the scores of alternate assessments, be included in the state accountability system. In December 2015, Congress passed the Every Child Succeeds Act (ESSA), which reauthorizes the Elementary and Secondary Education Act / No Child Left Behind (ESEA/NCLB). Modifications that affect children with disabilities include ensuring access to the general education curriculum, to accommodations, and to concepts of universal design for living; the right to evidence-based interventions; and the right to improved conditions for learning, for example, reduction in use of restraints, discipline, bullying.

Current law allows students with disabilities to be assessed in several ways. They may take part in the regular testing, with or without accommodations. Or they may take an alternate assessment that is aligned either with grade level achievement standards or with alternate achievement standards. Determination of whether a special education student participates in the standard or alternative testing rests with the student's IEP team. Without the demonstration of "adequate yearly progress" at the local school level, funding will be adjusted. In some cases, parents may be given the opportunity to change schools or access tutoring assistance for under-achieving students.

What types of schools do children with special needs attend?

For children with special needs there are many different kinds of educational programs housed in various types of schools. There are schools specific to the child's disability, such as schools for students with hearing impairments or schools for students with orthopedic disabilities. Depending on their specific needs, many attend their neighborhood schools, where they are "included," or "mainstreamed," in a classroom with children who do not have special needs. The child who has a disability may have an aide in the regular classroom; this is decided by the IEP team.

There are also programs in which children receive their instruction in a self-contained classroom for children with disabilities. Alternatively, some children are instructed part time in learning support classrooms and receive various necessary therapies during the school day but are included in the regular classroom for selected learning situations, such as music or social studies. Children with very mild physical disability may only be separated from their peers for an adaptive physical education class.

The type of school situation in which a child does best varies. Educational placement is dependent on many factors, including the child's disability and age, where required services are available, the requirements of managing the disability, prioritization of goals, the IEP, and, in some circumstances, the parent's advocacy. In order to determine where your child will go to school and what kind of services he or she will have access to, an assessment of your child's development and abilities must be made.

What should I do if I think my child has special needs?

Begin your quest as soon as you suspect that something is unusual. Intervention should begin as early as possible. You will need to arrange to have your child assessed to determine what kind of help she or he needs. Sometimes the parents are not aware of their child's needs, or they do not realize that the school system can provide special services. In these cases the school, or an individual teacher at the school, may ask that the child have an assessment.

In short, there are three ways that a child can be identified for an assessment:

1. Parents can request an assessment.
2. If your child is in school, the school may ask parental permission to assess a child based on a screening.
3. An individual teacher who knows your child well may ask for an assessment.

What is an assessment?

An assessment involves gathering information about your child and his development. It generally includes determining what kind of help your child needs. Information comes from a variety of sources: parents, the assessment team, the child's doctors and medical history, and reports and results from developmental tests. This assessment forms the basis for the IEP, as well as the services to be provided to the child.

Who does the assessment?

An assessment may be performed by a team of professionals that includes a special education teacher, an occupational therapist, a physical therapist, a speech and language specialist, medical specialists, and a psychologist. Individual state policies determine what types of professionals make up the team. To perform the assessment, these professionals observe and test the child and determine her strengths and weaknesses.

Who should I contact for information on early intervention programs and special education programs?	You can call your local elementary school or school district office and ask for the contact person who is in charge of these services. Or you can obtain technical assistance through one of six regional Parent Technical Assistance Centers or state-specific guidance through your state's Parent Training and Information Center. All can be accessed from the Center for Parent Information and Resources (http://www.parentcenterhub.org), the Native American Parent Technical Assistance Center (www.naptac.org), or the Branch Military Parent Technical Assistance Center (https://branchta.org/).
What is Child Find?	Child Find is a duty imposed by IDEA requiring that states and school districts identify and evaluate each resident child or student with a disability as a precursor to provision of IEP services. Child Find makes a special effort to identify children from birth to 6 years, but its goal is to identify all unserved children. Anyone residing in a school district can request Child Find screening. Criteria for determining who is screened and at what age are determined by the district.
What are early intervention services?	These are programs designed to identify and treat potential developmental delay as early as possible. Once it has been determined that your child is eligible for early intervention services, you will be assigned a case manager, who will help develop an Individualized Family Service Plan. The IFSP describes the services the child will receive, when and where he will receive these services, and how his progress will be evaluated. The case manager is involved with your family until your child's third birthday. The case manager then helps you move on to programs for children aged 3 through 5.
What does "free and appropriate public education" mean?	This provision, originally from Public Law 99-142 and now in IDEA, means that special and related services are provided at all educational levels, preschool, elementary, and secondary. These services are offered free to children because they are provided under the state education agency or in conjunction with other state agencies and are funded with public monies. This education must meet the needs of the child as identified by the IEP.
How are related services obtained?	Related service needs are identified during the evaluation process of the child with special needs. The IEP will identify the related services the student needs. The IEP serves as a written commitment for the delivery of services to the child with special needs.
What if I don't agree with my child's IEP?	If the school determines that your child does not need certain services and you think she does, you can appeal the decision of the team. If you choose to appeal the IEP, be certain to get some professional advice on how to proceed.
Who should I contact for help?	Get in touch with your local school district, your state Parent Training and Information (PTI) Center, or a regional Parent Technical Assistance Center (http://parentcenterhub.org/ptacs). The Parent Training and Information Centers are federally funded agencies that provide parents with the knowl-

edge and know-how needed to become partners in their child's education. They can provide you with the information you need for the appeal process if that becomes necessary.

Can I get an independent evaluation of my child's abilities and strengths?

You can always obtain an independent evaluation of your child. Sometimes the school agrees that there is a need for a second opinion and sets up the evaluation. If the arrangements are made through the school, the school pays for the independent evaluation. If you wish to make the appointment and seek the second opinion independently, you will be required to pay for it.

In any case, the school district must provide you with names of other professionals who can provide the assessment. Parent groups are good sources of information and can recommend specialists too. Local hospitals often have specialists on staff who get together as a team to provide assessments.

What happens at an IEP meeting?

The people who provide educational services for your child explain their findings, the assessment measures they used, and your child's rate of progress. The meeting should be interactive. You share your observations about your child with these specialists. The IEP meeting should not reveal any surprises about student performance. Ongoing communication as well as progress updates (report cards) are to be provided for students with IEPs at the same intervals as for all other students of the school district. At the meeting you will be asked to sign an attendance document. This does not indicate agreement with the proposed IEP. It documents attendance and participation at the meeting. Parent participation is critical. In-person participation is preferable; however, parents may participate by phone.

The IEP is an individualized document that provides goals that are measureable and designed to be accomplished in a year's time. Specially designed instruction is a vital part of the IEP. It describes the specialized supports, techniques, and equipment the student requires to achieve success in his or her goals. Every year, within the anniversary date of the current IEP, the school must schedule a meeting with you to review your child's progress and to develop the next year's IEP.

What is included in the IEP?

Included in the IEP are statements of the student's current baseline performance (present levels of academic and functional performance), measurable annual goals, and short-term objectives (if required), developed by the teacher and related service providers. The frequency and duration of related services, as well as specially designed instruction, are stated in the IEP. Additional planning is required if a student requires assistive technology or has a hearing impairment. Also included in the IEP are additional statements about what percentage of time the child will participate in regular educational programs, specialized transportation needs, supports provided for school personnel, participation in state assessments, target dates for the initiation and duration of special services, criteria for Extended School Year services, and criteria for evaluation, which will measure progress. For students 14 and older, a transition component is included in the IEP. All parents are offered information about procedural safeguards at the IEP meeting.

What if I'm not able to attend the IEP meeting?

The law and regulations governing the development of the IEP require that a meeting of the parents and professionals be held at a mutually convenient time. Every effort should be made to work out a schedule. Sometimes meetings are planned for after school, but typically a meeting can be planned during school hours at a mutually agreed upon time. Parents may participate by phone or video-conferencing.

Is there anyone who can help me understand all of this?

There are federally supported programs in each state that support parent-to-parent information and training activities for parents of children with special needs. The Parent Training and Information Projects conduct workshops, publish newsletters, and answer questions by phone or by mail about parent-to-parent activities.

Will these laws and rules change over time?

To a great extent, the basic emphases of these laws have stayed the same for more than forty years, though the laws may be interpreted differently from state to state. However, because IDEA needs to be periodically reauthorized, various groups lobby lawmakers for changes in these laws. Specific provisions requested by school districts or advocated by parent groups may be introduced at these times, and parent support groups will likely know which of these provisions might weaken the law to the detriment of children. It is important that parents and others concerned about the rights and services available in schools to children with disabilities lobby lawmakers and educate lawmakers about the needs of this vulnerable population.

What can I do to keep abreast of issues?

Keep in touch. Join parent support groups, in person or online, where information is shared. Get on the mailing list for the Center for Parent Information and Resources and the local or national United Cerebral Palsy. Contact the CPIR for information on federally funded parent programs. These programs provide information and training to enable parents of children with disabling conditions to participate more knowledgeably in their child's care. Phone the school districts and the Developmental Disabilities Council in your area for information.

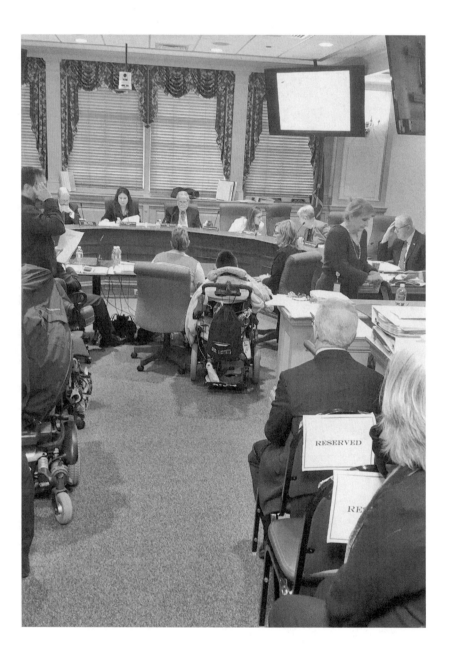

Being an Advocate for Your Child: Using the Legal System

FOR MANY PEOPLE, any discussion of the legal system evokes images of complicated procedures and tense courtroom scenes. High costs also come immediately to mind. Although it's true that the legal system can be confusing and even intimidating, this is not necessarily so in the area of the rights of the disabled. People with disabilities, their family members, and their advocates can often effectively, inexpensively, and easily use the law to obtain services and benefits.

A series of lawsuits in recent years has served to raise society's level of awareness about the lack of services available to people with disabilities. Legislatures, both state and federal, have responded by passing broad-ranging laws recognizing that people with disabilities have the right to be fully integrated into US society. These laws, which are administered by federal, state, and local agencies, go a long way toward ensuring fair and equal treatment, and they make it easier for people with disabilities and their advocates to obtain services. The people who staff these agencies are generally conscientious; nevertheless, bureaucracy and budgetary concerns sometimes interfere with the process. As a result, some individuals with disabilities are wrongly denied services to which they are entitled. For this reason, it is important for people with disabilities and those who advocate for them to understand what the law requires, as well as how to go about obtaining rights under the law.

To be an advocate, or champion, for the rights of the individual with disabilities, a person must be willing to learn what the individual's rights are, understand how the system works, and use the system to obtain maximum benefits. Although most people think only of lawyers when they think of advocates, there are in fact many different types of advocates. We begin this chapter with a description of the various kinds of advocates who may be helpful to you and your child. We then take up specific issues pertaining to the law as it applies to people with disabilities. Other legal assistance agencies are listed in the "Resources" section at the end of this book.

The legal advocate, or lawyer. We usually think of a lawyer when we think of a professional advocate representing the child or parent in litigation, and there's no question that employing a lawyer trained in handling disability cases is generally a wise decision. Whether it is or is not *essential* to obtain the services of a lawyer is often determined by the specific problem that needs to be addressed. If there are complicated legal issues with respect to educational requirements, or if parents need to write a will that provides for the survivor with a disability, then parents need to consult a lawyer specializing in these areas. Your family's general practice lawyer can usually refer you to a lawyer who specializes in disability cases. In addition, agencies such as United Cerebral Palsy (UCP), school districts, legal service agencies, and social workers can provide referrals to lawyers who specialize in this area of the law. Bar associations also offer lawyer referral services to the public.

The legal system overall is moving toward alternative disposition resolution (ADR), in which mediation and arbitration are commonplace options. For example, IDEA regulations require states to offer mediation to resolve special education disputes. Such alternatives may be less expensive and intimidating options for parents to pursue.

Protection and advocacy (P&A) agencies. Every state has a P&A agency, which provides advocacy and legal services to persons with disabilities, usually for free. The National Disability Rights Network (NDRN) has background information and links to all state P&As on its website, www.ndrn.org. The P&A system has been expanding since its inception in the mid-1970s to include a number of discrete programs. The programs that would be of most interest to persons with CP would be those earmarked for developmental disabilities (PADD), assistive technology (PAAT), and Social Security Disability/SSI beneficiaries (PABSS). P&As engage in a wide variety of advocacy activities, including systemic litigation, individual litigation, legislative and regulatory advocacy, and provision of information and referral services. State P&As generally publish eligibility information and priorities on their websites.

The parent as advocate. As noted above, a lawyer is not the only advocate who can benefit your child. The most important advocates for most children are their parents. To be an effective advocate, a parent needs to become very well informed about the laws pertaining to disability and about how the system works. A good place to begin is government websites, which compile laws and regulations for online viewing or download. You should also read publications on self-advocacy, which are available online and in bookstores and libraries. Each state has at least one Parent Training and Information Center. These centers are sources of parent information, referral, and training with a historical emphasis on special education. The Center for Parent Information and Resources website (www.parentcenterhub.org) has a link to the centers in each state. It is virtually impossible to be an effective advocate without knowing the rules of the game. The scope of benefits parents obtain from the government and insurance companies may be directly related to how aggressively informed parents advocate on behalf of their child.

Because the parent is not only the child's advocate but also the child's caregiver, the parent must be aware of two risks involved in serving as the child's advocate. First, advocacy can become a full-time occupation in its own right. Second, parents can become overwhelmed with the time commitment and begin to feel that they are neglecting other priorities, such as parenting their other children. Parents should only spend as much time in their role as advocates as they are comfortable with and then accept that they do not have to do everything themselves.

Being an assertive advocate also requires a certain personality, someone who is willing to confront others and to be in the public eye. Parents who simply cannot manage this type of advocacy should seek help from other advocates and not feel guilty about doing so. Joining local councils (such as Developmental Disabilities Councils and special educational councils) and local branches of national organizations (such as UCP) can be very helpful for parents who cannot serve as their own child's primary advocate but who can nevertheless contribute time and effort to advocacy groups. Each state has a DD Council, which serves as a systemic advocate for persons with developmental disabilities. The National Association of Councils on Developmental Disabilities website (www.nacdd.org) has a link to councils in individual states. A list of councils in all 50 states is provided. Special education councils are required by IDEA regulations. Participation in such councils provides an opportunity to network and receive free training. Such organizations provide valuable information, and the collective power they wield is often impressive.

The citizen advocate. A citizen advocate is someone with experience or training who is willing to become a child's advocate on a voluntary basis. Many communities have a citizen's advocacy board, often organized by parents to help provide this type of service. Alternatively, the local chapters of nonprofit organizations, such as UCP or the Epilepsy Foundation of America, may offer citizen advocacy. Many of these volunteers have gained a great deal of experience by working with other children with disabilities and can be very effective in obtaining services and providing parents with a sense that the right services are being provided for their child.

The press as advocate. Newscasters and columnists are often interested in "human interest" stories and can be very effective in helping to obtain services for a child. It is important to provide members of the press with your story in a manner that gives them the facts but also conveys the emotional impact of your situation. It is not a good idea to write a letter to the newspaper that is a personal attack on those who have thwarted your attempts to get help for your child. Instead, provide a documented history of your phone calls, the responses or lack of responses, and the effect of the problem on your family. Do not lie or exaggerate. Consider whether it is a good idea to include personal names; the better approach is generally to use generic terms and to identify persons only by position or title ("a staff member," for example). Let the press know that you are available for a personal interview. Make copies of the letter you send to the press and send them to all the individuals who have been giving you the run-around. Consider writing a letter to the editor of your local newspaper or organizing a group of parents to write to the editor about an issue of broad interest that affects many children or adults with disabilities.

The case manager advocate. A case manager is usually a trained nurse or social worker who is employed by an agency or an insurance company. State social service agencies may provide a case manager to help a parent negotiate a complicated medical problem. Nonprofit organizations such as UCP and Easter Seals, as well as many private charities, will also fund case managers to provide these same benefits to the child and the parents. There are also volunteer case managers with specialized training in this area. In order to assess how effective the case manager will be—how strong an advocate he or she will be for your child—you must first know who the case manager's employer is and the reason the case manager was assigned to your child.

Case manager advocates employed by insurance companies are becoming much more popular. These individuals can coordinate care and make sure that resources are used effectively. It is important to remember, however, that these individuals are employed by insurance companies, whose underlying goal is to minimize the cost of care and thereby improve the profit margin. In spite of this potential conflict of interest, these individuals can be very helpful to parents, especially in teaching them how to use the complicated and often fragmented medical care system.

Parents may want to obtain the written standards that describe the case manager's duties. This should be public information if the case manager is a government employee or contractor. Since caseloads are often excessive, case managers may not uniformly offer all services to which the parent may be entitled. If the parent has the policy in hand, he will be able to "prompt" the case manager to offer the entire range of authorized services. The parent may also wish to diplomatically request information on the availability of grievance systems. Almost all social services agencies and insurers have at least internal grievance systems, which may or may not be well advertised. If the case manager knows that the parent is aware of the grievance system, the case manager has an incentive to "aim to please."

The child protection advocate. The government has a mandate to protect children from harm, including possible harm or neglect caused by parents. All states have child protection laws requiring certain professionals (such as doctors and teachers) and other individuals to report suspected abuse. This suspected abuse is then investigated by child protection advocates, who issue a report announcing their findings in the case. A child protection advocate may be assigned to monitor a child over a long period; in this situation, the advocate is usually a court-assigned individual. Such advocates are for the most part dedicated and interested in the child's welfare, and many of them are well-trained professionals with extensive experience. In many states, budgetary concerns have resulted in low pay for these individuals, however, as well as extremely heavy caseloads. In some areas, poorly trained individuals may be working in this capacity.

It's important for parents to understand that if they are involved with child protective service advocates, those advocates will primarily be considering the interests of the child. If there are allegations that the parents have abused the child, then the parents may need their own advocate. This may be one situation in which advocacy for the child may need to be delegated to a professional.

Overall, federal law is clear on the point that these agencies should attempt to prevent unnecessary separation of families. The goal of most child protection advocates is not to remove children from the care of their parents or to punish the parents but to look out for the child's best interests. Families should be assertive about asking for support services that will benefit the child within the family unit. One method of guarding the child's best interests is to identify problems or stress areas and help the family deal with these. The goal, whenever possible, is to help the family solve problems and stay together. If parents understand that this is the primary goal and accept that the child protection advocate is in fact attempting to look out for the child's best interests, then the alleged problems can often be resolved in a positive way.

The legislative advocate. Industries and large special interest groups have long hired professional lobbyists to advocate for their interests. For people with disabilities, however, the most effective advocacy is usually done by parents whose efforts are directed to members of the legislature. For a parent advocate to become an effective legislative advocate, he or she must spend some time learning the system. It is important not to be intimidated by position and titles, since legislators are people like you who want to please you and who are often very touched by personal stories. Most people serving in government really *do* want to make life better for the people who elected them and whom they are serving. You should operate under the assumption that they are interested in helping you.

You may directly contact either a state or a federal legislator and request an appointment or opportunity to speak with him or her. Inviting a legislator to meetings of parents' groups, to special school events, or to a camp for children with disabilities may present an opportunity for advocacy in which the parents and children don't have to travel to where the legislature meets. Legislators often welcome the chance to learn from seeing people in their own environment and to have direct contact with those who make use of the services of government agencies.

When you approach the legislator, present a specific problem that can be addressed. It is very difficult for a legislator to be helpful when he or she is approached with general anger and frustration and comments such as "Life is hard" and "No one is willing to help." If this is how you feel, you should first work on defusing your anger and focusing your general frustration by talking with other parents or professionals. Try to understand what your specific problems are. Then, when you address your legislator, you can be concise and thereby more effective.

For example, suppose that the company providing the health insurance you receive through your place of employment claimed that it would cover the cost of medical goods and orthotics, but when you went to purchase such items, you were told it would only cover one pair of braces in the child's lifetime. Naturally, you are frustrated. Upon further investigation you discover that although the insurance company advertised that it would pay for braces, the small print of the contract limited coverage to one pair during the child's lifetime. Unfortunately, such ploys are common. It is clear to everyone that one pair of braces suitable for a child at 2 years of age is not going to last a lifetime. You may take this specific frustration to your state legislator and ask him or her to introduce a bill that would make it illegal for state-regulated insurance companies to use this type of deceptive advertising or adopt lifetime limits on braces. Legislators are likely to be receptive to this type of specific request, and they can, in fact, initiate legislation to bring about a change in the law. This mechanism has been utilized to pass many laws—those providing access to public buildings, preventing discrimination against people with disabilities in the workplace, and providing for special education.

The Partners in Policymaking program originated in 1987 and is now available in almost all states. It is an innovative leadership training program for adults with disabilities and for parents of young children with developmental disabilities. The program trains people to serve as effective advocates, including legislative advocates. There is an online course on how to communicate with public officials. An example of recent training topics in one state included local, state, and federal policy and legislative issues; how to meet public officials and give legislative testimony; community organizing; and working with the media. The skills one needs to advocate effectively with elected officials can be learned through this program or others like it.

The self-advocate. Probably the most effective advocate, especially in the legislative arena, is the self-advocate. Teaching the child to advocate for himself within his capability will provide him with a powerful tool to carry throughout his life. You can begin by teaching your child that he needs to be verbal about his needs and his abilities. For example, an intelligent child with a speech disability needs to be taught that he should be direct with strangers, explaining that having a speech disability does not equal having intellectual limitations. As children become older and start driving, they can learn to advocate for their rights to accessible parking. They can also advocate for access to public buildings.

Many adults with disabilities find that they grow tired of constantly having to advocate for themselves and for other people with disabilities. But this is almost universally recognized as a necessary part of functioning in society. Teaching children this lesson in a gentle and socially acceptable way is important. An increasing number of programs teach children and young adults with disabilities to be self-advocates. Some DD Councils offer such programs, as do local chapters of private agencies, such as UCP. The Partners in Policymaking program also teaches self-advocacy skills. Some states offer a "junior" Partners in Policymaking program, open to teens and young adults.

What is guardianship?   Guardianship is the legal means by which a person is appointed to act on behalf of and protect an individual who is incompetent, that is, incapable of acting on his own behalf. Guardianship is regulated by state law, which varies from state to state. In all states, however, guardianship of a minor child is automatically given to the birth parents until the child is legally considered an adult, at either age 18 or age 21, depending on the state. At the age of adulthood, the person automatically assumes all rights of an adult unless guardianship is specifically assigned to another person.

An adult may benefit from having a guardian appointed if he or she is unable to manage financial affairs, make decisions concerning medical care, or direct or plan activities of daily living. Because the birth parents' guardianship is automatically terminated at the age of adulthood, they must petition the court to continue in that role. Even in cases in which an adult is obviously unable to participate in or manage his or her own affairs and guardianship assignment is fairly straightforward, the court must still be petitioned. Specific local mechanisms differ; ask a social service professional or your family lawyer for information about how to proceed.

Often the level of competency of the child or young adult is not clear cut. In these situations a guardian should be appointed with care. Appointing a guardian removes significant civil rights from the individual. Although this varies from state to state, guardianship often severely restricts an individual's ability to manage his own money, makes marriage illegal without the consent of the guardian, and may affect voting rights. For these reasons, the appointment of a guardian in a borderline situation should involve careful consultation with the child or young adult as well as social service professionals and lawyers familiar with this issue. Because of the serious implications of guardianship, the court often appoints an attorney to represent the individual independently of parents and applicants seeking guardianship.

A person with a mild intellectual disability does not automatically need a guardian. The issue of mental competence also varies with situations and circumstances and can change over time. States have increasingly recognized that there are gradations of competence, and some states have assigned three levels of competence: full competence; partial competence in specific areas; and complete incompetence. In the past, individuals were considered to be either fully competent or fully incompetent. Now, in situations in which the level of competence is uncertain, a full evaluation by a professional with expertise in this area is strongly recommended.

There are also alternatives to guardianship. For example, in lieu of appointment of a guardian of the property, there are corporate bill-paying services that will, for a small fee, manage a consumer's funds. Another option available in approximately half the states is an AARP-sponsored money management assistance program. States may also offer bill-paying assistance as part of an attendant services program. If the individual with a disability is capable of signing a health care directive or power of attorney, the individual may appoint a relative or friend to deal with health care or financial matters. There is also a growing movement known as "supported decision-making," in which an agreement is signed authorizing the assistance of an agent in making and implementing financial and health care decisions. (The most comprehensive version of a "supported decision-making" law was adopted in Delaware in 2016.) Finally, if the individual with a disability lacks capacity, some states have laws authorizing certain relatives to make health care decisions on their behalf.

What types of guardianships are there?

There are different types of guardianship in most states, with the major types being either *plenary guardianship*, which involves complete and full decision making for an individual, or *limited guardianship*, which only applies in certain circumstances. The birth parent is a plenary guardian of a minor child who can, if court appointed, continue to serve in the same role even after the child has reached the age of majority. For individuals who may be able to manage some of their affairs, limited guardianship in specific areas should be considered. Financial and estate guardians are examples of limited guardians.

A financial guardian may be appointed to help an individual manage his or her funds, which includes paying rent and dispersing income, such as Supplemental Security Income (SSI) or Social Security Disability Insurance (SSDI) payments. A guardian of the property or estate is usually appointed for individuals who have significant resources, such as property or income-producing investments. The guardian of the estate also is appointed by the court, which usually requires the guardian to be bonded and to operate under strict rules, limiting the types of investments that may be made to only low-risk investments.

There are also different mechanisms for a parent or family member to become a guardian. One can become a guardian by

- filing a petition with the court asking to be named guardian;
- being named guardian in a person's will (testamentary guardian) and having it approved by the court; or
- being appointed by the court based on a petition filed by someone else.

The most common way for someone to become a guardian is to file a petition. For example, a parent may petition to be named guardian for an adult son or daughter.

Because of the significant powers a guardian may have, parents may wish to name someone to become their child's guardian after their death. This provision can be made in the parents' wills, where the parents can specify a desired guardian. Court approval will still be needed, but the court will often defer to the "nomination" of the guardian, though it can reject the recommendation for cause. We suggest that parents give this matter considerable thought and discuss with the proposed successor guardian the concept of a guardianship and what actions the parents would like to see taken. If a guardian is not named in a parent's will, the court may select a consenting relative or even an unrelated person or agency as guardian.

In many states, specialized corporations are authorized to serve as guardians upon court appointment. They may be a good option for families who would prefer the stability of a corporate guardian, which fulfills the responsibilities of a guardian, including accounting and preparation of reports. However, such corporations typically charge fees for their work, and their values may different from the values of family members. For example, while families might prefer that the guardian arrange in-home support services through multiple vendors, the corporation may find it more expedient to simply seek nursing home admission, which requires issuing a single monthly check for all-inclusive services.

Typically, public guardians are appointed by the state in the event of a parent's or parents' death that leaves the child or incompetent adult without a caregiver. These public guardians are usually social workers, attorneys, or a state or local agency. Public guardians are professional individuals with training who have a keen interest in doing what is best for the person in question;

however, they typically deal with a very large caseload and consequently have extremely limited opportunities to get to know any one individual.

Who will make the best guardian if one is needed?

People who serve as guardians take on a very serious and large responsibility. To handle it well, they need to be personally familiar with the individual, understand the individual's condition and medical problems, understand the individual's family values, and be aware of all special needs. Parents, as long as they are able, often serve this function best. However, appointment of a sibling may avoid the necessity of a change in guardianship as the parents enter advanced age. The appointment of two individuals as "joint" guardians is a common approach that provides flexibility and continuity if one guardian dies or is unable to serve. These options need to be discussed with professionals familiar with the family and the individual in need.

What is the role of a guardian?

The typical guardianship order allows guardians to do almost anything for the person with a disability that the person would do for himself if he could. A plenary guardian exercises full personal rights for the individual. A financial guardian exercises authority over an individual's assets as outlined by the law of the state. Once a guardian is appointed, he or she must file a report with the state at some predetermined frequency. Some states require that guardians be bonded. One of the important roles of a guardian is to give consent for care, education, and medical treatment for the individual.

There are three types of consent. *Direct consent* is given by the individual who will be treated. *Substitute consent* is given by the guardian of the individual. *Concurrent consent* is a combination of consent by the guardian and consent by the patient. Professionals may use concurrent consent in a situation in which an individual's mental competence is uncertain or hasn't been determined. For example, if an individual with a moderate intellectual disability wishes to take birth control pills, not only the individual but also the parents may be asked to give consent before a prescription is written. If the parent has been given legal guardianship of the individual, then the individual may not give consent but can still give assent. (*Assent* refers to the agreement of a minor to a medical procedure or treatment in addition to the consent of the parent or legal guardian. This approach may also be used for treatment given to teenagers who are not of legal age to give consent but are very involved in their own treatment plan.)

Giving consent for medical treatment, especially for surgical procedures, is often a very difficult and serious concern for parents. Guardians of adults have the same concerns, since it may be difficult to determine what is in the individual's best interests. This is especially true for procedures that involve significant risks or procedures that make significant changes in the person's body.

Both state laws and the courts place limitations on a guardian's ability to give consent for another individual, especially in the area of birth control. In general, guardians may not give consent for irreversible birth control methods, such as tubal ligation, removal of ovaries, or hysterectomies, unless that treatment is needed to correct a pathological process and is not being done for birth control purposes only. Guardians *can* generally give consent for reversible birth control mechanisms such as birth control pills or injections.

What are the caregiving options when parents cannot care for the child at home?

There was a time when placement in an institution such as a nursing home was the only alternative to living at home for children and adults with disabilities. Today, however, most persons (especially children) with chronic disabilities are not in institutions. The Supreme Court's *Olmstead v. LC and EW* decision in 1999 accelerated the movement toward community placements. Based on the Americans with Disabilities Act of 1990, this decision mandates that individuals with disabilities live in the most integrated setting that is appropriate for their needs. As a result of the Court's decision, states are required to prioritize community-based options for persons with disabilities in their social services systems.

Based on this ruling, states have moved to expand home- and community-based services, including small group homes, supported apartments, and family support services. Funding for community-based services is available to states under Medicaid home- and community-based services waivers. A waiver, which refers to "waiving" Medicaid's previous requirement of funding care in institutions only, is designed to provide services in the community as an alternative to institutionalization. Typically, the individual must have a qualifying disability, meet a level of care standard, and require certain support services. Such services can include case management, homemaker assistance, home health aides, personal care, respite care, transportation, vocational options, assistive technology, and physical or occupational therapy, among others. There is a growing trend to allow relatives to be paid for providing some of these services, including personal care. In some states a flexible stipend may be paid to families to cover a variety of costs of care. In 2014, federal regulations were adopted that define the settings in which waiver services can be provided (79 Fed. Reg. 2948 [January 16, 2014]). These regulations have prompted states to assess and revise their programs to fulfill federal preferences for offering services in integrated settings.

Specific to children is the "Katie Beckett" waiver, adopted by Medicaid programs in most states. Essentially, states have the option of providing Medicaid to children (up to their 19th birthday) with significant disabilities regardless of parental income and resources. Children must meet an SSI standard of disability and level of care standards. The parents can then tap home health, private duty nursing, therapy services, and so on to support the child at home.

Apart from waivers, other Medicaid programs have been established in recent years to fund community-based supports. States can elect to participate in the Community First Choice (CFC) Option, which funds hands-on assistance, safety monitoring, cueing, training, and assistive technology. The Money Follows the Person Option funds supports to allow individuals to leave institutions in favor of community living (such as in an apartment).

Another alternative to institutional placement is placement with another family. This could be placement with extended family members, such as grandparents, or with an adoptive or foster family. In most situations, the parent continues to be the personal guardian, which means that the parent has to give consent for medical treatment, such as surgical procedures. Children who are in foster care may go to the parental home on weekends, holidays, or special occasions, depending on the parent's ability and willingness to be involved. This type of complicated caregiver arrangement needs to be carefully worked out among the various parties, with everyone, including the involved parent, understanding what's involved.

When it comes to foster care, in addition to legal and financial considerations, there are often significant psychological and emotional implications for the parents. When another family is able to take their child into their home, the parents may feel that they have failed in caring for their own child. This is one of the reasons why many parents resist foster care placement and often prefer to see the child placed in a group home or institution. Counseling for the parents may help them understand that foster care placement does not mean that they are failures but that each person and family has certain strengths. Recognizing that foster care parents are paid a salary and that it is therefore their job to care for children with disabilities sometimes helps parents deal with this.

Are guardianship issues different for adoptive parents than for birth parents?

Adoption is a legal procedure in which an adult becomes a legal parent and has the same relationship to a minor child as do birth parents. The adoption laws with respect to children with disabilities may, however, differ somewhat from the laws pertaining to children without disabilities. Because the laws vary significantly from state to state, we strongly recommend that you consult a general practice lawyer or a professional with expertise in this area if you are considering adopting or have recently become the adoptive parent of a child with a disability.

Prospective adoptive parents and their lawyer need to look into what benefits the child will receive before and after adoption. In the past, it was common for the adopted child, regardless of disability, to be treated exactly as a biological child, so that the parents' income had to be included in all means-testing federal and state programs, such as SSI and Medicaid. (*Means testing* is a system of determining eligibility for financial assistance that is based on parental income and other financial resources.) Because of means testing and the costs involved in raising children with disabilities, in the past many children with disabilities were not adopted and remained wards of the state.

The trend in many states recently has been to change the laws so that children with disabilities continue to be eligible for all the programs they were eligible for prior to the adoption, such as SSI and Medicaid, without means testing based on the adoptive parents' income. This area should be investigated and considered prior to going through with an adoption. As noted, because of the laws in some states, it's possible that a person may be better able to provide care for a child with a disability if he or she remains in the foster parent role rather than becoming an adoptive parent. However, the disadvantage is that the child could be taken out of a foster home by the state agency even if a strong emotional bond has developed between the child and the foster family, whereas an adopted child is permanently part of a family.

There are also adoption assistance programs, which vary from state to state, whereby individuals are given cash benefits as well as medical assistance and social services when adopting a child with special needs. For instance, adoptive parents of a special needs child may be eligible for a one-time payment of expenses incurred in connection with adoption of the child, such as attorney fees, court costs, and other expenses directly related to the adoption. A portion of adoption expenses may be tax deductible.

There are also federal and state subsidy programs, in addition to tax incentives, for special needs adoptions. The federal Title IV-E adoption assistance program provides monthly financial assistance to parents of eligible children to help meet the child's needs. The automatic Medicaid coverage available through this program is invaluable, since medical costs may be extremely burdensome and most private health insurance is oriented toward acute care and not toward treating developmental disabilities. Approximately three out of four children adopted from foster care have an adoption agreement that includes Medicaid coverage. Adoptive parents do not have to meet any financial eligibility criteria to receive assistance through this program. For children who are not eligible for Title IV-E assistance, there are state adoption subsidy programs. These may cover medical expenses, living expenses, and special or extraordinary expenses incurred by the adopted child.

How do guardianship concerns relate to foster parents?

There may be an option for a long-term foster parent to obtain complete guardianship of a child. Most foster parents, especially those with short-term placement, are given only custodial rights over the person with a disability. These rights enable them to provide care for the child or older person, usually in conjunction with a state-assigned professional child care worker or child advocate. But because the role and rights of the foster parent can range from broad decision making to only short-term physical care of the person, the prospective foster parent must fully understand the extent of his or her role regarding the child's care.

The specific level of responsibility should be put in writing so that when the child is brought for medical care or other emergencies, health care professionals are aware of the child's legal custody situation. It is not sufficient for the foster parent to say that he or she has medical consent authority; the foster parent should present a document confirming authority, such as a court order or power of attorney. Like foster parents, older siblings, grandparents, and aunts or uncles who care for a child with CP can generally consent to medical treatment only if that authority has been granted by court order or delegation from the person with the authority (such as power of attorney from a parent). Documentation of authority should always be available when caregivers other than the birth parents are securing medical care. If children receive most of their medical attention at one facility, a copy of this authorization should be included in the child's medical record.

Is adult foster care different from foster care of a minor child?	In an adult foster care arrangement, a family takes one or two adults with disabilities into their home and cares for them in the same way that another family does foster children. The issues of guardianship in this situation, however, do not differ from those in other adult situations. What's essential is for the areas of guardianship to be defined and assigned by the court—and then recorded in a legal document.
What other living arrangements are being developed?	The current view is that individuals with disabilities, just like all other people, prefer autonomy and self-directed services. This view is reflected in attendant services programs in which the person with a disability is given public funds to hire (and fire) support workers. There is also a "home of your own" movement, in which parents may join to purchase a residence for 3 to 4 adult children with disabilities. The state provides support services but does not own the residence. Consistent with the Americans with Disabilities Act, government-sponsored residential programs are expected to promote integrated housing options without unnecessary restrictions. Supported apartments and housing vouchers are becoming more prevalent than group homes.
What other legal concerns do people with cerebral palsy have?	Over the past few decades, laws have been passed that significantly affect people with major disabilities. These laws have for the most part arisen from an increased awareness by the general population that people with disabilities should be incorporated into the community as fully as other citizens. Many laws have been passed regulating the educational setting for children with disabilities, and similar laws have been passed regulating adults' access to public facilities and preventing discrimination in the workplace.
How do the laws affect education for the child with cerebral palsy?	Although it is hard to believe, until the early 1950s children with major disabilities were often completely excluded from public education. In the 1950s and 1960s there was a resurgence of interest in establishing locally operated special schools exclusively for children with disabilities. Many of these schools were segregated, so that children with visual handicaps, orthopedic handicaps, or major cognitive disabilities, for example, were taught in schools that were separate even from one another. Many of these schools were very large facilities, often understaffed and with few resources. Some of these so-called schools were in fact full-time boarding institutions where little education took place.

This situation was dramatically changed in 1975 with the adoption of Public Law 94-142, also known as the Education for All Handicapped Children Act. This federal law (as well as state laws that have been patterned after it) is based on the dual principles of inclusion and integration of all children. In terms of inclusion, the law requires that a free and appropriate education be provided for all children, no matter how severe their disabling condition. In terms of integration, the law requires that children with disabilities be educated in settings where they are integrated with children who do not have disabilities to the maximum extent possible. This aspect of the law is known as placing the child in the least restrictive setting and has resulted in removing many children from special schools and returning them to regular classroom education. |

The Education for All Handicapped Children Act (renamed the Individuals with Disabilities Education Act, or IDEA) is an extensive and detailed law that defines many of the aspects of the education to which children with cerebral palsy are entitled. (Children with CP are not automatically eligible but must meet specific criteria.) The law sets age limits for children who must receive educational services; defines which services the children must receive; defines a specific mechanism by which this program must be carried out, including evaluations and written responses of which the parent must be aware (the Individualized Education Program, or IEP); and states what related services are required. There are also specific mechanisms for resolving conflicts between parents and professionals, or between professionals who hold differing views. The full details of this act are discussed in Chapter 11. A valuable and highly respected source of parental information on special education is www.wrightslaw.com.

What laws apply to adults with cerebral palsy?

For adults, the workplace is the main setting in which they interact with others and with society in general. Just as children with disabilities formerly were segregated in the school setting, historically people with disabilities were almost entirely excluded from employment opportunities. Congress took the lead in prohibiting job discrimination against persons with disabilities with the passage of Section 504 of the Rehabilitation Act of 1973, which makes it illegal for agencies and institutions that receive federal funding to discriminate against persons with disabilities. After extensive publicity and lobbying by numerous advocacy groups for individuals with disabilities, the job-related rights of these people were greatly expanded with the passage of the Americans with Disabilities Act in 1990. Features of the Americans with Disabilities Act include the following:

- Employers must assess the qualifications of an individual with a disability applying for a job based on the same criteria as those used to assess an individual without a disability.
- Employers must make reasonable accommodation for the hired person.
- Employers must provide access to nonwork areas provided to employees, such as lounges and cafeterias.
- Places of public accommodation (stores, hotels, theaters, gyms, etc.) cannot discriminate based on disability.
- State and local governments must reasonably modify policies and practices to accommodate persons with disabilities.

The employer cannot discriminate even in advertisements for jobs. For example, an employer may not advertise for "able-bodied" persons. Moreover, the employer may be required to provide accommodations in the interview and assessment process. For example, if a typing test were required for a secretarial position and an applicant asked to use his adaptive keyboard, this would be a reasonable accommodation. The employer could not insist that the applicant use the standard keyboard used by all other applicants. While in general terms the laws relating to the workplace primarily tell employers what they *may not* do, there are exceptions. For instance, Section 503 of the Rehabilitation Act includes an affirmative action obligation for employers who have contracts with the federal government amounting to $10,000 or more. It requires that such companies contracting with the government "shall take affirmative action to employ and advance in employment qualified individuals with disabilities." Many large employers have such contracts, and persons with disabilities may wish to focus their efforts on soliciting employment with such firms.

The Rehabilitation Act was amended in 2014 by enactment of the Workforce Innovation and Opportunity Act (WIOA). The WIOA promotes competitive integrated employment opportunities for individuals with disabilities. The new law places restrictions on sheltered workshops paying workers less than the federal minimum wage. Final regulations implementing the law were issued in August 2016.

What specific restrictions are provided for by the Americans with Disabilities Act?

Part of the Americans with Disabilities Act incorporates concepts from Section 504 of the Rehabilitation Act, which specifically prohibits employment discrimination against qualified people with disabilities in federally funded programs. Specifically, Section 504 states that "no otherwise qualified individual with disabilities in the United States shall solely by reason of his disability be excluded from the participation in, be denied the benefits of, or be subjected to discrimination under any program or activity receiving federal financial assistance." Disabilities are fairly broadly defined as any limits an individual has that impact "major life activities," which include caring for himself or herself or performing tasks such as walking, seeing, hearing, speaking, breathing, or learning. Recently adopted federal regulations have reinforced a liberal interpretation of eligibility under the ADA and specifically include cerebral palsy as a covered "physical or emotional impairment."

The Americans with Disabilities Act extended this prohibition against discrimination to all private and public employers. Congress reaffirmed and strengthened the law by enactment of the Americans with Disabilities Amendment Act (ADAAA) of 2008, which "rolled back" some adverse court decisions limiting the scope of the ADA.

The ADA states that "no employer shall discriminate against a qualified individual with a disability because of the disability of such individual in regard to job application procedures, the hiring or discharge of employees, employee compensation, advancement, job training, and other terms, conditions, and privileges of employment." In other words, the employer must assess an individual with a disability who is applying for a job using the same criteria that would be used to assess an individual without a disability. The employer is required to make reasonable accommodation for the person with a disability who is qualified for the job. This "reasonable accommodation" has been interpreted to mean removing job obstacles that would prevent the otherwise qualified person with a disability from working. This may mean removing physical obstacles, providing for movement in the workplace, modifying equipment so that it can be used by a person with a disability, and restructuring the job setting and schedules as well as training and policies to accommodate the person's disability. Failing to make these accommodations is a violation of the law; however, the employer is not required to hire the person with a disability if doing so would impose "undue hardship" on the employer. Undue hardship is determined based on the net cost to the employer. An employer should determine whether funding is available from an outside source, such as a state rehabilitation agency, to help pay for all or part of the accommodation. In addition, employers should determine whether they are eligible for certain tax credits or deductions to offset the cost of the accommodations.

Another part of the ADA provides access to government settings and services by prohibiting discrimination against people with disabilities. This means that all forms of public transportation, such as publicly operated trains, subways, and city buses, must gradually become accessible to those with disabilities. This means, for example, "phasing in" accessible buses while some older vehicles that may not be accessible are still in use. Architectural barriers such as stairs and narrow doors in terminals and stations must also be removed or bypassed to the maximum extent feasible, and all new buildings and facilities must be constructed without these physical limitations. The ADA applies different standards to private companies providing transportation services, such as bus companies, airlines, and taxi companies.

Another important aspect of the ADA is its prohibition of all discrimination in public accommodations against people with disabilities. This applies to almost every business or place frequented by the public, including restaurants, bars, theaters, stadiums, concert halls, hotels, inns, bakeries, grocery stores, gas stations, professional offices such as those of doctors and lawyers, bus and airport terminals, libraries, galleries, and physical exercising facilities, such as gyms and bowling alleys. Businesses are required to make reasonable accommodations, for example, by making doorways passable for someone in a wheelchair. Again, the law allows the business to plead unreasonable cost and thereby avoid making the structural changes necessary to provide access. Nevertheless, this aspect of the ADA should provide greater overall access and freedom of movement and opportunity for people with cerebral palsy to move in the public sector.

How does the ADA affect life or health insurance?

Another part of the ADA prohibits discrimination by life and health insurance companies, which are not permitted to deny coverage based on an individual's or a family member's disability. The practical effect of this provision is uncertain, however, because it continues to allow insurance companies to deny coverage if the denial is based on "sound actuarial principles" or "reasonable anticipated experience." This means that while an insurance company is not allowed to reject an applicant for insurance based on the disability, it may reject the applicant based on experience that shows that a similar person utilizes more services than the average person applying for insurance. Because of this uncertainty, many individuals and families find it very difficult to obtain life or health insurance unless it is in the context of a mandated group plan through employment. Some states are attempting to further tighten the prohibitions against discrimination by insurance companies with respect to people with disabilities.

Does the federal Affordable Care Act help with access to health insurance?

Several provisions in the federal Affordable Care Act promote access to health insurance. First, most covered insurers are barred from denying health insurance based on preexisting conditions, including cerebral palsy. Second, most young adults (under age 26) can receive health insurance through their parents' health insurance plans if the plans cover dependent children. Third, the act restricts covered insurers from imposing lifetime caps on the dollar amount they will spend on benefits. A useful overview of the act's impact on individuals with developmental disabilities is available at http://autisticadvocacy.org/policy-advocacy/reports-and-brief-materials/the-affordable-care-act-and-the-idd-community-an-overview-of-the-law-and-advocacy-priorities-going-forward/.

Can a person with cerebral palsy get a driver's license?

For individuals who are able, one of the major opportunities for developing independence is the ability to drive a motor vehicle. The laws regarding the specific driving requirements for persons with disabilities vary from state to state, but all states have four general rules. First, the individual's eyesight must be good enough to allow him or her to read road signs. The level of corrected vision must be well defined and documented before a person can obtain a driver's license. Second, an individual with a physical disability must document his or her ability to manage the controls of the vehicle to be driven. All states provide for limited licenses that prescribe modifications to the vehicle the individual will drive (hand controls and specific mirrors are examples). Some automobile companies or dealers will modify a vehicle to make it possible for the person with a disability to drive it. Third, individuals must have sufficient cognitive function to understand the laws, to read signs, and to be able to understand the use of a motor vehicle. Fourth, all states have specific laws regulating the circumstances under which a person with seizures may obtain a driver's license. These laws vary widely, so if you have seizures, you'll need to obtain a copy of the law in your state before proceeding. Some states require doctors to report all seizures of a patient with a driver's license. If the patient has well-controlled seizures, the state will issue a driver's license. The individual needs to work with the state licensing agency and the physician treating the seizures.

If a driver's education course is offered in the public school system, a qualified student with a disability must be given the opportunity to participate and offered reasonable accommodations. States may also offer special driver's education training, in which a person's individual disability is evaluated and driver's training is given in a specifically modified vehicle. The specialized driving instructor then assesses whether the individual is skillful enough to continue with the training. A license is usually only granted after the person has demonstrated driving competence to a state officer. Special education specialists or vocational rehabilitation professionals can provide further information about driver's education training for people with special needs.

What are the legal provisions for financial care for a person with cerebral palsy?

All parents must consider how they will provide financial protection for their dependent children, but financial considerations for parents who have a child with cerebral palsy may be more complicated than those for parents of a child without a disability. It is crucial for these parents to consult a professional who has a strong background in financial planning, accounting, and law and understands how these areas apply to the family's specific situation. In planning both for the family's financial security and for the financial care of the child, many areas should be examined, such as family assets, expected retirement income, the appropriate amount of life and disability insurance, and the amount of federal funds for which an individual is eligible.

The last area—identifying and obtaining federal funds—is complex. Parents should certainly obtain professional advice and assistance from a financial adviser and an attorney. Several of the federal programs administered by the Social Security Administration are briefly described below. See also Chapter 10, "Financing Care for the Child with Cerebral Palsy."

When is an individual with cerebral palsy eligible for Social Security and Medicare?

If an employed person with sufficient work history becomes disabled, he is eligible for disability insurance, and his spouse and children are also eligible for Social Security Disability Insurance (SSDI). Eligibility for SSDI is determined by the amount of the individual's prior Social Security contribution and by the number of years worked. Those eligible for SSDI are the spouse, minor children, and adult children whose disability occurred before age 22. These same individuals are eligible for survivor's insurance (upon death of a parent with qualifying employment history). The benefit received (either by the adult or the child with a disability) is not determined by assets or income level, but solely on the basis of whether the person has met the federal standard for disability. The National Organization of Social Security Claimants Representatives (NOSSCR) is made up of attorneys who specialize in Social Security. It provides a resource to persons seeking expert assistance on Social Security issues.

Medicare is a medical insurance program available to individuals qualifying for SSDI. Medicare eligibility begins two years after the date of initial SSDI entitlement. Medicare is also available under SSDI's Disabled Adult Child program to adults disabled before age 22 whose parent is deceased or is currently receiving SSDI or Social Security retirement benefits. This health insurance is for acute and chronic health management and can cover costs of wheelchairs and other assistive technology. Prescription drug coverage is also available to Medicare beneficiaries.

The other major federal program administered by the Social Security Administration is Supplemental Security Income (SSI), which is available to individuals with disabilities based on their financial need. SSI is available to children with significant disabilities if their parents' income and resources are low enough. SSI benefits can be paid even to parents of infants and toddlers. Some individuals start receiving SSI at age 18 because once a person turns 18, the law no longer regards parental income and resources as also belonging to him. In other words, children of "poor" parents may receive SSI from an early age.

Children of more affluent parents probably will not qualify (due to deeming of parental income and resources) until their 18th birthday. If the beneficiary is over the countable resource limit (generally $2,000), he is simply not eligible for SSI. Certain types of homes, household furniture, and clothing are excluded, up to certain limits, from the calculation of a person's countable assets.

There are many provisions for how assets and the living situation are considered. For example, SSI benefits are generally reduced by one-third if the person lives with someone else who provides both food and shelter. Also, SSI benefits are reduced to a minimal amount if the person lives in a facility paid for by Medicaid, the medical insurance program associated with SSI. The benefit amount is also affected (and may be reduced) by countable income.

The eligibility rules for Medicaid are generally similar to those for SSI. The major benefit of Medicaid is that in addition to acute health care, it provides for long-term chronic care. Medicaid will pay for ongoing long-term nursing home or institutional placement care for an individual or, often through its waiver programs, in-home supports such as personal care.

In addition to these federal programs, there may be other programs administered by other federal agencies—such as the Bureau of Indian Affairs and Armed Forces Retirement Benefits programs, as well as private pension survivor benefits—that need to be investigated. Any and all appropriate assistance for which a person is eligible should be pursued.

Do parents of children with cerebral palsy need wills?

In addition to considering the issues of guardianship and financial planning, parents should also provide for the distribution of their estate, whether they have children with cerebral palsy or not. If parents die intestate—without a will—the estate will be distributed as required by the state code. If parents want to make specific provisions for their child with disabilities that are different from those for their children without disabilities, they can only do this through a will or trust. Parents should seriously consider how they want to divide funds between children without and children with disabilities so that the child with a severe disability will be protected. A special needs trust or a group trust is often the best way if significant funds are involved.

Under certain circumstances, it may be necessary to consider disinheriting a child with a disability (discussed in detail below). This may be the best provision for the whole family, because it may maximize eligibility for needs-based public programs. This is an important consideration in future financial planning, and especially in preparing a will, in which the needs of the whole family are considered and not just those of the individual with the disability. Because of the complexity of the circumstances, it is advisable to consult an expert in estate planning for people with disabilities.

For parents of a child with cerebral palsy, what considerations are important in drawing up a will?

If the extent of the disability or the age of the child is such that the parents are complete guardians of the child, then they should state who they wish to act as the ongoing guardian of the minor child over whom they have guardianship. This is called *nominating a testamentary guardian*. The guardian named in the parents' will must still be formally appointed by the courts. Courts usually give weight to the parents' choice of guardian as stated in their will and often appoint that person as guardian. When making these provisions, parents should seriously consider which level and type of guardianship is most appropriate. This part of the will must be reviewed periodically, since individuals and their circumstances change over time. These provisions of testamentary guardianship apply to both minor children and adults over whom an individual holds guardianship. An alternate approach is to ask the court approving the parental guardianship order to identify a *successor guardian* in the order. Upon the death or inability of the parent to continue to serve as guardian, authority would vest in the successor guardian.

What are the advantages of disinheriting a child with a severe disability?

Though it sounds cruel, there are several reasons why disinheriting the child with a disability might be in the child's best financial interests. A child with a severe disability, especially one who also requires guardianship, usually is eligible for all the means-tested government programs, such as SSI and Medicaid. As soon as this individual acquires a certain level of countable assets or income, these means-tested program benefits are reduced. This is the government's way of allocating scarce resources to those most in need. This means that money inherited by the disabled child at the time of the parents' deaths will simply be used to replace government benefits. In essence, when the child receives the inheritance, his government benefits will be cut off until all the inheritance is spent, at which time the benefits will begin again. The result would be the same if all the inheritance were given to the government and the means-tested benefits to the individual were continued. Therefore, instead of allowing the individual with a disability to inherit equally and by the same unrestricted mechanism that a child without disabilities inherits, a parent may consider several other options, including completely disinheriting the child, establishing a trust fund with specific instructions regarding how the money may be spent, or leaving the child a significantly reduced sum at a level that will not diminish the means-tested government benefit.

In the case of a large estate, a court might decide to require the guardian of the estate to obtain a bond, hire an accountant, or file more comprehensive financial reports. The cost of implementing such requirements could deplete the assets of the disabled child or adult.

Another consideration is that if individuals who are incompetent or only marginally competent inherit funds, this often makes them targets of unscrupulous people who will try to take advantage of them. Providing the funds in the context of a trust fund may in fact be a better method of protecting the individual.

Finally, most states do not allow an incompetent person to make a will, which means that the estate of this person upon his or her death will be distributed according to state laws. Although a competent person can bequeath assets to a specific charity or to specific persons, an incompetent individual cannot.

All the above are reasons why you might consider disinheriting a person with a disability. But before taking this step, you should carefully discuss it with lawyers, accountants, and financial advisers familiar with this area of planning.

What are the disadvantages of disinheriting the child with a severe disability?

It is important to consider the feelings of the person with a disability. The idea of being disinherited may make the individual feel unloved or uncared for. This feeling may be prevented by bequeathing the person an amount that will not have an impact on means-tested income or assets. Parents may also wish to explain the reasons for the specific inheritance and to include with the will letters that express love and concern and explain the special care that the person will receive.

What is an ABLE Account?

A recent federal law offers a new option for an individual with a disability to acquire savings without affecting eligibility for means-tested programs. In 2014 the Achieving a Better Life Experience (ABLE) Act was adopted. It allows eligible individuals with disabilities with onset before age 26 to set up an ABLE account. The account can have up to $100,000 without affecting SSI or Medicaid eligibility. There is an annual contribution limit, which is adjusted for inflation. Funds can be used for a "qualified disability expense," including education, housing, assistive technology, personal care services, and health care. Relatives should be cautious about contributing large sums to such accounts, since funds remaining in the account upon the death of the individual with a disability may be subject to government "claw back" to repay Medicaid outlays. State laws are being adopted to implement the new federal law.

What is a trust?

Trusts hold money or property that the grantor (the person who sets up the trust) leaves for the beneficiary's economic benefit. Unlike an outright gift or inheritance through a will, trusts usually contain carefully written instructions on when and how to use the trust's contents. Parents (or others) can set up a trust while they are alive or as part of a will. If parents set up a trust while still alive, they can be the trustees (the persons who manage the trust). They can also assign someone else to be the trustee. A trustee can be a person or a financial institution.

There are many different types of trusts, serving different purposes. Laws that affect trusts differ from state to state. An attorney who specializes in special needs trusts should be consulted in developing a trust in this context. For example, states may have different standards for determining whether a trust is a "Medicaid qualifying trust" so as to authorize disregard of income and principal. These standards may be quite complex.

Most Medicaid programs have financial eligibility caps. The caps vary widely by program. Each Medicaid waiver has different caps. Some caps cover countable income only; others cover both countable income and countable resources (e.g., savings). Suppose an individual has a general trust (e.g., from a medical malpractice settlement) with $150,000 principal that pays out $1,000 a month, which is treated as "income" to the individual. If the individual applied for eligibility to a Medicaid program with a $50,000 resource cap, he or she would be disqualified since the $150,000 in principal exceeds the $50,000 resource cap. If the same individual applied for eligibility to a Medicaid program with no resource cap but an income cap of $900 a month, he or she would be disqualified since the $1,000 in income exceeds the $900 cap. If the trust were a Medicaid qualifying trust, both the trust's principal and its income would be disregarded, so the individual would be eligible in the above scenarios since the resource (trust principal) and income are disregarded (not counted). The actual numbers vary based on the size of the household and a percentage of the amount of the federal poverty level, which is adjusted annually. Therefore, consulting with a lawyer who is knowledgeable in this area is crucial.

What kinds of trusts are most commonly used for children with special needs?

Supplemental, discretionary, or cooperative master trusts are common options in most states. These kinds of trusts are usually recommended when parents want to protect their child's governmental benefits.

Supplemental trusts. Supplemental trusts are designed so that the principal and its earnings supplement the beneficiary's care but do not replace the funds required to pay for this care. This kind of trust is good for the recipient of SSI and Medicaid, whose assets cannot exceed certain levels. The trust grantor can carefully direct the trust not to replace the cost of services covered by Medicaid. Instead, the trust would require the trustee to only provide funds for certain items, services, or expenses not covered by SSI or Medicaid. As an example, a supplementary trust could be established providing income that allows a certain individual to spend money on entertainment, such as going to the movies, traveling to visit friends and relatives, and purchasing small gifts for loved ones. Because this money is restricted to specific uses, the income from such a trust, if it is not too large, will not be considered income in a means-tested program. Because the principal of the trust is not an asset of the individual beneficiary, it also cannot be considered in means testing for federally funded programs.

Discretionary trusts. Some states allow the grantor to give the trustee full discretion in how much or how little of the trust to distribute. This kind of trust can also contain provisions that limit distributions so that the person remains eligible for government benefits. The trustee must be careful not to distribute money from the trust for goods and services or outright to the beneficiary in a manner that will disqualify the beneficiary from receiving government benefits. There are drawbacks to this kind of trust. The trustee must be very knowledgeable about the benefits a person is receiving and the related eligibility requirements. Also, the trustee has total power over distribution of funds and may hold back trust distributions to the detriment of the beneficiary.

Some other potential dangers exist in establishing a trust in which the trustee is given full discretion on how to spend the funds. For example, the government may attempt, through legislation or the courts, to direct the trustee to fund or reimburse public outlays such as Medicaid, or count the full amount available for trustee disposition as a resource. The problem is that a trust established under today's legal standards must anticipate changes in the law 20 to 40 or more years from now. It has been suggested that an in terrorem clause be inserted in trusts such that if the government successfully breaks, or invades, the trust, the principal and proceeds revert to other relatives. This would be a disincentive to the government trying to break the trust.

Master cooperative trust. Also called "pooled trusts," these are special trusts established and managed by a nonprofit organization to help disabled individuals and their families. These trusts allow families to pool their resources with other families rather than set up individual trust accounts. A group trust allows a parent to fund a trust for a child without affecting eligibility for public benefits, while specifying support services and allowable uses. Such trusts are available in many states. Because the funds are pooled, there is greater potential for higher returns. Another advantage of this form of trust is that individual parents who lack sufficient funds to meet the minimum requirements of a commercial financial institution can do so by pooling their funds with those of other parents. Group trusts often have lower minimum trust amounts. In addition, because the pooled account is usually managed and invested as one large account, the administrative fees are lower. Beneficiaries of these trusts usually receive earnings based on their share of the principal.

How do I set up a trust?

There are basically two ways to set up a trust: It can be *testamentary* (as part of a will) or *inter vivos* (living).

A testamentary trust is part of a will and does not take effect until after the person who drew up the will dies. Such a trust can be funded by life insurance proceeds, which do not normally pass through the will. This is a way to fund a fairly large trust if a parent lacks significant assets to leave through a will. Parents can change the trust's terms any time the will is changed. So if the intended beneficiary should die first, the will and trust can be changed.

A living trust is set up and takes effect before the person dies. Parents and others can make regular gifts to such a trust. Grandparents can make testamentary bequests from their wills to such a trust. Parents can be the trustees and manage it at their own discretion, or they can assign someone else to be the trustee to see how that person would manage the trust. Living trusts are either revocable or irrevocable. A revocable trust can be changed or ended by parents before they die. In the case of an irrevocable trust, parents set up the trust and give up most power to change or end it. Either type has tax advantages depending on the size of the parents' estate, the family situation, and other factors. Remember to consult with an attorney who specializes in special needs trusts.

What happens when the beneficiary dies?

The trust must spell out what happens to the trust when the primary beneficiary dies. For example, a $50,000 trust may be established, with a specific bank as the trustee, with instructions to distribute income to a child with a disability as the beneficiary. The beneficiary may use this income for a specifically defined purpose as indicated in the trust. The trust may provide that when the beneficiary dies, the money will be divided among relatives of the beneficiary or the grantor. In this way, parents set aside money that benefits the child with a disability and that is then passed on to their other children or grandchildren, for example, upon the death of their child with a disability.

In establishing a trust, it is important to consider who will be the trustee. A large trust should probably have a corporate trustee, usually a bank. Although an individual trustee can be established, many states require a bond in those circumstances. The trust may also be established as a mandatory trust, which requires the trustee to pay a fixed amount of money to the beneficiary at predetermined intervals.

How do I obtain legal help to collect damages for an injury that may be the cause of my child's cerebral palsy?

It is your legal right to bring a lawsuit to collect damages for injuries resulting from medical malpractice or other injuries the child incurred because of the actions of someone else. There are many scenarios in which injuries to children occur that may cause cerebral palsy and permanent disability, such as falls, near drownings, smoke inhalation, overdosages, or adverse effects of drugs or surgery before, during, or after birth. Injury during birth as a cause of CP has been a major concern for many years but is now understood to be a cause in only a small percentage of cases.

Some lawyers specialize in evaluating injuries and preparing suits for medical malpractice. Usually your family lawyer or a general practice lawyer can help you find such a lawyer. Bar associations, referral services, and parent groups can also be good sources for recommendations. A competent lawyer will evaluate the evidence and then discuss with you whether he or she feels there is legal evidence sufficient to pursue a malpractice claim. These lawyers usually work on a contingency fee, which means that they will receive a specific percentage, varying from 25 to 50 percent, of the amount recovered. Therefore, they will probably tell you if they don't think you have a good case, because they do not want to spend their time and money unnecessarily. Some attorneys will ask the parents to pay their out-of-pocket expenses.

If my child has cerebral palsy due to a birth injury, doesn't that mean that I am entitled to a malpractice insurance settlement?

Medical malpractice, especially with respect to a birth injury, may be very difficult to prove. A malpractice claim requires proof that the medical care your child received was in some way below the ordinary standard of care in the community. The occurrence of even significant injury in the course of medical treatment does not automatically establish that malpractice has occurred if that medical treatment is deemed to meet the community standard of practice.

In addition, there must be harm or damage suffered by the individual as a direct result of this deficient practice. As an example, if your child was accidentally given a drug dose that was ten times the recommended amount, this clearly falls below the community standard of practice. However, if this error did not lead to any harm or damage to your child, then there may be no malpractice recovery.

Just because your child has cerebral palsy does not mean that there has been some kind of medical negligence. CP most often occurs because of damage suffered in the mother's womb unrelated to any issues of medical care. On the other hand, there are certainly incidents in which inadequate medical care during pregnancy, delivery, or shortly afterwards was responsible for the child's CP. For most children, cerebral palsy caused by such injuries does not become apparent until the child is at least 6 months old.

What's the best thing to do with a large settlement resulting from a malpractice lawsuit?

It is often a good idea to place large settlements from medical malpractice lawsuits into a trust fund for the child. Sometimes the trustee can be the parent, but often the trustee is a corporate entity, such as a bank. The court may define how the trust is to be used, such as for medical care or perhaps for housing. Spending money from the trust for certain items, such as specially modified vans, is usually allowed. Parents may receive a certain amount every month to help them care for the child.

Another, simpler option for protecting funds received by the child from a malpractice case is an annuity. This is an insurance policy that can be structured to pay out varying amounts at different times in the child's life (for instance, more as the child ages), with the principal to be distributed to designated persons in the event of the child's death. Because annuities generally earn tax-free interest, they can grow substantially during the early years, when needed payments may be small. Then by the time the child requires greater funding for housing or supportive services, the annuity can be structured to pay out at a higher level. The terms of an annuity are usually determined by the parents and the attorneys involved. The information above on structuring funds so as not to displace public program (SSI, Medicaid) eligibility applies here as well. Malpractice attorneys sometimes are not expert in this context and may need to consult colleagues who specialize in this field to structure the settlement in the way that is most beneficial to the injured child.

Are there special programs that pay damages for medically caused injuries?

Some states, such as Florida, have established birth injury programs in which benefits may be obtained outside the malpractice legal system. The federal government has also established a program for children sustaining injuries due to vaccinations, in which the insurer is the federal government. Benefits are paid out of this program if it is shown that the immunization caused the child's injury without the family having to go through a lawsuit.

How can I use the law to help my family member who has a disability?

The legal system exists to provide protection for individuals, including people with disabilities. Recent legal developments have provided much more opportunity for individuals with disabilities. To take advantage of this new legal and social climate, it is important to be an advocate for yourself and for the individual with a disability. Part of this advocacy work involves lobbying your state and national legislators so that the ability of the person with a disability to participate in society will continue to expand.

Being an able advocate also means educating yourself and others about both the specifics of the law and the arrangements for obtaining help from professionals. It is this combination of understanding the individual's rights and legal standing and understanding how to contact the appropriate professionals that allows the individual with the disability to take full advantage of the legal system.

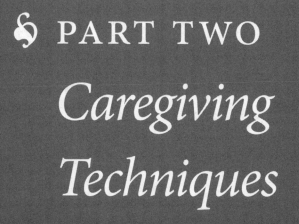

PART TWO

Caregiving Techniques

Taking Care of Yourself When You Care for Others

Taking care of any child requires a good deal of work, time, and patience, and taking care of a child with special needs requires an abundance of all three. It is widely recognized that being a caregiver can be a stressful and demanding job. Parents often feel overworked and frustrated, and they are concerned about and distracted by the emotional and financial struggles they face as they raise a child with cerebral palsy.

Stressors

Beginning with the birth of the child, and sometimes even before, parents have periods of anxiety and a great deal of uncertainty. Parents and other caregivers are faced with finding answers to questions that can't always be answered. They will often need to make important decisions quickly, since conditions can change swiftly. They must find professionals who can meet their child's needs—and can communicate with the family. This process, as well as the many other things caregivers do, requires a lot of time and effort.

There are a number of stressors commonly faced by parents and caregivers of children with disabilities. Some parents will experience symptoms of depression, which is a very common result of dealing with a child with disabilities. These symptoms may manifest as difficulty sleeping (trouble falling asleep, sleeping too much), over- or undereating, impatience, irritability, anger, guilt, or a profound sense of sadness. The physical health of caregivers is also at risk because caring for their children can present such heavy demands. Lifting children who have grown into adults can pose a tremendous physical strain, for example. Some parents find the needs of the child so overwhelming that they neglect their own health, either because it seems insignificant or because it is too costly to eat well and get proper rest and respite from caregiving responsibilities.

Marital discord can also result from the enormous stress of having a child with disabilities. Many feelings—including guilt, fear, anger, and anxiety—can cause people to lash out at each other. Sometimes a parent finds it difficult even to get in touch with his or her personal feelings, because the day-to-day activities of caring for a child with special needs while simultaneously holding down a job and caring for the rest of the family are overwhelming.

It's not uncommon for parents to react differently to the child's problem: one may become outwardly emotional, while the other withdraws and even appears uninterested. Parents may disagree on treatment options, or they may treat the child with disabilities differently than their other children, which can cause stress in the marriage. Partners often discover that they have less time for each other or seemingly less interest in the relationship than they used to. While a single parent might not have this type of conflict, he or she will have to make decisions alone, which is also stressful.

Siblings can also be affected by having a child with special needs in the family. A child with special needs often requires a great deal of parental attention and support. Siblings may respond to this by engaging in attention-seeking behavior, or they may become jealous of the child with a disability. They may experience worry and/or fear about their sibling. Younger siblings can sometimes believe "impossible" facts, such as that they caused the difficulties the child with special needs has or that they could "catch" the disability themselves. The sibling of a child who is unable to walk may feel overwhelming guilt about his own ability to run, jump, and skate. Additionally, siblings may have difficulty dealing with their peers' reactions to their sister or brother who has a disability.

Although it used to be thought that the impact on typically developing siblings was largely negative, more recently awareness of potential positive effects of having a sibling with special needs is being investigated. Many children cope pretty well with life's surprises, as one little girl named Colleen shows in her story "A Special Sister":

All my life I wanted to have a sister! I imagined her to be my best friend. I always wanted to have somebody there when I needed them. I wanted somebody to hug, to laugh with, and to be myself with. I wanted a special closeness with my sister. Kind of like we always had a secret together. A sister would be with me all my life.

My dream came true!!! I did get a baby sister. Her name is Kathleen. She fooled us all by being born on April first. I was so happy my insides were jumping all around. I made a big colorful picture for her to look at in her crib.

When I held her for the first time I felt my heart melt because we loved each other so much!

In a short time we found out that Kathleen has cerebral palsy. It's only on her right side. Her arm and leg don't work too well. So we do therapy with her! I am learning a lot about how our body works so I will be able to help her! She and I work well together. She listens to me, so I listen to her. And that's the way it will be all our lives.

Kathleen is more special than I ever thought she could be. I hug her, I laugh with her, and we already have secrets together! She is very special!!

As a child with a disability grows, parents need to deal not only with the increased time commitment necessary to care for the child but also with whatever prognosis the doctor has provided. Needless to say, the responsibilities of running a household coexist with these special responsibilities. Parents may find themselves making a multitude of visits to different physicians and therapists and spending untold time and money.

Children frequently need surgical procedures that require a parent to spend increasing amounts of time away from family and job, which can make life very difficult. Additionally, the financial cost of purchasing wheelchairs, braces, and various other equipment can be staggering.

How to Cope

All parents have dreams for their children. Some children with mild disabilities are able to live normal lives. However, there are many children whose parents must accept that they will never walk and may never be able to feed themselves or speak. It is therefore essential that caregivers—be they mothers, fathers, grandparents, siblings, or unrelated individuals—recognize their stressors and develop and maintain coping mechanisms. They must learn, for example, to ask for advice and help, and they must come to terms with the fact that not all of their child's needs can be met. Other parents who are now or formerly were in a similar situation can be of great comfort and help. Often they can provide more assistance than well-meaning friends and relatives who don't have any experience in this area.

Caregivers need to be in tune with their feelings and on guard for signs that they might need some help maintaining their own emotional health. Sometimes parents get so caught up in the day-to-day routine and needs of the child that they forget to consider their own health. Parents need to communicate with each other and with health care professionals as much as possible so that decisions are based on their true feelings. Couples need to be aware of the stress on their relationship and then avail themselves of opportunities for help. They may simply need to set aside more time for talking, or they may want to arrange for special times alone with each other, such as a weekend away or a "date night," even just grabbing a quick cup of coffee together. Marriage counseling can often help couples who are having trouble coping with stress of various kinds. Counseling can help couples recognize their feelings, their fears, and the stressors impacting the family, as well as help them communicate more effectively with each other.

Caregivers must acknowledge that they cannot be effective unless they take care of themselves. They must acknowledge their needs and seek out the resources to address those needs. "Resources" come in many shapes and sizes. You may develop a pool of friends who can provide respite or some time for yourself without the children. To reduce the time and strain of numerous appointments and errands, you can coordinate appointments and, if possible, obtain many services at the same facility. The various Ronald McDonald Houses throughout the country are a wonderful resource for families who have to travel away from home for specialized treatment or surgery. Minivacations, even a day trip to the country, can provide enormous relief. You also need to cultivate individual stress-reducing techniques, such as exercise, reading, hobbies, or prayer. Religious institutions and community groups may offer support. Finally, you may want to find a formal support group specifically for parents. There are professionals who can help guide you to a support group that fits your needs.

In some cases, you may decide that the best option for your child with disabilities and your family is to have the child live in a group home or a similar facility so the major responsibility for day-to-day care is put in the hands of people who are able to handle the nuances of nurturing a child with a disability. This is often a good idea as caregivers grow older or if siblings are being neglected or otherwise suffering from the experience. Ultimately, the caregiver needs to care for himself or herself in order to be able to continue to care for another person.

Protecting the Caregiver's Back: Basic Body Mechanics

Many tasks in caring for a child may place the care provider's back at risk for injury. Most of these tasks involve performing the activities of daily care, such as dressing, bathing, feeding, and moving the child. This section describes good body mechanics that can be used by the care provider to decrease the risk of back injury.

Dressing

Newborn to age 3. Use a surface that is at a comfortable working level, such as a changing table. The parent should not be forced to lean over the surface in order to dress the child. At this age the crib surface should also be at a comfortable level (keeping in mind that the mattress must be lowered when it is anticipated that a child will soon be standing up), and the crib mattress may provide a good surface for dressing the child.

Ages 3 to 10. If the child is able to, he ought to be encouraged to stand up and hold on to furniture while being dressed. In fact he should be encouraged to participate in the dressing process as much as possible. An occupational therapist can provide strategies and techniques involving the child, who will perform dressing skills at the level he or she is capable of, with assistance from the parent as needed. If timeliness in completing these tasks is an issue initially, having the child practice skills on a weekend or a day when there is not a deadline to "get out of the house" is a good start. This is good therapy and progress toward an adult style of dressing, and it involves less lifting than is involved when the child is dressed lying down. If the child must be dressed lying down, and the child's bed is used for dressing, then the mattress surface should be at a comfortable level for the parents to work. This can easily be achieved by placing the bed on blocks, but care must be taken to use side rails so that the child does not fall out of a high bed. If the bed is on the floor, the caregiver ought to place one or both knees on the floor rather than bend over from the back.

The older child and teenager. The same advice applies at this age, but now, because of the child's larger size, it is especially important to dress her while she is standing if at all possible. In preparation for transitioning to adulthood, if the child is physically unable to perform a dressing task, having the ability to direct a caregiver (someone other than the parent) to perform the task is essential.

Bathing

Bathing can involve a great deal of lifting and bending over in positions that are very stressful to the caregiver's back. Before bathing a young child on a changing table, the caregiver should adjust the level of the table to the level of the caregiver's mid-abdomen. Children from age 2 to age 10 especially enjoy being bathed in warm water and are usually bathed in a bathtub. There are several different kinds of bathing chairs that provide trunk support for the child

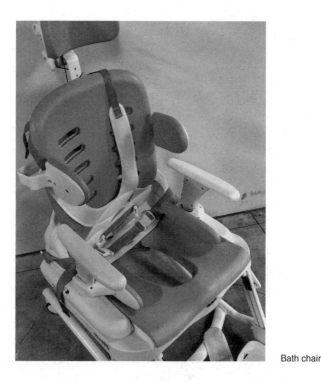

Bath chair

who has poor trunk control; an occupational therapist can help you select one that is appropriate for your child.

The main problem in tub bathing for caregivers, however, is lifting the child into the bathtub. Before he reaches about age 10, this may be difficult but can still be managed. After age 10 it becomes more difficult. Whenever possible, the child should be lifted or helped into the tub in a standing position onto a non-skid surface; then he can sit down from the standing position. This is much easier for the caregiver. Also, sitting on the edge of the bathtub and placing one foot in the tub before lifting the child reduces the stress on the caregiver's back. For the child who can stand, use a shower with a handrail for him to hold on to. This is an excellent way to bathe an older child who can stand. It is important to take into consideration that changes in the air and the water temperature can impact a child's tone and therefore change his ability to maintain an upright stance. A "dry run" of standing in the tub without water is a good way to assess any challenges that tone changes may present.

As the child approaches puberty and adult height, it is no longer wise to continue to lift her into a bathtub. This is hard on the caregiver's back, and it usually is unsafe for the child, because there is an increased risk that the caregiver will slip and drop the child when she is heavier. If she will continue to be bathed in a bathtub, a mechanical lift device that attaches to the bathtub or the ceiling should be used. Or she can be wheeled into a shower if the proper home modifications are made. There are a number of different shower chair alternatives. Ask your child's occupational therapist to evaluate her and determine the best way for her to be bathed—that is, the best way for the child, the care provider, and the housing situation.

Moving

The small infant and child is primarily moved about his environment by being carried. As the child grows but does not begin to walk, caregivers must begin to protect their backs and not simply continue to carry the child until they are physically unable to do so. This requires planning for a home environment that is accessible to a wheelchair; this planning should take place when the child is between the ages of 4 and 8. Another option is to use a rolling stool and push yourself, with the child on your lap, along the floor. Alternatively, if the child can hold on securely to the stool, he may be pushed along alone. This will only work if the house is not carpeted, however.

As the child gets larger, transferring from bed to wheelchair becomes difficult. If he may be capable of bearing his own weight so that standing transfers can take place, this needs to be encouraged even at the age when the child is still small enough to be lifted. If you wait to start doing standing transfers until he absolutely cannot be lifted, then it's harder for both the child and the caregiver to learn the technique, and it causes much more anxiety. Both of these factors make it more likely that attempts to learn the technique will be unsuccessful. If a child cannot bear weight and is to be cared for by one adult alone, then mechanical lifts are usually needed to improve the safety of the transfers and to protect the caregiver's back.

Feeding

Most infants are fed while being held by the caregiver. By 9 to 12 months, however, the child should be fed while sitting in a seat, with the caregiver doing the feeding sitting in front of the child. This frees both arms and allows the caregiver to position herself at a comfortable height and have a better view of how the child is doing.

General Guidelines for Protecting Your Back

1. Always get your body as close to the child to be lifted as possible before starting to lift.

2. Whenever possible, lift by bending the knees, not by bending through the back.

3. When working standing up, adjust the height of the work surface to place the child at the level of your navel (mid-abdomen) so that you don't have to bend over while bathing or dressing him.

4. If you are working with a child sitting (such as feeding a child), the child's face should be almost even with yours when you sit up straight. This prevents you from leaning forward and putting strain on your spine.

Making Things Easier for You and Your Child: Home Modifications

There are various ways to modify the home environment so that your child will have more independence and things will be easier on you. The cost of these modifications varies, from inexpensive to very costly. The desired mod-

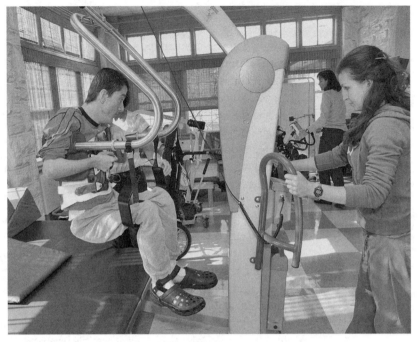

Lift system

ifications may involve more available space and current resources than the caregiver has, however.

Any modification must be consistent with the cognitive level of the individual for whom it is planned. In the case of individuals with significant cognitive impairment, the ability to be more independent in the home could remove a barrier that is a potentially useful safety net. In other words, it is undesirable to modify the home in a way that would allow the person more freedom of movement if the person might inadvertently hurt himself or herself.

Here are several suggestions for modifications. Some involve merely placing objects differently, some involve making purchases, others involve construction. Those that involve construction range from relatively simple projects that the caregivers might do themselves to modifications that will need to be contracted out.

- Rearrange furniture in order to remove obstructions from pathways to rooms as well as to allow for a wheelchair to turn within a room. This latter requires a space at least 60 inches by 60 inches square.
- Rearrange kitchen cabinets and the refrigerator to put necessary items within reach of your child. Do the same with bathroom accessories. Pull-out drawers and lazy Susans can increase accessibility.
- Remove plush wall-to-wall carpeting. Finish wood floors with a nonslip finish or install industrial-type carpeting.
- Widen doorways.

- Replace doorknobs with lever door handles.
- Replace entrance steps with ramps.
- Install a hinged arm support for help with toileting. A high-rise toilet is particularly helpful, as is a bidet.
- Install single mix faucets with levered handles and include an anti-scald device.
- Adjust the height of light switches and plugs to put them within reach.
- Program portable telephones or cell phones to allow your child full-time access to others.
- Install an intercom system that can be used between rooms as well as at entrances.
- Replace bathtubs with wheel-in showers.
- Install an adjustable-height sink and counter with an open front in the kitchen and bathroom.
- Install an angled mirror above stove burners to allow your child a view of the contents of pots from his or her wheelchair.
- Buy a home automation system that allows your child to control the TV, intercom, and thermostat from a central device.
- Buy a lounge chair with electrically powered positioning and lifting ability.
- Install a fire extinguisher at an accessible level and plan for emergency access (such as ambulance personnel entering) and emergency exit routes (such as in the case of fire).
- Make use of various adaptive devices such as bath chairs, lifts, corner chairs (which provide support on two sides rather than only in the back), hospital beds, and eating and writing utensils.
- Increase accessibility with a properly trained service dog.

A "backdoor" way to approach home modification is one that allows the child to remain in the home and the caregiver to "age in place" while taking care of the child over his lifespan, as opposed to planning to transition the child to a group home or community living arrangement when he gets older. To do this, the caregiver should investigate geriatric ("age in place") modifications and funding, not disability specific ones. One needs to be aware, however, that some modifications for the aging caregiver or parent may not be appropriate or helpful for the child. It is another option, however.

There are agencies that help plan for and carry out changes to accommodate the needs of individuals with disabilities. There are four with a national focus:

- ABLEDATA, a database of products, devices, and equipment for people with disabilities (800-227-0216; www.abledata.com)
- The National Rehabilitation Information Center (800-246-2742; www.naric.com)
- The National Council of Independent Living (703-525-3406; www.ncil.org)
- The Americans with Disabilities Act Information Hotline (202-514-0301; www.ada.gov)

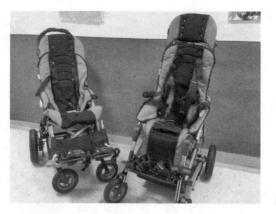

Medical strollers

Another helpful website is ucp.org, the website for United Cerebral Palsy. The local chapter of UCP may have information on agencies in your area.

Choosing Appropriate Seating

Special needs strollers, wheelchairs, feeding chairs, premolded soft foam chairs, seating supports, and corner chairs are forms of adaptive seating that may benefit children with cerebral palsy. Many companies make different types of seating in several categories.

Strollers are a universal method of seating—almost all infants and young children are wheeled about in a stroller by their parents or other caregivers. For most children with cerebral palsy who are younger than 1 or 2 years, the standard strollers that can be purchased at any department store are adequate. A 2-year-old who is having a great deal of difficulty with head control, however, and even the 1-year-old who is not able to provide any trunk support or head control needs more support than standard strollers provide. One good temporary alternative to buying a special stroller or a wheelchair is to have an insert fabricated for the existing stroller that can provide stability, head and trunk support, and more safety. But with the advances in technology, more special needs strollers are available to fit the smaller child.

Most of the nonmedical strollers that are available on the market are not strong enough for the slightly bigger child, between the ages of 3 and 5. At this point, how much support a child needs should be determined based on an assessment of how much head and trunk control he or she has. If the decision is made to purchase a special needs stroller, the parent may be pleased to learn that there are a number of such strollers on the market that look very much like the standard baby stroller.

Larger stroller-type chairs are useful for quick transportation, such as going to the grocery store. Most of these chairs, however, have a significant drawback for a child who is able to push a chair, since there are no wheels that the child can reach to push. In addition, many of these larger chairs have a fairly narrow base and can tip over easily on an uneven surface. Unlike these strollers, which usually have small wheels, there are strollers designed for outdoor use,

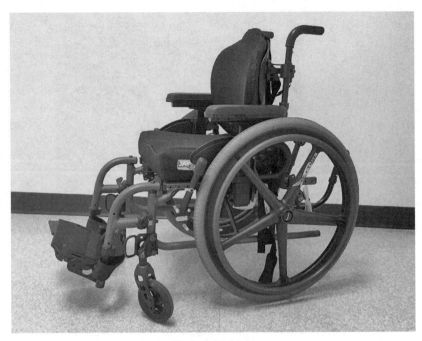

Medical wheelchair

which have larger wheels. They are especially useful for parents who want to take their children on outdoor walks. These large-wheeled strollers are very stable and are easier to push on uneven terrain. There are also a few specialized wheelchairs that can be used at the beach, over sand and even by the water.

For the child who isn't walking and needs more support, strollers generally are not a good idea for long-term sitting past age 2 or 3. All of these strollers continue to have the form and shape of the infant baby stroller. This is a factor that appeals to parents because the public tends to pay less attention to these strollers than they do to a wheelchair. From the child's perspective, however, continuing to be pushed around in a stroller type of device is undesirable, especially when the child is bright and interested in interacting with his peers. Moving to a regular large-wheeled chair or a more standard-appearing medical wheelchair gives him the sense that he is now growing up and is into a "grown-up's" wheelchair. Also, as awareness catches up with technology, these wheelchairs are becoming more attractive and colorful, thus more appealing to a child and more acceptable to his or her peers. Such a chair also allows the child to push himself if his arm strength and coordination permit. The earlier we can provide the child the opportunity to move, the greater the potential they will have to learn and develop.

There are many other advantages to having a standard type of medical wheelchair. The customizable adaptive seating—including trunk support, solid supported seats and backs, headrests, neck supports, and chest straps—is designed to match your child's individual needs. The large wheelchair is much easier to push over many kinds of terrain, and it is more stable. For this reason, certainly by the age of 5 or 6, since mobility is so important, the child should move out of the stroller into a regular type of wheelchair, perhaps a power wheelchair. If a power chair is purchased, a stroller might be an acceptable backup if you already own one. It certainly is not necessary to order a fully adapted secondary wheelchair if a power chair has been ordered. On the other hand, it is a good idea to have a secondary type of wheelchair available, both because power chairs break down and because there are many places where power chairs can't be transported or may not be usable due to the space required for maneuvering.

There are many adaptive chairs used to improve the child's sitting posture and especially for feeding. Generally, an adequately arranged wheelchair with good trunk support, head control, and a lap tray can be used as a feeding chair for the child. Some parents or therapists prefer to have a separate feeding chair. Frequently used types are the Tumble Forms chair and the Special Tomato chair, which are molded foam chairs that promote an upright seated posture for feeding. For the child who has a tendency to extend the head and spine, these chairs may provide short-term solutions for feeding and positioning. However, they provide very poor postural control for the child who tends to collapse forward and should not be used as wheelchair inserts or for a significant portion of the child's sitting time during the day. For the child who requires more postural control and pelvic positioning, the Rifton Activity Chair can provide adjustable positioning components to promote more aggressive postural control. Corner chairs help the very young child develop sitting balance. These are very simple and excellent seating devices to allow the child to develop sitting coordination and balance on the floor.

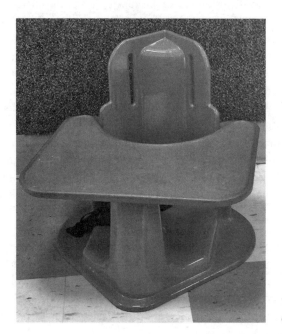

Corner chair

Purchasing a Wheelchair

Parents should never walk into a medical supply store and tell a salesperson that they would like to purchase a wheelchair for their child, because even well-intentioned salespeople have received little training in assessing the child's needs. Generally the child's physical therapist or the orthopedist or physiatrist who is seeing the child will provide guidance about purchasing a wheelchair based on the child's needs. Many pediatric hospitals have wheelchair clinics, where physical therapists, rehabilitation engineers, and physicians discuss the family's and the child's situation and determine what type of chair will meet the child's, the family's, and the school's needs and then advise the parents accordingly.

Before purchasing a wheelchair, the child's need for postural control and support, the child's ability to push his or her own chair, and the need for any adaptive devices must be considered. In addition to these issues, which directly involve the child, it is also important to consider the child's home and school—the settings where the wheelchair will be used. This will determine how important it is to have a lightweight chair and will have a bearing on the size of the chair purchased. A chair to be used in a country environment, where there are no sidewalks or paved streets, needs to be extremely stable. Consider using larger rear and front tires for the manual wheelchair to be used on rough terrain. Consider a front-wheel-drive system for a power chair.

The availability of service and repairs should also be considered (see "About Wheelchair Maintenance" below). Although manual wheelchairs need repair less often than do power chairs, eventually wheelchair parts will wear out or break and need to be replaced. Another issue that is important for many children and for their families is the appearance of the chair—its color and structure, as well as how the child looks when seated in the chair. Certainly a child who has a colorful, well-constructed chair in good repair is more likely to receive the same kind of positive response from friends, acquaintances, and strangers as the child who is well dressed and clean. A child in a drab, poorly maintained, and poorly constructed wheelchair often elicits the same type of response as the child who is taken into public wearing clothes that are worn, dirty, and badly coordinated.

Insurance companies and government agencies will usually purchase one wheelchair every three to five years for a growing child. For this reason, growth needs to be considered when selecting a chair, and parents and the child must understand that the wheelchair will need to last for three to five years. Some families who purchase a power wheelchair as their child's primary means of mobility seek alternate funding to purchase a backup manual wheelchair or special needs stroller for transport reasons. Insurances typically only cover one primary mobility system for that three- to five-year period. Social services personnel can be helpful in locating funding for purchasing chairs, but occasionally purchases will need to be organized through community groups such as the local UCP chapter or the Variety Club or possibly by community fundraisers.

Another important aspect to consider when purchasing a wheelchair is how it will be transported. If the only transportation available is an automobile, the size of the trunk needs to be considered. All chair inserts need to be removable. If your child goes to school on a school bus and rides the bus seated in his wheelchair, you need to make sure that the wheelchair is equipped with a transit tie down system. Only a few wheelchairs have been crash-tested, and as soon as a customized seating system is added, each one becomes unique. Be sure that a headrest and an automotive-style seatbelt (not Velcro) are added to the wheelchair for safety. Chest harnesses, abductors, and other positioning components are not substitutes for a seatbelt but can be used with the seatbelt for added trunk support and positioning. It is also important to understand that a wheelchair seatbelt is not certified to be a primary restraint when traveling in a vehicle. An additional seatbelt connected to the vehicle that goes around the passenger is necessary for safe transportation.

As mentioned, most wheelchairs for children can be expected to last approximately three to five years. However, a number of wheelchairs are marketed as being able to serve from age 3 to age 30, in other words, to take the child from infancy to adulthood. The reality is that it is virtually impossible to manufacture a wheelchair that fits adequately and is not overwhelmingly large and bulky for the 3-year-old that would not be inadequate by the time he is even 8 or so years old. It is extremely unusual for a wheelchair to last more than five years in childhood. Plan on making a wheelchair purchase every three to five years until your child is fully grown.

A child should be checked every six months or as needed to make sure the fit of the wheelchair meets his or her positioning needs. There are several ways growth is built into a wheelchair:

1. Most wheelchair frames are expandable in depth, and a few in width. Expansion requires replacing parts and seating components if a new wheelchair frame is not recommended.

2. Inserts (seat and backrest) for a wheelchair should be measured to allow for adjustments in seat depth and back height so that only adjustments—not replacements—are needed as the child grows.

3. The wheelchair base should be 2 to 3 inches wider than the hip width to allow for some growth. If the base is wider than this, a child who self-propels will not have the best access to the rear wheels and will lose stability. Remember, although provision for some growth can be built into the chair, significant changes in the child's size, such as significant weight gain or a growth spurt, can't always be anticipated.

Choosing and Using Car Seats

Most states have passed laws requiring that children under certain ages be transported on roads only in approved car seats. The purpose of this regulation is to provide a means of restraining children for their own safety during motor vehicle accidents. Car seats protect children with disabilities as well; in fact, they can be vitally important for children with cerebral palsy, since many of them do not have natural protective mechanisms because of poor muscle control

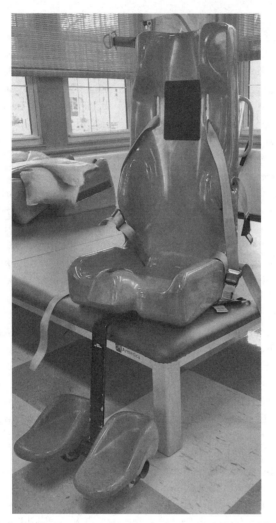

Medical car seat

and coordination. For many young children with CP, the standard approved commercially available car seats, using a 5-point harness system, provide adequate protection, typically for children weighing from 25 to 120 pounds. But they can be costly. For the child with poor head and trunk control who needs supportive seating, however, special needs car seats approved by the US Department of Transportation should be used if the child cannot be transported in his or her own wheelchair. Special needs car seats can provide improved postural support within a 5-point harness system and accommodate weights up to 108 pounds. These car seats are often heavy and difficult to move from car to car, so it is best that they remain in the vehicle in which the child travels.

The alternative to using a car seat is to use the child's wheelchair by placing it in a van and tying it down. With approved wheelchair tie-downs and adequate restraints in the wheelchair, the child is extremely safe. If the child is evaluated in a wheelchair clinic, the issue of vehicle seating should be addressed with respect to the child's specific needs and the vehicles in which the child will usually be riding. Obtaining funding to purchase special needs car seats may be difficult, because insurance companies expect a commercially available car seat to work.

Here are several things to think about when considering vehicular transport:

1. Standard car seats available at department stores should be used if the child meets the size and weight criteria. *Do not use strap covers, blankets, cushions, or padding under the harness straps or the child unless these materials are provided by the manufacturer.*

2. If the child exceeds the weight limit for a standard car seat, a number of car seats available through durable medical equipment dealers hold a child weighing up to 108 pounds. Only additional supports provided by the manufacturer should be used.

3. If a child has good head control and fair trunk control, an option might be to supplement the standard lap or shoulder belt with a harness specially available for transport. These harnesses should not be used by the child who requires total positioning, however, since their primary function is to provide lateral and anterior trunk support.

4. The child's own wheelchair, with the proper tie-downs, may be the best alternative if a wheelchair accessible van is available. Remember, for additional safety and positioning, some type of chest harness, as well as an approved seatbelt and headrest, should be added.

About Wheelchair Maintenance

Like an automobile or a bicycle, a wheelchair, whether it is motorized or manual, requires routine maintenance and care. Several parts of the wheelchair must be checked regularly to ensure the best use. In order to maintain a wheelchair, it's important to use the recommended tools and cleaning supplies. Here are some products that you'll want to keep on hand:

- auto paste-type wax for metal frame
- mild soap
- vinyl and upholstery cleaner
- tire pump
- flat and Phillips screwdrivers
- adjustable wrench (or socket set), ⅜", ⁷⁄₁₆", and ½" common
- spoke wrench
- set of standard Allen wrenches, English and metric, ⅛, ⁵⁄₃₂", and ³⁄₁₆" common
- hammer
- lithium grease (spray)

The guidelines presented below provide a general overview of preventive maintenance. You'll want to consult your owner's manual for specific information about how to care for your model.

Manual Wheelchairs

Monthly. Check tires for proper inflation (proper inflation specifications are usually recorded on the sidewall of the tire). Most tires require between 50 and 65 pounds per square inch; high-performance tires may need as much as 120 psi. Check tires for cuts, flat spots, and wear. Many tires are now filled with a solid inner tube, eliminating the need for maintenance.

After checking the tire pressure, check the wheel locks. They should engage and disengage easily. Over time, they tend to loosen and slide away from the tire (especially solid tires), and some tips that contact the wheel may also wear, so the wheel locks no longer hold. *Do not use wheel locks as brakes!*

If wheels are spoked, check to see whether spokes are loose or bent. They can be tightened with a spoke wrench or replaced. Bike shops can also repair spoked wheelchair tires. Loose spokes often are the main cause of wobbly wheels.

Clean metal parts to remove dirt and to avoid rusting. Tighten nuts and bolts, especially on moving or swing-away parts. Remove dust and hair that commonly collects in front tires.

Every six months. If the wheelchair has a cross-brace, lubricate the center bolt and tube. Typically, axles use self-lubricating bearings and do not need lubrication. Check the bearings; remove dirt, hair, and other materials from nuts and bolts (especially on removable or moving parts). Check for rust.

Battery-powered Wheelchairs

Power wheelchairs should be inspected by an authorized dealer once or twice a year for a "tune-up." An authorized dealer can also check the voltage at the posts to determine whether the batteries need to be replaced.

Wheelchair batteries should be deep cycle. They generally last for 300 to 500 charging cycles, which may be equivalent to between 10 and 18 months. Typically, power wheelchairs use gel-sealed batteries, which require no maintenance. Batteries do not have memory and therefore can be charged daily. When replacing batteries, replace both of them at the same time.

Seating Inserts (Cushions and Backrests)

If you are using a solid seat insert that attaches to the frame of the wheelchair, you need to check it every 3 to 6 months to make sure all the attaching hardware is in place and tightened. You should also check for rips and tears. Be sure that the insert can be easily removed, that it secures to the wheelchair properly, and that the wheelchair folds smoothly when the insert is in place.

Pressure Management Awareness

Most of us don't think about repositioning ourselves while sitting at our computer or getting up from our chair to simply move around; we do it automatically. We all need to change positions to manage the pressure points throughout our bodies. For some, changing positions is not that easy. For children who use wheelchairs, the need to change positions or relieve pressure, particularly on their buttocks or ischial tuberosities, is critical. If pressure is not relieved, skin breakdown or pressure sores can occur.

A primary factor contributing to pressure sores or skin breakdown, particularly as it relates to positioning in a wheelchair, is immobility, or the lack of movement within the chair. Poor distribution of pressure across the seating surface or seat cushion can contribute to skin breakdown, as can shearing or friction forces as the child transfers in and out of the wheelchair. Denervated tissue (the loss of sensation) can also contribute to skin breakdown secondary to reduced blood flow to that area of the body, though this is not a common problem in children with CP. Far more common in children with CP is the lack of subcutaneous tissue due to poor general nutrition, meaning there is no "padding" on the child's buttocks or legs to provide cushioning. Another contributing factor is postural changes in the body that alter the pressures distributed throughout the body. In a typical seating and mobility system, the seating components are not dynamic. In other words, as one's posture changes, the seating components do not accommodate automatically. Consideration needs to be given to adjustment of the seating and positioning components within the mobility system to accommodate for changes in the body following orthopedic surgery or a growth spurt. Another factor to consider is moisture. If a child is incontinent, the added moisture against the skin can cause the skin to be more sensitive to friction and pressure, resulting in increased skin irritation and possible skin breakdown.

When a child in a wheelchair has skin breakdown and the wheelchair is considered a likely culprit, seating specialists use tools to help determine the precise cause. Among these tools are several pressure-mapping systems, which provide pressure information relative to posture. These systems involve a mapping surface consisting of thin, resistive semiconductive polymers sandwiched between highly conductive fabric. The changes in resistance that result from the different pressures on the semiconductor are interpreted by the interface module and relayed to the computer, where they are displayed as an array of colors and pressure values. This provides immediate information to the clinician, who can use it to determine whether the seating surface is contributing to skin breakdown.

Pressure-mapping systems provide the clinician with the ability to compare different seating surfaces or cushions in an objective manner. In addition, they provide education to the user by graphically showing the effectiveness of weight-shifting interventions. Pressure-mapping systems can serve as a tool for configuring a seating system for the child who is prone to skin breakdown. Keep in mind that this is only an assessment tool. It is not something that is required on every evaluation or with every recommendation for a new seating system.

Ultimately, good pressure distribution and pressure relief techniques will greatly reduce your child's chances of skin breakdown. The successful management of skin and pressure sores depends on many factors, including peak pressure, friction, impact injury, heat, moisture, posture, immobility, sensory loss, body type, nutrition, infection, incontinence, and disease. One or more of these may be the reason for skin breakdown in your child. These are better dealt with in advance of an actual breakdown.

Choosing a Stander

A stander is a device that helps a child stand. If the child is not standing at between 18 and 24 months, it is necessary to help a child stand even when she does not have adequate head or upper body control to stand alone. Standing is important because it allows the child to bear some weight through the legs, which in turn helps make the bones stronger and stimulates the development of motor coordination and head control. It also allows the child to adopt a position different from sitting or lying, and many children interact better with their environment and their peers when they are standing up. Standing is strongly encouraged for all children, regardless of how severely involved they are. The benefits may be seen in many areas. They include improving bone size and strength, posture, breathing, and bowel function, as well as preventing muscle tightness that results from sitting too long.

The length of time in the stander will depend on how the child responds to it. You might start out by placing the child in the stander for 10 to 15 minutes a day and then try to gradually increase the time to an hour twice a day if the child tolerates it. The child should not be left in the stander if he is fatigued, crying, or uncomfortable. Music or television can often make a child's standing experience more pleasurable.

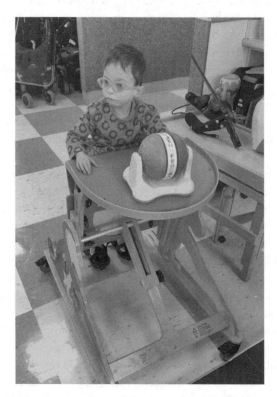

Prone stander

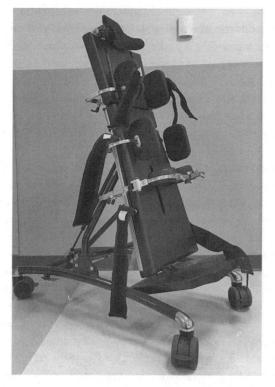

Supine stander

If the child has very poor control of her feet, a pair of ankle-foot orthoses (AFOs) will help support her ankles. Other bracing is not necessary, since the legs can be strapped into the stander.

Each of the different types of standers—prone, supine, sit-to-stand, and parapodium—is used in a specific situation. Most have the ability to adjust the angle of the stander and thus add or eliminate levels of support. Many also have some type of wheeled base. A base with small wheels allows a caregiver to move the stander from place to place, while a base with larger wheels allows the child to propel the stander himself. It is important to remember that the stander ideally should be used in the most upright position and with the least amount of support the child can tolerate. An angle of more than 30 degrees from the vertical position allows very little weight bearing. An upright position allows the child to work with his or her head and trunk in the most functional position.

A prone stander has pads and support in front of the child. The amount of support can vary, coming up to the child's chest or only up to her waist. The child leans forward in the prone stander. Often a tray is attached at the front of the stander, where the child can put her arms and play with toys. In prone standers the angle of standing can be adjusted from very low to nearly upright. The child who does best in the prone stander has at least partial head control. This child often has some difficulty with upper body support, but a prone stander helps her support her upper body.

In contrast to the prone stander, the supine stander has pads and support behind the child. The supine stander may be beneficial to caregivers of large or heavy children. The supine stander often allows for easy transfers from bed to stander when placed in the horizontal position. Once the child is secured, the caregiver can adjust the mechanism to get the child into the most tolerated vertical position. The supine stander is a good option for the child with poor head control whose head often falls forward in the prone stander. The supine stander is also a good choice for children whose knees do not straighten completely. With some padding placed behind the knees, the supine stander works well for this type of child.

A sit-to-stand stander is a newer type of stander. It allows a child to be transferred into the stander from a wheelchair or bed in the sitting position. Once the child is strapped in, a mechanism is used to transform the stander from a sitting position to an upright position. Sit-to-stand standers are excellent for heavier individuals.

A parapodium stander has a base in which the child's legs can be strapped up to the waist. The child stands straight upright; although the stander may provide slight support around the chest, most of these standers support only the waist or the bottom of the chest. In general, this type of stander is a poor choice for children with cerebral palsy because it provides only minimal upper trunk support. Children with CP have poor upper body control and end up falling forward and leaning against a strap or the tray.

Standers are expensive to buy from a medical equipment dealer. However, many health insurance companies will pay for standers. Parents may wish to investigate the different designs that can easily be made out of small stepladders, plywood, and upholstery. Physical therapists can often give parents excellent advice on the best type of stander for their child, and they often have a demonstration unit. Trying out various units before deciding which one to purchase can be extremely beneficial.

About Walkers and Gait Trainers

In a child with cerebral palsy the muscles of the body and extremities lack the coordination, strength, and stability needed to help keep the body upright while stepping. A walker can often help the child begin walking. There are no absolute indicators for when to initiate the use of a walker. However, a few motor control activities seem to be necessary. Among these activities are holding up one's head independently, sitting in a chair with minimal support, and standing and accepting weight through the legs. The child also needs to be able to guide the direction of the walker using his hands and to see where he is going for safety reasons. It is also helpful if he demonstrates an ability to maintain some weight on one leg while stepping with the other. As with standers, the goal is for the child to walk with minimal support and, at the same time, support some of his body weight while being properly aligned. Therefore, the child's skills need to be matched to the appropriate walker. This is best done by having the child evaluated in the proposed piece of equipment. There are many styles of walker, as well as accessories to maximize the child's ability to use the walker.

The most supportive type of walker is the *gait trainer*. The trainer is most often used as a rear-facing walker. The design is based on the idea that the child will stand more erect if he cannot push the walker too far in front of him and if he has to push up on the hand supports to keep his body upright. The trainer can be made into a forward facing walker by adjusting the foot pieces. This type of walker offers several levels of trunk and pelvic support. It may have a sling or a seat for a child who tends to collapse into flexion and/or guides to keep the legs from crossing and to control step direction and step length. Using the supports at the trunk and pelvis as well as the seat option can also help the older child who is large and difficult for the parent to control but who has the desire to walk. These options offer trunk stability to align the pelvis over the feet. The wider base makes it less likely that the walker will tip over, but it is more difficult to maneuver in the home. For the younger child these types of support may be assistive in bringing the child upright over her feet and beginning the action of stepping. To maximize the walker's usage, it is crucial that the child have the desire to walk and the ability to initiate stepping with a weight shift. The walker can also be used with just the pelvic guides and special arm supports for minimal alignment assistance. There are a few hand and forearm styles to choose from for support and guidance. There are multiple wheel features to control direction and speed. There are many different ways for your child to use the gait trainer, and it has many accessories that can be added or deleted as needed to fit your child's ongoing needs.

The more standard walker also helps a child walk, but with less assistance for alignment and more help for balance and weakness in the legs. This type of walker is similar to the older person's walker that you may be familiar with. It can have either 2 or 4 wheels and may be made of metal. Many children with cerebral palsy use the walker in the rear-facing position to help keep their hips straight and their bodies upright. The gait trainer can have a pelvic guide that assists in keeping the pelvis centered over the feet. It can have a seat for a child with limited endurance, though it will not prevent her from collapsing. This seat is posterior in the walker frame and must be manually adjusted. A variety of wheel options help to control the walker's stability, speed, and direction. The wheels can have drag to decrease the walker speed for the child who relies on its stability while stepping, or it may have wheels that prevent the walker from moving backward when the child pushes on it to step forward. Increasing the number of wheels from 2 to 4 may help the child who needs increased speed and efficiency. The walker can have swivel wheels to enable the user who has good balance and weight shift control to turn and adjust the walker simultaneously while walking.

Once the child is able to bear weight on her legs and demonstrates a desire to step, a walker evaluation, whether for a gait trainer or a standard walker, is appropriate. Finding the appropriate walker for your child is crucial for her success. It involves determining your child's specific needs and finding the equipment that matches these needs. Selecting the correct walker and accessories will maximize the support, efficiency, and usage of the walker.

About Braces

When your physician prescribes a brace (also referred to as an *orthosis*) for your child, be sure to find out its intended purpose. This will help you explain to your child why he or she must wear the device or, if the need is not severe, will help you decide on occasion to let your child go without it. Ask the doctor how many hours each day it is to be worn and exactly when during the day—for instance, in the daytime, at night during sleep, when standing, when sitting, or when engaged in physical activity. Ask the orthotist who made the brace to tell you how to clean it.

Other questions you may want to ask your doctor include the following: How is the orthosis to be applied? Where in relationship to the joint is the orthosis to be positioned? For instance, if my son has a knee brace, specifically where should the brace be positioned relative to his kneecap? Can the device be worn when exercising, or might that be a problem?

Skin care is very important for someone who uses an orthosis. You'll need to check your child's skin periodically for any sign of pressure, such as redness, blistering, or an open sore. Notify the doctor or the orthotist if skin problems occur. Generally if this happens the child must be examined by the doctor, who will evaluate the orthosis's fit. Because some problems that require the use of an orthosis change over time, it's possible that the child has outgrown the appliance. Sometimes the materials in the orthosis break down after longtime use, which means that the orthosis is no longer capable of doing what it was initially intended to do. Skin problems or problems with the brace itself need to be evaluated by the physician.

Insurance companies vary regarding how many orthoses they will pay for in the life of an insurance policy. To keep replacement costs to a minimum, some braces are designed to grow with the child to a limited extent. Parents can help by keeping the brace clean and in good working order.

Care and Maintenance

Cleaning and lubrication. A brace may be made of metal, leather, certain plastics, or a combination of these. These different materials require different kinds of care. Your child's orthotist and physician will give you instructions for keeping the brace in good working order, but here are some general tips to help you out.

To keep metal parts in smooth running order, keep them free of dust and dirt and lubricate them periodically. Leather parts also require periodic cleaning. Ask your child's orthotist what cleaner he or she recommends.

Plastic braces should be washed with mild soap and cool or lukewarm water. Some plastics change shape when they are exposed to heat, so it's important to keep the brace in a cool place. It should not be left in an automobile in the summer months, because the inside temperature of a closed-up automobile in the summer may be high enough to soften the plastic brace and cause it to change shape, thereby making it useless.

Labeling. Orthoses are very expensive. Therefore, in addition to keeping your child's braces clean and in good working order, you need to make sure that they are carefully and indelibly labeled with the child's name. This is especially important if your child participates in activities with children who have similar assistive devices. You should also indicate which part of the body the orthosis will be used on. Use labels like "inside left foot," "outside right wrist," "top of back," and so on.

Instructing others. If you know that someone else is going to apply the orthosis to your child, give that person instructions. Explain how the brace is supposed to fit and how it is to be applied. Do not assume that anyone else has been given information about your child's brace. No one knows as much about your child's particular brace as you do, so you need to share this information to be certain that your child is benefiting from wearing the brace.

Choosing the Correct Shoes

When choosing a shoe that is appropriate for the child with cerebral palsy, parents have many options. They will want a shoe that is as attractive as possible, of course, and one that takes the child's special needs into account. Many children with CP need to wear orthopedic shoes (also called corrective shoes), but many do not. An orthopedic shoe is usually made of heavy leather and extends above the ankle. It typically has a rigid sole and sturdy construction to provide support to the foot. It may have a straight last, which means that it does not have the normal inside curve. Some orthopedic shoes are made with special arch supports.

An extremely heavy, rigid, sturdily built shoe was considered essential footwear for all young children until about the 1980s. The theory was that these shoes would ensure that children developed well-balanced feet. It has subsequently been shown that children without disabilities have no need for special shoes or foot support. This severely reduced sales for manufacturers of orthopedic shoes. To compensate they have targeted the population of people with disabilities. The well-built athletic or running shoes on the market today, however, provide equally good support to the foot. They are well constructed, with soft arch support and very adequate ankle support.

The main reason for a child to wear heavy orthopedic shoes is to permit him to wear a metal brace attached to the shoe. These shoes are built of very sturdy leather and can be disassembled or have lifts and other devices added very easily. If a decision is made to use metal braces instead of the more com-

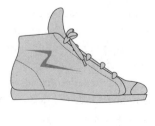

monly used plastic, then the orthopedic shoe is usually necessary. Except for use with a brace, there are few reasons today to prescribe orthopedic shoes or any other corrective shoe for children with cerebral palsy. In fact, the shoes that are best for these children are the same shoes that are best for other children, primarily athletic shoes that have soft soles made of rubber to prevent slipping and a moderate arch support that is soft so that it won't hurt the foot.

When choosing an athletic shoe for your child, consider that the upper shoe may be made of soft leather, a synthetic material, or a nylon fabric, all of which provide adequate support to the foot. These shoes very nicely accommodate inserts, which may be specially made in some circumstances to fit completely inside the shoe, as well as the more commonly used AFO. If you are searching for shoes to fit over AFOs, it is important to look for shoes with a tongue that goes as far out as possible on the toe box. Shoes can be laced out as far as possible to allow the shoe to be opened up and provide much better accommodation for the brace to fit into. This makes it much easier to put the shoes on and take them off with the brace. Extremely lightweight canvas shoes are ideal for this.

The main problem with standard orthopedic shoes is that they are very heavy. Also, they usually have leather soles, which do not provide the kind of traction that rubber soles do, and they look unattractive as well. They tend to draw attention to children with disabilities and make them stand out as being different. Regular shoes help promote an appearance of normalcy, which is especially important for children who are in regular schools, where wearing the latest style or fashion can provide a significant boost in self-esteem. Personal appearance also contributes to the public impression of a child who is not walking but is in a wheelchair.

It is important that children's shoes have plenty of room at the toes. The shoes should not cause the child pain or discomfort when he or she walks. Whether they are orthopedic shoes, athletic shoes, or high-top hiking boots, the main reason for wearing shoes is to keep the feet warm and provide a stable foundation so the child can walk without hurting his or her feet.

Increasing Independence with Service Dogs

Well-trained service dogs provide physically challenged individuals such as those with cerebral palsy with increased independence, as well as an emotional outlet. These dogs are trained and supplied by a number of organizations, most of them nonprofit organizations. A person receiving a service dog is asked to make a contribution, but the cost of training the dog is far more than the contribution—the nonprofit organization makes up the difference.

Most organizations provide dogs to children as well as to adults. The recipient must be able to accept the responsibility of owning a service animal. The organizations providing dogs are very careful to select healthy dogs that are well suited for their role.

To prepare a dog for service, the organization first gives the dog lessons in obedience. Once the dog has been obedience-trained, it receives general service training, including training in retrieving dropped objects, taking items from shelves, opening doors, and paying cashiers with a specially designed wallet.

Many recipients have very special needs, such as a dog that can follow commands given through an electronic communicator. After an individual has been matched to a specific dog, the dog undergoes additional training to enable it to accommodate the recipient's special needs. The dog's soon-to-be owner undergoes training in how to handle and care for the dog. The organizations that supply dogs provide counseling to help the animal's owner cope with the separation that accompanies the dog's need for retirement or the dog's death.

Several organizations provide and train dogs throughout the United States. Look online for "service dogs" or contact the United States Dog Registry (usdogregistry.org).

Managing the System

Caregivers can be either victims of the system or survivors of the system. By *system* we mean any organization whose rules and regulations may on occasion interfere with your ability to protect your child's interests. The system might be an insurance company, your state's Medicaid policies, the school system, a community service organization, or even a local sports league. Individuals with disabilities have different needs for services, and their caregivers' ability to obtain those services varies greatly.

Availability of services can differ even between neighboring states. One insurance company might cover new braces for a child every six months, while another claims to allow reimbursement for one set in a lifetime. One school might inform a parent that there are no services available for a child who by federal law must have services provided, while another might be providing an aide for a child with barely discernible hemiplegia. People with disabilities often have to contend with discrepancies such as these.

The first step in managing these problems is to identify the specific system that must be addressed and to represent your child wholeheartedly. If you cannot personally be an advocate for your child, find someone who can. The individual need not be a person with a special education or a prestigious position in society, but he or she does need to be persistent and patient with ongoing attempts to frustrate his or her best efforts. No matter who represents a person with a disability, good organizational skills and hands-on experience make the task easier. For children who are cognitively able, this is a responsibility they may assume as they reach adulthood.

Here are some tips that will help you as you learn to manage the system:

Never make a phone call without a pencil and paper in hand. When asking questions about an issue, find out and record the name of the individual who gives you information, as well as his or her title. Record the date of every phone call made, and write a brief description of the information exchanged. If the answer to your inquiry is not acceptable, persist until you are allowed to speak with the individual's supervisor. Make it clear that you are not going to give up. Try to do this calmly, because shouting only makes it appear that you are losing control. Instead, speak firmly and in a way that demonstrates that you will never get so frustrated that you'll give up and go away.

Don't stop calling. The old saying about the squeaky wheel getting the grease is extraordinarily appropriate when it comes to acquiring services. If you believe that your child's rights are being violated, do not hesitate to get legal help.

You can also use e-mail for communications, especially if you are communicating with your child's school. If your e-mail goes unanswered, you can always resend the original email and copy the person's supervisor or principal, which usually will prompt a response. This way you will have a record of the communication.

Keep an ongoing list of individuals who have been helpful and their phone numbers. Send a note to thank those who have been helpful and, when appropriate, a letter of commendation to their supervisor.

Network with other parents and other caregivers, and help one another by sharing strategies that have yielded results. It is particularly helpful to have one designated person with whom to discuss issues and strategies. This may be a therapist, a physician, a friend, or a relative.

Make use of community and church service organizations and local newspapers. Often the problem you are tackling is one that another child is facing, and the publicity you get can help others. For example, if the school system alters its treatment of your child because of your efforts, and then the local newspaper carries a story about this, other parents can learn about your efforts, the school system's response, and the rights of their own child.

More than anything, don't give up. Over and over we have experienced a situation in which an absolute no becomes a yes through persistence.

Working with a Case Manager

The case manager is the person who is responsible for coordinating and facilitating the procurement of services from different provider agencies in both the public and the private sector. This person can serve as a single point of contact in helping families obtain the services and assistance they need to care for the child or adult with cerebral palsy. The case manager may be a social worker connected to a school or agency, a public health nurse, or a nurse connected to an insurance company. He or she may be appointed by the state, by a county agency, or by the insurance company covering the child's medical expenses, or the case manager may be on the staff of a hospital caring for the child. When the case manager is a government child welfare manager, she or he may sometimes have to be an advocate for the child to make sure that the child receives appropriate medical attention.

While the case manager works to be sure that necessary care is obtained, he or she also regulates care to avoid duplication of services or provision of unnecessary services. Case managers have a good deal of control over the medical care arrangements made by many people today. For example, suppose that John Doe's company provides XYZ health insurance and that XYZ health insurance assigns a case manager to each individual and each family enrolled in the plan. If John's spouse hurts herself when she slips on the ice, the case manager will direct her to an orthopedist whose services are approved for payment on the XYZ plan; refer her for special studies, if necessary, at an appointed facility; and direct her to provider-approved therapists if physical therapy is suggested by the doctor. The goal for this type of manager is to manage health care to ensure cost containment.

Letters of Medical Necessity

In order to pay for the purchase of equipment or other durable medical goods such as braces, standers, seats, communications aids, toileting aids, and adaptive feeding devices, or for home nursing care, insurance companies or other funding agencies almost always require a letter of medical necessity from a physician or therapist. Such a letter must include the child's diagnoses and an explanation of why the equipment or nursing care is needed, or the request will be automatically rejected.

Because the letters written by physicians who are not familiar with insurance company requirements sometimes don't include all the necessary information, we've provided a sample letter here. To help avoid delay or hassle over reimbursement, you can make sure that the physician who writes a letter of medical necessity for you includes the kind of information indicated in this sample. If the physician follows this format, you will at least get a fair hearing from the funding agency. You might want to photocopy this sample letter and give your doctor a copy.

It is also very helpful for you to explain to the physician writing the letter how and why the equipment will be used. For instance, if you have developed a back problem and can no longer lift your child, that information should be included when you are requesting a lift for use at home or for your van. To obtain home nursing, there must be specific skilled nursing needs, such as giving medications or G-tube feeds at a time when the parent cannot (at night when parents need to sleep or when they are away at work). The letter should be sent on hospital or office stationery.

[Date]

To Whom It May Concern [or, better, to a specific employee of the funding agency]:

John Smith is an 8-year-old male with a primary diagnosis of cerebral palsy. He was seen recently at the Seating Clinic at the Nemours/Alfred I. duPont Hospital for Children in Wilmington, Delaware, for the prescription of a new seating system to meet his positioning needs.

John presents with the following: generally decreased tone in upper and lower extremities, and fair head and trunk control. He is dependent in transfers and mobility. He is cognitively severely delayed. He is incontinent in bowel/bladder. He has frequent respiratory complications and is subject to bronchitis and pneumonia, and he receives chest therapy. He occasionally aspirates, he has increased skin sensitivity, and he has seizures, but they're generally under control with medication. He must have a tilt-in-space wheelchair with appropriate positioning to provide safety and support and to facilitate breathing and feeding.

His current seating system is a Zippie tilt-in-space that is 5 years old. It no longer meets his positioning needs, because he has outgrown it, and the seating insert needs to be changed to meet his current positioning needs. Since receiving his previous wheelchair, he has grown 6 inches and gained 35 pounds, and the seat can no longer be expanded.

The goals for John for seating are to maintain posture, protect skin, provide comfort, and enhance function. Upon evaluation, the Seating Team has recommended that the following equipment be prescribed for John:

Action Tiger, desk arms, swing-away detachable elevating leg rests, semi-reclining back, special seat depth, stroller handles, custom positioners and lateral hip guides, high brackets, solid seat with attaching hardware, solid back with attaching hardware, shoe holders, heavy-duty straps.

The Action Tiger is prescribed because it is a manual wheelchair for total positioning and because he is dependent in mobility. The tilt is needed because he is hypotonic in head and trunk. He also has difficulty breathing, and it will help aid in feeding. It will help with low endurance and pressure relief. The adjustable-height arms are needed to support the tray at the right height, for upper body support and balance and for ease of transfers. The I-back will bring side supports in close to the trunk, and the insert will fit the full width of the wheelchair. The laterals will encourage midline trunk position, compensate for lack of trunk control, provide safety, and contour around the trunk for better control. The chest harness is needed for safety in transport by providing anterior support, preventing forward flexion, and retracting the shoulders. The headrest is needed for poor head control due to low tone, active flexion of the head, posterior lateral support, safety in transfers, and facilitation of breathing. The clear tray is needed as a functional surface for schoolwork, for stimulation, for upper arm and trunk support, and as a base for augmentative communication devices. The shoe holders are needed to control increased extension or spasms in lower extremities, excessive internal rotation, and external rotation and to prevent aggressive behavior for safety. The anti-tippers are needed for safety.

Should you have any questions regarding these recommendations, please do not hesitate to call me at (302) 651-4000. We hope that you will be able to accommodate these needs in an expedient manner. Thank you for your cooperation and assistance in this matter.

Sincerely,
Freeman Miller, MD
Pediatric Orthopedic Surgeon

Make a note of the date the letter was mailed, and if after three or four weeks you haven't heard anything, it might be a good idea to telephone the insurance company or funding agency and gently inquire about the status of the claim. Make sure to find out the name of the person you speak with, and write it down. The person will probably tell you that the claim is being processed; you can ask when you might expect to receive notification of payment and then call again if that date passes and you still haven't heard anything. It's not generally a good idea to be seen as a nuisance or, worse, an irate client, but you will want to stay on top of the situation and let the agency know that you are doing so. If the agency remains unresponsive, you can enlist your doctor's assistance.

Occupations for Adults with Cerebral Palsy

There are many options for teenagers and adults with cerebral palsy who wish to work. Options will vary depending on the degree and type of disability. A vocational rehabilitation evaluation should help determine the type of vocation or job for which the teenager or adult is best suited. For the high school student, vocational counseling is frequently offered through the school system. Many communities offer vocational rehabilitation programs for adults who are physically or intellectually challenged. People with diplegia whose legs are affected but who are able to use both hands effectively have many options, while those with hemiplegia or quadriplegia will be limited in jobs requiring bilateral manual dexterity.

About Hospitalization

A child—or anyone—may be admitted to the hospital on either an elective basis or an emergency basis. For an elective admission, you decide to admit your child to the hospital so that he or she can undergo tests or have a procedure or surgery done. You have some part in deciding when the admission and procedure will take place, taking into account the demands of your own life as well as the physician's schedule. An emergency is something over which we have little or no control—such as appendicitis or a heart attack. In an emergency your child would be admitted immediately to the hospital for treatment. Overseeing your child's care likely will be a pediatric hospitalist, a physician specializing in the care of hospitalized children.

Before Admission

Whether your child's admission is an elective admission or an admission as a result of an emergency, your child's physician will tell you why he or she wants to admit your child to the hospital. In addition to getting a detailed description from the doctor, you might also ask for any literature on the procedures to be performed, or ask for a reference list so that you can read about the procedures or tests in the library or online. You should find out what is involved for your child and what your responsibilities will be before, during, and after the treatment, so you will feel comfortable with the treatment plan. Be sure to ask your doctor the following questions:

- Will my child be in pain during or after the treatment?
- What measures will be taken to control my child's pain?
- How long will my child be in the hospital? Will he or she be in intensive care?
- Will my child need medication after discharge?
- Should I arrange for a hospital bed, wheelchair, potty chair, or anything else before admission, or will I have enough time to get these things while my child is in the hospital?

This information will help you to prepare your child for the hospital admission and to care for him or her at home after the test or surgical or other procedure. Your child's doctor must also explain the procedure so that you may give informed consent—to sign hospital forms saying that you are willing for your child to undergo the procedure and that you understand the possible risks and complications.

Preparing Your Child for Admission

Whether going to the hospital is a new experience for your child, or whether he or she has been to the hospital many times before, you must prepare the child in advance for what is going to happen. The hospitalization will be a more positive experience—less frightening and less traumatic—if the child has been told what to expect.

For most children, the more they know about the details of their hospitalization and, generally speaking, the more positive a parent or significant other is about the experience, the better the experience will be. With that in mind, you should inform your child about the hospitalization in the way that he or she can best understand and accept.

Ask if there is anyone responsible for patient education in the hospital where your child will be admitted who can advise you on how to best prepare your child for admission. Your child's physician may know professionals who can assist you, and the office nurse or clinic nurse may have advice or may be able to direct you to others who may be able to help. Pediatric hospitals often have a child life department, which can suggest the appropriate approach to take with your child. Nurses and social workers may be able to give you information well in advance of the admission date to help you prepare your child. You should plan to take your child's wheelchair, braces, walker, and some outfits of clothing and pajamas to the hospital. Your child may feel more comfortable in his own clothing, and he will need his bracing, walker, and wheelchair when he is allowed to be up and out of bed.

Online ideas should come only from a reliable source. KidsHealth (http://kidshealth.org) and the Nemours Get Well Network are two such pediatric health resources. There you can find information and videos for both children and parents regarding what to expect during a child's hospital stay.

The following guidelines for different age groups are guidelines only. Based on your knowledge of your own child, you can tailor them to help your child through this experience.

The young child. For a young child, preparation for hospitalization should take place as close to admission as possible, preferably only a few days before. Typically, children between 1 and 5 years of age can handle only simple explanations of what is going to happen. These children learn best by imitation, so a good approach is to use dolls as models to talk about the part of the body that will be affected. Play with puppets and "play" hospital equipment such as a stethoscope and a blood pressure cuff. Read books about hospitals and medical personnel, and look at pictures with your child. Sometimes, simply answering your child's questions is the best way to approach the experience.

If available, a tour of the hospital the day before admission may be beneficial for everyone. A call to the hospital's public relations department may provide specific answers to your and your child's questions, including whether there is a program for touring the facility. Arrangements for this kind of tour must be made ahead of time. Young children fear separation from their family and need to know that their parents will be waiting during their surgery or hospitalization. If you must leave your child, tell your child when you will be leaving and when you plan to return. Never tell a child that you will be right back when you know you will not. No matter how you approach communication, be honest with your child. For example, tell him or her, "I will not be back tonight, but I will be back tomorrow to have lunch with you."

The child aged 6 to 8. Verbal explanations can be given to a child of 6 to 8 years about one week before admission. Children in this age group are better able to tell you what they think will happen and better able to understand when you correct any misconceptions they may have. At this age children will likely ask questions and will expect their questions to be answered honestly. Parents can provide more details for them than for younger children. Children at this age are better able to grasp concepts such as the length of stay and separation, as well as postsurgery issues such as limits on activity. This age group may also benefit from the use of dolls or puppets, "play" hospital equipment, books, and/or a hospital tour.

The preadolescent child. The child 9 to 12 years of age can handle explanations given as much as two weeks before admission. Children in this age group learn by logical thinking. They benefit from clear verbal explanations and from a variety of visual cues: videos, diagrams of body outlines with minimal detail, and books. This group tends to enjoy handling technical equipment, and they can more easily formulate a question about something they do not understand. Children this age benefit from more detailed information about expected procedures, surgery, and specific treatments. They want information about how they can participate in their own care, and they should be told about limitations of activities that might be imposed after treatment. They often benefit from visits by family and friends.

The adolescent. Children between the ages of 13 and 18 years benefit from having all types of information shared in a variety of ways as soon as the admission is scheduled. This age group learns well in peer groups. They are able to understand many directions and rules. Use of correct medical terminology and detailed information is important for this group. Questions should be encouraged and should be answered in detail. Older children most fear disability and a loss of body parts. They miss their friends and are worried about death.

For all ages, try as much as possible to keep routines the same as at home, and encourage the hospital staff to do the same. Encourage your child to bring a favorite toy or other object from home, and if possible allow him or her to wear his or her own clothing in the hospital.

The Preadmission Process

Most hospitals have preadmission counseling that will answer your questions about the admissions process, insurance issues, and accommodations. Many insurance companies require preadmission testing to be performed at specific in-network locations. When you are planning for an elective hospital admission, an admission counselor will let you know if that is the case for your child's surgery, test, or procedure. Ask specifically about arrangements for parents who wish to stay overnight with their child and the circumstances under which you might not be able to stay at your child's bedside. If you plan to be absent from work during your child's hospitalization, your employer may require a letter from the hospital explaining the reason for your absence. If your employer requires Family Medical Leave Act paperwork, a preadmission counselor should be able to tell you who can provide the medical information necessary.

Your child's school should also be notified regarding his or her anticipated absence so the staff can plan accordingly. The child's teachers may want to schedule homework and exams with your child's hospitalization in mind or assign work for your child to complete during the hospital stay. The school may ask about any expected restrictions of your child's activities in order to prepare for his or her return to classes.

The Hospitalization

The hospital stay can be bewildering for both you and your child as you encounter unfamiliar people and experiences. Many different people will be taking care of your child, working together as a team with various supporting roles. The senior physician, ultimately responsible for the care of your child, is known as the attending physician. Generally, he or she will be a physician who is board certified in his or her area of expertise, with many years of training and experience. Sometimes other senior physicians with different medical specialties will be consulted to help manage your child's illness. The medical team may also include nurse practitioners or physicians assistants. At teaching hospitals, your child's care team may include residents—physicians who have graduated from medical school and are still learning under the watchful eyes of hospital attending physicians—as well as medical students. There are many other hospital staff members who might help take care of your child. Nurses provide the direct bedside care for your child. If you have a concern regarding your child's well-being, the nurse is usually the first person to call. He or she will do a bedside assessment to help determine the next course of action. Other staff who might be involved in the care of your child include physical, occupational, feeding, and respiratory therapists. Children's hospitals may have child life specialists, who can help your child cope with stressful events in the hospital. Finally, hospital chaplains, dietitians, and social workers may also provide support to you while your child is hospitalized.

Since hospitals run 24 hours a day, all staff members have colleagues who ensure round the clock care. All staff should introduce themselves by name and explain their role in helping care for your child. The medical team should see your child at least once every day in a formal bedside visit called "rounds." In a teaching hospital, the attending physician, nurses, residents, medical students, and other staff will examine your child and discuss your child's condition. At a nonteaching or community hospital, the team will be smaller, but it should include at a minimum the attending physician and the bedside nurse. You should ask what time the team comes for rounds. If you cannot be present at that time, ask to be included via telephone. The team should discuss with you the anticipated medical plan for the day and give you the opportunity to ask any questions or express any concerns. Occasionally, staff may use medical terms or jargon during these discussions. You should ask the medical team to explain anything that is not clear. Sometimes you may think of questions at times when the medical staff is not present. Be sure to write these down or let the nurse know so he or she can ensure that your concerns are addressed.

Anticipating Discharge: What You Need to Know

Discharge from the hospital can be a happy occasion, but it can also create stress for the families of children who need more care than their parents are used to providing. The hospital likely has a system in place to provide counseling regarding what the child will need after being discharged. The person providing the discharge instructions might be a resident physician, a social worker, or a nurse, any of whom can help you with the transition from hospital to home. As your child's discharge date approaches, ask this person or your child's doctor some of the following questions:

- Will my child require any special equipment (hospital bed, wheelchair, potty chair, braces or a walker) that I will need to learn about? Will the hospital be providing this equipment and training to use it?
- Will my child be more dependent on me than he was when admitted to the hospital?
- Will my child need specialized care upon discharge that I can provide at home? Who will teach me how to provide for my child's new special needs? Am I permitted to invite other family members to training sessions?
- Will my child require any specialized nursing care when she returns home from the hospital? Who will help me arrange for this care?
- If special therapy is required while my child is in the hospital, will this therapy be required at home? For how long? How will I arrange for home therapy?
- Will special lab tests ordered during the hospital stay be required at home too? How will I go about getting these tests completed?
- Will my child be able to walk or sit or move as she did before? If not, how long will it be before she returns to her prehospitalization state? If that is not expected, how long will it be before we know how much difference there is?
- How long will my child's activities be limited?

- When can my child return to school? Will he require any special accommodations or assistance? Will she be able to use the usual mode of transportation to school, or will special transportation be needed?
- Who do I call if my child is experiencing pain, fever, or other unexpected medical problems? What is the phone number I can use to reach this person?
- Who will need to see my child for follow-up after discharge, and when? Will these appointments be made before I leave the hospital?

Hospitalization is stressful. Your child's medical condition is the most obvious and important concern, but stress also comes from worries about other family members, pets, work responsibilities, and financial considerations. Being prepared is the best way to anticipate and decrease stress from these sources.

Keeping Medical History Records

One of the major changes in the area of health information in the past few years has been the use of electronic medical records. Electronic records allow a provider within a hospital or hospital system to view information from all the visits to other providers in the same system, as well as all laboratory and imaging studies, phone calls, and other communications. With a parent's consent, your child's provider can see records from selected hospital systems around the country that use similar electronic systems, thus hoping to avoid duplication of studies and giving valuable information to the physician who is currently evaluating your child.

Many of these electronic systems also have a mechanism for patients themselves or their guardians to see much, if not all, of their own records. They also allow patients and parents to see results of laboratory or imaging studies and to communicate with their doctors or other providers via the electronic system, which then records the communication. Such systems make it possible for parents to ask for refills of medications and for prescriptions to be sent electronically to their local pharmacy. All these innovations are intended to improve communication and improve medical care.

Nevertheless, it is still important for parents to maintain records of their own containing key information, as there will be times when the electronic record is not available or when you are in an emergency room that does not have the capability to see your child's records at another institution. A child with disabilities generally has a great deal of contact with health care personnel and may have undergone a series of surgeries and other procedures. The child may be on multiple medications, and the medications may need periodic dose adjustments. Keeping an up-to-date description of your child's medical care is extremely valuable in helping new providers assess your child and understand his or her condition. A brief "parent medical record" will also provide important information to emergency room personnel in the event your child needs to be taken to the emergency room. Because of the need for accurate, readily available medical information, the American College of Emergency Physicians, in collaboration with the American Academy of Pediatrics, developed an "Emergency Information Form for Children with Special Needs." This form (see pages 336 and 337) contains essential information emergency personnel need in order to make appropriate medical decisions. If you create your own brief record, it should include the following information:

Parent's Medical Record
1. Immunizations: list of immunizations given (include dates).
2. Allergies to medication, foods, pollens, etc.
3. Medical problems (for example, CP, seizures, cardiac, gastrointestinal, diabetes, asthma).
4. As applicable: current medications and dosages; size and type of tracheostomy; gastrostomy tube, supplier, and type and amount of feedings. This list may be lengthy but is essential.
5. Current pediatrician and other medical or surgical specialists (for example, neurologist or orthopedist) and therapists.
6. Most recent height and weight (include dates).
7. School assessments (most recent).
8. Documents to confirm legal guardianship; insurance cards.
9. Record of surgeries (most recent first).

Example:	Date	Procedure	Surgeon	Hospital	Complication
	2/2/2014	spine fusion	Miller	duPont	none
	5/9/2010	tonsillectomy	Stone	County	bleeding

10. Record of hospitalizations.

Example:	Date	Reason	Physician	Hospital
	2/6–2/11/2013	pneumonia	Bachrach	duPont
	3/5–6/5/2000	premature birth	Smith	Jefferson

11. List of names and addresses of individuals to whom you wish a copy of your child's most recent health report be sent. For example, when your child is seen by his neurologist, the pediatrician should receive a report.

You should carry the parent's medical record or emergency information form at all times so it will be available during scheduled appointments as well as in an emergency.

Although it's a smart idea to carry a brief record with you, we recommend that you keep a more extensive file at home. This file should include copies of reports from medical, psychological, and developmental tests done throughout the child's life arranged in chronological order.

The file should also include copies of the Individualized Education Program (IEP) and the Individualized Family Service Plan (IFSP), as well as notes and reports from teachers and therapists and copies of any correspondence written on the child's behalf, such as to insurance companies or schools. Without your written permission, such reports cannot be given to you or anyone else. In April 2003, privacy and confidentiality regulations of the 1996 Health Insurance Portability and Accountability Act (HIPAA) were implemented. The US Department of Health and Human Services announced changes in January 2013, called the Omnibus Rule, to provide the public with increased control over personal health information as a result of enhanced enforcement by the Health Information Technology for Economic and Clinical Act (HITECH),

Emergency Information Form for Children With Special Needs

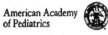 American College of
Emergency Physicians®

American Academy
of Pediatrics

Date form completed	Revised	Initials
By Whom	Revised	Initials

Name:	Birth date:	Nickname:

Home Address:	Home/Work Phone:

Parent/Guardian:	Emergency Contact Names & Relationship:
Signature/Consent*:	
Primary Language:	Phone Number(s):

Physicians:

Primary care physician:	Emergency Phone:
	Fax:
Current Specialty physician:	Emergency Phone:
Specialty:	Fax:
Current Specialty physician:	Emergency Phone:
Specialty:	Fax:
Anticipated Primary ED:	Pharmacy:
Anticipated Tertiary Care Center:	

Diagnoses/Past Procedures/Physical Exam:

1.

Baseline physical findings:

2.

3.

Baseline vital signs:

4.

Synopsis:

Baseline neurological status:

*Consent for release of this form to health care providers

Diagnoses/Past Procedures/Physical Exam continued:

Medications:	Significant baseline ancillary findings (lab, x-ray, ECG):
1.	
2.	
3.	
4.	Prostheses/Appliances/Advanced Technology Devices:
5.	
6.	

Management Data:

Allergies: Medications/Foods to be avoided   and why:

1.

2.

3.

Procedures to be avoided   and why:

1.

2.

3.

Immunizations (mm/yy)

Dates						Dates					
DPT						Hep B					
OPV						Varicella					
MMR						TB status					
HIB						Other					

Antibiotic prophylaxis: Indication: Medication and dose:

Common Presenting Problems/Findings With Specific Suggested Managements

Problem	Suggested Diagnostic Studies	Treatment Considerations

Comments on child, family, or other specific medical issues:

Physician/Provider Signature: Print Name:

enacted as part of the American Recovery and Reinvestment Act of 2009 and other rule-making proceedings since 2009. The privacy rule protects all "individually identifiable health information" held or transmitted by a covered entity (which includes providers and health care organizations) or its business associate, in any form or media, whether electronic, paper, or oral. No information can change hands without proper authorization. Consent forms must comply with the language in the privacy and confidentiality regulations. Parents therefore must sign appropriate HIPAA-compliant consent forms and state the names of individuals who will be allowed access to their child's health information, and specifically what information they may access. Authorization forms are required to indicate when they will expire. This can be determined by the parent. If the parent wants information released after the expiration date, a new authorization form must be signed. Similarly, a parent would have to sign an authorization form to allow his child's electronic medical records to be shared between hospitals or doctors.

In your file, include a list of contacts that includes phone numbers, the nature of your interaction with them, plus the outcome of the interaction. Also keep a list of all health care and school contacts. This list should include addresses and phone numbers, as well as information about insurance carriers and equipment vendors. Include a letter authorizing release of reports dealing with your child that you might wish to have sent elsewhere. If you leave spaces for the addressee, a description of the report, and where it originates, you can photocopy this letter and fill in the blanks as needed.

There are several ways to keep all this information in order. Many parents use their computer for record keeping. You do not need sophisticated computer skills to enter this information. You can easily list medications in a simple Word document and update this list whenever changes are made. Medication allergies, feeding schedule, supplies, procedures, and appointments are easily entered into the computer and can be printed out before a doctor's visit. Your cell phone can be especially helpful when making follow-up appointments. If you do not have access to a computer, you can use a file card system for telephone numbers, supplemented by a loose-leaf binder containing reports. Or you might want to keep records in a file drawer. If you take the time to set up the system properly, adding new information will be easy. This kind of record keeping will help you as you advocate for your child.

Life Planning Process

"What will happen when I'm no longer here?" This question keeps many parents up at night, and rightly so. It's important to know there are ways to prepare for your child's life without you and professionals who can help you do so. The process can seem daunting. It is best done in stages, keeping in mind that as your child grows and matures his needs will change. Regardless of the age of the child or the severity of the disability, creating a plan is critically important. Often, parents are not aware that financial decisions made early in the child's life may prevent their offspring from being eligible for government benefits as an adult. There are ways to avoid this outcome, but steps must be executed proactively, which is why working with a certified special needs estate planner is strongly encouraged.

Here are some key steps to take now:

1. *Register with your state intellectual/developmental disabilities (I/DD) agency.* Even if your young child doesn't have any need for services or supports now, register her so she is counted in the anticipated numbers for future services. The systems change dramatically once the child becomes an adult; also, the service delivery system is strapped for finances. Having your child included in the numbers gives the state a more accurate idea of the need for services in the long run. There may be also respite services you can access through your state agency.

2. *Meet with a certified special needs estate planner.* These professionals know all about government benefits and eligibility. They can help you make sure your child's financial situation does not keep her from being eligible for state or government programs such as Medicaid or SSI.

3. *Consider a special needs trust.* In order to qualify for government benefits like Supplemental Security Income (SSI), an individual cannot have more than $2,000 in assets in his name. Many people with disabilities need more than $2,000 in any given month to pay for housing, food, and other necessities. The only way a person who receives SSI can save more than $2,000 and not have it count against her eligibility for SSI is through a special needs trust. This trust can be created by an estate attorney or an elder law attorney. The special needs trust can have unlimited amounts in it. It's important to consider creating a special needs trust early in the estate planning process. You or loved ones can leave life insurance policies, retirement accounts, property, and stocks to the trust, ensuring that your child will have additional resources beyond what SSI can pay for. You should work with an attorney who specializes in drafting special needs trusts, because the laws and regulations change frequently. (For more information on this topic, see Chapter 10.)

4. *Create a blueprint guide for your child.* Consider looking at models of Essential Lifestyle Plans (ELPs), Making Access Possible (MAP), or People Active to Help (PATH) for ideas. A special needs estate planner can help you create a *letter of intent* as well. In a letter of intent you can write down the important things in your child's life whether positive or negative (for example, he hates it when someone sings to him in the bathtub) so a caregiver can smoothly assume responsibility for him if something happens to you. Think of important family traditions, events, or cultural holidays that may not be known to someone outside your immediate family. This guide can and should be updated regularly as your child grows and his preferences and experiences change. Consider photographing or videoing routine events. If your child uses certain expressions, gestures, or signs that you know the meaning of, take pictures and put them in an easy-to-access place (such as on a ring on the arm of her wheelchair) so other people can communicate or assist your child quickly without misunderstanding, for example, that when her lips quiver, it means she feels sick, not that she's scared. You know the most about your child, and others need a way to learn those things.

5. *Create a will.* Most adults know they should create a will, but many never get around to it. Having a child with special health care needs makes creating a will more urgent. Should something happen to you, who is going to be responsible for your child? Will she continue to live in your home, or will she move in with the caregiver? Does your family want to consider a residential support program (group home or facility based)? All these questions should be answered in your will.

6. *Research long-term care options.* You do not have to make a decision for your young child, but investigate the different types of adult long-term care. Some families plan on having their adult child live at home with them forever, while others plan for their child to move into a residential support program, such as a group home. It's important to know what options exist and how to access them. Typically you can find the answers through your state I/DD agency. There are waitlists for these residential support programs, sometimes with waiting periods of longer than ten years! Knowing the options and keeping up to date on new residential programs and new models and designs for homes positions your child for the best adult life you can imagine for him or her. Talk with your child's case worker about how to get on lists for residential and vocational programs, waiver funding, and other services not covered by traditional Medicaid.

7. *Plan for your when your child becomes an adult.* When your child turns 18, he becomes his own legal guardian, and HIPAA takes effect. Before he turns 18, look into options such as powers of attorney, conservatorship, and legal guardianship so you can decide what is best for your child. Also find out if your state has a health surrogacy law, which would allow you to make medical decisions if your adult child cannot. Talk with your state I/DD agency. Most services recognize that the family of an individual needing supports will have to be involved in decision making. Understand that guardianships are permanent and cannot be revoked, whereas a power of attorney can be changed as necessary.

8. *Use a life-plan binder.* Place all documents in a single binder and tell caregivers and family where they can find it.

9. *Hold a meeting.* Give copies of relevant documents and instructions to family and caregivers. Review everyone's responsibilities.

10. *Review your plan.* At least once a year, review and update the plan. Modify legal documents as necessary.

About Casts

Before taking a child in a cast home from the hospital or doctor's office, parents should receive detailed instructions in how to care for the child (and for the cast) from the child's doctor or another health care professional. For example, the parent should find out what physical limitations this cast will impose. If the child is normally ambulatory, for example, will she be permitted to walk with the cast? If she normally can sit on the toilet, will she be able to do so in the cast, or will a bedpan be needed? Other questions parents need to have answered include:

- Do I need to arrange special transportation home from the hospital, such as an ambulance?
- When can my child return to school in the cast?
- Will I need to provide special care for my child and the cast? Who will train me in how to perform this care, and when will the training begin?
- Will I need special equipment to help me position my child? Who will provide this equipment?
- What are some problems a cast can cause that I can look for?

The following care tips might be useful after you bring your child home:

Bathing. The skin under the cast should not get wet. If your child can walk to the bathroom for a sponge bath, let him do so. If you need to bathe your child in bed, here are suggestions:

1. Gather towels, a washcloth, a basin with water, soap, a soap dish, and protective towels or flannel-covered plastic bed protectors for the bed and the cast. Use a bath sheet (a large towel) to keep your child warm during the bath.

2. Wash the head, ears, and face first, then all other exposed skin, beginning with the chest and moving to the arms, trunk, back, and legs. Wash the genitals and buttocks last. Cover exposed areas with a bath blanket or dry towels.

3. Make sure that you remove all soap residue and dry the skin. Be careful not to get soap under the cast, since this may cause itching. Do not use lotions or creams under the cast or near the edges of the cast.

Tooth care. If your child can walk to the bathroom, allow her to brush her own teeth. If not, you will need a spit cup or emesis basin so she can spit out the contents of her mouth after she brushes her teeth in bed. If you normally brush your child's teeth, you should continue with your usual technique.

Hair grooming and washing. If your child can get to the kitchen or bathroom, help him wash his hair over the sink or tub. Protect the cast with plastic to keep it from getting wet. A plastic barber's or hairdresser's cape might serve the purpose. If the child must be confined to bed for bathing and hair washing, you may want to invest in special equipment that is commercially available to allow water from hair washing to drain off the bed. Check with local department stores or home care companies for a listing of the products they carry that make it easier to wash hair in bed. It may be possible to wash your child's hair in bed by funneling a plastic drape from around his neck into a plastic container (a trash can or bucket), allowing the shampoo water to run from the head to the plastic to the container.

Clothing. No special clothing is needed. The child in a cast should not be dressed in a way that will overheat him, since he may perspire and begin itching. Loose, comfortable clothing is the best choice.

Cast checks and skin care. Casts should be checked daily. Report to the doctor any changes in the cast or the skin. To check a cast, you'll need to use a flashlight and your eyes, hands, and nose. Note the general condition of the cast and look for any cracks, breaks, weakness, or damp areas. Observe whether the cast is getting tighter, either because of swelling under the cast or because your child has grown since the cast was applied. A tight cast can be very dangerous and must be reported to the doctor at once.

If your child is in a large cast such as a hip spica or body cast, you can feel the skin with your hands and look with a flashlight for any signs of secretions, drainage, or skin irritation. Check for odors coming from the area covered by the cast. Pay attention if your child complains of tingling and numbness, burning, or itching. Report any such complaints, as well as any sign of odor, secretions, or drainage to your child's physician.

Do not use lotions or creams under the cast, since they build up and can irritate the skin. Plain 70 percent isopropyl rubbing alcohol, with nothing added, is used by many physicians to clean older children's skin. It can be used sparingly on the skin at the edges of the cast, since it will dry better than soap and water. Rubbing alcohol should not be used on young children, since it dries out the skin and can produce skin irritation.

Neurovascular assessment. Probably the most important task you'll perform every day in connection with your child's cast is a neurovascular assessment. This involves observing all casted extremities (or in the case of a body cast or a hip spica, all extremities) for the following: color, temperature, swelling, any odor, sensation, numbness and tingling, range of motion, and circulation. Immediately report to the doctor any of the following:

- swelling
- extreme color change
- lack of capillary refill (indicated by the pink color returning to the fingertips after pressure is applied and then released)
- increased pain; strange feelings
- changes in skin or body temperature

Finishing or petaling the cast. This is a means of making the cast edges smooth and free from scratchy edges and of preventing pieces of the cast from falling off. If the cast is finished with stockinette pulled smooth over the edge of the cast, nothing more needs to be done. If the cast is not finished in this way, a variety of petaling materials may be used.

Cut moleskin or waterproof tape into strips an inch or two wide by three inches long. Place these strips on the edges of the cast in an overlapping fashion with about one inch of the tape inside the cast, sticky side against the cast, and the remainder pulled tight and placed on the outside of the cast. Carefully observe these cast edges daily, since they sometimes start to cause irritation. Some young children have a sensitivity to the adhesive material on the petaling strips, and even though the sticky surface is against the cast, there is enough sticky material at the petal edge to cause some irritation.

Positioning. If your child is capable of changing her position on her own, encourage her to do so. In any case, make sure that your child changes position at least every two to three hours during the day and every four hours during the night to relieve the pressure of the cast on the various skin surfaces and to avoid bedsores. This is especially important for the child in a body or hip spica cast.

Bedpan use. If your child is in a body cast and must use a bedpan, follow these steps to help your child use the bedpan successfully:

1. Elevate the head of the bed or use pillows to elevate the child's head higher than the hips so gravity can help drain urine and feces into the bedpan.

2. Cut pieces of plastic about 8 inches by 12 inches. Tuck these between the skin and the cast. Turn the child to one side and insert the plastic between the cast and the skin surface in the buttocks area such that the pieces of plastic overlap each other.

3. Place the rim of the bedpan against the cast. Center the child on the bedpan. Funnel the plastic into the bedpan to prevent fecal material from soiling the cast. Urine and fecal material will be diverted into the bedpan via the plastic.

4. When your child has finished, remove the plastic from the edge of the cast as you turn your child back to the side. Clean the genital area and dry it well.

For the incontinent young child in a spica-type cast, place a sanitary napkin or folded diaper for extra absorbency over the genital area, and then place a diaper over that. For a young child, the material must be changed every two hours; for the older child, the diaper must be changed every time the child eliminates.

Using Nutritional Boosters

Children with CP often have difficulty gaining weight and tolerating different textures. You can optimize your child's intake by providing higher-calorie food and beverage options (such as whole milk rather than skim milk) or by adding extra calories to the foods the child is already eating (such as extra oil to pasta or vegetables). In this way you can increase your child's calorie intake without drastically increasing the amount of food. Foods that have the most calories will also be highest in fat, because fat provides more calories per gram than carbohydrates and protein. Here is a list of high-calorie foods, arranged by food group, that can be added to your child's diet to improve energy intake and promote weight gain:

Dairy

- Whole milk and reduced-fat milk (2%)
- Pudding, yogurt, and ice cream
- Heavy whipping cream
- Cheese, cream cheese, and sour cream

Tip: Dairy items made with whole milk have the most calories.

Protein

- High-fat meats such as bacon, sausage, and ground meat that is 70 to 80% lean and 20 to 30% fat
- Breaded and fried meats
- Fish that is higher in fat than other fish, such as salmon, mackerel, and herring
- Nuts, nut butter, seeds, hummus, beans, and lentils

Tip: Fish and vegetable protein sources, such as nuts and seeds, provide the heart-healthy monounsaturated and polyunsaturated fats. Saturated fat comes from animal sources and can be harmful to health when eaten in excess.

Grains and starches

- Granola, ground flaxseed, wheat germ, bran, and chia seeds
- Bread, oatmeal, crackers, pasta, rice, and potatoes

Tips: Aim to make half of your grains whole grains. The grains listed above can be added to yogurt, cereal, or muffins, for example. Always top starches with a spread, sauce, or fat such as butter, oil, nut butter, hummus, cream cheese, or gravy.

Fruits and vegetables

Tips: Fruits and vegetables are high in nutritional value but naturally low in fat and calories, so they should always be offered with a food that provides more calories. Serve fresh fruits and vegetables with a dressing or spread such as salad dressing, yogurt dip, nut butter, or hummus. Top cooked vegetables with oil, butter, or cheese. Avocado is a stone fruit that is high in healthy oils and therefore a good source of calories. It can be mashed up and served with pita bread or blended with a fruit smoothie. It is a versatile food that can be used in many different dishes.

Fats and oils

- Canola, corn, cottonseed, olive, safflower, soybean, and sunflower oils
- Foods made mainly with oil, such as margarine, mayonnaise, and salad dressing
- Foods naturally high in oils, such as avocado, nuts, seeds, some fish, and olives
- Solid fats, such as butter, cream, coconut oil, and palm oil

Tips: Add extra fats and oils to foods as often as possible. Try to optimize intake of oils from plant sources to provide the heart-healthy unsaturated fats.

As a general rule of thumb, always try to add something to provide extra calories. If your child eats a pureed diet, use whole milk, gravy, or juice in place of water when blending foods.

When high-calorie foods aren't enough, nutrition supplements can be used. A wide selection of nutrition supplements are available. Many supplemental beverages are milk based and lactose free, but there are also specialized formulas for those with food allergies or intolerances and other dietary needs. Juice-based supplements are also available. Nutrition supplements can range from 30 to 60 calories per ounce. Formulas will differ for varying age groups. Many standard formulas can be found at your local pharmacy or grocery store, or they can be ordered online. They often come in a variety of flavors, such as chocolate, vanilla, and strawberry. For many children, taste is the determining factor when it comes to deciding which formula to use.

For those children who are supported nutritionally by a feeding tube, the appropriate formula can be determined with the help of your pediatrician or dietitian. Listed below are some products currently available:

Milk-based formulas

- BOOST Original / BOOST Plus / BOOST Very High Calorie / BOOST High Protein / BOOST Compact
- BOOST Kid Essentials / BOOST Kid Essentials 1.5 with fiber
- COMPLEAT / COMPLEAT Pediatric / COMPLEAT Pediatric Reduced Calorie
- Ensure Original / Ensure Plus / Ensure High Protein
- Fibersource HN
- ISOSOURCE 1.5 Cal / ISOSOURCE HN
- Jevity 1.0 / Jevity 1.2 / Jevity 1.5
- Nutren 1.0 / Nutren 1.0 Fiber / Nutren 1.5 / Nutren 2.0
- Nutren Junior / Nutren Junior Fiber
- PediaSure / Pediasure with Fiber / PediaSure 1.5 Cal / Pediasure 1.5 with Fiber
- Promote / Promote with Fiber
- Replete / Replete Fiber

Juice-based formulas

- BOOST Breeze
- Ensure Clear / Ensure Clear Therapeutic Nutrition

Specialized formulas

- EleCare Jr
- Ensure Original Pudding
- Neocate Junior / Neocate Junior with Prebiotics
- Neocate E028 Splash
- Neocate Splash Unflavored
- Pediasure Peptide 1.0 Cal / Pediasure Peptide 1.5 Cal
- Peptamen / Peptamen 1.5 / Peptamen AF / Peptamen with Prebio[1] / Peptamen 1.5 with Prebio[1]
- Peptamen Junior / Peptamen Junior 1.5 / Peptamen Junior Fiber / Peptamen Junior with Prebio[1]
- Vivonex Pediatric / Vivonex Plus / Vivonex RTF / Vivonex TEN

Other supplements

- Benecalorie
- Beneprotein
- BOOST Nutritional Pudding
- Carnation Breakfast Essentials
- Duocal
- Nutrisource Fiber
- Scandishake

Contact your insurance company to see if there is financial help for either oral supplements or tube feedings. You may also need a prescription for the supplements and/or a letter of medical necessity. If your child is eligible, the Special Supplemental Nutrition Program for Women, Infants, and Children (WIC) may provide some of the formula for you. In some states Medicaid or Medicare may help with payment as well.

Calories, which come from carbohydrates, protein, and fat, are essential for adequate weight gain and growth, but it is also important to make sure children with CP get enough vitamins, minerals, fiber, and fluids. These nutrients are also critical for growth and proper body functioning. Some children with CP need a multivitamin or mineral supplement or a specific vitamin or mineral supplement (such as vitamin D or calcium) if something is lacking in the diet or if there is a clinical deficiency. Fiber can be lacking if the child does not consume enough fruits, vegetables, and whole grains. Fiber is important for good bowel health and to promote regular bowel movements. Fiber can be supplemented if the child is unable to get it from food. Decreased fluid intake can occur if the child has difficulty drinking. Fluid is needed to maintain adequate hydration, which allows the body to function at its best. Talk with your child's pediatrician or dietitian to find out if your child needs a vitamin or mineral supplement and is getting enough fiber and fluid along with adequate calories.

Managing Tube Feedings

If your child is unable to gain adequate weight with oral feedings, or if your child is at risk for aspiration either because of poor oral motor muscle coordination or severe gastroesophageal reflux, tube feedings may be needed. Your child may begin with a nasal or oral tube feeding. With this type of feeding, a tube inserted into the nose or mouth passes through the esophagus (food pipe) and into the stomach or small bowel. This type of tube feeding can be used temporarily to help with weight gain and improve your child's nutritional status. Nasal and oral feedings are often used on a trial basis, before placement of a more permanent tube, to make sure your child will be able to tolerate this type of feeding method.

In contrast to these temporary tubes, the gastrostomy tube (G-tube), which is inserted directly through the belly into the stomach, and the J-tube, which is inserted into the small intestine, are more permanent. J-tubes are not commonly used. Placement of a GJ-tube, a tube that enters the stomach but then passes through the stomach into the jejunum, is preferred when G-tube feeding is not tolerated. A GJ-tube is placed by an interventional radiologist and must be changed every 3 months in the radiology department. All tubes can be skin-level tubes (commonly called "button tubes"), which lie flat on the skin, or catheters. A catheter can be secured to the undershirt by wrapping a piece of tape approximately 1 by 1 inch around a section of the tube and attaching a safety pin to the end of the tape. The safety pin can then be attached to the undershirt.

Before your child is discharged from the hospital, be sure that you understand and are comfortable with the care of your child's gastrostomy tube. There are many different types of tubes available, but you should be taught how to care for the specific kind of tube that your child is using. Health care specialists will teach you exactly how to feed your child through the gastrostomy tube, but here is an overview of gastrostomy tube feedings for you to refer to at home.

Types of Feedings

There are two basic types of feedings. One is the *bolus*. In this type of feeding, a specific amount of formula is given three or four times a day, much like regular meals. A syringe pump or gravity system is connected to the tube, and formula flows in over a period of between 15 and 60 minutes.

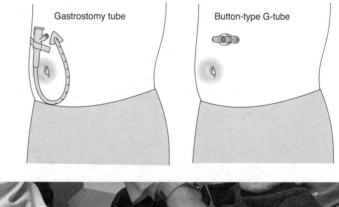

Gastrostomy tube   Button-type G-tube

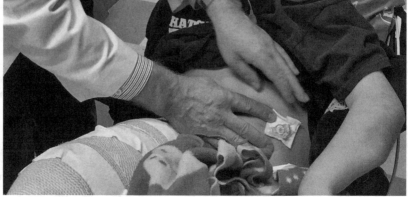

Gastrostomy tube

The other type of feeding is *continuous*. In this setup, formula flows slowly into the stomach or small intestine over a long period. A special pump is used to measure precise amounts of formula and to regulate the flow. J-tube and GJ-tube feedings are always given as continuous feedings.

You will need the following:

- Food at room temperature. It will most likely be a commercially prepared formula. Your physician or dietitian will determine which food is best for your child.
- tap water at room temperature (to rinse the tube)
- syringe
- feeding bag
- feeding tubing
- any special adapters specific to the tube used by your child

How to Give a Tube Feeding

1. Gather the equipment and be sure it is in working order.
2. Wash your hands.
3. Position the child so that his head is elevated. This can be done by positioning the child on your lap. If the child is older, you can elevate the child's head by raising the head of the bed with pillows, a rolled blanket, or a wedge under the child's head and shoulders. You may also position the child comfortably in his wheelchair.
4. If a feeding bag is used, run the feeding through the bag and the attached tubing.
5. Attach a syringe to the gastrostomy tube and flush with water to be sure that it is clear. (This preliminary water flush may or may not be recommended by your child's physician. Follow his or her instructions.) If the tube is occluded (blocked), consult your physician for further instructions. Do not force the flush.
6. Remove the syringe from the gastrostomy tube and attach the feeding bag and tubing to allow the bolus to go in or the continuous feeding to begin. Use the special extension tubing required by some button tubes for either type of feeding. You may use a 30–60 cc syringe without a plunger to allow the feeding to flow by gravity. Continue adding to the syringe until finished, or you should set the rate prescribed by your physician to run automatically on a pump.
7. When the feeding is complete, flush the tube with water in the amount specified by your child's physician.
8. Pinch or clamp the tube before removing the syringe or tubing. Clamp or cap indwelling tubes. Remove the feeding adapter from the button tube and snap the plug in place.
9. Observe the child for abdominal distention and vomiting. Notify the doctor if this becomes a problem. Certain venting procedures are required for some tubes; your child's physician will describe these to you.
10. Clean the syringe in warm soapy water. Rinse until clear.

Tube Feeding Information Card

Many parents find a feeding tube information card helpful. We suggest that you record the following information on a file card or on your computer and keep it handy. This way you'll be sure to have all relevant facts ready at a glance should you need them.

Child's name:
Tube specifications:
    size:
    type:
    balloon volume:
    button size:
    dates tube replaced:
Surgery date:
    surgeon: telephone number:
    specialist: telephone number:
Feeding:
    type:
    amount:
    water:
Feeding instructions:
    feeding times:
    amount of each feeding:
Pump setting or rate:
Flush with   cc water before/after every feeding

Providing Oral Care

Good oral hygiene begins before the child has teeth. At first you can simply wipe the inside of the child's mouth with a moist washcloth or gauze. If you do this regularly, the child will become used to having his or her mouth cleaned.

The first dental visit should be 6 months after the first tooth erupts or no later than age 12 months. X-rays are not done at this time. During this first visit the dentist will provide counseling about nutrition, including what foods to avoid to decrease the chance of dental decay, and answer any questions the parent may have. At this time the dentist will create an individualized dental home care program suited to the needs of parent and child.

To maintain good oral hygiene and prevent future dental decay and gum problems, the child's teeth should be brushed twice a day beginning at 12–18 months. Cleaning a child's teeth should not be a struggle for the parent or the child. As their child grows, parents will figure out when is the best time to clean the child's teeth each day. Eventually, tooth cleaning will become part of the daily routine.

If your child has problems with head and neck control, he or she can be positioned in the wheelchair, in a parent's lap, or lying down. If your child can tolerate a toothbrush and not gag, use a soft brush with circular motions. If your child cannot tolerate a toothbrush, you can brush with toothpaste on a cotton-tipped swab or soft washcloth.

If your child is able to brush on his own, you will still need to monitor his technique, as you do with other daily home activities, such as bathing. You will need to clean areas the child missed. By always giving positive reinforcement, you will assure better compliance and long-term success.

Fluoride is important for reducing the risk of dental decay. It comes as a flavored liquid, a chewable tablet, or a mouth rinse. The dentist can also apply topical fluoride at dental visits every 6 months. Whether there is a need for fluoride, and how much, depends on the amount of fluoride in the local water supply. You and your dentist can decide what method is best based on the water supply and your child's needs.

The risk of cavities can be reduced by watching the child's diet. When it comes to preventing cavities, fresh fruits are better than soft drinks, sticky snacks, cookies, and sugary fruit drinks.

Toilet Training Your Child

The most important factor in successful toilet training is the cognitive or developmental level of the child, regardless of his or her chronological age. Children can be successfully toilet trained if they have the developmental and cognitive abilities of a 2- to 4-year-old. Physical barriers can be overcome with adaptive seating so the child can be properly positioned on the toilet seat. The child will need the help of a parent at home or an aide at school to assist with transferring from the wheelchair to the toilet seat.

Another important factor in successful toilet training is the attitude of the parent, who must be relaxed and positive about the process of toilet training and must convey this attitude to the child.

Praising the child for success on the potty is crucial. But even before toilet training can begin, both the child and the parent must be ready. Your child may signal her readiness for toilet training in one of several ways. For example, while urinating or having a bowel movement (or just before), the child may become either fussy or quiet, wiggle and demonstrate the need to change position, suddenly lie or stand very still, go to the corner and squat, change facial expression, or say that she is wet. The parent needs to pay attention to these behavioral changes and be ready to interpret these gestures to mean that the child needs to eliminate. Only when all these signals and good intentions come together can toilet training begin in earnest.

Establishing a Pattern

One thing that will help establish a pattern of elimination is keeping regular mealtimes. Then the stomach, bowels, and bladder will be empty and full at regular intervals. Not only that, but food tends to stimulate the bowel, and many people go to the bathroom after a meal, usually breakfast or dinner. So you may be able to predict your child's bowel habits based upon mealtimes. Once you've determined the normal pattern of elimination, you'll know when to place your child on the toilet in order to achieve the best success.

Getting Started

Begin when your child is rested and in a good mood. You'll need a child-sized potty chair or potty seat.

When your child has indicated (by one of the signals mentioned above or something similar) that she needs to urinate or have a bowel movement, take her to the bathroom and explain in simple language what is to be done. Use very specific common words to describe the act of elimination. Place the child on the seat and stay with her until the training session is completed. After about five minutes on the toilet, the child should be wiped and rewarded with hugs and praise for the desired behaviors.

If the child was not successful in achieving the desired behavior, praise her for cooperating and sitting quietly on the toilet or potty chair. During training, the child should sit on the seat without toys or playthings, since these would divert attention from what she is supposed to be doing.

Repeat this process until the child is able to tell you in advance that she needs to go or is able to use the bathroom or potty on her own.

Bowel Training

If your child has an intellectual disability, it may be helpful to institute a bowel training program. This too involves establishing a regular pattern of mealtimes to help establish a regular pattern of elimination, but the difference is that routinely, about 15 to 30 minutes after one meal is finished, the child is placed on the toilet for 15 to 30 minutes. Choose either breakfast or dinner and stick with it, since the point of a bowel training program is to train the child to produce a bowel movement at the same time every day or every other day.

Make sure that the child is comfortable, with feet flat on the floor or supported by a stool. Use simple descriptive common words to describe the desired activity. Again, be positive. Praising the child, whether for the desired results or for sitting on the toilet as you wished even if there was no bowel movement. Be sure there are no distractions during this time.

Many children with CP have chronic constipation, which can interfere with bowel training. If your child does not have a bowel movement at least every other day, your child is probably constipated. The treatment of constipation is described in Chapter 3.

Adaptive Toileting

Special handling techniques are used for toileting the child with cerebral palsy who is physically challenged. To protect the child (as well as themselves) from injury, care providers need to learn these techniques. Ask a physical or an occupational therapist for tips in handling your child.

It may be necessary for a child with CP to use adaptive seating to be properly positioned on the toilet seat. Children with CP need firm support, with handrails and feet flat on the floor or a hard surface. Proper body mechanics while lifting a child to the toilet seat are necessary to decrease stress on the caregiver's

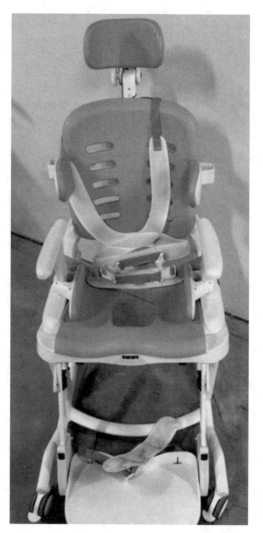

Toilet chair

back (see "Protecting the Caregiver's Back," above). Your child's occupational therapist can usually provide further information on adaptive seating.

Giving an Enema

You may have to give your child an enema either occasionally or on a regular basis. Enemas work by distending the rectum and making the child feel the need to have a bowel movement; in addition, they clean out stool that has been held in the rectum. You can buy Fleet or Pediatric Fleet enemas at the drugstore. Check with your doctor about what's best for your child. Before you give an enema to your child, be sure to explain what you will be doing and what will happen.

How to Give an Enema to a Child

    1. The enema should be warm—close to body temperature—not hot or cold.

    2. Position the child in one of three ways: sitting on the toilet or potty chair;

lying on a rug on the bathroom floor, face down with hips and knees bent toward the chest; or positioned on the rug on his or her left side, with the left leg straight and the right leg bent at the hip and knee and placed on top of the left leg.

3. *For a disposable enema:* Remove the protective cap from the enema bottle. Gently insert the tip about one inch into the rectum. Slowly squeeze the enema container until it is nearly empty (a small amount of the contents of the container will remain after squeezing). Remove the tip from the rectum.

For an enema bag: Put Vaseline jelly on the enema tip. Gently insert the tip about one inch into the rectum. Slowly squeeze the contents into the rectum. Hold the bag about one foot above the child's body.

4. Hold the child's buttocks together, if necessary, to keep the liquid inside the rectum until the child tells you he or she needs to have a bowel movement. This usually occurs after about three to five minutes.

5. Help the child to the toilet or potty chair or place her over a bedpan that has been placed in her bed. Or allow the enema to be expelled into a diaper, if necessary.

6. Keep a record of the results.

Giving Rectal Medications or Suppositories

For a variety of reasons, some medications may need to be given rectally. When a child is vomiting and it's important for her to take a medication, the medication can make its way into the child's system if it is administered rectally. Medications are also given rectally to children who have difficulty swallowing, who are unable to swallow, or who are actively seizing. Finally, a child who will be having surgery within a day often must refrain from taking anything by mouth. Some necessary medications can nevertheless be administered by rectum.

The medications most commonly given by rectum are antiseizure medications, sedatives, antipyretics (medications that help control temperature), antiemetics (medications that help control nausea or vomiting), and bowel-stimulating suppositories, usually composed of glycerin. Rectal medications are primarily supplied in suppository form (suppositories are shaped like bullets, with one rounded end and one flat end). You can lubricate a suppository for easier insertion by dipping it in water or in a water-soluble lubricant. Do not use an oil-based lubricant, since it may interfere with absorption of the medication.

How to Give Medication in Suppository Form to a Child

1. Before getting started, ask the child to try to move his bowels, since if there is stool in the rectum, this may interfere with absorption of the medication.

2. Position the child either on his left side, with hips and knees flexed, or on his abdomen with knees flexed and positioned toward the chest. Older children prefer to lie on their sides, whereas insertion is easier in infants if they are placed on their abdomen.

3. Put a non-latex glove on the hand you will be using. With a gloved finger, insert the medication beyond the sphincter. Use the pinky finger to insert the

suppository in infants and toddlers. In older children, use the index finger. The usual distance for the insertion of rectal medications is as follows:

- in infants and young toddlers, about 1 to 1½ inches
- in older toddlers and preschoolers, about 2 to 3 inches
- in school-age children or adolescents, about 3 to 4 inches

4. For the medication to be effective, it must be held in the rectum for 10 minutes. To prevent early expulsion of the medication—before it has been fully absorbed—it may be necessary to hold the buttocks together for 5 to 10 minutes. Older children are generally able to control their sphincter better than younger children. A suppository that has been administered to stimulate a bowel movement ought to be held for 5 minutes or until the child states a need to move his bowels.

How to Give Liquid Medications Rectally to a Child

The goal of the procedure is to deliver by rectum an appropriate amount of medication via a catheter. We recommend using a size 15 French (Mentor) catheter for this procedure.

The following equipment may be needed:

- size 15 French (Mentor) intermittent catheter
- the prescribed medication
- a syringe to deliver the volume of medicine ordered
- tap water
- a water-soluble lubricant
- a protective pad

1. Remove the syringe from the package and attach a needle to it.

2. Draw the medication from the bottle into the syringe, taking up a little more than the prescribed amount.

3. Flick the syringe with your finger to get rid of air bubbles and measure the amount of medication in the syringe again.

4. Remove the needle from the syringe and place the needle in a safe container for disposal. (Do not attempt to recap the needle because of the danger of sticking yourself with it.)

5. Draw up into the same syringe an amount of air equal to the amount of medication. The air will move to the top of the syringe when the syringe is held upright. When the medication is administered, the air will follow the medication into the rectum and assist in clearing the syringe and delivering the ordered amount of the medication.

6. Lubricate the catheter tip in a water-soluble lubricant and attach the catheter to the end of the syringe.

7. Position the child on his or her left side. Insert the catheter into the rectum. For a child weighing 22 pounds (10 kg) or less, insert it 1¼ inches; for a child between 22 pounds and 44 pounds (10–20 kg), insert it 1½ inches; for a child weighing more than 44 pounds (20 kg), insert the catheter 2¾ inches.

8. Hold the syringe upright so that the air bubbles rise inside the syringe

and are delivered last. Push the medication into the tubing and follow it with the air in the same syringe.

9. Remove the catheter and hold the buttocks together for 3 to 5 minutes to allow the medication to be absorbed.

Suctioning Techniques

Note: You must be trained in suctioning techniques by your health care professional or a home health professional before you try the procedure on your own.

Some children need help in clearing their airways of mucus. Suctioning will help clear the airways, but this procedure should only be performed when the child needs it. Suction your child under the following circumstances: (1) when you hear your child make wet breathing sounds, as if air is being pushed through wet mucus; (2) when your child is having difficulty breathing and is restless; or (3) when your child's color is paler than usual and the nostrils are flaring out. The child may gag and/or cough when you use a suction catheter.

The following description of the procedure for suctioning is provided only as a memory refresher for caregivers who have already been trained to perform the procedure by a doctor or another health care professional. If you do not feel comfortable performing the procedure, you should not attempt to do it alone. *Again, do not attempt to suction your child if you have not been trained to do so.*

You will need the following equipment for the procedure:

- a suction machine and tubing
- suction catheters
- salt water
- containers for storing salt water
- gloves

You can make salt water, or saline, solution by mixing ¾ teaspoon of table salt with 2 cups water in a pot. Boil this mixture for 5 minutes, turn burner off, place a lid on the pot or pan, and allow the salt water to cool to room temperature. After it has cooled, place it in a clean glass jar with a lid. Label each jar with the date and time when the solution was made, as well as the date and time when the solution should be discarded—usually 48 hours after it was made. Place the jar of solution in the refrigerator. Manufactured saline solution can be obtained with a prescription from your doctor.

How to Suction a Child

1. Gather the necessary equipment and make sure the suction machine is working properly. To prevent the risk of low oxygen levels or tissue damage, be sure the suction pressure on the machine is set appropriately. For infants the suction pressure should be 60–80 mm Hg; for children other than infants, 80–100 mm Hg; and for adults, 100–120 mm Hg.

2. Wash your hands thoroughly.

3. Connect the suction catheter to the suction machine tubing.

4. Determine how far to place the suction catheter into the nose by measur-

ing the catheter from the tip of the earlobe to the tip of the nose. Keep your fingertips on this mark.

5. Insert the tip of the suction catheter into the prepared saline solution to wet the catheter. Place your thumb over the suction port to check on the effectiveness of the suction.

6. Tell the child what you will be doing and what to expect.

7. Insert the tube into the nostril to the determined distance *without* applying suction. Keep your finger off the suction port opening in the catheter.

8. With the catheter in place, put your thumb over the suction port and rotate the tube as you slowly move it out of the nostril. This should take no longer than 10 seconds.

9. Rinse the catheter in saline. Let the child relax a moment.

10. Repeat steps 5–9 for the other nostril, if necessary.

11. After suctioning the nostrils, you may suction the mouth. Remember to rinse the catheter in saline first.

12. Insert the suction catheter into either side of the inside of the mouth *without* applying suction.

13. Once the catheter is correctly placed in the mouth, place your thumb over the suction port and rotate or twist the catheter out of the mouth for no more than 10 seconds.

14. Rinse the suction catheter and tubing by suctioning the saline through it until the catheter and tubing are clear.

15. Repeat oral suctioning if necessary.

16. Dispose of the suction catheter and any unused saline solution.

To clean the portable suction unit, follow these steps:

Daily

1. Empty the collection bottle contents into the toilet and flush.

2. Wash the connecting tubing, jar, and lid in warm soapy water (you can use dish detergent).

3. Rinse well under running water before re-using.

Weekly

1. Follow the steps for the daily cleaning.

2. Soak the tubing, jar, and lid in a solution of 1 part white vinegar and 1 part water for 30 minutes.

3. Rinse well under running water.

4. Hang the tubing to dry. Cover the rest with a clean cloth or paper towel and air dry on a clean towel.

5. When the parts are completely dry, put them back together and store in a plastic bag.

6. The connecting tubing (tubing between the suction machine and the suction catheter) should be replaced every two weeks.

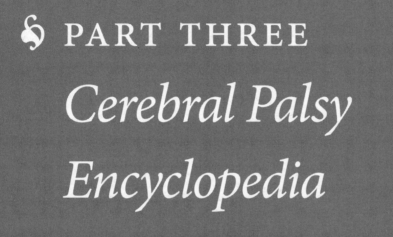

PART THREE

Cerebral Palsy

Encyclopedia

Achilles Tendon Lengthening

(TAL, tendon Achilles lengthening, Achilles tendon contracture, equinus contracture)

The Achilles tendon is the muscle that is most commonly contracted in children with cerebral palsy. Contracture of this muscle prevents the foot from being flexed up. For the child who is able to stand, this contracture prevents him from standing with his foot flat—instead, he is on tiptoe. He may try to place his foot flat, but he will have to bend his knee back to do this. The initial treatment for an Achilles tendon contracture usually involves physical therapy combined with brace use (AFO) during the day.

Indications: Achilles tendon lengthening is indicated for children for whom the brace no longer keeps the foot flat or for teenagers trying to discontinue the use of the brace. Also, if the muscle is too tight to allow the child to use an AFO, then Achilles tendon lengthening is recommended. Occasionally, tendon lengthenings are also done for people who cannot stand or walk but who want to keep their feet flat on a wheelchair rest. In this case, the procedure is done for cosmetic reasons and to enable the person to wear shoes.

The surgery: The Achilles tendon is located behind the ankle and is attached to the gastrocnemius and soleus muscles, which are located just above and behind the knee. There are three different techniques for surgical lengthening of the Achilles tendon. *Percutaneous tendon Achilles lengthening* involves making a small stab wound through the skin in two or three different places, then stretching the tendon. The goal is to nick the tendon in several places and have the tendon tear in such a way that it stretches itself out and heals back in place. The advantage of this procedure is that it involves very small incisions; however, it provides the least control over the amount of lengthening, so there can be too much or too little lengthening.

The second method, called *Z-plasty lengthening*, involves making an open incision that exposes the tendon; a Z-cut is then made in the tendon. The tendon ends slide apart and are sutured into place again. This procedure allows the most controlled lengthening of the whole tendon and muscle area.

The third method is called *Baker lengthening*, *gastroc recession*, or *myotendinous lengthening* and involves identifying where the gastrocnemius and soleus muscles come together in the middle of the calf to form the Achilles tendon. The gastrocnemius muscle is loosened and slid proximally over the soleus. The advantage of this procedure is that it has the lowest risk of *over*lengthening; one disadvantage is that sometimes it does not provide sufficient lengthening. This difficulty in obtaining sufficient lengthening with the Baker method explains why the Z-plasty is often the preferred procedure.

After-surgery care: After an Achilles tendon lengthening the child wears a short cast (from the toes to the knee). This cast typically has a sole, which allows the child to stand and walk immediately after the Achilles tendon lengthening has been done. Following removal of the cast in 4 to 6 weeks, the child returns to a stretching program for maintenance. An AFO may also be used to maintain correction, especially for the growing child. A hinged brace may also be used, allowing the child to raise the front of the foot but not to lower the toes to walk on tiptoe.

What to expect: The complications from Achilles tendon lengthening, especially in children who walk, may be very severe if the tendon is overlengthened. It is far preferable for the child to have a slightly tight Achilles tendon, so that the child tiptoes slightly, than to have a completely nonfunctional tendon. Another risk from

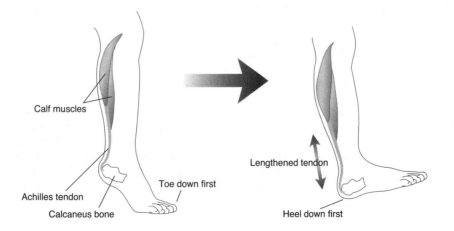

Calf muscles

Achilles tendon

Calcaneus bone

Toe down first

Lengthened tendon

Heel down first

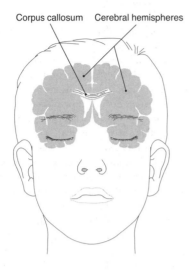

Corpus callosum   Cerebral hemispheres

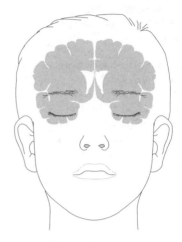

Without corpus callosum

Achilles tendon lengthening is the need to have the lengthening repeated. The child between the ages of 3 and 5 has a 25 to 30 percent chance of having the lengthening repeated between the ages of 9 and 12. Repeated lengthenings can be done three or four times, but it is seldom necessary to repeat more than once.

Agenesis of the Corpus Callosum
(Aicardi syndrome)

The corpus callosum is the structure in the brain that joins together the two cerebral hemispheres and provides a pathway from one side of the brain to the other. If a child does not have this structure, he may have seizures and mild to moderate intellectual impairment, as well as impaired visual and motor coordination. Sometimes children who don't have the corpus callosum are also deficient in cellular migration and proliferation, which essentially means that the brain wiring is not correct; this can be seen in a variety of chromosomal defects. Agenesis of the corpus callosum is an integral part of Aicardi syndrome, which appears to occur only in females and is characterized by severe intellectual impairment, generalized seizures that begin early in life, and specific abnormalities of the retina.

The absence of the corpus callosum is diagnosed with an MRI or a CT scan of the brain. Some individuals with this diagnosis are completely normal otherwise. However, children with many other congenital deformities of the brain are at higher risk for having this deformity. When it is seen by MRI or CT scan during an evaluation of a child for cerebral palsy, it suggests more underlying problems. This diagnosis by itself cannot be used to make a specific prognosis of what will happen to

the child, however. Because of their brain abnormalities, these children often have cerebral palsy.

Air Swallowing
(aerophagia)

Chronic air swallowing is predominantly a problem for children with intellectual disability. It is also commonly seen in children with Rett syndrome. Its main characteristic is a distended abdomen. If a child has had an operation to prevent gastrointestinal reflux, so that stomach contents cannot come back up to the mouth, then she is not able to release the air pressure that develops in her stomach by burping, which may cause significant abdominal distension and pain. If she has a gastrostomy tube, the air can be vented through the tube. If she doesn't, occasionally the pain becomes so severe that a tube is required. Usually children who have not had operative procedures to prevent vomiting or reflux are able to release the air themselves by burping. Aerophagia is usually worse when the child is agitated or is not engaged in an activity. Treatment is predominantly directed toward keeping the child comfortable and occupied with some form of activity.

Airway Clearance

Respiratory complications are often a significant problem for children with CP. Respiratory infections are the most common reason for repeated admissions to the hospital for these children. One of the reasons for their susceptibility to respiratory problems is that their normal airway clearance is often compromised by their limited mobility and a weak or ineffective cough. Children who have quadriplegic CP, resulting in their inability to walk, spend most of their day in a wheelchair. Thus, they do not have the opportunity to exercise and breathe deeply, which is one of the main mechanisms for clearing one's airways. In addition, many children with CP cannot clear their airways with an effective cough. They may be unable to take in enough air to have an effective cough, or they have poor coordination of the muscles of their throat, making their cough either ineffective or nonexistent. Without the ability to cough effectively, these children are unable to clear the secretions that are normally produced in the lungs, and such pooled secretions can lead to recurrent pneumonia or bronchitis.

The traditional technique for removing mucus from the lungs of a child who cannot cough effectively has been *chest physical therapy*. Typical treatments last 20 to 30 minutes and are usually required several times a day. The caregiver or nurse administers percussion to the chest wall of the child while having her lie in a variety of different positions. Many children with CP have scoliosis and/or contractures, making the proper position difficult to achieve.

Another treatment to help mobilize secretions in the lungs is use of the ABI vest. The ABI vest is an inflatable vest connected by hoses to an air-pulse generator. The generator rapidly inflates and deflates the vest, thus compressing and releasing the chest wall. The resulting chest wall oscillation generates increased airflow through the airways, creating forces that are like a cough and mobilizing secretions. It does not require any positioning or special breathing techniques.

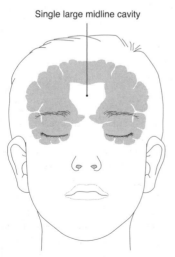

Single large midline cavity

Example of anterior midline defect

Anterior Midline Defects
(holoprosencephaly, septo-optic dysplasia)

A number of malformations fit into the category of anterior midline defects. The most common is holoprosencephaly, which involves failure of the midline facial structure and the brain behind it to develop. In the deficit's most complete expression, the brain has a single large ventricular cavity, with the inferior frontal and temporal regions of the brain often absent and the remainder quite rudimentary. The brain stem and cerebellum are present and fully developed.

Septo-optic dysplasia is a form of holoprosencephaly in which the optic nerves are underdeveloped, resulting in severe visual impairment or blindness. It also results in deficiencies of certain hormones produced by the brain. This can cause very short stature, frequent urination, and other abnormalities. Any of these brain malformations can be accompanied by cerebral palsy.

Arthrogryposis

Arthrogryposis is a congenital condition in which a child's muscles and joints are stiff, often causing the child to hold the affected limbs in extended positions. This condition may affect one, two, or all of the limbs and varies in degree from relatively mild to so severe that a person is unable to walk or to use his arms for functional purposes. There are four basic causes of arthrogryposis: muscle atrophy, lack of sufficient room in the uterus during pregnancy, malformation of the brain or spinal cord, and abnormalities of tendons, bones, or joint linings.

Children with arthrogryposis are not spastic, although their condition can be mistaken for cerebral palsy. They have normal mental development, and their surgical treatment is very different from that of children with cerebral palsy. Although the surgical treatment is different, other aspects of treatment and care are very similar. Aggressive physical therapy is the ideal treatment to maintain the joints in the best functional position and maintain the limited amount of motion that is often present.

Asthma
(reactive airway disease, wheezy bronchitis)

Asthma is defined as recurrent and reversible bronchospasm, meaning that the airways of the lungs go into spasm and narrow, obstructing airflow. This narrowing results from contraction of the muscles around these little airways, as well as from increased production of mucus and swelling because of inflammation. Both large and small airways can be involved and are responsive to a variety of stimuli, including pollens to which the patient is allergic, dander from cats or dogs, cold air, or noxious environmental agents such as tobacco smoke, aerosols, chemicals, or strong aromas. Some children develop symptoms when they exercise or when they laugh or cry. Overall, it is estimated that between 5 and 10 percent of children have asthma at some time during their childhood.

Asthma accounts for 10 percent of emergency room visits and 10 percent of medical hospitalizations in the United States and is the most frequent cause of school absenteeism and chronic illness in children under age 18. Boys are affected more than girls, by a 3:1 ratio. Though many children who develop asthma early in life tend to improve during mid-childhood and adolescence, a significant proportion continue to have symptoms into adulthood. There has been an increase in hospital admissions and in deaths from asthma over the past 20 years for reasons that are not clear.

Asthma does run in families, but it is not strictly a genetic disease. The fundamental abnormality seems to be a hyperreactivity of the airways. A history of bronchiolitis early in life is a risk factor for the development of asthma later in childhood, as approximately one-third to one-half of the children who have asthma in adolescence had more than one episode of bronchiolitis early in life.

The hallmark of asthma is recurrent wheezing, which is reversible with the use of specific medications. Wheezing is a high-pitched sound heard when the child breathes out. Some children have only occasional episodes of such symptoms, which can vary from mild to severe and may require medication just on those infrequent occasions. Others may have recurrent episodes every few months yet be free of symptoms in between. Still others may have chronic or daily symptoms that interfere with their lives, school attendance, and physical activity, with frequent visits to the emergency room and hospitalizations. Many of these children require multiple medications every day.

Not every child who wheezes has asthma. There are many other causes of wheezing, including tracheomalacia (a soft, floppy trachea), acute infections such as RSV bronchiolitis, cystic fibrosis, bronchopulmonary dysplasia, or aspiration of a foreign body. Children with cerebral palsy may have chronic or recurrent wheezing because they are aspirating their stomach contents, their food while eating, or even their own secretions and saliva. These items often get into their lungs rather than into their stomach and cause recurrent respiratory symptoms, such as bronchitis, pneumonia, or wheezing. Treatment of the underlying abnormality (such as preventing gastroesophageal reflux) may end the respiratory symptoms. In other children with CP and asthma, the asthma will require chronic treatment with medications because their asthma is similar to other children's asthma and is due to allergies or environmental irritants.

Ataxia

Ataxia means a lack of balance. Under conditions of normal development, the body's balance mechanism evolves from three separate systems: the eyes provide input to determine the body's position in space; the semicircular canals in the inner ear work like a gyroscope to tell the brain what position the head is in or how it is changing; the position sensors in the joints, particularly those in the neck, provide important information about where the limbs are. A child with ataxic cerebral palsy has limited balance capabilities, often expressed as an uncoordinated gait or difficulty standing in one place without moving. Ataxia continues to improve until the child is approximately 8 to 10 years old, at which time his balance and coordination system reaches maximum improvement. Because ataxia involves the hands, it makes activities requiring fine motor control, such as writing, difficult.

One of the ways a child may compensate for ataxia is to walk very rapidly, because balance tends to be better when the child goes fast, just as riding a bicycle is easier at a faster speed. The child may also adopt a very wide-based stance. Often it is easier for the child to stand with some joints immobilized by ankle braces. For many children, the main reason they cannot walk independently is severe ataxia. However, there is no surgery or medication to help this problem. The best way to reduce ataxia is by practicing movements similar to those taught in ballet or gymnastics. A physical therapist can structure balance activities and exercises to maximize a child's abilities. These usually involve walking on a balance beam, learning how to fall, and working on a therapy ball.

Athetosis
(movement disorder)

Athetosis is a movement disorder characterized by gross movements, often with fanning of the fingers. Athetosis is usually most prominent in the arms, where it causes slow, irregular, writhing involuntary movements at or around the long axis of the limb, which become more intense with attempted voluntary movement. In another movement disorder, called *dystonia*, movements may involve more rotation or torsion. In some people it is hard to clearly separate athetosis, dystonia, and spasticity, because the person may have all three—in which case it may be called a mixed movement disorder. Athetosis may make it difficult for the person to speak clearly. Athetosis does not cause contractures to develop, although often both athetosis and spasticity are present in the same person, and the spasticity may cause contractures.

Care and treatment: Treatment for a child with athetosis involves finding postural positions that allow her to control her movements. Weighted vests or weighted sleeves may help to suppress the movements. If spasticity coexists, the spasticity dampens the athetosis. For this reason, suppressing spasticity in the presence of athetosis must be done with caution, because it may bring out athetosis. Although initially the use of the baclofen pump was felt to be contra-indicated in people with athetosis or mixed movement disorders and spasticity, it is now recognized as one of the best treatment options available. For reasons not well understood, the intrathecal baclofen reduces the abnormal movements. Rhizotomy is not indicated, because it is permanent and not reversible. Generally, surgical muscle releases are very unpredictable with athetosis, but operations that stiffen joints, such as spinal fusions and foot fusions, work extremely well.

Most children with athetosis are initially very floppy and often have very good cognitive function but poor upper body control. The gross movements are not present at birth but slowly develop after the first year and increase in severity by ages 6 to 8. With the child who has normal cognitive function, communication problems, because of the impact of athetosis on speech, are the most difficult problems to overcome. Early use of augmentative communication devices should be encouraged if the child is not speaking. Power wheelchairs are also recommended for the child who is unable to walk by age 5, since the child who is unable to walk due to athetosis is seldom able to propel a manual wheelchair.

Augmentative Communication

Augmentative communication is a term used to describe the technology and services that help a person with complex communication needs interact with others. The technology used for augmentative communication is similar to a prosthesis, which is used for a person who is missing a limb; in that sense, this technology could be considered a communication prosthesis. There are many different levels of augmentative communication. The best technology is determined by the child's age, cognitive level, and level of disability and by the environment in which she lives. Augmentative communication techniques may involve the use of sign language by one's hands; symbol boards or picture boards; or computer-generated speech devices, which may be accessed through keyboards, screens, switches, or eye movements. Assistive writing devices such as comput-

ers with speech-recognition software are important aids for written communication, especially in the school environment and in social relationships.

Indications: A child who is unable to speak or communicate by 2 to 2½ years of age should be evaluated by a speech-language therapist or an augmentative communication specialist with the goal of trying to establish the most appropriate communication system. A total communication system may comprise spoken words or word approximations, sign language, picture and symbol boards, simple speech output switches, and more complex and flexible speech output systems. A child's nonverbal gestures, eye contact, and eye gaze can be important elements of such a communication system as well.

Speech output augmentative communication devices can enable nonverbal 3- and 4-year-olds to actively participate in communication turn-taking and in reading books and singing songs with adults, classmates, and siblings. Early participation in such activities provides children with a foundation for later learning of language, literacy, and communication skills. Appropriate technology choices may require the combined efforts of an occupational therapist, a speech-language therapist, an augmentative communication specialist, and a wheelchair specialist. Choosing appropriate augmentative communication options requires sensitivity to and knowledge of an individual's cognitive, visual, and motor capabilities.

Such early learning and literacy experiences also can provide important foundations for entering kindergarten, when vocabulary, syntax, and communication skills become important for active participation in the classroom. This may be when children who have neuromuscular disorders and/or developmental delays can start to benefit from assistive and augmentative technology devices to support their speech sound awareness and speech development, as well as their expressive spoken and written language development.

Writing aids may be based on tablet or laptop computers, which often include the same type of word prediction software used on smart phones, which predicts words after one or two keystrokes or based on word sequences occurring in a person's writing.

Benefits and risks: The effects of augmentative communication device use on the speech development of children with cerebral palsy and other complex communication needs are difficult to measure, because oral and fine motor involvement, visual skills, and cognitive skills or impairments vary greatly from person to person. It also is of questionable ethics to withhold this option from a matched control group of children, who might otherwise benefit from this intervention. The most helpful lit-

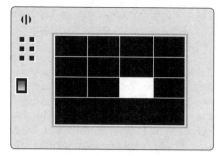

Simple communication device

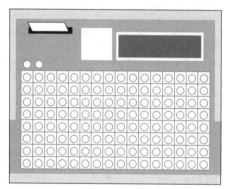

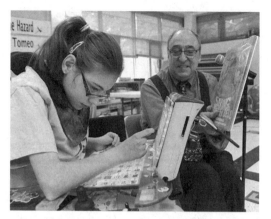

Augmentative communication device on wheelchair tray

erature is based on *meta studies* that combine data from multiple studies of small numbers of individuals. The meta studies consistently show that perhaps 75 percent of children who use augmentative communication devices increase their speech attempts, more than 20 percent show no change in their speech attempts, and fewer than 5 percent exhibit decreases in their speech attempts.

Online resources, including social media, provide much excellent information about apps for tablet computers and other augmentative communication options that people have found helpful for their children. Unfortunately, such information rarely compares different options in ways that help parents and professionals decide (*a*) which options are appropriate for children who have complex profiles of motor, sensory, developmental, and social strengths and challenges; and (*b*) which options are easy or difficult to customize to fit a child's skills, needs, and home and school settings. Speech-language therapy evaluations, along with other professional services, may help parents determine which options are best for them. *The evaluation process should always include parents' and family members' active and detailed input.*

Finally, integrating such low-tech or high-tech tools into a child's life requires collaboration among family members, caregivers, teachers, therapists, and others. Failing to plan with and train team members from all

parts of a child's life often leads to frustration for the child and others and the possibility of "technology abandonment," which likewise can be frustrating for everyone.

Maintenance and care: Unanticipated problems with any technology can quickly lead to frustration and anger. Key features that have an impact on maintenance and care of augmentative communication technology include battery life on a single charge, durability of touch screens, resistance to wetness (whether from rain or drooling), and cost, if any, of software upgrades that improve features or correct glitches. The levels of support provided by manufacturers of apps and "dedicated speech output devices" range from none to shipment of a loaner device while a child's device is being repaired. (The latter service typically is provided only for devices that are under initial or extended warranties.) These considerations can be as important as the appropriateness of a specific device for an individual child.

Autism Spectrum Disorder
(ASD)

According to the latest edition of the *Diagnostic and Statistical Manual of Mental Disorders*, published by the American Psychiatric Association, *autism spectrum disorder* is the term now used to encompass disorders that used to be labeled autism, Asperger's syndrome, and pervasive developmental disorder not otherwise specified. ASD is a neurodevelopmental disorder whose characteristics include difficulties with social interactions and social communication, as well as restricted, repetitive patterns of behavior or interests. Children and adults with ASD do not necessarily have intellectual disability.

The cause of ASD is unknown, and no medication has yet been found to treat this condition, although there are some medications that can treat some of the more severe symptoms associated with the diagnosis. There are children who display symptoms of ASD and have cerebral palsy or motor problems, but ASD and cerebral palsy are separate problems even when they occur in the same child.

Autologous Blood Donation
(blood transfusion)

It is not unusual for children with cerebral palsy to require corrective orthopedic surgery. Such operations, including correction of scoliosis or hip abnormalities, may require support in the form of blood transfusions. Because these are likely to be planned or elective operations, patients have the option of donating their own blood. That is, in the weeks prior to surgery patients can donate their own blood, to be stored for use during their operation if the need arises. This type of donation is called a preoperative *autologous* blood donation. Donation of blood for use by those other than oneself is called *allogeneic* blood donation.

To qualify for preoperative autologous blood donation, patients must be old enough to understand the procedure and cooperate fully. Hospitals and blood centers that collect donations typically require the patient to be of a certain weight to ensure a good-quality sample. While these criteria vary, a realistic weight standard is 65 pounds or greater.

It is preferable to collect autologous blood during the weeks before surgery. Blood collected more than 6 weeks prior to surgery must be frozen. The last collection should occur at least 72 hours before the scheduled surgery to allow the patient time to replace his or her own blood. The number of units donated depends on the anticipated surgical blood loss. Patients should take iron supplements during the weeks before surgery.

The main purpose of autologous donation is to prevent the transmission of blood-related infections to the patient. However, the current blood supply is very safe from the standpoint of infections caused by viruses like hepatitis and HIV. In fact, the most common causes of transfusion-associated infections are bacteria. The risk of a transfusion-associated bacterial infection is the same for both autologous and allogeneic transfusions. Thus, if a patient is not capable of donating his own blood for surgery, blood from an alternative donor can be safely provided.

Despite significant efforts to maintain a very safe blood supply in the United States, transfusion is not without risks. Minor complications of transfusion include fever, nausea, or hives (allergic reaction). Rare complications include (1) transfusion of a different blood type, causing blood cells to break (hemolysis);

(2) patient intolerance of the fluid volume, causing heart failure; (3) difficulty breathing; and (4) severe infection.

Although blood transfusions can carry risks, when children must undergo major surgery such as spinal fusion, blood transfusion can be lifesaving.

Back Knee Gait
(knee hyperextension)

A back knee gait, in which the child's knee bends back when she steps on her foot, is usually due to a tight Achilles tendon and an overlengthened hamstring or weak hamstring muscles. Children with cerebral palsy and children with muscle weakness or severe hypotonia who do not have good control of their knees often have a back knee gait. The primary treatment of a back knee gait is to use an ankle-foot orthosis (AFO), which may be hinged to allow for the ankle to be lifted, but blocked so the knee cannot bend backward without lifting the toes off the ground. There is almost never a need to use a long leg brace for this condition. It does not harm children to walk short distances without their braces if they wear their braces the majority of the time. Another treatment for a back knee gait caused by very tight Achilles tendons is surgical lengthening of the Achilles tendon followed by the use of an AFO.

Indications: The indications for surgical treatment vary; generally, however, as long as the back kneeing can be controlled with an AFO, surgery is not indicated. If the Achilles tendon is tight and does not allow the ankle to

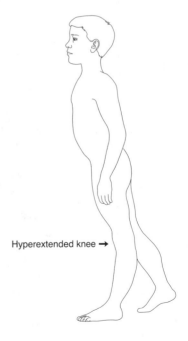

Hyperextended knee ➡

come to neutral or to be held in an AFO so that both the front and the back of the foot touch the ground, surgery should be performed to lengthen the tendon. For an adult, an attempt should be made to discontinue the AFO by lengthening the tendon. Care must be taken not to overlengthen the tendon, which may cause further instability while standing and more difficulty in walking.

A back knee gait can result in a gradual stretching of the knee structure. In young adults, severe back knee gait often becomes uncomfortable and can significantly limit the amount of walking that can be done. In rare cases, in children with significant weakness, a back knee gait is the only stable gait pattern; following surgical lengthening of the Achilles tendon, they may be unable to walk without braces.

Baclofen Pump
(intrathecal baclofen, ITB)

Spasticity is the most common motor disorder in those with cerebral palsy, seen in approximately two-thirds of cases. While some spasticity may be necessary for function in children with CP, it is often a problem that can be difficult to treat. Treatments include physical and occupational therapy, oral medications, Botox injections, orthopedic surgery, and neurosurgical procedures such as selective dorsal rhizotomy.

Baclofen is a muscle relaxant. When taken by mouth, it is not always helpful in treating spasticity in children with CP. However, when given to patients intrathecally, that is, injected into the spinal fluid, it works much more consistently and efficiently to reduce spasticity, with fewer side effects. The goals for treatment with intrathecal baclofen should be realistic and individualized, and they need to be agreed on by the patient, the family or caregiver, and the medical team. Ideally, a multidisciplinary team should be involved in the decision making.

Patients with dystonia have also responded to this treatment, often at higher doses. Patients with athetosis, ataxia, and myoclonus may also show improvement. ITB can help with spasticity-related pain during the day and at night.

A trial of baclofen by mouth is not a prerequisite for patients with spasticity and CP to receive the pump. When a patient is felt to be a potential candidate for ITB therapy, a screening trial may be scheduled. This involves a lumbar puncture and injection of an intrathecal baclofen test dose. Spasticity scores are recorded before the injection and at 2-hour intervals postinjection for up to 6–8 hours. If the trial dose is felt to have benefited the child, and if the parents agree, then placement of the pump is the next step. However, this test dosing is now done much less often, because the test dose is often

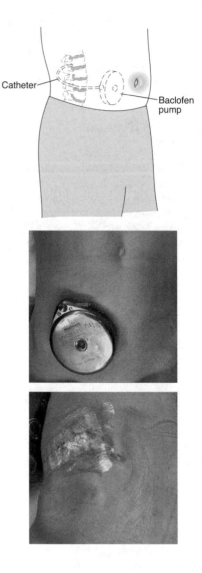

a poor predictor of how the child will respond to the pump after it is implanted, when doses can be adjusted in small increments until just the right dose is reached. Patients who have had a spinal fusion cannot undergo a trial, but they can have the pump implanted.

The ITB delivery system consists of a programmable subcutaneously implanted pump with a reservoir attached to an intraspinal catheter. The pump is inserted under general anesthesia. Postoperatively, the patient remains flat in bed for 48 hours.

The pump reservoir is refilled approximately every two to six months through a port located directly under the skin of the abdomen. Dosage adjustments are made via an external computer or programmer and transmitted to the pump by a handheld computer mouse. Doses can be programmed to deliver the baclofen in several ways. Examples include: the same dose all day long ("continuous"); the same dose all day long, with occasional extra boluses given when spasticity is highest ("intermittent bolus"); or continuous doses that vary throughout the day based on when spasticity is highest ("complex continuous").

Important issues to consider include:

- A history of seizures does not contraindicate intrathecal baclofen therapy.
- The presence of a ventriculoperitoneal shunt is not a contraindication. Patients with VP shunts may require a smaller dose of baclofen.
- The patient must be big enough and have enough room in his abdomen to accommodate the pump. We like to see the child weigh at least 35 pounds.
- The patient and family need to understand and accept the look of the pump. Typically the pump can be felt under the skin, although now it is inserted between the muscles of the abdomen and is much less visible. It is about the size and shape of a hockey puck.
- The entire team must agree on appropriate goals.
- The patient and family must be motivated to achieve these goals and be committed to the follow-up required to maintain the pump treatment.

Success of the intrathecal baclofen therapy seems to be related to appropriate patient selection, setting of achievable goals, patient and family motivation and compliance, and the help of a dedicated multidisciplinary team.

Behavior Modification

Behavior modification may best be described as a series of learning-based interventions aimed at developing wanted behavior or decreasing unwanted behavior. Behavior therapists typically evaluate a child's behavior within the context of where the behavior occurs. Therapists develop a "functional analysis" of the behavior to determine how the behavior "functions" in the environment. In one example, a child with cerebral palsy screamed frequently at home but not in the classroom. The therapist made observations in the home and found that the child typically screamed when the child's mother was busy cooking dinner. Mom would stop and reprimand the child and then return to her chores. The screaming would recur, and mom would reproach the child again. Here, it appeared that the absence of mom's attention during cooking chores resulted in the child's screaming, and mom may have been inadvertently "rewarding" this behavior with her attention. The therapist recommended paying increased attention to the child when mom was cooking to "reward" positive behavior and ignoring the screaming.

Typical strategies for increasing wanted behavior include the use of praise and attention and tangible rewards. These positives tend to increase the frequency of the desired behavior when they are delivered following the behavior. Typical strategies for decreasing unwanted behavior include the removal of reinforcement, like "time out" (e.g., removing the child from the work table for a minute for hitting or spitting) or providing a negative consequence. Negative consequences like spanking generally should be avoided because of such unintended consequences as fear, avoidance of the punisher, or modeling the very behavior that therapists would like to see decreased. Ignoring is another strategy for decreasing behavior. When behavior is not dangerous, ignoring can be a powerful way of helping behavior to decrease. However, with ignoring, behavior typically "gets worse before it gets better."

Indications: Behavioral strategies are clearly indicated to develop particular behaviors, such as appropriate toileting or social behavior. The use of rewards to shape the development of new skills is key. Likewise, behavior management is indicated to increase desirable behaviors such as saying please or cleaning up after playing or to reduce unwanted behaviors such as hitting or biting. When attempting to increase or decrease the target behavior in the child's natural environment, the child's behavior should be analyzed to discover what in the environment is maintaining the behavior. Changing whatever is maintaining the behavior should help to change the behavior. Examples of common behaviors often maintained by the environment are biting, tantrums, and acting out in class.

Benefits and risks: The use of organized, data-driven, reward-based programs can be of great benefit. Keeping records of the incidence of the target behavior and how it changes with intervention allows the parent or teacher to determine whether the program is working and to make changes if needed. Punishment-based programs, including behavioral programs that emphasize the removal of positives, should be used sparingly and monitored closely to prevent "negative side effects." When behavior management is applied to self-harm situations such as self-injurious behavior, it is important to work with an experienced therapist who is familiar with the use of behavior modification approaches for that behavioral issue. It is always important to reward small steps, progress toward a clear goal, and be flexible about changing a program that is not effective.

Maintenance and care: When beginning a behavior modification program, it is important to use a consistent approach across environments (e.g., home and school).

Reward often, reward immediately after the behavior occurs, and reward specifically (not "you were good"). As the behavior changes, begin to reward intermittently to maintain the behavior change. Always adapt the behavioral program to the child's developmental level. Find a way of rewarding parents and teachers for their good efforts as well.

Biofeedback Devices
(auditory feedback, augmented feedback, behavioral training helmet)

Biofeedback devices operate based on the theory that if a child is given feedback about an unwanted position or behavior and then rewarded for changing it, the child will learn to use the more normal behavior. Biofeedback has been used in an attempt to control drooling, to encourage head control, to improve sitting posture, and to decrease toe walking. Many behavior modification techniques use devices with electric switches. For example, a helmet is fitted with a level so that when the child allows his head to drop, a switch activates and turns off his television set. When the child holds his head up straight, the television set turns on again.

Similar types of devices have been developed for many other functions. For example, another biofeedback device is the small bib or cup held under the chin. When a child drools and wets the cloth, an electric switch is tripped and the child's television set is turned off. Therefore, if he does not control his drooling, he is unable to watch TV. In still another example, a small switch may be inserted in the heel of an ankle brace and operated in such a way that if the child steps on her toe but does not step on her heel at the same time, a loud noise will be generated. In this way a child can be trained to walk with her foot flat so as not to activate the negative reinforcing noise.

Indications: At this time, there are no established clinical indications for the use of biofeedback devices, although many people continue to explore their use, especially in research environments. They have been evaluated predominantly for control of drooling, for head control, and for attempts at improving gait.

Benefits and risks: The main benefit of biofeedback devices such as the helmet, the drooling cup, or the ankle switch is that they can change behaviors without the use of medications. The major risk is that the desired behavior may not continue after the device is removed. This may establish a false hope in parents and other caregivers that a certain activity can be learned, when in fact the child may never be able to make it automatic. In a sense, this situation is similar to that of the person who can sit erect with good posture when he is reminded to "sit up straight" but slouches as soon as he relaxes and stops concentrating on maintaining the correct position.

Maintenance and care: Most biofeedback devices are electrical and therefore require ongoing maintenance. Some of these devices may be difficult to maintain, such as the drooling-control devices, which require wetting a cloth to make an electrical connection. Since most of these devices are used in a research environment, the person fitting the device is usually quite familiar with their maintenance. If devices are purchased from a commercial vendor, it should be clear who will provide the service and maintenance needed in addition to the normal cleaning the caregiver would provide.

Bone Densitometry
(DXA)

The mineral content of the bones can be measured by using a low dose x-ray called dual energy x-ray absorptiometry, or DXA. Low bone mineral content increases the risk of fracture (broken bones).

In bone densitometry, the whole body or a part of it (leg, hip, spine) is scanned with the x-ray while the patient lies on a table. The time needed for the study

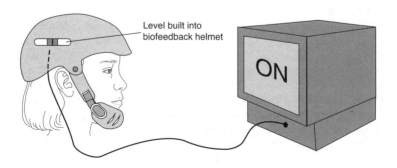

Level built into
biofeedback helmet

ON

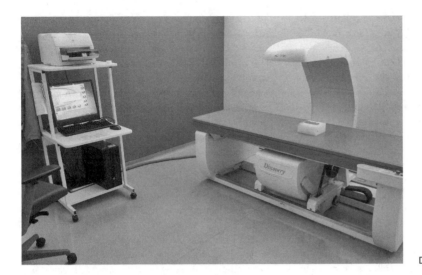

DEXA table

varies from 30 seconds to five minutes, depending on the scanner used and what body part is scanned. Movement during the scan affects the result. Nothing touches the patient, and the table is padded.

Indications: Children with CP are frequently found to have low bone mineral density, especially when they are non-ambulatory and/or have difficulty getting a nutritious diet. In many, minimal trauma results in fractures (broken bones). A bone densitometry study may be done if a child has had one or more fractures or if it is suspected that the child is at risk for low bone density based on his or her clinical condition.

Benefits and risks: Once one knows one has low bone density, it can be treated with nutritional supplements and/or medication. Treatment that raises bone mineral density may reduce the number of fractures or prevent fractures. The only risk of the test is minimal radiation exposure from the x-ray, which is not considered significant. If the child needs sedation to hold still for the study, then that adds the risk associated with sedation, and the child will need monitoring while sedated.

Botulinum Toxin Injections
(Botox, Myobloc)

Botulinum toxin is a drug that may be injected into the muscle to weaken or temporarily partially paralyze very spastic muscles. There are two commercially available types: Botox (botulinum toxin A) and Myobloc (botulinum toxin B). The drug is injected through a very small needle and causes little pain. Unlike alcohol and phenol injections, both now uncommonly used, botulinum

toxin injections do not cause scarring. Botulinum toxin lasts four to six months and can be given multiple times. It can be given in up to four to six involved muscles at a time, with the total medication given limited by the body weight of the patient. It does not seem to prevent contractures but may delay their development.

Indications: The main indication for botulinum toxin is spasticity. Injections are most commonly given in the hip adductor, hamstring, and gastrocnemius muscles. In the upper extremity, the biceps, pronator, wrist and finger flexors, and thumb adductor are also commonly injected. An excellent indication is a circumstance in which the underlying spasticity is expected to improve significantly or there is concern about the impact of permanent weakness. In a situation in which a child is improving, such as after an acute head injury or near drowning, injection of botulinum toxin provides a six-month window to see how much recovery and natural diminishing occurs in the spasticity. However, spasticity in the child with cerebral palsy does not change significantly, and it is almost certain that six months after the injection the problem will be the same as before. In these children, injections are used primarily to delay surgery or to make therapy more effective and achieve some short-term goals.

Another indication is *dystonia*, which is a movement disorder often affecting one or two muscle groups. Dystonia may cause very severe contractures of one muscle or muscle group for a short period of time and then switch and cause the opposite deformity. For this reason, surgical lengthening may be performed, but it is more unpredictable. Using botulinum toxin decreases the high risk of the opposite deformity occurring.

Another use of botulinum toxin for children with CP is as a treatment for drooling. A single injection of botulinum toxin into the submandibular glands has been effective in reducing drooling, with the maximum effect occurring from three to six months after the injection.

Benefits and risks: The main benefit of botulinum toxin injection is that it allows the physician time to observe how much natural recovery of spasticity is taking place.

The risks of botulinum toxin injections are rare but can be severe. The most frequent is temporary muscle weakness for up to 24–48 hours and mild fever. Acetaminophen (Tylenol) can be given to relieve any discomfort. Rarely, temporary excessive localized muscle weakness and temporary generalized weakness, including difficulty breathing and loss of bladder and bowel function, have been reported. In the United States, botulinum toxin is not approved for use in children. A special black box warning states that children with cerebral palsy are at higher risk for complications, including death. Allergic reaction is extremely uncommon. In addition, it is not uncommon for patients to eventually develop a tolerance to botulinum toxin, requiring an increase in dosage or making the drug ineffective. This is occasionally due to true antibody formation against the drug.

Although botulinum toxin injections have clearly shown a reduction in spasticity of the injected muscle three months after the injection, there is no evidence of long-term gain from the injections, since the benefit tends to be lost by six months and repeated injections are usually less effective. New studies show increased muscle scarring (fibrosis) that continues for a number of years. This has raised the concern that there may in fact be long-term negative effects from muscles' becoming more scarred and stiff. Therefore the risk-benefit balance, especially for long-term effects, has changed due to these concerns in the last several years. There seems to be no evidence of long-term benefit but more evidence of long-term negative effects.

Maintenance and care: After botulinum toxin injections, normal activity may resume immediately. If the injections are performed for contractures such as of the hip or ankle, it is important to continue splinting and stretching to maintain the correction for as long as possible. Usually these injections will need to be repeated in four to eight months if the gain is to be maintained.

Brace, Ankle
(ankle-foot orthosis, AFO, MAFO, DAFO)

Ankle braces are the most common type of brace used in children with cerebral palsy. The brace begins just below the knee, crosses the ankle, and includes the foot. Although some physicians may still prescribe a leather shoe attached to a metal upright, most up-to-date ankle-foot orthoses (AFOs) are made of a lightweight, high-density plastic and are custom molded (MAFO) to the patient's foot and ankle. More recently, a wraparound style of ankle-foot orthosis with "tone reducing" features molded into the foot plate (DAFO, Cascade, Inc.) has been very popular. Most braces fit well inside a sneaker or shoe, although a larger size is usually required to accommodate the brace. Removable inlays helps sneakers accommodate the AFO.

Indications: The most common indication for this type of brace is a child who toe walks or back knees due to a tight gastrocnemius muscle or Achilles tendon. The muscle or tendon cannot be so tight, however, that the foot cannot be positioned into the brace without causing excess pressure. This means that a child who has a fixed ankle deformity that is unable to be ranged into a neutral ankle position cannot use an AFO. Varus or valgus foot deformities may require a MAFO if the foot cannot be controlled with a shorter brace. Occasionally, the child with a crouched gait may require a MAFO to keep the ankle from collapsing into a dorsiflexed position.

There are many types of MAFOs, some of which are described here.

1. Solid ankle MAFO. This brace is fixed at the ankle and gives maximum ankle support. It is best for the young child who is just beginning to walk and requires ankle stability for balance or for the severely involved child (quadriplegic) with poor ankle control or severe foot and ankle deformity. There is typically a strap around the ankle and one just below the knee.

2. Articulated MAFO. This brace has an ankle hinge and typically allows dorsiflexion but stops at 90 degrees to prevent toe walking. It is best for the child who is ambulatory and able to voluntarily dorsiflex the ankle. A child who crouches at the knee should not use it. Due to the extra bulkiness of the hinge, it may be more difficult to fit into a shoe.

3. Plantar flexion block MAFO. The indication is very similar to that for an articulated MAFO. However, movement does not occur at a hinge. Instead, it allows the ankle to dorsiflex forward out of the brace, because there is no strap below the knee holding the leg in the brace. Plantar flexion is blocked at 90 degrees. This MAFO is best for the child who cannot tolerate a hinge due to rubbing or the child who requires maximum control to correct a severe varus or valgus foot deformity.

4. Ground reaction MAFO. The indication for this brace is the child with a severe crouch. The foot slides into the brace from behind. With each step the child

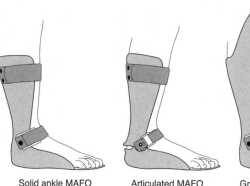

Solid ankle MAFO   Articulated MAFO   Ground reaction MAFO

takes, forces are generated up to the front of the lower leg just below the knee to help push the knee into extension.

5. Leaf spring or plantar flexion resist MAFO. This brace is best used by the child without significant contractures who has mild toe walking due to spasticity of the gastrocnemius muscle. It resists plantar flexion but will allow for some pushing off at the ankle. It also helps to spring the foot back up into dorsiflexion. This is especially important for children with weak dorsiflexion due to tibialis anterior muscle weakness. These patients have a foot drop when their heel strikes the ground during walking.

Benefits and risks: A MAFO gives the ambulatory child a more stable base of support to walk on by controlling the foot and ankle deformity while the brace is on. In the nonambulatory child, the brace can provide stability in a stander or gait trainer. It also helps to delay fixed muscle contractures. There is a risk that with a more rigid deformity, the brace may cause pressure sores. Also the more rigid the brace as it crosses the ankle, the less exercise the gastrocnemius muscle gets. An increasing concern for long-term and full-time brace wear is weakening of the muscle. To stimulate muscle strength development, attempts should be made to encourage the child to spend some time walking without the brace.

Maintenance and care: Most of these braces are made of high-density plastic. They will occasionally break if the brace is used to correct too rigid a deformity. In general, a growing child requires a new brace approximately every 12 months. Pressure areas may develop during rapid growth spurts, requiring adjustment of the brace. The brace should be checked every 6 months for the need for adjustments. The parent should check the child daily for pressure areas.

Brace, Back
(thoracolumbosacral orthosis [TLSO] spinal brace, body jacket, scoliosis brace, Boston brace, Milwaukee brace, Wilmington brace)

Back braces are used to help straighten a child who is having trouble sitting up and, in some cases, to straighten the spine, which may be developing a deformity or already have one. The correct medical designation for back braces that extends from the top of the chest down across the pelvis is TLSO. If there is an extension including the neck, or cervical area, the proper designation is CTLSO, for "cervical thoracolumbosacral orthosis." These are very unusual and are rarely prescribed for children with cerebral palsy. *Spinal braces*, *body jackets*, and *scoliosis braces* are general and older terms for these braces. There are many different designs for them.

The majority of current braces are made of molded plastic and open in the front or back. Some have a separate front and back that are held together with velcro straps. Design variations in different geographical areas have led to names such as the Boston brace, the Milwaukee brace, and the Wilmington brace. The Boston brace is a factory-made brace modified by orthotists. The standard off-the-shelf plastic brace is not particularly useful for children with cerebral palsy, since they are very difficult to fit. The Milwaukee brace is an older design that was used for bracing scoliosis. It is made with a plastic mold around the pelvis, metal uprights and pads pushing against parts of the trunk, and a circular extension around the neck. This brace is seldom used today and rarely has a place in the care of children with cerebral palsy.

There are many local braces such as the Wilmington brace, which are made with minor design changes by a local orthotist. Most of these require a cast to be made of the child's body. The cast is filled to make a mold, over which the brace is then made. Most of these custom-molded braces fit much better. They may be made of very soft plastic, which helps reduce skin irritation, or they may be made out of a more rigid, thinner plastic that can be concealed under clothing. The process of molding and brace construction generally takes at least 24 to 36 hours.

Indications: Although there is no consensus among physicians about the benefits of back braces for children with cerebral palsy, there are two primary indications for ordering a brace. The first is for a child who has difficulty controlling his body, so that when he is sitting he collapses either sideways or forward. The brace may thus be ordered for children for postural control. In this way it is used in place of a custom-designed and tightly fitted wheelchair insert, which serves the same function.

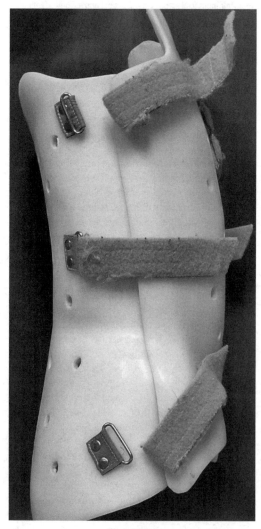

Body jacket

Using spinal braces for children with CP to maintain postural control, provide better head control, and provide better use of the arms is one option; using an adequately designed wheelchair is another. The benefits of the brace are a close fit to the body and concealment under clothing. Additionally, when the child is moved from one chair to another the brace goes along with the child. Clothes such as winter coats can be placed over the top of the brace. The advantage of wheelchair supports is easy application to the child. However, because a wheelchair is tightly fitted when the child is wearing regular clothes, it will not fit when the child wears a heavy winter coat. Also, a modified wheelchair is only useful when the child is sitting in the chair.

The second use of a back brace—in our view a misguided use—is to treat spinal deformities, such as scoliosis. These braces were initially designed for children with idiopathic adolescent scoliosis, a condition in which a normal preadolescent or adolescent girl develops a spinal curvature. This type of scoliosis is entirely different from the scoliosis that occurs in children with cerebral palsy. There continues to be controversy concerning how effective these braces are in the control of scoliosis in children with idiopathic scoliosis, but there is almost no controversy about their lack of effectiveness in children with CP. Braces have no significant effect on the development or progression of scoliosis in children with cerebral palsy. There is a general, but not universal, consensus that the use of any kind of spinal brace in the treatment of scoliosis provides no impact on its eventual outcome in the child with cerebral palsy. Likewise, treating kyphosis is generally not felt to have any long-term impact.

Benefits and risks: The primary benefit of a well-fitted brace is that it provides better postural and head control and is less cumbersome and noticeable than a wheelchair. The primary risk is that a brace that is not fitted adequately causes skin irritation leading to blisters and subsequent skin sores. The skin needs to be checked every day; whenever pressure areas are found, the brace should be modified.

Many of the children who need these braces for postural control either have feeding problems or have difficulty coughing. The use of these restrictive braces further restricts their lung function and may put them at higher risk for developing repeated pneumonia because they are unable to clear their lungs when they develop minor viral infections. The chest wall in a growing child is flexible; tight braces can deform the chest wall, causing protruding ribs or flattening of the chest. Likewise, the application of a tight, constricting abdominal brace may increase nutritional problems, such as GE reflux, poor stomach emptying, or constipation. Generally, because of these complications, which are most likely to occur in children who need the postural support, the adequately fitted wheelchair is a better option.

When a brace is needed for postural control, a brace made of a soft foamlike material is more comfortable and less likely to cause complications than the more rigid plastic brace.

Maintenance and care: At first, these braces should be used for short periods—at most, several hours during the day, while the child is closely monitored for skin irritation. Areas of pressure underneath the brace may be toughened by being cleaned with alcohol after the braces are removed. There is no need for a child with CP to use the brace at night. It will only increase pulmonary and abdominal constriction and will not benefit the child in any way, since lying in bed does not require any postural control.

If the brace is made of a low-temperature plastic, it must be carefully protected from direct sunlight and must not be left in a car in hot weather, because the brace may melt. It should not be cleaned with harsh detergents, since they may also damage the plastic. Usually, a T-shirt or an undergarment needs to be worn underneath the brace so the plastic does not directly touch the child's skin.

Brace, Foot
(heel cup, UCB orthotic, arch support, SMO)

Foot braces and special shoe inserts cover part of the foot up to the ankle or slightly above the ankle. Foot braces, heel cups, and arch supports are smaller than the ankle-foot orthosis (AFO), which extends from the toes to just below the knee. These braces, called supramalleolar orthoses (SMOs), are at the highest just above the anklebone. They vary greatly, including those that are custom molded from casts, and range from the AFO to the simple arch supports that may be sold over the counter (such as Dr. Scholl's arch supports).

Heel cups are manufactured by a number of companies as off-the-shelf products. They are made of either hard or soft materials that cover the heel. They are meant to help control the tilt of the heel and to keep it flat inside a shoe. Generally, they are quite inexpensive and don't provide much support.

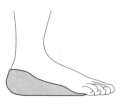

There are many different kinds of arch supports. They range from those made from casts, costing from $700 to $800, to those that may be purchased off the shelf for $5 to $10. These are constructed of leather, plastic, or metal.

A special type of orthotic that has received a lot of publicity is the University of California at Berkeley (UCB) orthotic, a foot orthosis made from a cast. A close mold of the heel is made and then extended forward to the base of the toes or under the toes. In some circumstances, this brace is brought up over the anklebone to help provide further stability for the heel so it doesn't twist. Because the UCB orthotic is very tightly molded, it is supposed to correct rotation of the heel and is usually used to improve flat feet. A number of proponents of the UCB orthotic recommend that various pressure points be molded into the braces to decrease spasticity. Although there may be regional advocates of these special braces, there is very little scientific evidence that any one of these special orthotics has a significant advantage over the others.

Indications: There is no recognized standard of care or application for shoe inserts. Often an individual practitioner or geographical area may seem to favor a particular brace, while the preference of a neighboring practitioner or community may be entirely different. Heel cups are usually utilized for people with painful heels in an attempt to stabilize the heel fat pad; they are often made of soft material to provide extra cushioning.

Some practitioners prescribe heel cups to improve flat feet, but in general arch supports are used. Arch supports are frequently prescribed for knee pain in runners. This is not relevant to the CP patient, and certainly no arch support will reduce knee pain in the child with cerebral palsy. The UCB type of orthotic, with its multiple variations, is the foot orthosis most commonly prescribed to treat flat feet in children with cerebral palsy. It is probably the second most popular brace after the full-length AFO, which provides much better support.

The specific indications for foot braces are diverse, and none of them have well-documented scientific support. Certainly, in normal children the use of arch supports or any shoe inserts has been shown to make absolutely no difference in long-term outcome, since the foot tends to progress along whatever course the child's genetic predisposition has determined. In children with cerebral palsy, it is not certain whether arch supports make any long-term difference, and there is currently no scientific evidence to suggest that they do. However, there is no good evidence to suggest that they don't make a difference. The natural history of flat feet varies in children with cerebral palsy; for this reason, the main indication for shoe orthotics ought to be those that make the patient's feet feel more comfortable and improve the patient's ability to walk. If shoe inserts or braces detract from either of these daily necessities, then there is very little indication for continuing their use.

Benefits and risks: The immediate benefit is comfort to the wearer. The main risk is pain and discomfort, especially if the insert or brace is incorrectly fitted. This is particularly true of tightly molded braces that try to make a lot of correction in the flat foot. Frequently the foot looks nice in the brace, but the child complains that his feet hurt when he walks. Because of the uncertain benefit of these braces, any brace that causes the child pain or diminishes his ability to walk should promptly be removed or at least modified in an attempt to alleviate the discomfort.

There is never a good reason to use a brace or shoe insert that rubs the foot, causing blisters or breakdown of the skin. If these skin breakdowns are ignored, they may become infected, leading to long-term periods of "feet up" rest. Obviously, the inability to walk is very detrimental to a child's continued progress in gaining mobility.

Maintenance and care: When new shoe inserts are obtained, the child should get used to them gradually, wearing them for only one to two hours at a time at first. As they become more comfortable, as long as they are not causing any blisters, they may be worn for longer periods of time, comparable to a normal day's "shoe wear." The care of the brace depends on the material it is made of. Braces made of leather should be kept as dry as possible, and plastic braces, depending on the material, need to be protected from high temperatures.

Brace, Hip
(hip-knee-ankle-foot orthosis [HKAFO], pelvic band, hip brace, hip abduction brace, A-frame brace, abduction pillow)

There is a whole family of braces that extend across the hip joint from the pelvis to the thigh, across the knee, and attach to a foot brace. The designation hip-knee-ankle-foot orthosis, or HKAFO, covers all of these areas. Older terms include *long leg brace with a pelvic band* and *pelvic control brace.*

The typical long leg brace with a pelvic band is constructed with metal uprights that are attached to shoes. There is a metal joint at the knee. The uprights extend again to the thigh cuff and then cross the hip on the outside, having a hinge at the area of the hip joint. This metal upright bar is attached to a metal, leather-covered band that goes around the pelvis. This typical long leg brace with a pelvic band was used extensively during the polio era of the 1920s to 1950s. Many older people who had polio continue to use these braces.

Other types of hip braces sometimes used for children with cerebral palsy include twister cables. The cables, made of a type of flexible material (usually plastic or flexible metal), attach to a an AFO brace below the knee. There are also braces that are constructed to prevent the legs from crossing. Frequently these hip abduction braces do not extend below the knee; they may have hip hinges or may be rigid, simply holding the legs apart. The standard brace has a metal band around the hip that extends to metal braces along the outside and thigh cuffs just above the knee.

Some braces are constructed to fit on the inside of the legs, where they push the knees apart. Often these have the appearance of A-frames. They may extend below the knee and usually do not have hinges at the knee. This type of A-frame brace is usually constructed of a soft material and has the appearance of a pillow with velcro straps; the straps hold the knees against the side of the "pillow."

Indications: There are a number of indications for the use of braces across the hip joints. One of the indications is to improve a child's ability to walk or to allow a child to walk. For children with cerebral palsy, the use of braces above the knee is seldom helpful. Most of these long leg braces with pelvic bands or the standard HKAFO are used today for children with spinal cord dysfunction (such as spina bifida, meningomyelocele, or spinal cord injuries). These children have normal upper body strength, motor coordination, and balance; when their lower legs are controlled, they are able to walk by using crutches.

Children with this degree of cerebral palsy in their lower extremities almost never have enough upper extremity strength, muscle coordination, or balance to be able to profit from this much bracing. It usually only weighs the child down, making him look good while standing and taking a few steps but blocking him from functional walking. These braces may also be used to control feet that turn in, and frequently a lighter version or a twister cable brace as described above may be prescribed for this purpose. These twister cable braces frequently make the child look better standing but in no way improve his function. They usually greatly diminish how far and how fast he can walk and may injure the knee joints. The use of these long braces is seldom recommended for children with cerebral palsy.

Another indication for these braces is to prevent the adductor muscles from becoming tighter. These muscles, in the inner thigh, make the legs cross over each other. Because this process causes the hips to dislocate, there has been some sense in the past that using braces to keep the knees apart might help prevent this dislocation or keep the muscles from becoming tighter. Cur-

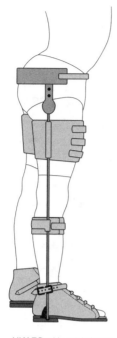

HKAFO with pelvic band

Abduction brace

rent guidelines, however, are not to use hip abduction bracing in any child with cerebral palsy unless muscle surgery has been done to release the tight muscle first. There is some indication that bracing against very tight muscles only injures the hip joint further, which may cause abnormal growth in the hip joint or cause it to dislocate more quickly than if no bracing were used.

Opinion continues to be divided with respect to the use of braces following hip muscle surgery. There is some evidence that diligent use of night braces to keep the hips apart may help the hips develop more normally or at least avoid dislocation. If this is done, however, the opposite deformity may occur: the hip may become stuck in the outward direction, which is even more disabling for sitting. The consensus seems to be that there is little indication for long-term rigid bracing for hips after muscle releases. The efficacy of short-term bracing is also debatable, although maintaining the child in a good position during sleep and sitting is important, and hip braces are one means of achieving this goal.

Finally, the use of hip abduction braces, A-frame braces, or abduction pillows to treat the problems of hip subluxation or tight adductor muscles after muscle surgery continues to vary greatly. It is a fairly well established opinion among physicians treating patients with CP that bracing before muscle release surgery has no efficacy and is probably more detrimental than effective.

Benefits and risks: The benefits and risks of using abduction braces, pillows, and A-frames for the child with spastic hip subluxation are uncertain, and there is no agreed-upon community standard of practice. Generally, the trend is that the risks and complications in bracing outweigh their benefits.

The primary complication of the use of bracing to improve gait is that it diminishes the ability of the child to walk by decreasing speed and distance at the expense of better cosmetic appearance. Any brace that is attached to a pelvic band makes sitting more difficult. It is also cumbersome to constantly apply and remove these braces; consequently, it is not practical for a child to wear such a brace constantly if she is sitting for long periods of time. Nor is it practical to apply the brace every time she wants to get up and walk.

The complication of using hip abduction braces to improve hip subluxation or treat tight muscles can be dislocation of the hip if braces are used before muscle release surgery. If an abduction brace is used after muscle release surgery, it may create a deformity called the *windblown deformity*, in which one hip abducts, or becomes more "stuck away from" the midline of the body, while the other hip tends to drift in toward the midline. This deformity tends to make sitting and standing very difficult. Also, children who have very tight muscles or who are becoming more contracted are frequently very uncomfortable in these braces and find them almost impossible to sit in. Many of these braces also are stuck in hip flexion (legs drawn up) either because the hinge is fixed in flexion or because there is no hinge, which may contribute to the development of hip flexion contracture.

Occasionally, the very young child (less than 6 years old) with low muscle tone (hypotonia) and a hip subluxation will benefit from a hip abduction brace. The hip should be less than 50 percent subluxated, and the brace should be worn at night time to maintain hip stability until the child's acetabulum develops and his hypotonia improves. The child's hips require close observation and may require surgery when the child is older.

Maintenance and care: The majority of hip braces are made of metal and plastic. The plastic may be cleaned with a gentle detergent, but it is important to keep it out of high temperatures, such as in direct sunlight. Braces made of leather or with leather components should be kept dry, and the leather should be cleaned with a leather-cleaning agent. Most of these braces have joints that should be lubricated with a small amount of lubricant such as WD-40 or the lubricant recommended by the orthotist. As children grow, these braces need to be adjusted. They should be seen by a physician or an orthotist at least every six months to check on their fit. Parents should check the skin daily when the brace is removed for any red areas or skin breakdown. If skin breakdown is noted, they should check for wrinkles in the stockings underlying the brace; if the same area is persistently red, the brace needs to be evaluated by the physician or orthotist.

Brace, Leg
(knee-ankle-foot orthosis [KAFO], long leg brace, twister cable, circular wrap, knee brace)

A knee-ankle-foot orthosis (KAFO) is any brace that starts just below the hip and extends to the ankle, crossing the knee joint. There are a number of variations. A very common older brace has a metal hinge that often has a drop lock at the knee to prevent the knee from bending. When the patient wants to sit down, she can pull the drop lock up, which allows the knee to bend. This device may be called a drop lock, a double upright, or a long leg brace—which is its older name. Yet another leg brace is a twister cable, which has cables attached to a short leg brace but extends above the knee and often above the hip. A circular wrap is a soft device that is wrapped around the leg and tied above the hip to control rotation about the hip.

Indications: These braces are rarely used for children with cerebral palsy. Most children with CP who have trouble controlling their knees also have much difficulty with balance and motor coordination. The addition of long

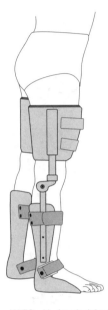

KAFO with drop-lock knee

braces may make these children look better standing or walking, but in fact the braces make them walk more slowly because they have a great deal of difficulty handling the extra weight of the braces.

The metal knee hinge brace is primarily for children with spinal cord dysfunction such as meningomyelocele, spina bifida, or a spinal cord injury. These children have excellent upper body strength and have no control or very little control of their legs. Using the brace to control their legs often allows them to walk because of the rigid support, but they often have a decrease in their function because of increased energy needed to handle the braces. Additionally, there is no long-term benefit.

A long leg brace, often a knee immobilizer, is often used temporarily after surgery. During the period after surgery, patients often have difficulty developing control of their muscles. These temporary braces may be used to help patients learn to control their muscles. These braces should only be used for one to two months at most, however, and should *not* become permanent means of locking the knees.

Benefits and risks: Although these long leg braces have clear benefits and indications for selected patients, as mentioned above, invariably for children with CP the risks created by the braces are far greater than any benefits they bring. The primary risk in using KAFOs for children with cerebral palsy is typically a decreased functional ability to walk. These braces generally create an improved cosmetic appearance while the child is standing, but at the expense of a greatly diminished functional ability. Children who have a great deal of difficulty walking only short distances with walkers usually cannot walk any farther when they are encumbered with long leg braces. Additionally, they have difficulty sitting, because these long leg braces are usually rigid under the thigh. If they are not properly fitted, they may cause skin irritation as well.

Using braces such as twister cables or wraps for rotational control can also lead to the possible complication of twisted stress through the knee joint, which may become painful. Certainly, the joints are much more susceptible to overstretching than the bones, and a child usually complains of pain when too much rotational stress is applied.

Maintenance and care: Some leg braces are constructed with a plastic AFO foot section, although some of them are attached to rigid orthopedic-type shoes at the foot. In some newer models, the metal uprights and metal hinges at the knee have been replaced with plastic uprights and hinges attached to either leather or plastic cuffs at the thigh. Care must be taken to ensure that the braces continue to fit a growing child—they should be checked every six months by the physician or therapist. After the brace is removed, the skin needs to be checked daily for pressure areas or blisters. Hinges should be kept dry.

Bronchopulmonary Dysplasia
(BPD, chronic lung disease [CLD])

BPD is a chronic lung disease seen primarily in premature babies who require ventilator support and oxygen therapy after they are born. (Many children who have cerebral palsy were premature.) Occasionally a baby who never required ventilation will develop chronic lung disease as well. In general, the lower the birthweight and the gestational age of an infant, the higher the incidence and severity of BPD. In premature and low birthweight infants, hyaline membrane disease (respiratory distress syndrome) is almost always present before they develop this condition. It is possible, however, for term infants to develop a BPD-like illness or chronic lung disease after neonatal pneumonia, meconium aspiration, or another severe illness in the neonatal period.

The specific criteria for the diagnosis of BPD are subject to opinion and debate. However, BPD is considered in an infant who was treated during the first two weeks of life with mechanical ventilation, continuous positive airway pressure (CPAP), or oxygen and who continues to have respiratory difficulty at the age of 28 days after birth or at 36 weeks postconceptional age. Respiratory difficulties include at least the need for supplemental oxygen therapy (some infants with severe BPD may require even more respiratory support) and symp-

toms such as requiring increased work to breathe. Chest x-rays will show characteristic changes, including cystic changes in the lungs, and in some cases the lungs will generally appear cloudy instead of clear.

In some children with BPD the lungs develop areas of fibrosis, or scarrin atelectasis, areas of the lung that do not fill with air; and small cysts, not unlike emphysema in an older person. In other children with BPD, the lungs remain underdeveloped and lung growth is not normal, but scarring and other changes are less prominent. In severe cases of BPD, oxygenation and ventilation are more severely impaired and increased pulmonary fluid may be present. Infants with BPD may be discharged home from the nursery with oxygen, monitors, and other technological supports. In infants with BPD, growth and nutrition are extremely important to promote lung healing and the growth of new lung tissue, which occurs most dramatically during the first two years of life.

As new lung tissue grows, BPD symptoms improve. However, infants and young children with BPD remain susceptible to respiratory viral infections, particularly RSV (respiratory syncytial virus), and readmission to the hospital for pneumonia, respiratory distress, or other problems during the first two years of life is not uncommon. It is important that the appropriate vaccinations and other strategies to protect against infection be maintained. Other challenges that may require medical intervention include the development of asthma symptoms, including chronic coughing and wheezing, and feeding difficulties, including aspiration, oral aversion, gastroesophageal reflux, or failure to thrive.

Bronchoscopy

Bronchoscopy is a procedure in which a physician places a flexible or rigid telescope into the back of the throat and down the airway, allowing him or her to look into the airway and assess whether it is inflamed or floppy or has any other problems that are causing difficulty in breathing. The test is generally done under heavy sedation or under general anesthesia and can be performed on an outpatient basis.

Indications: Children who have difficulty breathing and possibly have some anatomical obstruction in the trachea or bronchi must have this area directly visualized with the bronchoscope. Children who may have breathed in a foreign object that cannot be dislodged must also have a bronchoscopy. Occasionally, a child may develop fixed secretions and form a plug in one of the large airways in the lung; the bronchoscope can be used to go into the plugged tube and remove the obstruction. Bronchoscopies are performed by physicians with special training in this technique. They are pedia-

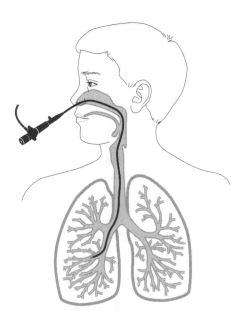

tricians specializing in pulmonary diseases or are ear, nose, and throat (ENT) surgeons.

Benefits and risks: Bronchoscopy allows the direct visualization of the airways, so that anatomical problems such as obstructions or collapses of the airways can be directly seen. Sometimes scar tissue has formed from having an endotracheal tube in the trachea for long periods of time. Scar tissue can also be directly visualized through the bronchoscope. With rigid bronchoscopy, there is a small risk of dental injury. Rarely, swelling from manipulating the airways can cause a crouplike picture. The major risk of this procedure is that it requires significant sedation and is occasionally done under general anesthesia. The airways must be carefully maintained because the child must continue to breathe during this whole procedure. In general, when this procedure is performed by physicians who are trained in its use, the risks are very small.

Care after the bronchoscopy usually centers on the child's recovery from the anesthesia or sedation. If there is a risk of postoperative airway swelling, steroids may be used, along with close monitoring to make sure that breathing continues without difficulty. The procedure may be repeated, especially if it was performed for removal of obstructions such as thick secretions.

Bunions
(hallux valgus, cocked-up great toe, flexed great toe, great toe arthritis)

A bunion is a prominence that develops on the inside of the foot where the big toe joins the foot. Children with spastic cerebral palsy often develop bunions, especially

if they have flat feet and tend to walk on the inside of the foot. A bunion may become sore as it rubs against the side of the child's shoe. It is usually associated with a toe that has slipped over or started bending toward the inside of the foot, often overlapping or underlapping the second toe. This deformity is called *hallux valgus*. It may also be associated with a cocked-up great toe that becomes stiff and painful. The big toe may also become flexed down and curl inside the foot.

In all of these deformities, as the toe gets stuck, arthritis develops in the great toe joint. Not only can the arthritis cause a significant amount of pain, but the deformity makes wearing shoes problematic. These deformities also occur in patients without cerebral palsy, but it is important to note that the treatment differs significantly when no spasticity is present. Treatment in patients without CP often involves attempts at rebalancing muscles and correcting the alignment of the toe, but this approach almost always fails in the patient with spasticity. The natural history of these deformities in children with spastic feet who are more than 7 years old is that they gradually get worse and continue to become more problematic. Some young children around 2 or 3 years old develop severe bunions and flat feet, but as the child grows, both the flat foot and the bunion improve.

Indications: The child should be treated if there is pain with shoe wear or with activity. If the primary problem is irritation from the shoe, initially some modification of the shoe may be attempted. If this is not successful, a surgical correction is indicated. The surgical correction performed for almost all of these types of deformities is a fusion of the joint between the great toe and the metatarsal, called a great toe metatarsal phalangeal joint fusion. Often it is fixed with one or two pins or screws after the joint cartilage is removed, which places the toe in a good position. The correction lasts a lifetime and eliminates pain.

Benefits and risks: The benefits are relief of pain and the ability to wear shoes comfortably. The main complications

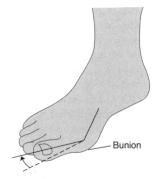

Bunion

of this surgery are the possibility that the bones will not fuse properly or difficulty with healing. Although non-fusion is rare, it requires a second procedure, because pain usually persists if the bones do not heal together. Following a fusion of this nature, the child is placed in a cast that covers the lower leg from his toes to just below the knee; the cast is worn for six to eight weeks. If a pin is used and is left sticking out of the joint, it is usually removed at the time the cast is removed. Usually no bracing or therapy is needed after this procedure.

CPAP; BiPAP

(continuous positive airway pressure; bilevel positive airway pressure)

When a person breathes in, the respiratory muscles create a negative (below atmospheric) pressure in the chest cavity, causing air to flow into the lungs. Exhaling (breathing out) is normally a passive process that does not require any muscular force.

Although normal breathing depends on the development of negative pressure, occasionally it becomes necessary to apply positive pressure to the respiratory system (the airways and lungs) to assist breathing. For example, this can be needed during surgery, acute illnesses in which breathing becomes ineffective (respiratory failure), or if the airway is obstructed, as occurs in obstructive sleep apnea. Positive pressure can be applied to the respiratory system via a tightly fitting face mask in what is called noninvasive ventilation or via a breathing tube in the airway (either an endotracheal tube or tracheostomy tube) in what is called invasive ventilation.

Positive pressure respiratory support is a form of respiratory assistance that is used when the pressure of air entering a person's lungs needs to be higher than normal atmospheric pressure. Positive pressure respiratory support should be used in the case of unacceptably low levels of blood oxygen, unacceptably high levels of blood carbon dioxide, or unacceptably high levels of respiratory distress. With positive pressure respiratory support, air is pushed into the lungs by a machine rather than, or in addition to, being pulled in by the respiratory muscles. There are a variety of strategies to facilitate this process, but two are described here: CPAP and BiPAP.

Definitions and indications: CPAP, continuous positive airway pressure, can be administered either invasively or non-invasively. CPAP applied invasively is also called PEEP (positive end-expiratory pressure). CPAP is used to provide positive pressure at a constant level throughout the respiratory cycle, in both inspiration and exhalation. It is used acutely to support breathing for several reasons, one of which is helping to keep the alveoli (the very small air sacs in the lungs) open. The alveoli have a tendency

to collapse during illnesses such as severe pneumonia and respiratory distress syndrome (seen in premature infants), which often cause unacceptably reduced blood oxygen levels. CPAP can be used to support the respiratory muscles when the work of breathing is increased and to keep the airway open in conditions such as tracheomalacia, in which the trachea has a tendency to collapse, or in cases of upper airway obstruction. Conditions such as these can be associated with unacceptable increases in the carbon dioxide level or unacceptable levels of respiratory distress due to labored breathing. Conditions requiring a more chronic use of CPAP include obstructive sleep apnea, for which positive pressure is applied to the airway during sleep to stent it open. In some very severe cases of tracheomalacia, CPAP is applied via a tracheostomy tube to keep the airway open. A final example is in cases of muscle weakness, in which extra support is needed to assist the respiratory muscles.

BiPAP, bilevel positive airway pressure, is another form of positive pressure respiratory support. It involves the application of a constant level of airway pressure during exhalation (CPAP) but a higher pressure during inspiration. Bilevel positive airway pressure support provides a boost of pressure either to assist the respiratory muscles or to push the airway open during inspiration. During exhalation, continuous positive airway pressure at a lower level is applied to help keep the lungs or airway open. BiPAP is applied with a mask that fits over the nose or, occasionally, over both the nose and the mouth.

The acute indications for BiPAP are generally similar to those for CPAP, although since it is an increased level of support, patients who require BiPAP may be sicker than those who need only CPAP. Patients who are recovering from surgery or other severe illnesses and who needed invasive mechanical ventilation with a breathing tube may be placed on BiPAP for a short time as they recover. The most common chronic uses of BiPAP are for obstructive sleep apnea and muscle weakness requiring more support than CPAP can provide.

Benefits and risks: Positive pressure ventilatory support, either invasive or noninvasive, is used to address significant abnormalities with airway or respiratory muscle function and gas exchange. The risks of leaving these sorts of problems untreated are almost always greater than the risks of the therapy. Positive pressure ventilation allows for improved oxygen absorption and carbon dioxide elimination by the lungs and provides needed support to the airway or respiratory muscles without having to use a breathing tube and invasive ventilation. The major acute risk of all positive pressure ventilation is the development of a pneumothorax, a condition in which air escapes from the lung into the chest cavity, causing the lung to collapse. This complication is extremely rare with noninvasive ventilation and even with CPAP applied via a tracheostomy tube. A pneumothorax is easily identified with a chest x-ray, and a tube can be inserted into the chest cavity to drain the air if needed.

Although mask ventilation is preferable to invasive ventilation for many reasons, both CPAP and BiPAP can be challenging therapies in both the short and the long term. Tight-fitting masks are sometimes difficult for people to tolerate, and care needs to be taken to find a mask that fits correctly and maximizes comfort and tolerance. The sensation of air being forced into the nose and/or mouth can also be difficult to adjust to, and various strategies may be necessary to enhance acceptance. Nasal drying and irritation and sinusitis are possible consequences of nasal mask ventilation, and excellent skin care is needed to minimize irritation or even breakdown at the site where the mask comes into contact with the skin. Each of these problems is treatable and in the vast majority of cases does not preclude the use of these therapies.

Maintenance, care, and discharge planning: When CPAP and BiPAP are used acutely in the hospital, the maintenance, care, and administration are primarily the responsibility of the medical team. It is important for the family to attend to patient comfort and tolerability of the mask and to regularly evaluate the underlying skin. When CPAP and BiPAP are used chronically in the home, the maintenance, care, and administration are primarily the responsibility of the family. Although this responsibility may seem overwhelming at first, with the appropriate training it can become routine. The care team should provide supervision and medical follow-up on an ongoing basis. It may also be beneficial for the patient to bring his own mask to the hospital when testing or hospitalization is required.

Carpal Tunnel Syndrome
(finger numbness, hand pain)

Carpal tunnel syndrome is a common problem that occurs most often in people who use their hands extensively in repetitive tasks, such as knitting, typing, or using hand tools. It sometimes occurs in younger individuals, especially in women during pregnancy.

The median nerve is the major nerve that travels to the hand through a very narrow area called the carpal tunnel, located at the wrist. The area is occupied by this nerve and eleven tendons. If the tendons are used extensively, they may become inflamed and swollen and thus cause tightness, thereby constricting the nerve and causing numbness, usually in the thumb, the index finger, and the long finger. The feeling is often worse at night, when the fingers are not moving. It may be a dull ache or

a sensation of needles or pins in the fingers. Sometimes the pain also shoots up toward the elbow. In teenagers and young adults with cerebral palsy, carpal tunnel syndrome may occur as a result of using the hands for pushing manual wheelchairs or for using walkers or crutches for weight bearing.

Indications: The use of anti-inflammatory medications such as naproxen, ibuprofen, or other antiarthritic medicines is the first line of treatment. Splints should be worn at night to hold the wrist extended. If this intervention does not relieve the symptoms or if they return immediately after discontinuing splinting, the tunnel in which the nerve runs can be surgically released with a procedure called a carpal tunnel release. This is a simple outpatient procedure that can be performed on adults under local anesthesia. It requires only a soft bandage for ten days. However, individuals would be restricted from weight bearing with walkers and crutches and from wheelchair use for three weeks.

What to expect: Complications and risks of the procedure are minimal and mostly relate to possible recurrence as the tunnel heals and tightens up again. The main instructions for preventing recurrence include ensuring proper hand use with wheelchair wheels, crutches, and walkers.

Cerebellum

The cerebellum is the upper back part of the brain. It consists of two hemispheres and is located in the posterior cranial fossa portion of the brain. The cerebellum coordinates the action of muscle groups and times their contractions so that movements are performed smoothly

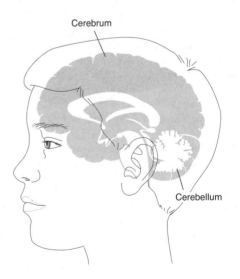

Cerebrum

Cerebellum

and accurately. The disorder characterized by clumsy and disorganized motor skills caused by damage to the cerebellum is called *cerebellar ataxia*. Sensory information may also be integrated through the cerebellum.

Cerebrum

The cerebrum is the major front and upper part of the brain, where active coordination and voluntary muscle movement is controlled. This is also the part of the brain where consciousness, thought, and psychological functions reside and are organized (called the executive function). This part of the brain is extremely vulnerable to injury and is the area in which scars occur that lead to cerebral palsy.

The cerebrum is divided into two halves, the right and left hemispheres. The right side controls the left side of the body, and vice versa. Injuries to one hemisphere cause dysfunction of one side of the body, called *hemiplegia* (motor involvement of one arm and one leg on the same side of the body). Injuries to both sides cause *diplegia* (motor involvement of the lower extremities with difficulty in trunk control and fine motor skills) or *quadriplegia* (motor involvement of all four limbs).

In each half, or hemisphere, specific areas control specific functions. Specific areas such as the frontal lobes predominantly control emotion; speech is controlled primarily on the left side of the brain; and specific areas of the brain control the hands, while others control the feet. The different areas of function have been mapped out very well—largely by careful observation of known areas in which injury has occurred, followed by recording the deficits that patients subsequently exhibit.

Injury to specific areas of the brain explain why some children with cerebral palsy exhibit behavior difficulties or have specific problems with motor control. Children with cerebral palsy may have entire areas of the brain missing (revealed when scans are performed), but because their brain is still developing, the function ordinarily performed by a part of the brain that is missing may be taken up by another, healthy part of the brain that doesn't ordinarily perform that function. This is known as *brain plasticity*. This plasticity in the young brain is the major reason why the outcome of head injuries in children differs greatly from the outcome of head injuries occurring in adults.

Child Abuse
(child neglect, shaken baby syndrome)

The key federal legislation that addresses child abuse is the Child Abuse Prevention and Treatment Act, first enacted in 1974. This act has been amended and renewed a number of times, most recently in 2010. In addition, each state has responsibility for prevention and evaluation of possible child abuse. Child abuse is defined as "an act or failure to act on the part of a parent or caregiver which results in death, serious physical or emotional harm, sexual abuse or exploitation, or an act or failure to act which presents an imminent risk of serious harm."

There is much about the abuse of children that is not understood. We do know that child abuse is more likely to occur in families in which the parents themselves were abused or were exposed to family violence as children. Children with disabilities, especially severely involved children with cerebral palsy, are at higher risk for child abuse than children without disabilities. These children may be unusually irritable or difficult to comfort, which can become frustrating for parents and caregivers. Parents of children who are very difficult to care for may neglect or physically harm them as a way of dealing with their own frustration. Any stress can precipitate striking out, and parents of children with disabilities often experience a great deal of stress related to their child's care.

Parents of children with disabilities need to have someone whom they can call for help. This may be a grandparent, a friend, a neighbor, or a social worker. Parents should learn to call and admit that they are unable to handle the situation, especially when they have difficulty controlling their emotions and when their frustration level is very high.

Shaken baby syndrome occurs when a caregiver tries to quiet a baby by shaking her back and forth. If this maneuver is done too roughly, it can cause bleeding inside the baby's head and injury to the brain, which can cause long-term brain scars and cerebral palsy. This too is a form of child abuse. In addition to shaking, infants can suffer abusive head trauma or brain injury from being struck.

The complications from child abuse can be very severe, from bruises and broken bones to neglect, such as not being given needed medication or adequate food, and can even lead to death. Very few parents intentionally abuse their child, but it can become the only form of reacting to the environment that the parent is capable of at the time.

By law, suspicions of child abuse must be reported by school, child care, and medical personnel to the appropriate state agency, which will investigate the situation. Responses may include support for the family or, in severe situations (in which the child's safety or health is felt to be threatened), removal of the child from the home on a temporary or long-term basis. The vast majority of reported suspicions of child abuse are handled by child and family services workers or children and youth services workers, who are able to provide education and supportive help to the parents so they can deal with the situation.

Chromosomal Disorders

Each human cell contains a full complement of genetic information that is encoded in 46 chromosomes, which are actually made up of 23 pairs of chromosomes, with one set of 23 donated by each parent. Chromosomes are composed of genes, which are themselves composed of DNA. Each chromosome pair contains genes coding for similar traits; we have 2 of almost every gene, one from our mother and one from our father. One chromosome pair is made up of the sex chromosomes, consisting of the XX chromosome pair in a female and the XY pair in a male.

Trisomy is a condition in which there is an entire extra chromosome, meaning that there are three copies of a particular chromosome rather than the usual two copies. Most people recognize Down syndrome (also known as trisomy 21), in which there is an extra chromosome number 21. People with Down syndrome share certain physical features, such as a flat profile, eyes slanting up, hyperextensible joints, and varying degrees of cognitive impairment. Heart defects and defects of the intestines are also frequent.

Another chromosome anomaly is the deletion, or absence, of a small piece of a chromosome (so that a number of genes are missing), a duplication in which a piece of a chromosome is present in three copies rather than two, or a translocation whereby a small piece of a chromosome may be attached to another chromosome. These can be identified by examining the chromosomes under a microscope. Depending on the specific genes involved, these children may have multiple physical and cognitive problems as well. Rarely, one healthy parent of an affected child may have a rearrangement of his or her chromosomes, which predisposes the child to a (micro) deletion, duplication, or translocation. Thus, when any chromosome deletion, duplication, or rearrangement is identified, parents are often tested.

Very small submicroscopic (too small to be seen with the standard microscopic techniques) chromosome deletions can also be identified. They are referred to as *microdeletion syndromes*. Once again, depending on the specific gene or genes involved, features may vary and patients may have a diagnosis of cerebral palsy early on until the genetic abnormality is found. These microdeletions will not be found through standard chromosome studies, but instead require more complex DNA tests. Identifying patterns of physical and behavioral features is important for the physician trying to decide which syndrome, if any, should be tested for in any individual child.

Subtelomeric deletions or rearrangements involve the very ends of the chromosomes. Features of the specific chromosome abnormality vary. It is estimated that a subtelomeric rearrangement will be identified in 4 to 7 percent of children who have developmental delay and are small in size.

The field of genetics has been changing rapidly. It is now possible to sequence the entire genome or a subset of the genome called the *exome*. This testing has become faster and less expensive but often is not paid for by medical insurance. Exome sequencing identifies the sequence of the genes in the genome that code for proteins (these are known as exons and account for 1 percent of all the genes). Mutations in these sequences are much more likely to affect the health of an individual than are mutations in the other 99 percent of the genes. Therefore, rather than sequencing the entire genome, whole exome sequencing is being used to identify mutations likely to have health consequences.

In children with CP, when the usual testing has not identified a cause, whole exome sequencing has been used. This sequencing has sometimes identified a chromosomal mutation that may explain the child's disability. The significance of these abnormalities is not always clear; they may sometimes be the cause of the child's disability, or they may create a susceptibility that leaves the child vulnerable to environmental stresses, whereas another child without this susceptibility, even when exposed to the same environmental stress (for instance prematurity), may not develop CP. As this new testing becomes less expensive over time, it will likely be used more frequently and decrease the number of cases of CP whose cause is unknown (though there likely will remain a certain percentage of cases in which the cause cannot be identified).

Clonus

Clonus is a symptom of spasticity. It is a special reflex from the spinal cord that is not being controlled by the normal mechanism in the brain. Rapid stretching of a muscle, such as pushing hard against the sole of the foot, causes the foot to make rhythmic movements. As the muscle is held under tension, these rhythmic movements may gradually die down, but in some people they are persistent. Constant clonus is noted to be present when a certain pressure causes a constant beating of the muscle. Clonus activity that causes a beating motion at the ankle joint is very common in children with cerebral palsy. This can cause a problem for children who are sitting in wheelchairs, because their legs may jump. AFO braces used on the ankle may suppress this reflex.

Cochlear Implants

A cochlear implant is an auditory rehabilitation option for children with sensorineural (nerve) hearing loss that

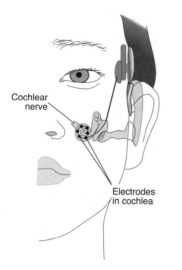

Cochlear nerve

Electrodes in cochlea

cannot be treated with conventional hearing aids. In this situation, the hearing aids are not powerful enough to bring the hearing thresholds into the normal range. Because most types of sensorineural hearing loss involve disorders of the cochlea (the organ of hearing) but spare the nerve of hearing (the cochlear nerve), it is possible to directly stimulate the nerve of hearing electrically and carry sound information to the brain.

The cochlear implant is a surgically placed device that takes sound information from a microphone and transforms this information into pulsed electrical signals that are sent along an electrode array in the cochlea to directly stimulate the nerve of hearing. Not all children with profound sensorineural hearing loss are candidates for cochlear implantation. An experienced cochlear implant team made up of audiologists, speech pathologists, deaf educators, language scientists, ear surgeons, and social workers evaluates each patient individually to help with this important decision. The success of the cochlear implant in restoring hearing depends upon intensive therapy after the device has been placed. This therapy includes additional counseling, education, and training to teach the brain to process the new input from the implant. A patient who is unable to participate in this therapy is unlikely to be a candidate for surgery, as the implant on its own, without accompanying therapy, usually will not rehabilitate the hearing.

Complementary and Alternative Medicine
(CAM)

The term *complementary and alternative medicine* (CAM) describes a group of diverse medical practices and products that are not presently considered part of conventional medicine. While some CAM therapies

have been studied scientifically, most have yet to be investigated through well-designed scientific studies, and questions remain as to whether these therapies work for the medical conditions for which they are used and whether they are safe. Although it is often assumed that natural products such as herbs must be safe, this is not necessarily true, as many have significant medicinal properties and may have significant side effects. Because the US Food and Drug Administration does not have jurisdiction over these products (they are considered a food rather than a medicine), they are not tested for safety or effectiveness and may include harmful contaminants, or they may not contain the ingredients they say they do.

Complementary medicine is used together with conventional medicine, whereas alternative medicine is used in place of conventional medicine. A third category, integrative medicine, combines mainstream medical therapies and CAM therapies for which there is good scientific evidence of safety and effectiveness.

The federal government has established the National Center for Complementary and Alternative Medicine to explore these practices in the context of rigorous science. The center has sponsored research into many alternative medical treatments and disseminates authoritative information to the public and to medical professionals.

Chiropractic is an example of an alternative medical system. Chiropractors use manipulative therapy as a treatment tool. Another alternative medical system is homeopathic medicine, which uses small quantities of very diluted medicinal substances to cure symptoms, when the same substances given at higher doses would actually cause those symptoms. Dietary supplements are products taken by mouth that contain a dietary ingredient that is meant to supplement the diet. These may include vitamins, minerals, herbs, amino acids, and substances such as enzymes. Dietary supplements can certainly be used as complements to conventional medicine, but they have also been used as an alternative to conventional medicine.

Patients and families need to weigh the cost versus the benefit of using these products and, as with many other treatments, discuss with their medical practitioners both whether these products are effective and whether they are safe.

Computerized Axial Tomography
(CT scan, CAT scan)

The CT scan is a special type of x-ray. The computer makes pictures using information from x-rays taken on all sides of the body. A CT scan can be made of any area of the body and gives excellent definition of bone and soft tissue. Scans of the brain can define major abnor-

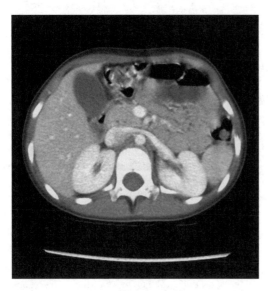

CT scan

malities, such as tumors, increased fluid in the brain, and major congenital deformities.

The dose of radiation is higher than for conventional x-rays, but a single scan is not considered harmful. The patient lies on a table and must hold still. Contrast material is sometimes injected into the bloodstream to help define the blood vessels. CT scans cannot, however, detect all deformities or scars.

Indications: For children with cerebral palsy, CT scans are utilized mainly to define possible deformities in the brain. Often a CT scan may be used in the initial evaluation to see if there are any abnormalities that would explain the child's cerebral palsy or any treatable conditions of the brain, such as hydrocephalus, or increased fluid on the brain. Another common reason for obtaining a CT scan is to check the functioning of a shunt in a child with hydrocephalus.

Benefits and risks: The benefit of the CT scan is that it provides a good view of the brain and can often be done much more quickly than an MRI (magnetic resonance imaging) scan. The machine also is a smaller tube and does not make the person being examined feel as enclosed as an MRI scanner does. There are a few minor risks related to CT scans. First, there is a minimal risk because a low dose x-ray is used. There is also a very small risk of allergy or kidney problems if an IV contrast injection is used, although these risks are extremely small for most children. Because the scan requires a child to hold still, some children may require sedation. Another problem with the CT scan is that it is limited to defining only major deformities of the brain. This means

that there are subtle brain deformities that the CT scanner cannot define.

Maintenance and care: If a child is sedated, care must be taken to monitor the child until the sedation has worn off.

Congenital Infections
(cytomegalovirus [CMV], toxoplasmosis, syphilis, rubella [German measles], herpes simplex virus, varicella [chicken pox], Zika)

A number of infectious agents can infect a pregnant woman and then infect the fetus she is carrying, causing a variety of physical abnormalities and sometimes brain damage resulting in cerebral palsy. These infections may be acquired during pregnancy, during delivery, or occasionally following birth. Frequently, these infections are subclinical (meaning that they do not show any symptoms), and yet they can later result in neurological damage.

The infections listed here are known to cause brain damage in the fetus or young child. Fortunately, two of these, varicella and rubella, can be prevented with immunizations. Most young people should have received these immunizations well before they were of childbearing age. All pregnant women should be screened for syphilis, a sexually transmitted infection, with a blood test early in pregnancy and preferably again toward the end of pregnancy. If a pregnant woman is known to be infected with syphilis, she can be treated with antibiotics, which should eradicate the infection.

Toxoplasmosis is an infection that can be prevented by avoiding handling the feces of cats (ask someone else to clean the kitty litter) and avoiding eating raw or undercooked meat. CMV, or cytomegalovirus, currently is the infection most likely to cause brain damage in the fetus. It is a common virus that will cause typical cold symptoms, and there is no immunization to prevent it. A woman who experiences her first infection with CMV while pregnant has a risk of infecting her fetus, and 5 percent of the fetuses who are infected will have significant brain damage, which can cause CP, cognitive impairment, hearing loss, microcephaly and other abnormalities. Zika virus is a newly recognized cause of brain damage in infants. Like CMV, it causes microcephaly and other abnormalities of the brain. We do not know the long-term consequences yet, as it has only recently been described, but it is likely that many of the newborns born with microcephaly due to infection with Zika virus will have neurological problems, including cerebral palsy.

Herpes simplex infection of the newborn can result in hepatitis, pneumonia, meningitis, or encephalitis, which can result in permanent brain damage and cerebral palsy. Other infected newborns may have more localized infection of the skin, eyes, and mouth. New-born infants with a herpes infection have a high risk of dying from the infection or living with severe brain damage. Antiviral drug therapy with acyclovir improves the prognosis. If a woman in labor reports signs of genital herpes infection, then delivery by cesarean section is recommended, because this method of delivery reduces the risk of transmitting the infection to her baby.

Contracture, Elbow

Elbow flexion contractures are present in children with severely involved quadriplegic or hemiplegic cerebral palsy. In the severest form, the elbow is tightly flexed, and it is impossible to extend the elbow enough to clean the elbow crease. This causes a foul-smelling moist area. When the elbow cannot be extended, it is also difficult to dress the child, especially to put sleeves on the arm. Elbow flexion contractures in children with hemiplegia are cosmetically unappealing, especially when the child walks, because the elbow is held flexed up.

Elbow flexion contractures occurring in children between the ages of 3 and 6 with quadriplegic CP have a tendency to get slowly worse. For the young child under age 8 with hemiplegic CP, the flexed elbow tends to improve during adolescence as the child become more self-aware. If good elbow motion is maintained until adolescence, generally it can be maintained throughout adult life. However, there is a tendency for muscle stiffness to increase with aging, and further contracture may develop in the late teenage years or adulthood.

Care and treatment: Children with a tendency to develop contractures may use night resting splints as well as physical therapy exercises to maintain range of motion. Since it is not certain whether contractures can be avoided in certain children, opinion varies widely on how aggressive the medical professional should be about splinting and stretching.

The majority of children continue to work with some combination of stretching and bracing; only in rare cases do the flexion contractures become so severe that cleaning the flexion crease or dressing the child becomes extremely difficult. In these circumstances, release of the biceps and the brachial muscles at the elbow is recommended. This is a relatively minor procedure and is frequently combined with other procedures that address specific functional care problems. For some children with severe hemiplegia, cosmetic concerns are such that release of the muscles to let the arm extend greatly benefits the child's self-image.

Benefits and risks: The benefits of a successful procedure are greater ease in cleaning and dressing the child and an enhanced appearance. Surgical release is a rather simple procedure with few complications. There is a risk that brace wear may cause skin breakdown, so the skin needs to be monitored daily after the brace has been removed. Also, stretching, if done too aggressively, may cause fractures of the arm. Surgical release of the elbow, if it is too aggressive, may result in the elbow's being stuck in an extended position—which is even more cosmetically objectionable and more functionally debilitating than a flexed elbow. The goal should be to have the elbow at approximately 90 to 100 degrees if the child is wheelchair bound or approximately 120 degrees if the child is ambulatory.

Maintenance and care: The main instruction after surgery is to work with range of motion. For parents, this may involve gentle work with range of motion during bathing or at dressing time. It can often be done in the context of the normal activities of daily living, without having to set aside special exercise times. Braces used may be quite flexible and variable. If surgical release is performed, it is recommended to continue with exercise and occasionally with a bracing program for at least six months to a year.

Contracture, Finger
(flexor tendon lengthening)

Tightness of the finger flexion muscles often coincides with another problem: wrist drop and tightness of the muscles that pull the wrist into flexion. Two groups of muscles cause the fingers to flex. One is the profundus muscle, extending from the forearm all the way to the tip of each finger. This muscle does not cross the elbow and is usually the least likely to have significant shortness. The other is the flexor sublimis muscle, which starts above the elbow and goes to the first joint (PIP joint) of each finger and is primarily involved with contractures.

Often the finger flexor muscles are not tight when the wrist is in the flexed position, but if surgical procedures are done to correct the fixed flexion and put the wrist in a better position, at times the finger muscles become

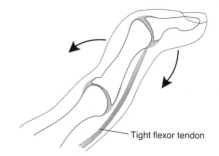

Tight flexor tendon

so tight that the fingers cannot be straightened out. The tendency over time is for these muscles gradually to get tighter, although they seldom become so tight that the fingers are clenched into the palm.

Care and treatment: The primary treatment is splinting, which is usually used in addition to the wrist drop splints that are described in the wrist contracture section. It is seldom necessary to treat the finger flexors or to brace the finger flexion contractures without also addressing the wrist flexion problem. If a decision has been made to treat the wrist flexion contractures and the finger flexors are tight, they should be treated surgically at the same time.

The surgery: There are two surgical approaches. One involves loosening the muscles at their insertion above the elbow and allowing them to slide toward the fingers; this is referred to as the muscle slide procedure. The other involves identifying and lengthening each finger tendon with a Z-cut. The first procedure, the muscle slide lengthening at the elbow, involves less exact lengthening. The more commonly used procedure at the wrist is more exactly controlled, and only the sublimis tendons may be lengthened. In severe deformities, the profundus tendons may need lengthening as well.

Benefits and risks: The benefits are both cosmetic and functional. Overlengthening, which removes the strength from the muscles and decreases the ability to close the fingers or to grasp objects, may be a significant complication that is best avoided by conservative, controlled lengthening. If both the sublimis and the profundus tendons are lengthened, major weakness is a higher risk. If only the sublimis tendons are lengthened, there is a risk of developing swan-neck deformities, which means that the first joint (the PIP joint) of the finger may go into extension, while the joint at the end of the finger (the DIP joint) flexes. This causes the fingers to lock and makes it difficult for a person to use them for grasping.

Another possible complication involves scarring of the tendons, resulting in decreased motion. This can usually be treated with occupational therapy through motion exercises. Occasionally, surgery is needed. Following lengthenings, the fingers are usually immobilized, slightly flexed, in a cast, and the tendons are allowed to heal for four weeks before they are allowed to move again.

Contracture, Peroneal
(peroneus longus contracture, peroneal tendon lengthening)

The peroneal tendons and muscles are located along the outside of the leg (lateral side) and pull the foot out.

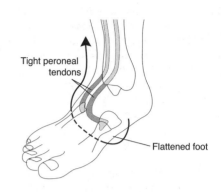

When they are spastic or too tight, they cause severe flat feet. These muscles are not commonly severely spastic, but some children do develop significant spasticity.

Care and treatment: If severe spasticity seems to be a significant cause of flatfootedness, lengthening these tendons may be necessary. The outcome of peroneal tendon lengthening, however, is unpredictable, with a high incidence of either recurrent deformity within several years or developing the opposite deformity if too much lengthening is done. Peroneal tendon lengthening is not a commonly performed operation because of its unreliability. Usually it is better to use a brace (AFO). If this is not possible, one should proceed with subtalar fusion, which involves fusing the bone in the back of the foot to correct a flat foot deformity.

Contracture, Pronator
(pronator teres transfer, pronator release)

A common contracture that develops in children with cerebral palsy is a pronator contracture, in which the hand is turned with the palm away from the face. The primary muscle involved is the pronator teres, which extends from just above the elbow to the middle of the forearm. This contracture occurs commonly in children with hemiplegia and is present in some children with moderate to severe quadriplegia. The deformity begins as the child's preferred position. As the child grows, the muscle frequently becomes tighter and more contracted.

Care and treatment: Exercises to stretch this muscle should be incorporated as part of the child's elbow and hand exercises. Splinting the muscle is difficult because torsional splints require tying up the hand from above the elbow all the way down to the wrist. Splinting is generally not useful because of the difficulty of keeping the arm in a fixed position. This deformity does not cause any significant hygiene or dressing problems; however, it does cause functional problems, because the palm and

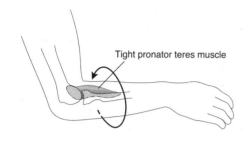

Tight pronator teres muscle

fingertips are turned out of sight, making it difficult to manipulate switches and joysticks because the child cannot see how his palm and fingertips are moving. It also makes picking up utensils or other objects difficult. Pronation often becomes a significant cosmetic deformity, especially for the child with hemiplegia who is walking and participating in normal daily activities.

The surgery: The treatment for pronator contracture involves either releasing the pronator muscle from its insertion on the forearm or transferring it so that it winds around the bone in the opposite direction—making the hand supine, or turned up. Some surgeons believe that the transfer provides a better outcome. Opinions vary about whether to release or to transfer, and for most patients the two provide essentially the same results.

Benefits and risks: Benefits are the ability to see the palm and therefore to possibly use it better and a more pleasing appearance. The complications from pronator release or transfer surgery include the possibility of developing the opposite deformity, but this seldom occurs. The procedure is quite minor and is usually performed at the same time as a number of procedures to deal with other deformities.

After-surgery care: Following the operation, the patient usually wears a cast above the elbow for four to six weeks. Exercises are subsequently started; bracing is not used.

Contracture, Shoulder
(pectoralis contracture, latissimus dorsi contracture)

Shoulder contractures are common in children with severe quadriplegia. However, they seldom are a problem except for the child whose shoulder is pulled down to the side with the hand across the chest—or, alternatively, for the child whose shoulder may be pulled down to the side with the arm stuck straight out. If the arm is pulled across the chest, it is called an *internal rotation contracture*. If it is pulled out away from the body, it is called an *external rotation contracture*. Internal rotation contractures are usually due to the contracture of the

pectoralis major and minor muscles, and the therapy usually involves working at range of motion. External rotation contractures are often due to the contracture of the teres minor and latissimus dorsi muscles. Again, the treatment involves working on physical therapy and positioning.

The surgery: For severe external rotation contractures that cannot be stretched out with therapy, surgery may be necessary, usually an osteotomy (cutting the bone) just below the shoulder. The arm must be turned in and held in this position while the bone heals. For severe internal rotation contractures, a pectoralis release is occasionally necessary. This is a very small procedure done at the shoulder that allows the arm to rotate externally far enough to allow for personal hygiene and dressing.

Indications: The main indication for surgical procedures for internal rotation contractures is the need to improve the caregiver's ability to dress the child, especially to place the arms in sleeves, and to perform personal hygiene, primarily to clean the armpits. For external rotation contractures, the major problem develops in a larger child, whom it may be difficult to get through doors and who may be unable to sit well in a wheelchair.

Benefits and risks: The major benefit is improved range of motion, which allows the caregiver to clean and to dress the child, and increased ease of moving the child. The complications from either of these procedures may involve overcorrection. Overcorrection is a special concern with the internally rotated arm: release should not be overly aggressive, since the arm may become fixed in external rotation. Likewise, for the externally rotated arm that is surgically rotated in, too much internal rotation is possible.

After-surgery care: The postoperative treatment usually is immediate, aggressive physical therapy for the muscle releases. Three to four weeks of splint immobilization is necessary after the osteotomy to allow healing.

Contracture, Thumb
(adducted thumb, thumb tendon release, thumb fusion)

Thumb deformities are very common in children with cerebral palsy. The most frequent problem is a thumb that is drawn close to the index finger, making the web space between the index finger and the thumb very tight and narrow. This makes it difficult to get the thumb out away from the hand to grasp objects such as balls or glasses. Sometimes the thumb is flexed tightly into the palm. In some children this can make hygiene very difficult, with the palm becoming moist and foul smell-

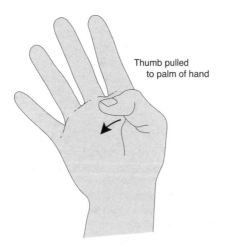

Thumb pulled
to palm of hand

ing. From a functional perspective, the problem of the thumb in the hand makes grasping objects more difficult; pinching from the tip of the thumb to the index or the long fingers may also be difficult. In some children the first thumb joint (the IP joint) may also become extended, and the joint at the base of the thumb (the MCP joint) may be flexed or extended.

Care and treatment: As long as the hand can be cleaned and the palm does not become moist and smelly, treatment for thumb deformities is not needed. If the thumb is tightly drawn into the hand and flexed into the palm, then hygiene is a problem, and the appropriate treatment is almost always surgical. The most common technique involves fusing the joint at the base of the thumb (the MCP joint or the IP joint), with release of the thumb flexor tendon and the adductor tendon in the palm. Sometimes a tendon transfer to help pull the thumb out of the palm is needed. These fusions are minor procedures in which the cartilage and the joint are removed and the thumb joint is held with a pin for four to six weeks as the bones grow together. This is a permanent correction.

Initially, hands that are functional but cause difficulties should be splinted. Either rigid plastic splints to deepen the space between the index finger and the thumb or a splint that is made as part of a hand or wrist splint should be used. There are soft splints that hook over the thumb and pull it back. These are useful for pulling the thumb out of the palm to improve use of the hand and prevent development of contractures. This type of splinting is especially useful for children aged 2 to 10. Adolescents almost never accept splinting because of the attention it draws to the hand's appearance. Functionally, the splinting usually is more of an impediment to the teen than a benefit. If thumb deformities continue to be a functional problem, they are generally best handled with surgical correction, which is usually done along with multiple other procedures either on the same arm or on the legs. The timing is related in part to the timing of other procedures.

The surgery: The simplest surgical procedure is the release of the thumb adductor muscle by means of a small incision in the palm. The incision often needs to be followed by transfers to help increase the strength or power of the thumb-extending muscles. Usually, the muscle in the palm called the palmaris longus is transferred to help pull the thumb out of the palm. Multiple other muscles, such as finger flexor muscles or wrist flexor muscles, may be transferred to assist in thumb control. In the case of a severely involved hand, fusion of one of the thumb joints may also be indicated.

The procedures used to treat thumb deformities vary among surgeons. The same surgeon may use many different combinations, because thumb deformities differ from one hand to the next. Which muscles to transfer and whether fusions are indicated are determined by physical examination and the surgeon's specific experience.

Benefits and risks: Benefits include improved use of the hand and better hygiene. One risk is that bracing thumb deformities may cause skin irritation. Regular observation of the skin and well-fitting braces can prevent this complication. The surgical complications are related to overcorrection of deformities, the severest being the thumb stuck far out of the palm, which creates significant cosmetic problems and difficulties with dressing, such as getting a hand through a sleeve. Although complications are rare, the most frequent complication is the deformity that is not completely corrected. It is much better to have some residual tightness with the thumb in toward the hand than to have the opposite problem.

Maintenance and care: After surgical correction, casting is usually required for four to six weeks, sometimes followed by splinting. In a functional hand, some occupational therapy aimed at achieving the maximum benefit from the surgery is usually necessary for one to three months.

Contracture, Wrist
(wrist tendon transfer)

Wrist flexion is a common deformity in children with hemiplegia and severe quadriplegia. The wrist is dropped in position and is sometimes referred to as a *dropped wrist*. Occasionally, the child is able to bring the wrist up to a neutral position. In this flexed position it is difficult to get good finger grasp because the wrist position makes the finger flexion muscles much weaker. This flexion contracture develops between the ages of 3 and 6. Initially, the wrist is flexible and does not cause any problems, but tightness develops as the child continues to grow into the early teens; during the adolescent growth spurt, the muscles become shorter relative to the bone.

At this point, correction of the deformity becomes more difficult. In its severest form, the hand may be folded completely onto the forearm, making skin care and hygiene difficult and creating a moist area that may start to smell. For those children who have a mild case of cerebral palsy and are more functional, as the wrist flexion becomes more contracted, they encounter more difficulty with hand use, especially with finger grasps.

Care and treatment: The primary treatment for wrist flexion contracture is an exercise program of gentle stretching and the use of resting splints. If splints are used to cover the hand, the child may lose interest in using the hand, and its ability to stay limber diminishes. For this reason, some combination of splint use and functional use is best. For wrists that are not developing significant contractures and can be brought completely into an over-corrected position, overtreatment with braces should be avoided. For the child with severe quadriplegia and no functional hand use, the goal should be to create sufficient flexibility to allow for good hygiene and ease of dressing. The development of some contracture in this situation is not detrimental.

For the child with functional use of the hand, attempts should be made to keep the wrist in a functional position. If this is not possible, as the child grows into adolescence surgical correction should be considered. Usually no earlier than age 6 and generally between the ages of 9 and 12 is the best time for surgery. Children with significant wrist flexion contractures and hemiplegia, even if they are nonfunctional, often have cosmetic appearance concerns and should be considered for surgical corrections. An awkward-looking hand draws much less attention if it is corrected, even if its function is not changed. The best age for the surgery is at or just before the adolescent growth spurt in the early teen years.

The surgery: Surgical treatment typically involves transfer of the muscle on the little finger side of the wrist called the flexor carpi-ulnaris. It is attached to the muscles that lift the wrist, usually the extensor carpi-radialis brevis. For children who have difficulty lifting their fingers, the muscle is transferred into the extensor digitorum communis muscle, which helps to extend the fingers. This transfer, along with tightening the muscles that lift the wrist, helps straighten both the fingers and the wrist at the same time.

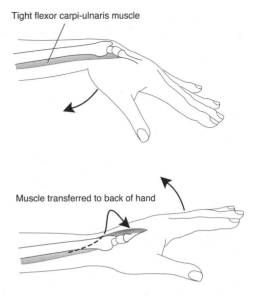

Tight flexor carpi-ulnaris muscle

Muscle transferred to back of hand

The tendon that is transferred into each muscle varies and is determined by clinical examination. There are laboratory tests available that use electromyographs (which involve inserting small wires into the muscle) and observation of the hand as it functions to determine which muscles are functioning and in what fashion. These tendon transfers are well established, not new or experimental.

Benefits and risks: Benefits include improved cosmetic appearance and better hygiene; often function is improved as well. The main problem associated with splints is the possibility of causing skin irritation and diminished function. Overly aggressive stretching of very tightly contracted muscle may cause fractures and should be avoided. The major surgical complication is overcorrection or undercorrection. A mild undercorrection is preferable to an overcorrection in the opposite direction.

One severe complication is a backward overextension of the wrist. This could result from too much tendon release at the palm side of the wrist or a too tight tendon transfer on the wrist. This is especially detrimental if the transfer is into the finger-extending tendons, which means the fingers cannot be bent. It could also make grasping difficult. These problems can be corrected by lengthening the transfer tendons, but it is best to avoid them by less tight transfers. Occasionally the transferred tendons may tear out, leaving the person with essentially the same deformity he started with.

After-surgery care: After surgical transfers to correct wrist contracture, the person usually has to wear a cast for four to six weeks, followed by a positional brace, usually worn at night. After one year all bracing is stopped. Intense occupational therapy aimed at improving function and mobility is recommended after the surgical healing period is over, usually beginning at four to six weeks after surgery.

Cord Blood

There are research trials in progress to test whether infusions of a child's own cord blood, banked at birth, can be used to treat his or her cerebral palsy. It is too soon to know whether this can work, but studies in animal models have given positive results. Other studies are using stem cells in children with cerebral palsy. It will likely be a few years before we know the outcome of these studies.

Cortical Visual Impairment
(CVI)

Cortical visual impairment may occur in up to approximately 70 percent of children with cerebral palsy. CVI is defined as a deficit of visual function caused by damage to the parts of the brain responsible for vision. Some children with CVI remain significantly impaired, while visual function in other children may improve over time. Regardless of the level of function, interventions are directed at improving function so a child may use the vision he or she has to reach his or her full potential.

Crouched Gait
(tight hamstring, tight hip flexor, overlengthened Achilles tendon)

A crouched gait is commonly seen in children with diplegia: they stand with their knees and their hips flexed and often with their ankles dorsiflexed, so that their weight is resting on the heels. Children with a crouched gait may also stand on tiptoe. When it is mild, this natural pattern works quite well, and there is no need to correct it. However, if the crouch becomes severe, for example, with knee flexion of 45 degrees when standing, then the gait consumes a lot of energy and it is extremely difficult to walk. When a child gains weight, often the crouching becomes more severe, especially during a growth spurt.

A crouched gait is usually caused by a combination of factors, the primary one being a tight hamstring muscle. Tight hip flexor muscles are another cause, and often an overlengthened Achilles tendon may be a contributing factor.

Care and treatment: The treatment of a crouched gait initially involves physical therapy, with therapist and child working at stretching the hip flexors and the hamstring muscles. In younger patients, botulinum toxin injections into the hamstring muscle and the hip flexor muscle (iliopsoas) may be helpful when the tightness is due pri-

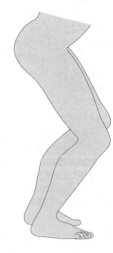

marily to tone. If the crouched gait gets worse in spite of therapy, a ground reaction ankle-foot orthosis that locks the ankle may be necessary. If this fails and the crouching continues to get worse or the hamstring and hip flexors are very tight, lengthening the hamstring muscles and hip flexors, especially the iliopsoas muscles, should be considered. If the Achilles tendon is tight, it may need to be lengthened, but with extreme caution, since an overlengthened Achilles tendon will certainly make the crouching worse.

The complications of a long-term crouch are knee pain and the gradually reduced ability to walk. The knee pain is caused by increased pressure on the kneecap and may become severe enough to prohibit walking. If muscles are lengthened early in a child's life (before age 8), this often needs to be repeated at adolescence, since growth will again cause shortness in the muscle. If the degree of crouching is mild as the child reaches full maturity, it generally will not get worse. If it is severe, however, it will tend to get slowly worse. Overlengthening the muscles, which may cause the knee to bend backward, may be another complication of treatment. This gait pattern is even worse than a crouched gait, and it should be avoided by conservative lengthening of the muscles, with the risk of needing repeat lengthening.

After surgery, some surgeons use long leg or hip spica casts for three to six weeks, followed by physical therapy exercises for stretching and teaching an improved gait pattern. Many surgeons don't use casts but instead use removable splints that are worn part time in conjunction with physical therapy that is started immediately, usually on the first or second day after surgery. Braces, either standard nonhinged or ground reaction AFOs, are often used to help reduce the crouch for the first 6 to 12 months after surgery.

Crutches
(canes, quadcanes, Lofstrand crutches, walking sticks)

Crutches is the common term for a group of devices that may be used to help a child with mild cerebral palsy walk. The standard crutches that go under the armpits, which are often used by people with a broken leg, are seldom used for children with cerebral palsy, because there is a tendency for the child to hang on the crutches by the armpit. This incorrect use usually leads to very poor standing posture. If crutches are recommended for a child with CP, most physicians prefer the Lofstrand, or forearm, crutches, which have a ring through which the arm goes and a handle for the child's hand. This discourages leaning on the crutches and requires the child to hold on to the crutches, putting the weight on the hands.

Indications: Crutches are most useful for children who have a great deal of difficulty balancing. Children with severe leg involvement but excellent arm function can also become excellent crutch users. The child who tends to lean forward when using crutches might try one of the many different kinds of canes that one holds on to only with the hand, with the arm not touching the cane. The quadcane has small feet and stands on its own but isn't much more helpful than a standard cane. A good choice is the use of a straight stick, which the child can hold slightly higher, giving her extra balance. Canes are used less for leaning against the floor than for the additional weight they provide for the child to hold in front of herself.

The resulting bent posture should not prevent a child

from trying crutches or canes. For most children with cerebral palsy, the use of crutches or canes is temporary, and most children who are able to walk eventually abandon all assistive devices. However, a few children do permanently need the extra assistance for balance, and the device that they are most comfortable with is generally the correct one. Trying out multiple devices, such as Lofstrand crutches and different types of canes, allows the child to find the one he is most comfortable with. If a child refuses to use a specific crutch or cane, it usually is his way of telling you either that he doesn't need it or that he is uncomfortable with it.

Benefits and risks: Greater balance is the most obvious benefit of using crutches or a cane, but often there are risks involved when a child is moved from a walker to one of these devices. The child may initially have a cosmetically poor forward-bent posture, sometimes crouching further with his knees bent. It is best for the child to have the aid of a therapist work from the outset of this transition at the outset and then move to using the new device around the house.

Moving from a walker to a cane or crutches often makes the child more unstable, so the child should practice in a safe environment. The child may also feel less efficient and slower with crutches than with a walker. If there are any concerns that an injury might occur from the child's frequent falling, the use of a helmet should be encouraged to avoid head injuries. Practice falling should be strongly encouraged and rehearsed under the guidance of a physical therapist in a safe therapy environment.

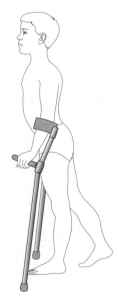
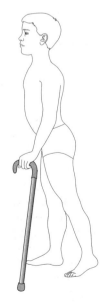

Maintenance and care: All crutches and canes should have rubber tips where they contact the floor to prevent slipping. These rubber tips should be inspected frequently to make sure that they have not worn through; as soon as there is significant wear and the rubber starts slipping, the tips should be replaced. Every six months while the child is still growing, the length of canes and crutches should be evaluated by the therapist or physician who is following the child so that adjustments appropriate to the child's growth can be made. Most crutches and canes have a fixed life expectancy of two to three years, especially if they are used heavily by an active child. As soon as connections become loose or start to slip, the device should be repaired or replaced.

Cyanotic Extremities
(blue hands, blue feet)

Cyanosis is characterized by skin that is light to dark blue in color and somewhat cool. This blue discoloration may be due to poor oxygen saturation in the blood and may indicate heart and lung trouble. In the child with cerebral palsy, cyanosis in the hands and feet is almost always due to poor regulation of blood flow rather than to heart or lung problems.

Because of nervous system difficulties and poor circulation, the extremities are often cold to the touch and can show marked changes in color. These circulatory problems are not the same as those seen in individuals with diabetes or cardiac abnormalities or in elderly individuals. The feet of the individual with CP should be kept as warm as possible with appropriate socks and shoes. They are not at risk for skin breakdown due to this poor circulation. In the child with cerebral palsy, these changes in color and temperature are only cosmetic and do not cause discomfort for the child. Except for making sure that the feet don't get too cold, there should be no other restrictions or concerns.

Decubitus ulcers
(bedsores)

Decubitus ulcers, or bedsores, are breaks in the skin that occur due to pressure or friction over areas of bony prominences. The most common sites for these ulcers are over the sacrum, or tailbone area, from lying or sitting; over the ischial tuberosities, or the prominences on the bottom of the pelvis, where one puts most of the pressure when sitting; or over the side of the hip, from lying on one side too much. Other places that may develop ulcers are over prominent areas of metal rods or plates that have been used to correct alignments of bones. Also, the bony areas about the ankle or knee can occasionally

develop skin breakdown. Bedsores are caused by lying in one position for too long.

The best treatment for decubitus ulcers is prevention. Prevention requires that the skin be inspected daily. Any areas that are red or appear to be developing increased pressure need to be carefully protected. This means these areas should be carefully padded to avoid pressure and that the position in which the child is lying needs to be avoided. In prevention, the most important element is the length of time involved. In other words, while a child lying on an area at risk for developing skin breakdown may be able to do so safely for five minutes, if the child lies on this area for eight hours during sleep, skin breakdown will occur rapidly.

If the breakdown has started, then the primary treatment is to keep the area clean and dry and avoid placing pressure on it. This may mean lying in a different position or avoiding sitting, if that was the cause. Often, changes in wheelchairs or mattresses are necessary. Careful attention must be paid to the seating system when this problem starts to occur. Pressure mapping may be used to assess the child he is seated in his wheelchair.

If the skin breakdown becomes very deep (which occurs only rarely), using special medicated creams and avoiding pressure on the area sometimes will allow the wound to heal. Some deep wounds need surgical treatment, which involves removing all of the dead tissue and adding new tissue with a good blood supply. This procedure is usually performed by a plastic surgeon.

Children with cerebral palsy usually have good sensation and are at low risk for developing decubitus ulcers. However, children who have more severe involvement and are very thin may have prominent bones and are thus at high risk, especially if they are wearing a cast or if they are very ill and lack their normal ability to move or respond. For such children, it is essential that the caregiver inspect the skin every day during bathing and diapering to make certain that no skin breakdown is occurring.

Deep Brain Stimulation
(DBS)

Deep Brain Stimulation (DBS) is a technique in which a wire electrode is surgically implanted in the brain to control unwanted movements such as dystonia, athetosis, or mixed movement disorders. This technique was developed and is most widely used for progressive neurological conditions like Parkinson's disease and congenital dystonia. Over the past 10 years a few centers have tried to use this technique in people with nonprogressive but difficult to manage movement disorders, mainly those with CP or adult-type brain injury. After the wires are implanted in the brain, they are connected to a pacemaker that is implanted in the upper chest, similar to a cardiac pacemaker. The electrical dose can then be adjusted to get the best result in terms of decreased movement and better function. It usually takes 6 to 12 months to arrive at the optimal electrical dose.

Although good results have been reported in several cases, the results in persons with cerebral palsy have been uniformly less dramatic than in people with congenital dystonia or Parkinson's disease. At this time DBS can be considered an option for very difficult to manage movement disorders in children with CP. However, there are not good data to guide decisions about which patients might benefit most or at what age. The implantation requires drilling a hole in the skull and placing the wires directly into the brain. In children with CP, where to place the wires is not clear at this time. Because of the very significant complication risks and many unknown factors, DBS should be considered only in the most difficult cases and only after all oral medications and the intrathecal baclofen pump have been tried. It is possible to use the baclofen pump and DBS at the same time.

Developmental Delay

A child whose development is behind that of the standard population is experiencing developmental delay. The delay may be in physical development (such as the ability to walk), in cognitive development (such as the ability to recognize shapes or stack blocks), or in language (both in speaking and in understanding language).

Many children who are developmentally delayed at a young age eventually develop physically and cognitively, so that by the time they enter school they are within the developmental norm. Thus, the term *developmental delay* does not generally imply a permanent condition. When properly used, the term indicates that there is some expectation that the individual may eventually reach normal developmental milestones. When the developmental lag continues into late childhood, then developmental delay should not be used as a diagnosis; instead, a specific diagnosis such as *cerebral palsy* or *cognitive impairment* should be applied.

Developmental Disability

Any disability during childhood that impacts on the child's normal development is considered a developmental disability. This is a very broad category that includes such diverse diagnoses as autism, cerebral palsy, cognitive impairment, and genetic conditions associated with delays (such as Down syndrome).

Developmental Dysphasia

The development of language and speech is delayed in many children with cerebral palsy. When this delay is due to neurological problems originating in the brain, it is termed *developmental dysphasia*. This is a common problem in children with athetoid pattern cerebral palsy. It is treated with speech-language therapy and augmentative communication.

Developmental Milestones

The typical development of a child includes a specific growth process that involves progress reaching specific milestones. A child's development is assessed in terms of when he or she reaches these milestones. These include a child's ability to crawl, to walk, to understand what is said to him or her, and to speak in sentences.

In a child with CP, however, the typical developmental milestones are often delayed. The specific age at which developmental milestones are reached is unique to each child with cerebral palsy. It is very difficult to predict how rapidly these developmental milestones will be reached or even whether they will be. (See Chapter 2 for an overview of child development.)

Diplegia
(paraplegia, bilateral cerebral palsy)

Diplegia and *paraplegia* are terms used to describe children with cerebral palsy who have difficulty using their legs. Generally the term *diplegia* is applied to children with cerebral palsy who, in addition to the leg problems, have some difficulty with upper body control, including use of their arms and fine motor skills. If the motor problem is secondary to a spinal cord injury or spina bifida, the term generally applied is *paraplegia*, which means that the child has minimal or no limitation of the arms above the area of injury. Most children with diplegic cerebral palsy walk either independently or with assistive devices, such as crutches or a cane. A more recent term preferred by some is *bilateral cerebral palsy*, which implies that both sides of the body have involvement. (See Chapter 6 for more details regarding diplegia.)

Discretionary Trust

This is a legal term. It means that the trustee (the person responsible for a trust) has the authority or the ability to use the funds from the trust toward the goals outlined in the definition of the trust. Specifically, the parent who has a discretionary trust in his or her child's name may

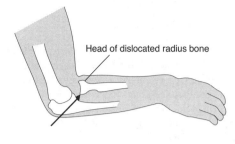

Head of dislocated radius bone

be required to use funds from that trust for the care and benefit of the child, but the parent is given the discretion to decide what constitutes care and benefits for their child.

Dislocation, Elbow
(radial head dislocation)

Dislocation of the whole elbow is rare in children with cerebral palsy but does occasionally occur in a child who has an extremely severe spastic pattern and whose function is limited. Although the dislocation causes a cosmetic deformity, usually the arm can easily be placed into a sleeve. An isolated radial head dislocation, in which the small bone just below the elbow becomes dislocated, is much more common. This deformity has the appearance of a lump on the outside of the elbow and may limit bending, but not enough to prohibit driving a wheelchair or using eating utensils. There is also significant limitation in the degree to which the hand can be turned palm up. Because the deformity is subtle, often these dislocations are not noticed for many months, sometimes years, and when they are noticed they are usually functionally well compensated for by the child.

Generally, the disability caused by a dislocated elbow is so minimal that risking a surgical procedure is not warranted. In the late teenage years or early adulthood, if pain develops from the dislocated radial head, it can be removed surgically, ending the pain while not limiting motion. After surgery, the elbow should be splinted for three weeks, and a program of gentle range of motion exercises should be completed. Complications from the surgery are rare, but there may be some persistent pain and a small loss of movement.

Dislocation, Hip
(spastic hip subluxation, spastic hip dislocation, acquired hip dislocation, congenital hip dislocation, migration index, Reimer's migration index, developmental hip dislocation, CDH, DDH)

The terms *congenital hip dislocation* and *developmental dislocation of the hip* (DDH) refer to conditions in which the hip has already started to come out of the joint or is already out of the joint when the child is born. If these conditions are treated early and aggressively with splinting, usually a normal hip develops and is functioning perfectly by 6 to 9 months of age. If the hip dislocation is discovered later in a child's life, it can be quite a difficult problem, often requiring surgery, especially if it is not discovered until 18 months of age or later.

The exact causes of congenital hip dislocation are not known, but evidence suggests it is related to the mother's pelvic anatomy, family history, and especially how the child is lying in utero. These factors are further influenced by how the child is positioned and cared for as an infant.

Congenital hip dislocation is an entirely different condition from the hip dislocation developed by children with cerebral palsy. It is possible for a child with CP to have congenital hip dislocation as well. Usually, though, hip dislocation related to CP occurs in middle and late childhood, from age 2 to 10 years. Almost always these children have normal hips until 18 to 24 months of age, but then, under the influence of bone growth and short, spastic muscles, the ball of the hip joint is gradually pulled out of the socket. The process occurs slowly, taking from many months to years.

There are many different terms for hip dislocation in children with cerebral palsy. The most widely used is *spastic hip dislocation* because this term conveys the idea that spasticity causes the dislocation. Another widely used term is *acquired hip dislocation*, which distinguishes it from congenital hip dislocation—*congenital* implying that the child is born with the problem.

The term *subluxation* means that the hip joint is partially out of the socket but still in contact with it. Because this is a slow process, a child's hip goes from being a normal or reduced hip to a subluxated hip, and at the point of severe subluxation the ball moves completely away from the socket. It is then dislocated.

Indications: Spastic hip dislocation is a common and physically disabling muscle and bone condition in children with cerebral palsy. The first signs of hip subluxation are an increasing spasticity in the legs and the inability to spread the legs. Because hip subluxation cannot be detected by physical examination alone, especially in its early stages, by 2 years of age all children with CP should have an x-ray of their hips. As the child grows or the spasticity gets worse, the legs often become tighter; at some point, it may be difficult to diaper the child because of the tightness. As the hip starts to migrate out of the joint and becomes more subluxated, this tightness generally increases.

Hip dislocation occurs much more frequently in children who are unable to walk, and it progresses more quickly in children who cannot walk. Hip dislocation

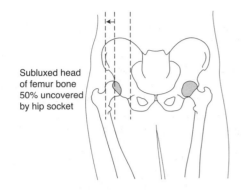
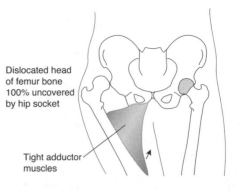

Subluxed head
of femur bone
50% uncovered
by hip socket

Dislocated head
of femur bone
100% uncovered
by hip socket

Tight adductor
muscles

occurs most commonly in children 2 to 8 years old, but it can occur at any age while the child is growing.

By the time the hip has become dislocated, it is extremely tight; often the dislocated leg appears to be shortened. Because of the tight contractures, perineal care, diapering, and wheelchair seating are difficult, especially if both hips are dislocating. During the time in which the hips are becoming subluxated and dislocated, there may be some mild to moderate discomfort for the child, especially when the parents attempt to diaper or bathe the child, which is often the first sign of any problem with the hip. Frequently the child does not indicate discomfort until late in the subluxation phase and perhaps not until the hips are actually dislocating.

After the hips become dislocated, they are no longer in a nice smooth cup, and there begins to be abnormal wear on the end of the bone. Arthritis sets in and over a number of years gradually becomes worse. Children with cerebral palsy who have an untreated dislocated hip can expect a 50 percent or higher chance of developing severe pain from degenerative arthritis by their early twenties. Seating and nursing care are also more difficult. For children who are walking, the pain from arthritis often significantly limits their ability to walk.

Not all children with CP are at equal risk for developing hip subluxation. Children with hemiplegia, except those with severely turned in feet, have almost no risk of developing it, but those with moderate or severe diplegia have approximately a 20 to 25 percent risk of developing hip subluxation or dislocation. Therefore, this group needs to be closely observed. Because these children are walking, hip subluxation or dislocation is especially debilitating for them. As they become young adults, it frequently limits or diminishes their ability to walk. Children with quadriplegia are at the highest risk of developing hip dislocation, with both moderately and severely involved children having a 75 to 80 percent chance of developing this condition.

Hip dislocation in children with cerebral palsy can be avoided by early close monitoring coupled with ap-

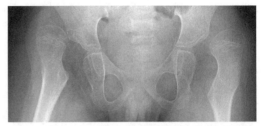

Dislocated hips

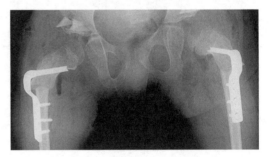

Dislocated hip osteotomy

propriate treatment for the young child, with the goal of the child's having normal hips by the time he is a teenager. Almost all hip dislocations in children with CP are preventable.

Care and treatment: Care and treatment options for spastic hip subluxation in children with cerebral palsy are still somewhat variable but are becoming more standardized. The primary treatment is early detection, and the standard early detection method involves a physical examination and an x-ray of the hips. We recommend that all children with CP who are not able to walk independently (without a walker or crutches) have a hip x-ray once a year from 2 to 8 years of age and every two years from age 8 until they are finished growing. If the x-ray shows more than 30 percent subluxation, surgical treatment or more frequent x-ray follow-up should be considered.

Most experts agree that bracing for the prevention of hip subluxation prior to surgery is not helpful. There is a subgroup of children who do not have spasticity, are extremely floppy, and develop hip subluxation or dislocation. These children have what is called *hypotonic hip dislocation.* They may benefit from bracing to allow the development of normal hips, but even this is uncertain at this point.

The standard measurement of hip subluxation on an x-ray is the *migration index.* It defines how much of the ball of the hip joint has moved out of the socket. Generally children whose migration index is between 30 and 60 percent should be considered for surgery to lengthen the adductor muscles (the muscles on the inside of the thigh). For higher migration indexes or older children, varus osteotomies, or cutting and redirecting the bone, should be considered. These surgical procedures reliably prevent hip dislocation and are far superior to anything available to treat hips that are dislocated and painful. Once the hips have become dislocated and painful,

the treatment requires either resection of the hip joint, which frequently does not alleviate the pain, or a total hip replacement, which is often difficult.

The complications of hip dislocation arise in three areas. Fifty percent of children who develop hip dislocations develop significant and debilitating pain at some point in young adulthood. The treatment of this disabling pain is extremely difficult and unrewarding. The dislocated hip becomes contracted, which often makes nursing care, specifically perineal care and diapering, difficult. Dislocated and contracted hips often put the body in positions that make seating difficult. Although seating difficulties may be addressed with wheelchair modifications, they often continue to present problems. Some dislocated hips cause the pelvis to tilt and thus may initiate scoliosis because of the posture required for sitting. Professionals differ on whether a sitting position might cause scoliosis.

Dislocation, Shoulder
(shoulder subluxation, shoulder instability)

Shoulder dislocation means that the shoulder is coming out of its joint. The humerus is the bone in the upper arm that can completely come out of its socket at the shoulder joint. This is a fairly common occurrence in teenagers and is frequently associated with athletic injuries. Children with cerebral palsy who have significant spasticity and have vigorous physical therapy for mobilization of the shoulder can suffer a shoulder dislocation as a result of aggressive therapy. Picking up children who have abnormal muscle control by their arms can also cause a dislocation; children should be picked up by the chest instead. Another group of children with CP who have frequent trouble with shoulder dislocations are those with significant athetosis, whose movements involve pulling the arm out and back. These movements stretch out the shoulder joint capsule, as well as the muscles that hold the bone in joint.

Children with cerebral palsy who have shoulder dislocations often have specific postures that lead to the dislocations. One common posture particularly in children with significant athetosis is holding the arm overhead during sleep. If the circumstances under which the shoulder dislocates are removed, the joint will frequently tighten up again and resolve without further treatment. The caregiver should consider tying the child's pajama sleeve to a waist belt if the shoulder is dislocating during sleep. During waking hours, it may be necessary to use straps to hold the arm down by the side, especially if athetosis is part of the problem. Keeping the arm in place may also be accomplished by placing lead weights in the arm sleeve to keep the arm on a wheelchair tray. If there is sufficient muscle control, working with exercises

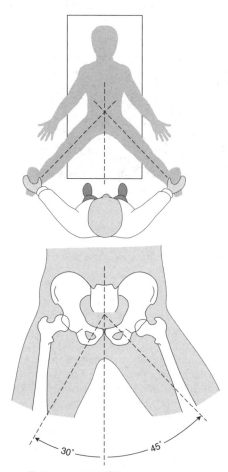

Tight muscles if <45° leg spread on each side

to strengthen the muscles that pull the arm down to the side of the body and to the midline are helpful.

Shoulder dislocations are seldom significant long-term problems for children with cerebral palsy. Usually the discomfort is minor and temporary, and when the activity has been eliminated for a period of time, the dislocation is resolved. It is uncommon for a shoulder to become dislocated and stay dislocated; in those cases in which it does remain dislocated, the shoulder is not usually painful. However, the shoulder should not be left in a dislocated position if it can easily be corrected. In the rare cases in which recurrent dislocations become painful, the muscles around the shoulder joint should be surgically tightened. Surgery to reduce a dislocated shoulder should only be considered if the shoulder is painful.

Disorders of Cellular Migration
(schizencephaly, lissencephaly [agyria], macrogyria, micropolygyria)

During the first seven months of fetal life, the brain and central nervous system undergo both growth of new cells and migration of these cells to their correct location. Failure of these cells to reach their proper location results in various abnormalities of the brain that are termed *disorders of cellular migration*. They can cause cerebral palsy.

The failure of brain cells to migrate correctly can be caused by chromosomal defects, fetal alcohol syndrome, or fetal hydantoin syndrome (the exposure of the fetus to hydantoin or Dilantin, a medication used to treat epilepsy in the pregnant mother). However, most cases have no known cause.

There are a number of types of defects in this cat-

egory. They can be distinguished on CT scans or MRI of the brain. One type of migrational disorder is schizencephaly, characterized by clefts within the brain extending from the surface of the cortex to the underlying ventricles. The region of the brain that has a cleft is usually underdeveloped. This can result in cognitive impairment and/or cerebral palsy, specifically hypotonia (decreased muscle tone—see Floppy Infant), hemiparesis (weakness of one side of the body), or spastic quadriplegia (affecting all four limbs), and may be accompanied by seizures and microcephaly.

Another type of migrational disorder is lissencephaly (or agyria), which literally means "smooth brain." The surface of the brain ordinarily has indentations called gyri. Their absence results from defects that prevent the migrating nerve cells from reaching their proper location. In about half the patients, lissencephaly is characterized by severe cognitive impairment, marked hypotonia, and microcephaly. Seizures tend to be difficult to control.

Other types of migrational defect include macrogyria, in which the indentations on the surface of the brain are very coarse and too few, and micropolygyria, in which the brain has an excess of indentations, which are both too small and too numerous. Macrogyria clinically resembles lissencephaly but is usually unilateral. The clinical picture in micropolygyria is one of cognitive impairment and spastic or hypotonic CP.

Double Hemiplegia

The term *double hemiplegia* is used to describe children who have a weakness in all four limbs, with more involvement on one side of the body than on the other. It is also applied to children who have more arm involve-

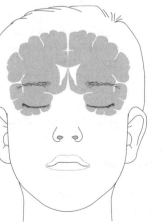

Normal, bumpy brain with gyri

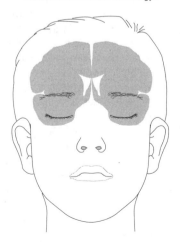

Smooth brain surface without gyri

ment than leg involvement. The use of this term can be confusing. In general, *double hemiplegia* as a term for a pattern of involvement should be avoided, and more specific terms such as *quadriplegia, diplegia,* or *hemiplegia* should be used. The current favored terms are *unilateral CP* if it involves one side of the body and *bilateral CP* if it involves both sides.

Drooling
(sialorrhea)

Drooling, or sialorrhea (which is the medical term for drooling), results from a lack of coordination of the oral, facial, and neck muscles. An extremely common problem in younger children with cerebral palsy, it may improve as a child grows. Drooling causes the face to be frequently wet and often results in wet clothing as well. Many parents use colorful bandanas or bibs around the neck to keep clothing dry, changing them throughout the day as they become wet.

Although bibs keep the child's clothes dry, they do not protect the face and chin from getting wet. Wetness can cause chapped facial skin, especially in cold weather. As the child gets older and goes to school, drooling often becomes a barrier to social interaction with other children.

Treatment: The first level of treatment is behavioral. Some children can be taught to swallow their saliva more often or to wipe their mouth with a tissue or an armband when they begin to drool.

The next level of treatment should be directed at the child's sitting posture. The child should be in a well-supported seat so that his head does not droop forward. If his head is tilted back, he will drool less. Attention to good oral hygiene and correcting severely malaligned teeth, which may prevent the mouth from closing comfortably, is important. Elimination of very large tonsils and adenoids, which may prevent the child from swallowing his secretions, is occasionally necessary.

Some medications that cause the child to become drowsy or increase secretions may make drooling worse. These medications might be discontinued if there has been a significant increase in drooling and it's safe to discontinue them. Biofeedback mechanisms in which the saliva triggers a switch that causes some unpleasant effect for the child, such as turning off his television, can be used to help control drooling. Studies of biofeedback suggest, however, that it only works when the biofeedback mechanism is in place and does not have any carryover effect.

Medications are often the next step. A variety of medications called anticholinergics have been used to successfully reduce drooling. These include glycopyr-

rolate (Robinul), atropine (Saltropin), benztropine (Cogentin), hyoscyamine (Levsin), and the scopolamine patch (TransdermScop). They have similar potential side effects, including constipation, urinary retention, behavioral changes, and facial flushing. Glycopyrrolate appears to have the lowest frequency of behavioral effects. Another medication is botulinum toxin (Botox), injected directly into some but not all of the salivary glands. This has been shown to be effective for up to 24 weeks after injection. Only minor side effects were seen, such as temporary pain while swallowing, but the injection is done under sedation, which has risks of its own. Repeated injections of Botox sometimes result in the glands no longer producing saliva, so that the injections can be stopped.

Surgery may be indicated for children who continue to have significant problems after the above attempts to control drooling have been exhausted or who experience significant side effects from the medications. Most of the surgical procedures to control drooling tie off some of the salivary gland ducts, reroute the drainage ducts from the glands to the back of the throat, or cut the nerve of the glands. These minor surgeries are usually done by ear, nose, and throat surgeons or by oral surgeons. As is true for Botox injections, not all the glands are removed or tied off, because the child needs some moisture in his or her mouth.

The major complication of surgery is that in some children its benefits are only temporary, and the child will begin to drool again. In rare instances, the child's mouth becomes too dry, which is uncomfortable and can also lead to dental caries (cavities).

Due Process Hearing

A due process hearing is a legal procedure established by Public Law 94-142 to allow the resolution of disputes arising between parents and their "special needs" children, on one side, and the educational system, on the other. The law allows for a hearing before an impartial person to review the identification, evaluation, placement, and services given the disabled child.

Dysarthria

Dysarthria is a term used for people who have difficulty with their speech, specifically pronouncing (articulating) words. This condition is especially common in children with athetosis. Sometimes spasticity also affects the vocal cords and causes dysarthria, and there is a dystonic type of dysarthria as well. Many adults who have dysarthria find it to be the most disabling impairment because it makes communication so difficult.

Because speaking is such an integral part of relating to others, any speech problem can make relating to others more difficult. People with dysarthria often find that others presume they have cognitive limitations because their speech cannot be understood. It is important to encourage them to confront this assumption and explain to others that their speech difficulty does not mean that they don't understand what is said but rather that they have problems forming the words to respond. All efforts should be made to teach the child to communicate as effectively as possible; for many children this may mean using an augmentative communication device, such as a speech synthesizer, or using writing, if their hand function is adequate.

Treatment involves speech-language therapy to assist in learning better articulation. In patients with dystonia the small muscles in the larynx may be injected with botulinum toxin.

Dyslexia

Dyslexia is a condition that interferes with a person's ability to read. It may involve the cognitive inability to recognize letters, difficulty in seeing the letters because of visual problems, or difficulty with processing visual information, such as the orientation of the letters.

Dyslexia is relatively common in children with cerebral palsy who are otherwise cognitively normal. It may involve some difficulty with information processing in the brain, or it may be related to motor coordination problems with their eyes. For many children there may be some combination of both. It is important that this disability be recognized by the educational system, which can usually structure an educational program to accommodate and/or remediate the learning difficulties.

Dysmetria

Dysmetria is poor coordination of the hands. The inability to follow a line or to write smoothly is a characteristic of dysmetria; indeed, a child first notices it when he is unable to stay within the lines when coloring. The condition may improve into late childhood or early adolescence, especially when aided by occupational therapy for fine motor control. Dysmetria can be commonly found in children with CP whose fine motor function is affected.

Dysphagia

Dysphagia is difficulty feeding. Just as a person with cerebral palsy may have abnormal posturing of the head and upper body and motor disturbances of the face, lips, and tongue, she can have abnormal mobility of the throat muscles that can impair her ability to eat. Dys-

phagia is more often seen in people who also have other problems with face and tongue control, including speech problems and drooling, and in those who have severe cognitive impairment.

People with dysphagia may have chronic respiratory infections, such as recurrent pneumonias, wheezing, or repeated bouts of upper respiratory infections (sometimes called bronchitis). Others may show signs of coughing and choking when eating, especially when drinking liquids, because liquids are more difficult to swallow than pureed foods or thickened liquids.

Addressing the problem of dysphagia for the child with cerebral palsy involves identifying the food textures the child can handle best, the best position for feeding, and any adaptive equipment needed to promote safe feeding. It may be necessary to thicken liquids or avoid food textures that may be difficult to handle. Different eating strategies should be evaluated and prescribed by a speech-language therapist. In some children with severe dysphagia it may be necessary to stop oral feeding and introduce a gastrostomy tube.

Early Intervention
(infant stimulation)

Early intervention means providing therapy for a child who is not reaching her normal developmental milestones. Children qualify for such services by demonstrating greater than a 25 percent delay in one or more areas of development. The types of services provided by early intervention programs vary. They can include helping parents care for their child's specific developmental needs, such as difficulty using utensils, feeding problems, or difficulty walking. Therapists work with parents to show them how to help their child develop her speech capabilities, or how to provide extra support to a child who is struggling with a specific disability. Early intervention is usually provided by a team that includes physical, occupational, and speech-language therapists; nurses; and physicians experienced in dealing with children with developmental delays.

Frequently, children with cerebral palsy have motor difficulties that preclude their developing normal movements as they grow. A 9-month-old child with CP who is still completely immobile continues to be very dependent upon others to stimulate him. Infant stimulation therapy is directed at providing the increasingly complex stimulation that the developing child needs. It often involves play therapy, providing the child with different sitting positions, movement, and visual stimulation. Another important component of infant stimulation therapy is working with the caregivers or parents of a child with CP and encouraging them to continue the stimulation process as part of their care at home.

Benefits and risks: The benefit of early intervention is the improved stimulation of the child by a team that continues to evaluate the child's progress. This includes close monitoring of the child's feeding, physical, language, and cognitive skills. A risk of early intervention can be seen in children who are medically fragile and unable to tolerate the significant degree of stimulation that early intervention may provide. Early intervention needs to be provided by a team approach with case management available so parents are not overwhelmed by many different professionals, some of whom may give different messages to the parents.

Early intervention usually continues until the child is 3 years of age, at which time he or she moves into a more formal educational setting.

Endoscopy

Endoscopy is the introduction of a thin, lighted tube into an area of the body in order to inspect it and sometimes to collect samples. For example, endoscopy may be performed by a gastroenterologist interested in inspecting various parts of the gastrointestinal system, either from above (an upper endoscopy) by introducing a tube through the mouth or from below (a lower endoscopy) by introducing a tube through the anal sphincter. An upper endoscopy may consist of esophagoscopy (inspection of the esophagus), gastroscopy (inspection of the stomach), and duodenoscopy (inspection of the duodenum, which is the first part of the small intestine). Lower

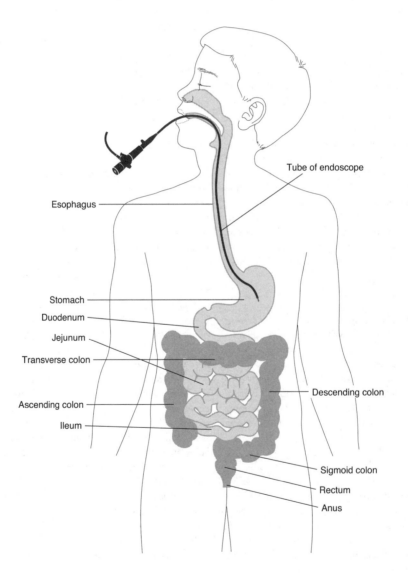

Tube of endoscope

Esophagus

Stomach

Duodenum

Jejunum

Transverse colon

Ascending colon

Ileum

Descending colon

Sigmoid colon

Rectum

Anus

endoscopy may consist of anoscopy (inspection of the anus), sigmoidoscopy (inspection of the sigmoid colon, which is the lowest part of the colon, just before it exits at the anus), or colonoscopy (inspection of the large intestine or colon).

During these procedures the physician is able to inspect the designated inside part of the body and record the findings on videotape or with photographs. Biopsies of the inspected tissue may be taken or samples for culture obtained. In addition, procedures such as the removal of a polyp or growth can be done via lower endoscopy, and placement of a percutaneous gastrostomy tube can be done via upper endoscopy, thus avoiding surgery.

Indications: The most common indication for upper GI endoscopy is concern about an ulcer or stomach acid refluxing into the esophagus. Another indication is the possibility that an infection is causing pain in the abdomen. The common indication for lower endoscopy is to evaluate blood in the stool.

Benefits and risks: The benefit of endoscopy is that in most children it can be performed with heavy sedation. If major internal procedures are to be performed, such as removal of a polyp or placement of a gastrostomy tube, general anesthesia is required. The risks, however, are much less than would be required for open surgery, and the recovery period is shorter.

Maintenance and care: After the procedure the child needs to recover from the sedation. It is often several hours before he is comfortable enough to start feeding.

Epilepsy Surgery

Epilepsy is common among children with cerebral palsy, especially children with hemiplegia. Antiepileptic drugs, the ketogenic diet, or the vagal nerve stimulator will be successful in stopping seizures in many children, but when none of these modalities is successful, uncontrolled seizures may delay development, interfere with education, and disrupt the lives of the child and the family. In such circumstances a variety of surgical options deserve consideration.

When seizures can be determined to arise in a restricted part of the brain, surgical removal of that portion may offer a cure. The process for identifying the location in the brain where seizures arise is complex, and confirmation based on two or more kinds of evidence is required. The initial steps are electroencephalography (EEG) and magnetic resonance imaging (MRI). EEG is a recording of the electrical activity of the brain with electrodes on the scalp. EEG can locate areas of brain irritability where seizures arise, and patients who are

being considered for surgery are often admitted for prolonged EEG recordings to capture the electrical activity of seizures themselves. High-detail MRI of the brain can identify areas of brain injury or abnormal brain development that may give rise to seizures. Another useful confirmatory test is positron emission tomography (PET) scanning. PET scanning provides pictures of the energy consumption in various regions of the brain. Between seizures, epileptic regions of the brain show lower energy consumption than do healthy regions and can be identified by PET. During a seizure, higher energy consumption is seen. Psychological testing can sometimes provide additional evidence about the site of the development of seizures, and it is necessary as well for assessing the potential benefits and risks of surgery.

For some children this evaluation is enough to support a confident recommendation for surgery, but in other cases more information may be needed. Precise identification of the site of the onset of seizures may require recording the electrical activity on the very surface of the brain. Identification of critical brain regions responsible for movement and speech may require direct stimulation, a process called *brain mapping*. When such needs arise, a preliminary operation is performed to lay a grid of electrodes on the brain's surface. Afterwards, in the epilepsy monitoring unit of the hospital, antiepileptic drug therapy may be reduced or stopped to allow a small number of seizures to emerge for recording. When over the course of several days all the vital information has been collected, the patient returns to the operating room for removal of the electrode grid and for the planned surgery to control the epilepsy.

There is not just one operation for epilepsy. Surgery must be planned carefully for each individual patient on the basis of the information collected in the presurgical evaluation. In a child with hemiplegic cerebral palsy, an operation to remove or to disconnect the damaged half of the brain can eliminate seizures without causing any new neurological disability. This operation is called *hemispherectomy* (removal) or *hemispherotomy* (disconnection). Other children may require removal of a limited portion of the brain that is causing seizures because of abnormal development or past injury. Most often the temporal lobe is involved, but abnormal brain development can affect any region of the brain.

If seizures arise in more than one region of the brain, or if the location of the origin of seizures cannot be determined, an operation that separates the two halves of the brain can be of great benefit. The large bundle of nerve fibers connecting the two halves of the brain is the corpus callosum, and the operation is *corpus callosotomy*. It can be very helpful for children whose seizures take the form of drop attacks, sudden falls to the floor that often result in injury, or in generalized tonic seizures, which are seizures in which the whole body becomes stiff.

A child who has had surgery for epilepsy spends the first hospital night in the pediatric intensive care unit to ensure comfort and safety. Parents can stay with the child. Transfer to a regular nursing unit is expected on the first postoperative day, and the entire hospital stay may last five to seven nights on average. Return to school is expected within two to four weeks depending upon the type of surgery, but physical education and athletic activity are restricted for at least six weeks to allow the surgical site to heal.

Antiepileptic drug therapy is continued after surgery. Under the supervision of the neurologist, doses are reduced, and medications eliminated, only very gradually over several months based on the child's response to surgery and the EEG. The ultimate goal of epilepsy surgery is to render a child free of seizures on medication without side effects or off medication entirely. This goal cannot be achieved in every case, and the likelihood of achieving this goal depends heavily on the underlying brain condition and the nature of the operation. The neurologist and the neurosurgeon will provide counseling on these matters, and parents must make their decisions carefully.

Esophagitis

Esophagitis is inflammation of the esophagus, the tube that leads from the mouth to the stomach. Esophagitis is often seen in the person with cerebral palsy because of gastroesophageal reflux, the process by which stomach acid comes up into the esophagus.

Since the esophagus cannot tolerate stomach acid, it is very easily damaged, and the result is heartburn, pain, and bleeding. A child with longstanding esophagitis may

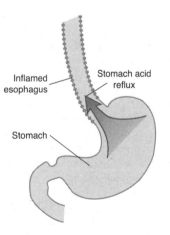

Inflamed esophagus

Stomach acid reflux

Stomach

simply refuse to eat, even if he has previously been a good eater. He may show signs of pain and weight loss, although the site of the pain may not be clear. While acute esophagitis can be treated with medications to ease the inflammation and pain, the underlying cause, such as GE reflux, needs to be addressed in order to relieve the problem for the long term.

Eye-Hand Coordination

Many activities, especially fine motor activities, require being able to get a visual fix on an object and then bring one's hand to that object. This is known as eye-hand coordination. Feeding oneself, for example, requires being able to fix visually on one's food, bring the spoon to the food, and then bring the spoon holding the food into one's mouth. Some children with cerebral palsy have difficulty coordinating daily tasks because they can only perform one of the two required actions: either they can fix visually on an object or they can attempt to bring their hand to an object, but they cannot do both. The lack of eye-hand coordination makes some activities, such as feeding oneself, brushing one's teeth, or using a computer, very difficult.

The treatment for this lack of coordination requires repeated training, usually by an occupational therapist, especially in finding the specific movements or techniques that allow the child to reach for an object while looking at it. Optimal seating is very helpful, especially systems that provide maximum trunk and head control.

Failure to Thrive
(FTT)

A child who is not gaining enough weight is said to be failing to thrive. By definition, a child whose weight is below the fifth percentile for his age and gender or a child whose weight crosses more than two major percentile groups (such as from above the 50th to below the 25th percentile) over a relatively short period of time is recognized by physicians as having trouble growing. A cause of failure to thrive can be almost any illness or condition of childhood, although it often reflects insufficient caloric intake. A child with cerebral palsy often does not grow adequately because he is unable to take in enough calories, mainly due to some of the swallowing problems that many children with CP have.

Before failure to thrive can be treated, the cause must be identified. In the case of a child with CP, the investigator needs to compile a careful record of how much the child eats. Often the parents keep a diary in which they record all the foods eaten by the child over several days. A nutritionist can calculate the average number of calories per day, as well as specific minerals and vitamins that the child consumed. In addition, for many children with CP a feeding evaluation by a speech-language therapist may be helpful in identifying specific textures or liquids that the child has trouble swallowing. These may be causing the child to gag, or the child may actually be aspirating into his lungs, causing respiratory problems.

Treatment modalities may include the use of high-calorie foods (for example, whole milk, butter, or oil), commercial nutritional supplements; the elimination of liquids or certain textures that may be difficult for the child to swallow; or the placement of a feeding tube, either to supplement what the child can eat by mouth or to take over feeding the child who can no longer be safely fed by mouth.

Familial Spastic Paraplegia (FSP)
(hereditary spastic paraplegia [HSP])

Although this is not a type of cerebral palsy, children with familial spastic paraplegia resemble children with spastic diplegic CP in having spasticity and increased reflexes in their legs. They often are delayed in walking. The way they walk looks much like the way children with diplegia walk. The spectrum of disability is wide, from exceedingly mild to severely involved—to the point where some young adults may need a wheelchair. The genes responsible for several forms of FSP have been identified, and more will likely be identified in the future. FSP is a descriptive diagnosis of a genetically diverse group of disorders. While patients within this group experience similar symptoms, the genetic causes differ. Researchers have reported autosomal dominant, autosomal recessive, and X-linked recessive inheritance patterns for this disorder. Genetic counseling is strongly recommended for families with this condition.

The treatment program is the same as that for spastic diplegic cerebral palsy, although children with spastic paraplegia have some risk of deteriorating function. For this reason, they may not make as much progress as the average child with diplegia. Some children, however, experience almost no deterioration over time. Spastic paraplegia is more common than many people realize; many children who are thought to have standard diplegic CP in fact have this inherited condition, but since they are the only ones in their families, familial spastic paraplegia is not suspected. It goes without saying that familial spastic paraplegia should be strongly considered as a diagnosis if two children in the same family have spastic diplegia or if a parent with spastic diplegia has a child with similar symptoms.

Femoral Anteversion
(in-toeing gait)

Femoral anteversion is a term that describes a twisted femur, or thighbone, with the knee turned in relative to the hip joint. This common twist is present at the time of birth; under the influence of normal muscle pull and walking in the early childhood years it slowly corrects itself. Children with spastic muscles, however, do not develop normal muscle pull; as a consequence this rotational malalignment is *not* corrected with growth.

An early sign of this condition is the child who prefers to "W-sit," that is, to sit with her legs in the W-position. There is no evidence that W-sitting causes femoral anteversion or that W-sitting causes any harm or prevents a naturally occurring correction of the anteversion. Thus, there is no reason to prevent the child from W-sitting if that is a comfortable sitting posture for her. In times past, W-sitting was blamed for causing in-toeing and dislocated hips. Now it is generally understood to be just another symptom of increased femoral anteversion and not its cause.

When the child starts walking, the anteversion causes her to walk with her knees and toes pointed inward. Obviously, if the condition is severe, it makes walking difficult. However, there are no braces that can correct this position. Short of surgical correction, continuing with physical therapy gait training as the child develops motor control offers the best chance of improvement.

If anteversion is a major detriment to the child's walking, is preventing her from improving her gait, or at adolescence is continuing to be a significant cosmetic or functional problem, it should be surgically corrected. At whatever age surgery is performed, the correction will most likely be maintained, although a few children develop recurrence. There are three methods of correcting femoral anteversion.

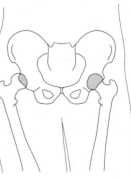

Subluxed head of femur bone 50% uncovered by hip socket

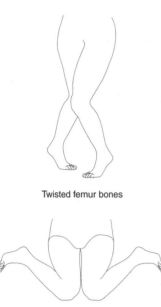

Twisted femur bones

Sitting "W" style

The surgery: Of the three methods of correcting femoral anteversion, the procedure performed at the hip end of the femur is the most significant with respect to surgical time and blood loss. The bone is cut just below the hip joint, and a plate is utilized to hold the osteotomy in place. This procedure allows direct visualization of the bone and the most accurate correction with the fewest possible complications, but it involves implanting a plate, which occasionally needs to be removed after healing. Usually casts are not necessary, and the child can immediately start walking after this correction.

The second method is to operate on the middle of the femur with a surgical saw that cuts the femoral bone from the inside out. A rod is placed to hold the bone in the corrected position. With this surgical procedure, it is hard to measure the exact amount of correction; this method is primarily indicated for adults and is not widely used for children.

The third procedure, which is widely used for children, involves cutting the femur just above the knee and inserting a plate. The outcome for any of these procedures is the same, and the method used depends mostly on the surgeon's preference.

What to expect: No matter which surgical option is chosen, the postoperative care and management usually requires intensive physical therapy. If the correction has been done properly, the knees may point slightly outward, placing the muscles in different positions. Intensive therapy can help the child learn the new gait pattern this calls for.

Femoral Osteotomy
(varus osteotomy, varus derotational osteotomy, hip osteotomy)

Femoral osteotomy is a surgical procedure that is often performed on children with cerebral palsy. The femur (thighbone) is cut, most commonly just below the hip joint, to make a change in the bone that will correct either of two categories of problems: hip dislocation (subluxation) and difficulties with walking.

The surgery: Osteotomies to correct hip subluxation or dislocation involve cutting and repositioning the femur in order to place the ball of the femur more directly into the socket. Often the leg is slightly shortened, which in turn makes the hamstring muscles feel looser. The procedure is usually combined with muscle lengthenings, such as adductor and iliopsoas lengthening in the groin.

The osteotomy performed to improve walking involves turning the leg so that it points in the correct direction, which is especially helpful for children who walk with their legs severely turned in. Some older children may have a hip flexion contracture, which causes them to walk very severely bent forward at the hips. This condition may also be improved by a similar osteotomy and muscle lengthenings.

An osteotomy can be done in many different ways, but it almost always involves implanting a plate to hold and fix the osteotomy. One of the most commonly used plates is a blade plate, which is placed into the bone and fixed with screws. The plate type used depends largely on the surgeon's preference. The operation is usually performed with the patient lying on his back under general anesthesia and can often be done on both right and left legs without any blood transfusions. The incision is made along the outside of the hip joint.

After-surgery care: After a hip osteotomy, with current modern fixation plates such as blade plates no cast is necessary, and children who were walking before the operation are able to get up after recovering from surgery. Undergoing this procedure without any casting makes after-surgery care much easier and rehabilitation much quicker.

After an osteotomy, a child's hips will appear much wider, generally because he started with abnormally narrow hips. In reality, however, they are only slightly wider than normal hips. The wide hips are especially good for children who are sitters, providing them with a wider base. Also, when the child is lying down, both hips should now lie flat, and the knees and feet should point slightly outward, much like a normal child's sleeping position. Getting the rotations correct is difficult; it

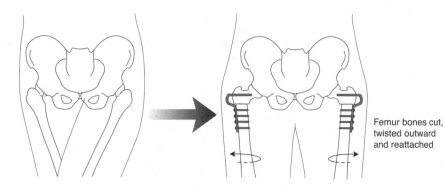

Femur bones cut,
twisted outward
and reattached

Femoral osteotomy

is important to make sure that the child can sit with his legs pointing straight down.

What to expect: Possible complications depend upon the plate that is used. When the plate is properly placed, the likelihood of the realigned bones coming apart is extremely low. However, it is possible that the child may twist his leg and break the bone just below the screws even months or years after the osteotomy has healed, especially if the child has low bone density.

There may be other changes over the long term (from one to five years). The wide hips that the child initially has after the femoral osteotomy gradually become less wide as the child grows. If the child has significant growing to do after the surgery, hip width relative to the width of the trunk decreases significantly. If the child is nearly finished growing, however, hip width does not decrease. In addition, the inward twist of the bone that may have been present usually will not recur in the nearly grown child. The straightening at the hip may return, however, if the child has significant growth time remaining. The child who had this surgical procedure at age 3 or 4 may have a recurrence of the hip subluxation and occasionally needs to have the femoral osteotomy repeated.

Flat Feet
(planovalgus foot deformity)

A person with a flat (or planovalgus) foot has an ankle that rolls in. At its worst the foot turns so much that the sole is not in contact with the floor but is pointed laterally or to the outside. When a child with flat feet walks, her weight bears down on the inside of the foot and on the great toe. This severe condition is unusual, but a mild to moderate flat foot deformity is extremely common in children with cerebral palsy, as well as in the general population. A mild flat foot has no arch and is

very wide. A moderate flat foot is clearly turned out but not to the point where the child walks on the anklebone.

The course of flat feet for a child 2 or 3 years old is difficult to predict, but almost all of them will improve. Some will become completely normal, while others will get better but still have flat feet. Normal children who have flat feet at this early age almost never have pain as they get older, and there are no braces or shoes for which there is documented long-term impact upon this condition. For children with cerebral palsy, the natural progression of flat feet is unpredictable, and there is no evidence that the use of braces or shoe inserts makes the feet better or worse in the long term.

Many children who have mild and moderate flat feet early in life develop better motor control as they get older, and their feet end up looking normal. In some cases the feet reverse and develop the opposite deformity, an arch that is too high. Many young children with CP have moderate flat feet that don't ever change, function well, are pain free, and need no treatment, especially no surgical treatment.

Indications: For other children, mainly at adolescence, the flat feet get worse: as the child gains weight and continues to walk, the foot seems to break down more. Bracing should be tried first, using arch supports in the shoes or AFOs. If the braces cause foot pain, it is much better to discontinue them and allow the child to wear shoes that aren't painful.

If the condition is so severe that walking becomes extremely difficult, and bracing is not tolerated, then surgical correction may be necessary if the child is to continue walking. If surgery is indicated for the child under age 9 or 10 years, the subtalar (or Grice) fusion, which involves fusing the calcaneus and talus bones at the back of the foot, is classically the operation of choice. More recently, a calcaneal lengthening (lengthening the heelbone) has shown promising results in less severely flat feet without the need to fuse joints. The older adolescent child with a more longstanding flat foot is often treated by a multiple arthrodesis, which involves fusing joints in the foot needed to support an arch. Arthrodesis provides a more reliable lifelong correction of the foot. However, it does decrease the mobility of the foot below the ankle joint and may lead to long-term ankle arthritis.

Floppy Infant
(hypotonic infant)

An infant sometimes seems limp or immobile, like a rag doll. Such children are often described as floppy infants. The three main features associated with hypotonia are unusual postures, diminished resistance of the joints to passive movement, and increase in the range of movement of the joints. In the newborn period, such an infant will usually display unusual postures and little active movement. The older infant is delayed in reaching motor milestones.

Hypotonia may be associated with a wide variety of conditions. It may indicate a neuromuscular disorder; it may occur in children who are cognitively impaired; or it may be the manifestation of a connective tissue disorder, a metabolic disorder, or the early phase of cerebral palsy. It may also occur as an isolated symptom in an otherwise normal child, with the symptom eventually disappearing.

The cause of hypotonia can be found anywhere from the brain, to the spinal cord, to the peripheral nerves, to the muscle, to the connective tissues of the extremities. Thus, the list of conditions that can cause hypotonia is a long one. In addition to conditions affecting specific parts of the nervous system, hypotonia can be seen in metabolic, nutritional, or endocrine conditions, such as rickets, hypothyroidism, or renal tubular acidosis. It can be found in genetic disorders such as Prader-Willi syndrome (in which hypotonia is associated with failure to thrive early in life) or Down syndrome. As already mentioned, it can be a part of nonspecific cognitive impairment, of hypotonic CP, or of metabolic disorders such as aminoaciduria or organic aciduria.

Hypotonia can also reflect a basic weakness in the muscle itself, such as is seen in various myopathies or muscular dystrophies. Lastly, it can be a normal transient condition known as benign congenital hypotonia (or essential hypotonia), which eventually disappears. Children with this condition have no underlying muscle weakness, intellectual impairment, or associated disease.

Although many children outgrow hypotonia, some children with cerebral palsy continue to be very floppy throughout their entire lives. Stimulating the child to develop and strengthen her muscles is an important part of treatment. Also, it is necessary to provide excellent supported seating postures to allow her to focus on controlling other parts of her body. For example, caregivers should provide good trunk and body support so the child with hypotonia can focus on head and hand control.

FM System

FM system is one among a wide array of "assistive" devices to help children with hearing loss connect with their sound environment. The FM system consists of headphones, or on occasion a direct link to a hearing aid, connected via a radio (FM) signal to a microphone worn by the speaker. These are typically used in the classroom and ensure that the child receives a consistent acoustic signal. This eliminates the vagaries of poor classroom acoustics and the problem of background noise. Because of this, FM systems have been noted to improve the school performance of children, not just those with hearing loss. They have been used especially to help children with attention deficit disorder focus on what is being said by the teacher.

Fusion, Foot
(subtalar fusion, Grice fusion, triple arthrodesis, planovalgus foot deformity, severe equino varus foot deformity)

A fusion is an operation that causes two bones to grow together to form one bone. In children with cerebral palsy, fusions are commonly performed on four bones in the back part of the foot, predominantly to improve the position of the foot. These individual fusions can be somewhat confusing, but it is important to understand the exact reason for performing them, as well as what motion will be lost after surgery.

Indications: If a child with spasticity has developed severe flat feet or the opposite deformity (a severe foot deformity with a high arch and the foot pointed down), then three joints in the foot are improperly aligned. If the child with severe flat feet is relatively young, the primary problem is between two of these joints. Initially this condition can be braced with a variety of different in-shoe braces such as arch supports or a full-length ankle-foot orthosis (AFO), especially for young children. However, if the child is unable to tolerate the brace or the deformity becomes so severe that he has a great deal of difficulty walking in spite of the brace, a foot fusion is usually necessary.

The surgery: The most common surgical procedure for the child older than 9 years is a subtalar fusion. This involves placing a bone block between the talus bone and

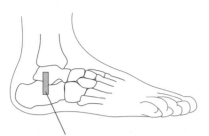

Heelbone fused with talus bone

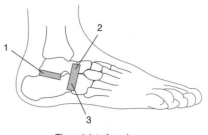

Three joints fused

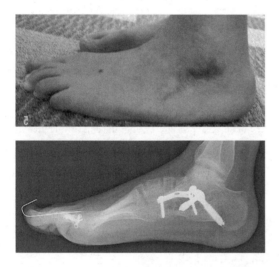

the heelbone in the corrected position. Often a screw is placed across the heelbone and the talus to hold the position. This procedure results in a nicely corrected foot, with only rare failures. In the adolescent with the same severely deformed foot, the multiple arthrodesis may be required for better realignment of the foot and permanent correction. However, the foot can move at the ankle joint. The arthrodesis is fixed with screws and plates to hold its position until bone healing occurs.

After-surgery care: Usually short leg casting, from the toes to the knee, is applied for 6 to 12 weeks. For some or all of this time the child may not be able to step on his foot. This is determined at the time of surgery by the specific surgical procedure performed, the strength of the bones, and the surgeon's experience. After the cast is removed, it usually takes approximately 4 weeks to get used to walking on the foot.

Benefits and risks: The primary complication from the arthrodesis is inadequate correction at the time of the surgery or the failure of one of the joint fusions to heal. Sometimes the metal is prominent and needs to be removed. Over the long term, the fused joint may cause earlier arthritis in the ankle; however, the chance of de-

veloping arthritis is probably less than it would be from walking on the deformed foot for many years.

Although there is the risk of eventual arthritis, the foot will be much more stable and will be able to support the person's weight during standing. These fusions are performed because the feet have a tendency to collapse. The real benefit of a fusion is that it is durable and will not give way over a person's lifetime.

Gait Analysis
(three-dimensional gait analysis, foot pressure measurements, gait videotaping, dynamic EMG analysis)

Gait has been analyzed visually by physical therapists and orthopedic doctors as long as patients with cerebral palsy have been treated. Visual gait analysis involves having the patient walk sufficiently undressed that the whole body can be carefully observed. An experienced physician identifies the major concerns, such as the alignment of the legs, bending of the knees, or toe walking. There are, however, no measurements to take and no numbers to record. For this reason, mechanical gait analysis was developed.

The simplest way to record gait analysis is by using a video camera. The videotape can be viewed in slow motion, forward and backward. The videotape itself can be very helpful for assessing very subtle problems, such as the symmetry of steps, how much knee bend is present, and how the feet are used for standing. The next level of sophistication involves using markers on the body, which allows the physician to measure the angles of joint motion as the child walks. Very simple analyses are two-dimensional, using only one camera. Markers are placed on the joints, and the angles between joints are calculated mathematically. For the child with cerebral palsy, this assessment is too simple and not very useful because of the high potential for error in the assessment.

The more common and most sophisticated analysis is three-dimensional. Reflecting markers are attached at multiple points on the body, and a series of cameras are utilized to record the person's movement patterns. This analysis defines all the joints in three-dimensional space and allows assessment of all joint motions in top-down, side, and front views. In addition, recorders with radio transmission are frequently used to record the activity of the muscle by means of small pads placed over the muscles. This principle is the same as for a cardiogram for the heart. A third component of the evaluation is an instrument in the floor that the child stands on and walks over to record the exact amount of force placed on each leg. An additional device may be inserted into the shoe to help define specifically how the foot surface takes pressure, or foot pressure can be measured by having the child walk barefoot on a walkway. For some children, the amount of oxygen they use for walking is measured by having them wear a mask while they walk.

The full three-dimensional gait analysis with EMG recording, force plate recording, and foot pressure recording yields an enormous amount of quantifiable, permanently recorded information. This information is important for determining specific orthotic prescriptions and making decisions about surgical corrections. The information does not in itself provide immediate answers, however, but must be interpreted by an experienced physician. These analyses can be quite complex and are often open to different interpretations.

After the gait analysis is complete, there is a final interpretation. This interpretation usually includes an assessment of the predominant abnormalities and some recommendation that the physician feels would benefit the child. The presentation includes a series of stick figures that demonstrate the visual appearance of the child's walking pattern and charts and graphs that demonstrate muscle function and the range of joint motion as components of the gait pattern.

Indications: Gait analysis is indicated for a child whose physicians and caregivers are considering a major treatment decision such as surgery. Full three-dimensional gait analysis is often required before surgery, especially if the gait problem is complex. However, if the child has a relatively simple condition, such as an isolated tight tendon, often gait analysis does not provide additional information, and simple videotaping with a standard format is sufficient.

Benefits and risks: Besides the obvious advantage of providing a full and complete analysis of a child's gait pattern, gait analysis also allows physicians to detect unknown problems early on. However, the gait analysis should be performed in a laboratory and interpreted by a physician with experience in treating patients with cerebral palsy. Because some gait analysis laboratories are run by people who, while they may be very experienced in gathering the information, do not have expertise in interpreting the information, a full-service lab with qualified physicians should be located.

Gait analysis is also expensive. The full three-dimensional gait analysis, including joint measurements and a physical examination, usually costs several thousand dollars or more. It is also time-consuming, usually requiring two to four hours. Any gait analysis that costs only a fraction of this amount and takes only about thirty minutes will by definition be much simpler and less complete. The simpler analyses do provide *some* information, but they are not comprehensive, and the laboratories that provide these services vary, so do your homework before enlisting a particular lab's services. There is currently an accreditation system. The most advanced laboratories have Commission for Motion Laboratory Accreditation. These laboratories provide comprehensive and accurate analysis.

What to expect: Gait analyses are often repeated following major surgical procedures, after the child's full rehabilitation has occurred. This usually means that approximately one year after the surgical procedure has been performed, the gait analysis is repeated to measure how much correction was obtained and also to set parameters for continuing to monitor the child. After the child has grown more, often four or five years later, if the deformity recurs, a repeat gait analysis should be performed in anticipation of a new surgical procedure or other major change.

Gastritis
(ulcers, *Helicobacter pylori*)

Gastritis is inflammation of the lining of the stomach, which can sometimes lead to an ulcer. An ulcer is an erosion of the lining of the stomach or the small intestine. Ulcers can cause abdominal pain and bleeding, which then can lead to vomiting of blood or dark "tarry" stools that contain blood that has been digested. Although many thought in the past that gastritis or ulcers were related to increased secretion of stomach acid or emotional upset, we now know that a large percentage are due to a bacterium called *Helicobacter pylori*.

H. pylori infection is best diagnosed by obtaining a stool specimen and testing for the *H. pylori* antigen. The infection may be confirmed by biopsy during an upper endoscopy. A special breath test for urease can be done to diagnose this infection, but this test is not commonly done as a means of diagnosing *H. pylori* infection in children. We do not know how these bacteria get into the body, but it has been suggested that we can pass this infection to one another, as we have seen groups of children that live together in institutions become infected.

Some people have these bacteria in their stomach but do not have any symptoms.

Some other causes of gastritis and/or ulcers are surgery and medications. During the immediate postoperative period, there is a surge in secretion of acid, which can cause inflammation of the stomach. Medications such as steroids, aspirin, and ibuprofen can irritate the lining of the stomach and result in gastritis as well.

Gastroesophageal Reflux Disease
(GERD, reflux)

Gastroesophageal reflux is the process by which stomach contents come up into the esophagus, causing inflammation. These contents may include acid as well as undigested food contents. It is a common problem in young infants and is recognized when babies "spit up" following a feeding. In most infants this problem does not require any treatment. It gradually subsides as children grow and usually disappears by the time they are between 12 and 18 months of age, when they are up and walking about. Many adults experience this problem as "heartburn" after a meal.

In a minority of infants, the problem causes symptoms such as failure to thrive, esophagitis, anemia, and irritability. If the reflux is more severe, the stomach contents may reach the back of the throat and be aspirated into the lungs, causing respiratory symptoms such as wheezing, congestion, or even pneumonia. Treatment includes modification of the infant's position (keeping him upright after feeding and not laying him down for at least 30 to 60 minutes after a meal), modification of the diet (thickening formula with rice cereal), medications, or surgery.

In children with cerebral palsy, GERD is very common and often does not go away by the time the child is 12 to 18 months old. The treatment is the same as noted above, primarily a combination of thickening foods, placing the child in an upright position after meals, and a variety of medications. If severe symptoms continue, especially episodes of pneumonia or chronic wheezing from aspiration, then surgery is often required to control the problem. The procedure, known as a *fundoplication*, can be done either endoscopically or via an open procedure (see Chapter 3 for more details).

Gestational Age
(small, appropriate, and large for gestational age [SGA, AGA, LGA])

Gestational age is the number of weeks of the pregnancy, calculated from the date of the woman's last menstrual period. Forty weeks, with a range of 38 to 42 weeks, is considered full term. A child whose birthweight is within the normal range for that length of pregnancy is considered appropriate for his or her gestational age (AGA). There are growth charts showing the normal expected weight for infants of various gestational ages ranging from very small premature babies to children born at full term. Any infant who is either below (small for gestational age, or SGA) or above (large for gestational age, or LGA) the expected weight may be showing signs of medical problems. For example, a child born to a mother with diabetes may be born LGA, weighing much more than normally expected, and is at risk for a variety of problems associated with being LGA (such as hypoglycemia). A baby born SGA may also be at risk for specific medical problems, such as poor nutrition due to placental insufficiency or an infection suffered in utero. Babies born SGA are usually followed as at risk in early intervention programs, as they have an increased risk for developmental disabilities.

Gingivitis
(gum hypertrophy, plaque)

Enlargement and inflammation of the gums is common in children with abnormal muscle control around the mouth. It may also be increased with the use of certain medications, such as phenytoin (Dilantin). The main cause of this overgrowth is gingivitis, or inflammation of the gums, which is caused in part by lack of routine dental care, such as brushing and flossing. In children with spastic cerebral palsy, such dental care can be very difficult because the child may involuntarily bite down every time something is introduced into the mouth, such as a toothbrush. The main method of preventing gingivitis is to practice good oral hygiene and receive routine dental cleaning every three to six months.

Indications: If the overgrowth becomes large with frequent bleeding when brushing, then surgical removal of the excess gum tissue is usually indicated. This procedure must be done in the operating room under general anesthesia. Often children have to stay in the hospital overnight in case there is excessive bleeding. The main

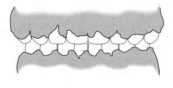

Overgrown, inflamed gums

complication, however, is recurrence if oral hygiene is not maintained.

Another cause of gum inflammation is plaque, a hard tissue that builds up on the base of the teeth. Plaque can cause inflammation and may eventually lead to decay of the base of the tooth, where the tooth is connected to the bone. Good oral hygiene is essential, and some individuals require frequent dental cleaning to control plaque.

Growing Spinal Rods
(Magec Rods)

Growing spinal rods are used for children younger than 9 to 10 years who have developed severe scoliosis and still have significant growth ahead of them. The evolution of this technique has been long, and the current reported outcomes show very high complication rates in children with CP. However, newer developments show some promise. Up to this time most systems implanted the rods and then every 4 to 6 months repeated a surgery to lengthen the rods. This led to high infection rates and bone failure in children with CP due to weak bones and other medical problems. The newer system is implanted and has a magnetic motor (Magec Rod) that can be used to lengthen the rod without surgery in the outpatient clinic. This allows for small, more frequent lengthenings. At this time there is no information on the use of this system in children with CP.

Growth Charts

Growth charts plot the normal growth of a child from birth to age 20. Several organizations, such as the World Health Organization, publish growth charts. The most commonly used in the United States are those published by the National Center for Health Statistics (NCHS). Separate charts are available for boys and girls from birth to age 3 and from age 2 to age 20. These charts plot the weight, length (and later height), and head circumference of the general population and show the distribution of values based on a percentile scale from the 3rd to the 97th percentile. Thus, a child whose weight is at the 5th percentile weighs less than 95 percent of children of his age and gender but is still within the norm, since someone has to be in the lowest 5 percent of the population. A child whose weight places him either below the 5th percentile or above the 95th percentile for his age is considered out of the normal range, and some medical investigation may be indicated.

These charts were generated using healthy children, and many children with CP do fall below the 5th percentile. It is extremely important to continue to monitor the growth of the child with CP even when he is below the 5th percentile for weight, because even more important

than the specific percentile is the progression and the weight gain over time. The child who remains at the 5th percentile over ten years is better off than one who falls from the 50th to the 5th percentile over the same period.

Growth charts for children with cerebral palsy are divided by gender into the five Gross Motor Function Classification System (GMFCS) categories. However, the information for the charts was gathered on children with CP who were fed in a variety of ways and experienced variable growth patterns, so clinicians don't know how helpful these charts may be for your child. The information on these CP growth charts is limited; it does not represent the ideal or even what should be expected for children with CP. Therefore, most clinicians continue to use the NCHS growth charts for typically developing children. For children who are very short for their age, most often those in GMFCS levels IV and V, the ideal weight is based on their height rather than on their age. Those with CP whose function is classified as GMFCS I through III would be expected to have a growth pattern similar to that of typically developing children.

Halitosis
(fetor ex ore)

Halitosis means foul or bad mouth odor. The foul odor may come from the lungs, the stomach, or the nose, although all of these sources are uncommon in children. Most halitosis comes from a source in the mouth—decayed teeth, ulcerated gums, or decomposed food in the mouth because of poor dental care. Children with cerebral palsy may be mouth breathers, which can dry out the mouth. This decreased moisture leads to less cleaning of the mouth tissues and thus to bad breath.

The treatment of halitosis starts with determining the cause. You should begin with a complete evaluation by a dentist, making sure the dentist knows that you are concerned about the child's bad breath. Filling all cavities and correcting gum problems should be the first priority. This needs to be followed by good oral hygiene. If this combination does not work, the dentist may refer you to a physician for a complete medical evaluation. Gastroesophageal reflux is another common cause of bad breath in children, including those with CP. Using antiseptic mouthwash may help for several hours but should not be considered the primary treatment. It can be used on a cloth to wipe the teeth and the inside of the child's mouth.

Hamstring Lengthening
(hamstring transfer, knee flexion contracture, crouched gait, tight hamstrings, hamstring contracture)

The hamstrings are a large muscle group located on the back side of the thigh. They comprise two muscle groups, one on the inside of the thigh, which includes the semi-tendinosus, semi-membranous, and gracilis muscles, and the lateral hamstring group toward the outside of the thigh, which includes biceps muscles. These two groups have a tendency to become tight and contracted and are especially problematic for children who spend most or all of their waking hours sitting. The muscles become tighter as the child grows because of decreased muscle growth due to spasticity.

The major problem these muscles cause for the walking child is crouching while both standing and walking. Often the knees are bent, so that the child's toes or ankle must flex upward. Children who develop severe hamstring contractures because they sit all the time eventually are unable to lie down with their legs straight. Also, when they sit in the wheelchair they pull their feet underneath the seat.

Indications: Hamstring contractures are treated because of a child's problems with walking, sitting, general positioning, and spastic hip subluxation. Hunched posture is another possible indication of the need to lengthen hamstrings. If the muscle in the front of the knee is very tight, it pulls the knee straight; then the tight hamstring rolls the pelvis back, causing the child to sit hunched over. In certain circumstances, the tight muscles may contribute to hip subluxation. In these situations it may be necessary, especially if the child can't stand, to loosen the muscles as much as possible. The main problem in walking for which hamstring lengthening is indicated is a crouched gait.

The surgery: To enable the child to stand up straight, the hamstrings may be lengthened. These lengthenings are usually done behind the knee; occasionally, the tendons are transferred to the femur. Currently, the transfer operation is not favored, because removing tendons often causes hyperextension (the knee bending backward). It is extremely important to be conservative in lengthening the hamstring tendons, because an overlengthened tendon can make walking much more difficult than does an underlengthened tendon. Occasionally the tendons may be lengthened at the buttock through an incision just below the hip. This is done less frequently, because it may allow increased hip flexion. In this case, often the iliopsoas muscle needs to be lengthened on the front of the hip to balance the muscle forces about the hip.

For seating problems, the hamstring muscle may be lengthened either behind the knee or behind the hip. Again, it is important when lengthening behind the knee not to lengthen too much or the knee will be stuck straight out. For problems in lying down, muscle lengthening behind the hip involves making cuts in the muscle and allowing the muscle to slide. Lengthening behind the knee ensures that the major muscles will not be overlengthened so they do not tear completely. This is usually done by cutting the tendinous part of the muscle and allowing it to stretch, although some surgeons make Z-cuts in the tendon, allow it to slide apart, and then suture it together again.

Benefits and risks: The benefits of hamstring lengthening are that the child can sit, stand, and walk more easily. There are two severe complications. The first is overlengthening the hamstrings, so the knees are stuck straight. This makes walking very difficult, and the knees eventually become painful from bending backward. It makes sitting very difficult, because sitting well requires bent knees.

In correcting severe hamstring contractures, stretching of the sciatic nerve may occur, most likely during a second lengthening. Repeat lengthenings are done when a child had a hamstring lengthening four or five years earlier and now with growth has tightened up again and needs another one. Although this is the highest-risk area, if the sciatic nerve does stretch, it is usually only temporary. It may cause some pain and discomfort, occasionally with numbness in the foot, but it almost always resolves.

The more common but much less problematic complication after hamstring lengthening is that the hamstring continues to remain somewhat tight. However, for

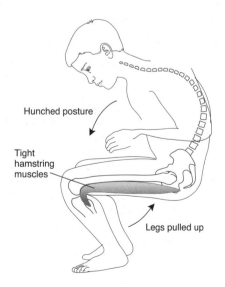

Hunched posture

Tight hamstring muscles

Legs pulled up

patients who are walking, it is much better to continue with a slightly crouched gait than to stand straight with the knee bending backward from overlengthening.

After-surgery care: The usual treatment after hamstring lengthening involves casts, splints, or just physical therapy to gain motion. Most of the time, at least some temporary splinting is used while the muscle heals in a lengthened position. If casts are used, they should not be worn for more than six weeks, as this will increase the possibility of overlengthening.

What to expect: Following the healing phase, continued stretching is important. An intensive period of physical therapy focusing on improving the crouched gait and occasionally using AFOs is necessary. AFOs are helpful interventions aimed at keeping the muscle stretched out while the child is relearning to walk. Additionally, night braces may be used for up to a year.

Hearing Loss
(hearing impairment, auditory evoked potentials)

Several things must happen in order for a person to hear sounds. The sound must get into the ear; the inner ear mechanisms must transmit the sound impulse to the brain; and the brain must be able to interpret what the sound means. At birth, the organs and mechanisms for hearing can be affected or damaged by low oxygen levels, prematurity, infections, or severe jaundice. Hearing loss is more common in children born with a very low birthweight, and the child with cerebral palsy is at much higher risk than the general population for hearing problems. Detection of hearing loss is critical for all children, especially those who show signs of other problems, in particular a delay in speaking. The child with severe neurological impairment may not be responding, and testing hearing will provide important information about the child's function at an early age.

Very young infants or children who can't respond can be tested by otoacoustic emissions and/or auditory evoked potentials. Otoacoustic emissions are sounds produced by the outer hair cells of the organ of hearing (cochlea) and can be measured in the ear canal, indicating cochlear health. These sounds can be evoked and give a picture of cochlear function and hearing level. For the auditory evoked potential, a sound is presented to the ear, and brain waves are recorded. The auditory-evoked potential detects the lowest sound intensity capable of producing a brain wave. This test indicates whether there is an alteration in the ear's ability to perceive sound, but it does not evaluate how the child interprets this sound. Conditions such as intellectual disability and attention deficit disorder may affect the child's

response to the sound. A very young child can also be tested by a well-trained pediatric audiologist if the child can be taught to respond to indicate that he is hearing.

In order for a child to speak normally and learn language, he must be able to hear correctly. Often, a language delay indicates a hearing problem. All children are screened in the newborn nursery. Children with cerebral palsy should have their hearing screened at least one other time, and hearing function needs to be maximized to help the child with CP get the best possible education.

Hemiplegia
(unilateral CP, monoplegia)

Hemiplegia means motor involvement of one arm and one leg on the same side of the body resulting from an injury to the brain. The newer term used by some medical providers is *unilateral CP*. This term is applied to difficulties caused by any injury to one side of the brain, whether the injury is caused by cerebral palsy, a head injury, a stroke, or a tumor. The term *monoplegia* is used for involvement of only one leg or one arm. In reality, this is usually an extremely mild hemiplegia—occasionally a child has such a mild involvement that it affects only one limb. The term *monoplegia* should be reserved for those difficulties caused in one limb by a brain injury and not by nerve injuries such as a brachial plexus palsy.

Hernia
(inguinal hernia, hernia repair, herniorrhaphy, hydrocele)

A hydrocele is a sac with a collection of fluid that comes out of the abdomen from an opening in the abdominal lining, which loops down around the testicles in the male. This opening in the abdominal lining normally closes at the time of birth but frequently does not; a boy who develops an enlarged scrotum or appears to have swollen testicles often has a hydrocele. The fluid flows back and forth from the area around the testicle into the abdomen, so that often the swelling seen in the scrotum increases or decreases depending on the time of the day and how much the child is crying or eating. If the swelling is not too large and the fluid does flow back and forth, there are usually no major problems with the scrotum or abdomen, and for the first six months of life an operation is seldom necessary.

If the abdominal lining opening and sac is large enough that part of the intestine falls down into the scrotum, it is called an inguinal hernia. Like the fluid, the intestine may come down into the scrotum and then disappear again. If this area develops redness, becomes swollen, or becomes very painful, it is an emergency, and a doctor needs to see the child *immediately*—he may have developed a twist in his intestine, which can quickly become life threatening. If the inguinal hernia is present where the intestine descends into the scrotum, it almost never disappears on its own, and a surgical procedure called a herniorrhaphy is necessary. Hernias and hydroceles are very common in children in general, but they are more frequent in children with cerebral palsy.

The surgery: A hydrocele that is present after 6 months of age and continues to be quite large often should be repaired surgically. A hernia in which the bowel descends into the scrotal sac should be removed to prevent entrapment of the intestines in the scrotum, which is a surgical emergency. The surgeries for the hydrocele and the hernia are similar in that a small incision is made in the lower abdomen, the sac that comes out of the abdomen is removed, and the abdomen is closed.

Benefits and risks: There are few complications from this surgery, but occasionally an infection may develop. Symptoms include a raised temperature, loss of appetite, and a very red and inflamed incision. Occasionally the hernia or hydrocele may recur; often all that is needed for it to close up is to draw the fluid out of the sac.

After-surgery care: Hernia repairs are often done as outpatient surgeries, during which the child has a general anesthesia. The child is taken home shortly after he awakens. The pain is usually minimal and easily controlled with Tylenol. The child may be somewhat uncomfortable in certain positions for a week or two but then usually recovers very rapidly. Children who undergo this procedure can be bathed after three or four days, depending upon the specific recommendations of the surgeon.

Hip Muscle Releases
(hip adductor lengthening, adductor lengthening, adductor transfer, iliopsoas release lengthening or transfer, obturator neurectomy, anterior branch obturator neurectomy, proximal hamstring lengthening)

Hip muscle releases include a number of similar operations on the groin to treat problems with walking, spastic hip subluxation, or both. The adductor area, which is the inside of the thigh in the area of the groin, involves a number of muscles. These muscle groups and the nerves that drive them are the primary causes of spastic hip dislocation. They also cause scissoring problems with gait. The many different operations are directed toward balancing the effect of these muscles with that of the far less spastic muscles on the outside of the hip.

Indications: There are three major reasons why children with cerebral palsy may require hip muscle releases. The

first is to prevent hips from dislocating. A child usually under age 8 will be examined, and when the hip muscles are noted to be tight and an x-ray demonstrates mild hip subluxation (the hip moving out of the joint), the spastic muscles should be surgically released. Children between the ages of 3 and 6 are the most likely to need this operation.

The second reason hip muscle release surgery may be necessary is to help a child who is walking but whose feet cross. Because the muscles are tight when the legs are spread apart, they work to keep the feet constantly crossed and tangled while the child is walking. This is a common problem that occurs when children with CP start to walk, but often it resolves itself without surgery. For some children, however, the problem continues, and the surgery is then necessary—mostly commonly between ages 5 and 10.

Third, hip muscles may become so tight and spastic that providing for toileting and perineal care becomes impossible. This is often a problem for young adult women, who find it difficult to take care of their menstrual period. Hip muscle surgery to improve the ability to provide for perineal care is most commonly performed between ages 12 and 20.

The surgery: The most widely used procedure involves lengthening selected groups of the groin muscles, most commonly the adductor longus and the gracilis. Generally these two muscles are completely cut and allowed to retract. They will scar back down again to their underlying muscles. For more severe contractures, partial lengthening of the adductor brevis is indicated. Additionally, cutting the anterior branch of the obturator nerve further weakens the muscles.

It used to be common procedure to cut the entire obturator nerve, but this weakens the muscles so much that frequently the legs become stuck in a spread-open position. Almost all surgeons believe that the posterior branch of the obturator nerve should be preserved. Some surgeons advocate transferring the heads of the adductor longus, gracilis, and brevis muscles more toward the rear to help extend the hip. This is a larger and more difficult operation, and current reports suggest that it is no more effective than a simple release.

The iliopsoas is a large muscle that contributes significantly to problems with gait and spastic hip disease. The most common procedure for releasing this muscle involves cutting the tendon and allowing it to retract. In children with severe involvement who are not going to walk, the goal should be to try to completely prevent the severed tendon from growing together again by allowing the whole tendon to retract. If the operation is done on children who are walking, only the tendon of the psoas muscle is cut, allowing the iliacus muscle to stay intact.

The psoas reattaches again but is lengthened. The importance of this is not fully understood or completely agreed upon.

Through the same incision on the inside thigh the proximal hamstring muscles may be lengthened or completely released. This procedure works well in relieving hip subluxation in severely involved children who cannot walk. However, many surgeons feel that it should not be performed on those who walk. Iliopsoas lengthening is by far the most widely used procedure for decreasing the force of the hip flexor muscle, although some physicians advocate transferring the tendon and suturing it to the pelvis or the hip joint capsule. Some surgeons advocate swinging the tendon around and inserting it on the outside of the femur bone, which has been done for patients with spina bifida but is not generally considered a good procedure for patients with spastic cerebral palsy.

Benefits and risks: The benefits of these operations include relieving hip dislocation, improving walking, and making it easier to care for the perineal area. The risks and complications of these procedures fall into the categories of either overcorrection or undercorrection. Determining how much lengthening is necessary may be difficult, and certainly the child may outgrow it with time. Whether there was insufficient release at the time of the first procedure or there was a sufficient release that the child outgrew, so that the muscles tightened again, insufficient release eventually causes the contractures to recur.

The more serious complication is over release of these muscles, which causes the legs to become contracted in a spread-open position. This is very detrimental for children who are walking, because it makes them walk with a wide-based gait and a large waddle. For those children who are only sitters, this abduction contracture is less detrimental, but it is cosmetically extremely unappealing. It also makes lying on one's side difficult.

A more common complication of the surgery is the combination of overcorrection on one side and undercorrection on the other, termed *windblown hip deformity*, in which one hip becomes contracted out to the side and the other hip becomes contracted across the midline. This misalignment is usually due to the asymmetry of the involvement, but the use of bracing may also contribute to the condition. Some patients will develop this deformity without any medical intervention.

After-surgery care: Several postoperative care techniques can be used following muscle releases. One form of management is to forgo casting or immobilization and start immediately with physical therapy. This approach generally makes it slightly harder to handle the child in the immediate couple of hours or couple of days after the

surgery, but she will be largely recovered and completely back to her daily routine by three or four weeks after surgery. This method of treating spastic hip disease result in a slightly higher incidence of repeat surgery later on, although this is not well documented. There is clearly a lower incidence of developing abduction and windblown deformities. Adductor lengthening for walking children should be immediately followed by physical therapy so that they can regain their walking ability.

Another common postoperative management technique involves placing casts on both legs, with a stabilizer between to keep the legs apart. Alternatively, the child may be placed in a full-body cast, reaching from chest to toes. Some combination of casting may be used for periods ranging from two to six or eight weeks. The advantage of casting is that the child is easier to handle in the immediate postoperative period, although she still may have many muscle spasms and need pain medicine and antispasmodic medication, usually diazepam (Valium). When the casts are removed, the child is very stiff and has a good bit of discomfort when she tries to move the hip and knee joints. The inability to move about easily is especially difficult for children who are walkers, because they often have a more difficult time regaining their walking ability. The development of the opposite deformity (a spread-open position) is increased by this casting.

Following the casting, some surgeons prescribe long-term abduction braces, which hold the legs apart, worn either at night, when the child is sleeping, or, occasionally, full time. The use of bracing after muscle releases, especially muscle releases done for the treatment of

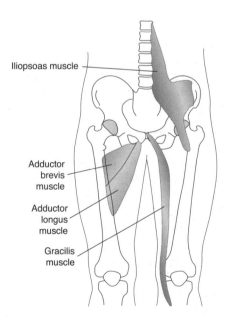

Iliopsoas muscle

Adductor brevis muscle

Adductor longus muscle

Gracilis muscle

spastic hip subluxation, continues to be controversial and is a likely cause of later windblown hip deformity.

What to expect: Pain may be quite severe for the first 24 to 48 hours due to muscle spasms, but by four weeks after the surgery it is very minimal, occurring only with extreme stretching. In the first 48 hours after surgery a good dose of Valium should be given to reduce muscle spasms. The muscles should be substantially looser after the surgery; however, it is very important to start an exercise program to maintain flexibility, because the natural tendency is for these muscles to retighten over time. This is especially true for a child with significant growth remaining, who may develop a repeat contracture over two or three years to the point that his condition is similar to what it was before the surgery was performed. Children who have had this procedure performed to improve their walking will need extensive therapy to gain the maximum benefit from the release.

Young adults who have the surgery performed to improve toileting and perineal care will see almost immediate benefits. In general, however, they will find that their hips do not open extremely widely but that their legs will spread much more easily and will stay moderately spread.

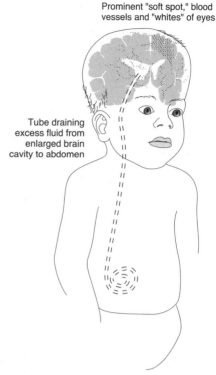

Prominent "soft spot," blood vessels and "whites" of eyes

Tube draining excess fluid from enlarged brain cavity to abdomen

Hydrocephalus

Hydrocephalus is the enlargement of fluid-filled spaces in the brain, known as ventricles, combined with signs and symptoms of increased intracranial pressure. This enlargement derives from an imbalance in the production and absorption of cerebrospinal fluid and is usually caused by blockage in the normal circulation of this fluid.

Hydrocephalus can be seen in children who have cerebral palsy. Because CP is the result of some scar in the brain, the scar may occur in an area affecting the natural flow of the fluid in the brain. When this occurs, a blockage may develop, and the fluid builds up. Extra fluid may also be present because the brain damage is so extensive that there is a decreased amount of brain tissue; if it is able to drain naturally, it does not need intervention. Most of the time, however, when increased fluid is present, a shunt, or drainage tube, must be inserted. Another option is to use a scope to look into the brain and open the blockage so a drainage tube is not needed. (See Chapter 3.)

Hyperbaric Oxygen Therapy
(HBOT)

Hyperbaric oxygen therapy (HBOT) is the inhalation of 100 percent oxygen inside a chamber that is pressurized to greater than 1 atmosphere. (The therapy is described as hyperbaric because the pressure is above atmospheric pressure.) HBOT is typically administered at 1–3 atmospheres of pressure.

For many years, HBOT has been successfully used to treat certain types of infections, carbon monoxide poisoning, and decompression sickness in deep-sea divers. A medical specialty known as undersea and hyperbaric medicine was developed, and indications for the treatment were outlined.

More recently, HBOT has been advertised as a treatment for traumatic brain injury and stroke, as well as for more chronic brain injuries such as those associated with CP. This treatment has received a great deal of publicity despite very little scientific evidence that it works. It is not clear from a scientific standpoint how HBOT could help overcome damage to brain tissue that occurred years before in a child with CP. When HBOT was studied in a scientific manner in two groups of children with CP, with a control group placed in pressurized room air and a treatment group in pressurized oxygen, both groups improved, without any difference between the two groups. Similar results were found in a second such controlled study of children with CP.

Ear pain or discomfort and bleeding from the ear are by far the most commonly reported adverse events during HBOT. In addition, there may be an increased risk of seizures in those treated with HBOT.

In summary, HBOT is a treatment that has long been known to work for specific medical problems and has recently been touted as a cure for CP. The limited number of controlled scientific studies do not support these claims, and one should proceed cautiously before embarking on this treatment, which is expensive in terms of both time and money.

Hypersensitivity
(tactile defensiveness)

The brain must receive or register stimuli in order for a response to occur. For this reason, individuals with cerebral palsy can experience a number of difficulties with the sensory system as a result of their brain abnormality. The problems frequently involve the senses of touch and equilibrium, as well as awareness of the body's movement and position in space.

Hypersensitivity to touch is called "tactile defensiveness." Normally, infants react to touch in a self-protective manner but become more comfortable as they learn to discriminate among degrees and varieties of touch. The individual who is unable to mature in this fashion remains highly reflexive and self-protective. The goal of therapy is to enable the child to develop an adaptive response to touch. The answer is not to avoid touching the child but rather to help the child gradually learn to handle the sensation of being touched. Therapists use a number of techniques, including introducing varied textures, to stimulate the desired responses.

Hypersensitivity to external heat or cold can present difficulty for the individual with CP because of the diminished ability to self-regulate body temperature in response to air temperature. What this means is that a child sitting in an excessively warm room will not automatically be able to discharge heat and can become seriously overheated. Similarly, the self-regulating mechanism that conserves body heat in cold weather can be impaired. Caregivers must be aware of external temperatures in order to monitor the individual's comfort and safety.

Difficulties with equilibrium and position in space result from malfunction of the vestibular and proprioceptive systems. Individuals most commonly display two problems: gravitational insecurity and an intolerance of spinning or circular movement. Because of gravitational insecurity, the child may react with intense anxiety to a simple change in head position. For example, he may become very frightened when placed on an examining table, not because he fears a needle but because he has the sensation of falling. Spinning or turning may cause excessive nausea and discomfort. Reassurance, combined with therapeutic intervention aimed at bringing about an appropriate response to these sensations, can help a great deal. Sensory integration therapy, in particular, is designed to overcome these hypersensitive reactions.

Inclusion
(mainstreaming)

Inclusion, or mainstreaming, is the practice of moving children with disabilities into regular classrooms or a regular school environment.

Indications: A child whose cognitive abilities are age appropriate, who is able to communicate, and whose medical problems do not necessitate specialized medical care can be mainstreamed. Specifically, if a child entering first grade requires a wheelchair for mobility but can speak and is at approximately the age-appropriate cognitive level, she should be mainstreamed in almost all environments.

Benefits and risks: The primary benefit of inclusion is that it exposes a child with a disability to children who do not have disabilities, and vice versa. This can expand her circle of friends and give her a broader, more normalized school experience. Through inclusion, children without disabilities have the opportunity to develop a better understanding of what it is like to have a disability.

The major disadvantage of inclusion is that frequently the staff are not as specialized, so that teachers without special experience or training will be providing education to the child with a disability. This is not a major issue if the disability does not greatly interfere with the child's regular functioning, but the child with severe motor or cognitive limitations may not be handled well by an educational staff without appropriate training.

Another disadvantage is that many public schools do not have specialized equipment that can benefit a child with a significant disability. At times, inclusion is supported by educational administrators because it is cheaper than sending a child to a specialized facility with more equipment and specially trained staff. Nevertheless, by law, the child needs to be in the least restrictive environment, so for many children with CP this will be the regular classroom setting.

Maintenance and care: The decision to mainstream a child is not made just once during a child's lifetime, to apply forever. Rather, it must continually be reevaluated as the child grows and develops. For example, a child may enter kindergarten, first grade, or second grade in a specialized educational environment where additional expertise in early childhood education and additional medical services and equipment are available. As this child continues to develop, a decision may be made in middle school that he can be moved to a regular environment for part of the day, and then as the child enters junior high, he may be ready for complete inclusion. For children for whom it is not entirely clear whether inclusion will be a positive or a negative experience, ongoing evaluation is especially appropriate.

Incontinence
(urinary incontinence, bowel incontinence)

Incontinence is defined as the inability to prevent the accidental loss of urine or feces. Incontinence is normal for the newborn baby, but most children are toilet trained by age 3. However, urinary incontinence (enuresis), especially at night while sleeping (nocturnal enuresis), is a common condition and usually does not need a medical evaluation until the child is close to age 6.

Generally, achieving normal bladder control requires the following steps: (1) an awareness of the bladder as it contracts; (2) the ability to realize the state of a full bladder and to plan ahead to go to the bathroom; (3) the ability to inhibit early contractions and postpone urination and to facilitate the emptying reflex when circumstances are right; (4) an awareness that the bladder has emptied completely; (5) the ability to hold urine when the bladder is overfilled or during momentary stress by voluntarily contracting the muscles of the pelvic floor; and (6) the ability to inhibit emptying during sleep. Thus, a child needs to be developmentally ready before he can be toilet trained, and the child with developmental delay or a cognitive impairment may be toilet trained at a later age than other children.

Incontinence may also be caused by physical problems, including a urinary tract infection or an abnormality of the urinary system. In the child with cerebral palsy, the nerves leading to the bladder may not be functioning normally and may cause either involuntary emptying of the bladder or abnormal retention of urine to the point that the bladder "overflows" and urine dribbles out. These two conditions aren't common but may occur in the child with cerebral palsy. They occur far more frequently in children with other neurological disorders, such as spina bifida.

A child who is incontinent during the day beyond the expected age of 3 or 4 and who otherwise is developmentally normal, should have a good physical examination, a urinalysis, and a urine culture. In the case of the child with CP who has normal cognitive function, the problem may lie in his physical ability to get to the toilet or his inability to sit up on the toilet. This latter problem is not just physical but also psychological: the child may feel as if he is going to fall, and thus he may

not be able to relax enough to cooperate in toilet training. There is equipment available to help support a child sitting on a toilet.

If tests show that the bladder and kidneys are normal, then behavior modification techniques may be used to teach the child bladder control. These should include a conditioning technique such as a reward system or an alarm system. In the older child, medication is sometimes used to control enuresis.

Incontinence of stool is not an uncommon problem. Constipation is very often the cause in a child who has previously been toilet trained and then begins to have fecal soiling. What happens is that the child builds up a large mass of dry stool that is difficult to pass, and then liquid feces flow around this mass past the sphincters. Fecal incontinence caused by such an impaction is often mistaken for diarrhea because the stool that is escaping is liquid.

Fecal incontinence may also occur when the toddler-aged child is stressed, such as following the birth of a sibling or a death in the family. If soiling begins at the time of toilet training, it is best to back off and stop the training for a while, as this is a sign that the child simply is not emotionally prepared to be trained. Incontinence of stool is commonly seen if the child has a cognitive impairment or has severe constipation. Cerebral palsy by itself is almost never the cause of failure to become continent. If the child is developmentally age appropriate but is still soiling, an evaluation is in order, looking for constipation or neurological problems as the cause.

Individualized Education Program
(IEP)

An Individualized Education Program is a written plan that outlines the educational program for a child in special education. It is to be reviewed annually and agreed to by the parents of the child after they meet with members of the school staff who are trained to develop the plan and explain it to parents.

The IEP for a school-aged child with CP (over the age of 3) will be based on therapists' and teachers' evaluations, as well as on a psychological evaluation. The process usually includes a physical therapist's assessment of the issues around gross motor problems and often also includes assessments by occupational and speech-language therapists if the child with CP has fine motor or speech problems too. The IEP should describe the child's level of development and should specify goals for the child with CP in terms of gross motor, fine motor, speech and language, social, and cognitive skills. It also should specify who will work on each of the goals (teacher, occupational therapist, physical therapist, etc.) and how often each week the child will receive each therapy. It should also specify the extent to which the child will be able to participate in regular educational programs. This should result in an educational program based on the individualized needs of the child. A suitable IEP requires parents' direct involvement and agreement.

Individualized Family Service Plan
(IFSP)

An Individualized Family Service Plan is a written plan that outlines early intervention services for a child under age 3 with disabilities and his or her family. It is similar to an IEP, but the focus is on the family as a whole, rather than just the child. It describes the services necessary to enhance the development of the child with disabilities and the ability of the child's family to meet the child's needs.

The IFSP for the child with CP who is younger than 3 years of age is based on evaluations by therapists and doctors. Like the IEP, it should specify an educational program and a therapeutic program aimed to meet specific goals for that individual child. It will be based on evaluations of the child's cognitive, gross and fine motor, speech and language, and social skills and should aim to meet goals in each of the defined areas. In addition, based on an evaluation by a social worker, it should also address family needs that are related to the child's disability, such as respite care or homemaker services for a parent who is working with the child.

Ingrown Toenail
(infected toenail, paronychia)

An ingrown toenail is a nail that has inflamed skin overlaying it. It is caused by either trimming the nail too close to the skin or having too much pressure against the side or corner of the nail. Once the tissue has become infected, it is difficult for the infection to heal. Once tenderness is felt, the primary treatment should be to prevent pressure and discontinue wearing shoes that put pressure on this area of the nail. It might be helpful to take an old pair of athletic shoes and completely cut out the top front of the shoe so there is no pressure on the toe with the inflamed nail.

A common cause of ingrown toenails in children with cerebral palsy is wearing braces that irritate the toenail or cause the shoes to be too tight for the toenail. A common cause in teenagers with CP is the development of flat feet, so that the pressure when walking is on the side of the toe, causing the toenail to be irritated.

To prevent ingrown toenails, the toenails should be carefully trimmed straight across, and the corners and cuticles should not be touched. To treat an ingrown nail, the inflamed toenail should be soaked twice a day in

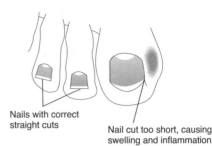

Nails with correct straight cuts

Nail cut too short, causing swelling and inflammation

warm water and dried well. Packing under the corner of the toenail with a small piece of lamb's wool helps avoid further irritating the inflamed tissue. If the skin is very red and extremely warm, antibiotics may be necessary.

If soreness does not improve within a week, occasionally surgical drainage or excision of the edge of the nail is needed to allow the toe to heal. This is often unnecessary for a first- or second-time inflammation; however, after a nail has become repeatedly infected, it often develops a significant amount of scar tissue, and the only way to eliminate the problem completely is to do a surgical excision of the edge of the toenail.

Inhibitive Casting
(tone-reducing cast, tone-reducing brace, serial casts)

Inhibitive casts are usually applied to the legs and sometimes the arms to inhibit a specific movement. Initially the cast may be used to stretch out a contracture, such as a tight Achilles tendon. In the case of a tight Achilles tendon, the cast is used to keep the foot in a position in which the sole and heel touch the ground. Keeping the ankle from plantar-flexing allows other movements to improve; the elbows flex better, fingers move more easily, and spasticity decreases in the hips or knees. The inhibitive ankle-foot orthosis (AFO) is useful in stabilizing the ankle for standing.

Indications: Indications for the use of inhibitive casts are not well defined. There is variable success when they are used for severe spasticity or in the attempt to stretch out tight muscles. Initially, the muscles may be stretched out, but as soon as the casting is discontinued the contracture recurs. Whether inhibitive casts can decrease unwanted movements or improve function also remains uncertain. Clearly, immobilization of the ankle does decrease abnormal posturing in some patients; however, as soon as the immobilization is removed, the posturing returns.

In general, the use of inhibitive casts for children with cerebral palsy is rapidly decreasing, but AFOs are widely used for inhibiting movement. The AFO may be worn to immobilize the ankle, and normal shoes can be worn over the orthotic, providing a much more cosmetically acceptable approach to casting.

Benefits and risks: The use of inhibitive casts, or alternatively an AFO, with the goal of inhibiting movement does improve positioning and function in some children, although the benefit is lost as soon as the immobilization is removed. Elaborate tone-reducing splints and casts with special pressure points have not demonstrated any benefit over comfortably fitting AFOs. Inhibitive casts are most beneficial after acute head injuries because the casts prevent short-term contractures. With time, as the brain heals, the tendency to contract decreases. In some clinics, serial casts are frequently used after botulinum toxin injection.

The purpose of both casting and the use of an AFO is to stretch tight muscles and provide positioning. Serial casting involves placing a cast that is removed after one to two weeks and replaced with another. When the replacement cast is placed, the position of the body part being casted is closer to normal because of the effect of the first cast. Theoretically, one can continue with this process until the desired position is achieved. The inhibitive cast is similar but is removable by the caregivers for bathing and any other functions for which the physician may recommend removing it. Serial casting can be helpful after Botox injections to the gastrocnemius muscle in a child who has had a recent growth spurt by maximizing the increased range of motion and getting the child back into a well-fitted AFO.

Maintenance and care: Serial casts often need to be changed every one to two weeks. If they are applied too tightly, they must be removed on an emergency basis. If a cast becomes very painful, then an emergency may occur, because the muscle may be in such spasm that it will not get enough blood flow.

One of the main reasons serial casts are used much less commonly now is the difficulty of maintaining a cast on a child. A child cannot be bathed while wearing a cast, and ongoing cast wear causes discomfort. A major side effect of casting is muscle loss and weakness, which

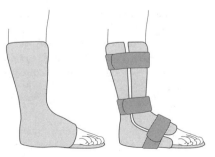

is hard to regain. As soon as the cast is removed, within several weeks to a month all its benefits can be lost without ongoing casting or splinting. Some physicians feel that using botulinum toxin with casts allows the gains achieved in stretching to be maintained longer—a view not supported by scientific research.

Intellectual Disability
(ID, cognitive impairment, intellectual impairment, cognitively challenged, mental retardation)

Intellectual disability and *intellectual impairment* are now the medical terms used for intellectual functioning that is at least two standard deviations below the norm; it is usually categorized as mild, moderate, or severe. Previously the term *mental retardation* was used, but this term has fallen out of use in the disabilities community due to its use as a derogatory term. *Cognitive impairment* and *cognitively challenged* are also felt to be more acceptable.

Intellectual disability may exist together with cerebral palsy or by itself, without a motor disability. It is generally diagnosed during the developmental period from 2 to 8 years of age. It is nearly impossible to make a firm diagnosis or determination of intellectual disability in the very young child, because tests of intellect are not valid until age 3. Even at age 3 or 4, an assessment of intellectual function is especially difficult in children with CP who can't speak or can't use their hands, as it may be difficult for them to show what they understand. Treatment involves recognizing the child's functional level and placing the child in an educational environment in which he is able to maximize his natural learning abilities.

Approximately two-thirds of children with cerebral palsy have some degree of intellectual disability (ID). One-third have mild to moderate ID, one-third have severe to profound ID, and one-third have normal intelligence. Intellectual disability is often the most disabling factor for the child with CP.

Intrauterine Growth Retardation
(IUGR)

Intrauterine growth retardation is a term used to describe a fetus that is not growing appropriately in the uterus. Infants born with IUGR are small for their gestational age, with a low weight, short length, and small head circumference, and they almost always have had some significant insult that explains their growth retardation. Causes for IUGR might include congenital infections, such as cytomegalovirus (CMV) or toxoplasmosis, or malnutrition, placental insufficiency, or a variety of other conditions. Infants with IUGR are at increased risk for developing cerebral palsy because the brain is dependent for its full-term development on normal intrauterine growth.

Jaundice
(hyperbilirubinemia, icterus)

Jaundice is yellow discoloration of the skin and eyes. While jaundice can be an early sign of liver disease, it is common in newborn infants and is not usually associated with any disease. This type of jaundice, called "physiologic jaundice," rarely leads to problems.

When babies are born, they have a high red blood cell count. As these red blood cells are broken down in the first few days of life, a breakdown product called bilirubin is generated. If the bilirubin is not excreted through the liver and the gastrointestinal system, the child will become jaundiced and appear yellow. This is common in the first few days after birth, when the liver is not yet mature enough to break down all the bilirubin. If the level becomes too high, the baby is put under special lights called "bili-lights," which help break down the bilirubin as it goes through the blood vessels in the skin. If the bilirubin level continues to rise even after treatment with bili-lights, then exchange transfusions can also be done. Such a transfusion is not often done in a full-term healthy baby but may be done in small premature babies, in whom complications can develop from a lower level of bilirubin than in a full-term baby with a higher birthweight.

Sometimes jaundice in newborns is not benign. For instance, a severe infection in the blood system can cause jaundice, as can defects of the liver and incompatibility of the blood type of the mother and the infant. This last, hemolytic disease of the newborn, was a common cause of severe hyperbilirubinemia in the years before phototherapy and exchange transfusions began to be used to prevent the complications of severe jaundice. The high levels of bilirubin caused kernicterus, a staining of part of the brain with bilirubin, causing brain damage. This resulted in lethargy, poor feeding, and a shrill cry.

While many babies with severe kernicterus died, many of those who survived eventually showed signs of the athetoid type of cerebral palsy.

Ketogenic Diet

The ketogenic diet is a treatment for seizures. The ketogenic diet is a rigid, mathematically calculated, physician-supervised diet that is very high in fat and very low in carbohydrates and protein. It usually has three to four times as much fat as carbohydrate and protein combined. Fluids and calories are strictly limited. This diet allows the body to primarily burn fat rather than glucose for energy. The ketogenic diet can be con-

sidered for patients experiencing any type of seizure, but it is most effective in treating absence, atonic, and myoclonic seizures. The diet should not be tried without the supervision of a health care provider and dietitian, both of whom must be knowledgeable in the diet.

Knee Immobilizers

A common problem for children with spasticity is the development of tightness in the hamstring muscles (back of the thigh). This can make standing upright and even sitting difficult. A knee immobilizer is a splint that is often used in this situation. The goal of this splint is to hold the knee completely straight. The splint, which is usually made of canvass or plastic, is wrapped around the leg and fixed with Velcro straps. This splint does not need to be custom fitted. It comes in a number of different standard lengths, one of which should be right for your child.

Knee immobilizers can be used to prevent or decrease contractures. They need to be worn approximately 8 hours a day. For most children, it is most convenient to wear them during sleep time, since the splint would prevent sitting and moving during wake times. A major side effect of the splints is that many children cannot tolerate them during sleep, and they severely restrict the child if they are worn during the day. Knee immobilizers are frequently used after surgery, especially after hamstring lengthening.

Kyphosis
(round back)

Kyphosis is the term for a rounded spine or a severely slouched body frame. Also referred to as forward bending of the spine, kyphosis is very common in young children with cerebral palsy who do not have good upper body control. Their kyphosis completely corrects itself when they lie down. In children with CP, the deformity is due to poor muscle control, but kyphosis may also occur in adolescents in the front of the spine as a result of abnormal growth. In this case, it is known as adolescent round back or *Scheuermann's kyphosis*.

Sometimes the bones in the front of the spine form abnormally during the child's development, in which case the child is said to have congenital kyphosis. The most common kyphosis occurs in older people, especially older women—their bones soften, and the spine collapses down, and they become severely roundbacked. This condition is termed *senile kyphosis* and is due to osteoporosis.

Care and treatment: Kyphosis in children with cerebral palsy is not well defined. It typically occurs between the ages of 3 and 8, when children with severe involvement have difficulty with trunk control. When treating a young child with kyphosis, it is necessary to modify the wheelchair so that the child sits up straight. At this age, often the best treatment is the use of an adequately contoured wheelchair with shoulder straps and a reclining seat. It is also important to have the lap tray in a high position so the child can lean on his arms and not flex the spine. When the child is sitting upright the lap tray should be at the nipple level. A prone stander that stimulates the child to pull her spine up straighter and lift her head is another useful device; a stander that does not support the child's upper body and allows her to slouch forward without any support for the chest should not be used. Chairs that are contoured with a round back, such as the plastic molded Tumble Forms chairs, should also be avoided, as they can make kyphosis worse. Special exercises are not very helpful, since the child mainly needs to mature.

As children increase their trunk control, this type of kyphosis is generally corrected, although a few children enter adolescence with the head drooped forward and shoulders rolled severely forward. Sometimes this posture becomes stiff, which makes sitting up and looking forward difficult. It is also very difficult for children to sit in a chair, especially if the kyphosis starts stiffening, and they are unable to lie down except in a ball shape. For the rare child whose deformity stiffens, a posterior spinal fusion and instrumentation to straighten the spine is recommended in order to allow the child to sit up straight, look forward, and interact with the environment.

Complications due to kyphosis are not well defined. Children between ages 3 and 8 with flexible kyphosis have no known complications, except that they roll for-

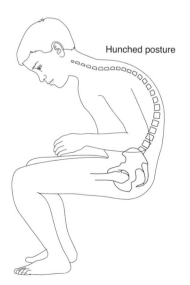

Hunched posture

ward and have difficulty holding their head up to participate in activities. For this reason a body jacket or a body brace may be used for positioning comfort and for better head control and arm use. As the large curve becomes stiff, however, children have difficulty lying on their backs. Often they end up lying on their sides. When they are sitting, they cannot hold their head back, and they end up with the head dropped forward. At present it is uncertain whether this posture has any effect on respiration or gastric function. For some children, breathing and eating habits improve when they can sit up or stand up straight.

Laryngeal Stridor
(laryngomalacia, tracheomalacia, inspiratory stridor)

Laryngeal stridor during the first few months of life is a harsh sound heard during respiration. It can be high-pitched when the child breathes in. There are many causes of stridor. The most common of these, laryngomalacia, is caused by weak cartilage in the airway and results in partial airway obstruction.

Care and treatment: Usually no therapy is needed, since the condition improves on its own by the time the child reaches 18 months of age. There may be difficulty feeding a child with stridor. Rarely, a child will need a tracheostomy or other procedure because of the airway obstruction. Most children with this condition seem more comfortable and breathe less noisily when lying on their stomachs.

If the child with cerebral palsy develops laryngomalacia or tracheomalacia in early or later childhood, it may be associated with severe gastroesophageal reflux. The underlying reflux is treated with either medication or surgery.

Other children with CP can develop upper airway obstruction and stridor because of low tone of the muscles of the throat and face. The low muscle tone causes the tongue to fall to the back of the throat, which intermittently obstructs the airway. This problem does not tend to disappear with time, although positioning the child on the stomach sometimes resolves the problem. If not, the child may need a tracheostomy to relieve the airway obstruction.

Laryngoscopy
(bronchoscopy)

Laryngoscopy is a procedure that involves inspection of the larynx and the upper airway. An indirect laryngoscopy is done with the aid of a mirror; a direct laryngoscopy, in the office, involves a small, flexible bronchoscope that is passed through the nose. *Bronchoscopy* is an examination of the lower airway, including the trachea and mainstem bronchi. Rigid bronchoscopy, with a metal telescope, requires general anesthesia.

Benefits and risks: Bronchoscopy and laryngoscopy are useful procedures for inspecting the airway and obtaining a culture or biopsy. Also, a foreign body can be removed via bronchoscopy. Complications of bronchoscopy can include transient hypoxia (a decrease in oxygen in the blood) and spasm of the larynx or bronchus. Less commonly, oral or dental injury can occur. A child can also develop post-bronchoscopy croup, which is usually short-lived and can be treated with medications and mist.

Latex Allergy

Latex is a natural rubber produced by the rubber tree. Some people develop allergic reactions after repeated contact with latex. Allergic reactions can be localized, such as rash and itching after wearing latex gloves, or generalized, such as sneezing, runny nose, or wheezing. Rarely, life-threatening reactions (anaphylaxis) can occur.

Latex allergy usually affects people who are routinely exposed to latex products, such as health care workers and people who have had multiple surgeries or medical procedures. This includes children with medical conditions, such as myelomeningocele or occasionally cerebral palsy, that result in multiple surgical operations or repeated bladder catheterizations.

Years ago, latex might have been encountered in medical equipment such as latex gloves, blood pressure cuffs, drains, tourniquets, urine catheters, and adhesives used for dressings. However, most health care products are now made with latex-free alternative materials, and most hospitals and many physician offices now have a latex-free environment, thus reducing the likelihood of developing a latex allergy. Latex can also be found in common household items such as rubber bands, computer mouse pads, and balloons. Several allergenic proteins have been identified, some of which are similar to and "cross-react" with proteins in certain foods, such as bananas, kiwi fruit, and avocados.

If a latex allergy is suspected, a blood test can be done that tests for latex-specific antibodies. Once the diagnosis is confirmed, avoidance is the best way to treat a latex allergy.

Least Restrictive Environment

If a child with cerebral palsy or another disability is found to need early intervention services or special education services, these should be provided in the least restrictive environment. This means that the child re-

ceives services in settings and facilities in which children without disabilities would participate, unless the Individualized Family Service Plan (IFSP) or the Individualized Education Program (IEP) indicates a need for a special setting.

An example of a least restrictive environment is the regular classroom, in which a child who can speak and has an age-appropriate cognitive level but requires the use of a wheelchair should be included with age-matched peers in almost all environments. On the other hand, a child who has severe intellectual disabilities along with a severe motor disability would not be expected to be in a regular classroom with age-appropriate children, because the least restrictive environment for this child would not be able to meet the child's needs as identified by the IEP.

For a significant group of children with CP, determining the least restrictive environment that best meets a child's needs may be challenging. In fact, there may be a combination of environments that would best meet the child's needs, and this would be determined by the IEP.

Lordosis
(swayback)

Lordosis is the spinal curvature that is normally present in the small of the back. In the swaybacked person, the spine arches to such an extent that it causes the abdomen to protrude. If a person spends a lot of time sitting, lordosis can be beneficial, because it projects the weight

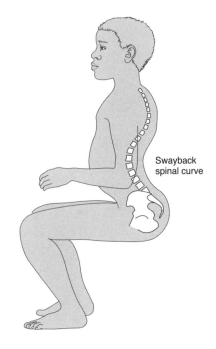

Swayback
spinal curve

of sitting forward onto the thighs, where there is less likelihood of developing pressure sores.

An abnormal degree of lordosis as an isolated problem is the most rare spinal deformity in children with cerebral palsy. Severe lordosis may be a long-term complication after a dorsal rhizotomy procedure. It is frequently associated with scoliosis, but usually scoliosis is the more predominant deformity and the lordosis is an additional difficulty. Some children with lordosis roll so far forward that their abdomens rest on their thighs; this makes seating almost impossible. It is extremely difficult to modify wheelchairs to correct for increased lordosis, although the main method is to recline the wheelchair to about 45 degrees.

Indications: Once increased lordosis becomes a significant condition, it tends to get slowly worse until a spinal fusion is performed. The indications for spinal fusion are rare in this deformity. Fusion should be considered if lordosis makes sitting difficult or impossible or if it causes intractable back pain. Unfortunately, bracing or wheelchair modifications do not benefit or reduce severe lordosis.

Low Bone Mineral Density
(osteopenia, osteoporosis)

Osteopenia is lower than normal bone mineral density that is not yet osteoporosis. The term *osteopenia* is now mostly used for adult populations; it is no longer recommended for use in reference to pediatric bone density.

Low bone mineral density (BMD) as measured by dual-energy x-ray absorptiometry (DXA) in children (and adults up to age 50) is defined as a bone mineral density value that is two standard deviations or more below the mean for age and gender. How BMD is reported for children differs from the way it is reported for adults. In adults over age 50, a T-score is used to estimate or to predict risk of fracture using the World Health Organization (WHO) criteria. To determine the T-score, a person's BMD is compared with that of a person at his or her maximum, or "peak," bone mass, typically around age 25. The T-score is the number of standard deviations above or below the mean for this reference population. In contrast, the BMD of children and young adults uses a Z-score, which is calculated by comparing the person's BMD value with the mean value for children of his or her age and gender; the Z-score is the number of standard deviations above or below the mean for the reference population. A BMD Z-score of −2.0 or lower is considered "low BMD" in children or "below the expected range for age" in adults under age 50.

A number of conditions can lead to low BMD in childhood: certain medical conditions affecting skel-etal development, medication use that negatively affects bone metabolism, lack of weight bearing, delayed puberty, compromised nutritional status, low intake of nutrients (such as calcium and Vitamin D) needed for bone growth. Children with CP who are nonambulatory are at increased risk for developing nontraumatic, or "fragility," fractures. Fragility fractures occur with minimal trauma and under conditions that do not typically result in a fracture. Osteoporosis in children is defined as a history of fracture combined with low BMD. Activities such as dressing a child, performing range of motion exercises, or even just picking the child up can result in a fracture in a child with severe osteoporosis. Once a child has sustained a fragility fracture, the child's likelihood of sustaining fracture again is very high. Bisphosphonates have proven to be an effective treatment for osteoporosis in children with CP.

Magnetic Resonance Imaging
(MR, MRI)

Magnetic resonance imaging is an imaging method used extensively to examine brain tissue, though it may also be used to image the spine or other areas of the body. It involves being placed in a very large magnet that magnetizes body water for a fraction of a second. Radiofrequency pulses are used to measure the properties of the water in body tissue. The computer uses this information to create a series of pictures. There is no x-ray radiation involved in the MRI scanner, but the child is required to lie very still, which often means sedation will be needed. Sometimes intravenous contrast material is injected to learn more details about the body tissue.

The MRI scanner is the most sophisticated imaging method available. It can detect most major brain problems, such as tumors, large congenital deformities, increased fluid, and many degenerative conditions. However, many children with cerebral palsy can have normal MRI scans. The reason is that MRI mostly picks up structural defects. Very tiny abnormalities or most functional problems present in the brain cannot be seen on MRI.

Indications: Many children with CP will have one MRI scan unless there is clear evidence for the cause of the cerebral palsy. The main purpose of this MRI scan is to rule out such problems as brain tumors, major vascular abnormalities, and other treatable conditions. Children with seizures may require more scans as their condition changes.

Benefits and risks: Of the imaging tests available, MRIs currently are the most likely to pick up structural disorders of the brain. The major risk is in requiring the child to

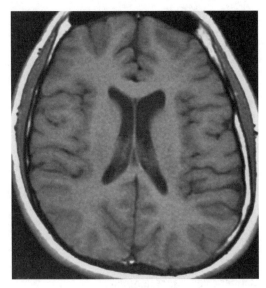

Brain MRI scan

hold very still for a prolonged period of time, from 30 to 90 minutes. For many children, this requires heavy sedation or general anesthesia, and there is some risk of breathing problems, so the child needs to be closely monitored. An MRI scan involves no pain, though patients who are uncomfortable in small spaces may feel very anxious inside the machine, which looks like a large tube. Because the magnet used for MRI is very strong, the scan may not be safe for some children, including children with implants such as pacemakers or cochlear implants.

Malformation of the Central Nervous System

Three percent of newborn infants have major malformations of the central nervous system. Some are caused by genetic conditions and others by environmental factors, including maternal infections or drugs. However, the majority do not have a known cause.

Such malformations can fall into a number of broad categories, including neural tube defects, anterior midline defects, spinal cord dysraphic states, disorders of cellular migration, and agenesis of the corpus callosum. The last two are often found in association with cerebral palsy (and are described in greater detail in entries devoted to them in this encyclopedia). Disorders of cellular migration are often a direct cause of CP, whereas agenesis of the corpus callosum frequently causes seizures.

Medical Home

A medical home is an approach to providing comprehensive primary care to children with special needs.

Ideally, such a medical home is defined as primary care that is accessible, continuous, comprehensive, family centered, coordinated, compassionate, and culturally effective. This concept was developed by the American Academy of Pediatrics in the hope that many pediatricians and family physicians will serve as medical homes for chronically ill and physically disabled children.

In a medical home, the clinician works in partnership with the family and patient to assure that all the medical and nonmedical needs of the patient are being met. Such services might include specialty care, educational services, family support, and other community services that are important to the health of the child.

Although the American Academy of Pediatrics proposed this definition of a medical home in 1992, efforts to establish such medical homes for all children have encountered many challenges. One of the major challenges is a lack of adequate reimbursement for the kinds of services that physicians provide to children with complex medical problems. In contrast to care provided in a medical home, care provided through emergency departments, walk-in clinics, and other urgent care facilities, though sometimes necessary, is more costly and often less effective. (For more on the medical home, see Chapter 3.)

Medical Marijuana
(cannabis, cannabinoids)

Marijuana (cannabis) for medical use has been approved in a number of states in recent years. It remains an illegal drug at the federal level, however, and is classified as a Schedule I drug by the Drug Enforcement Administration (DEA), making it very difficult even to do research on its use. Therefore, there is little research available to help guide patients and the medical community on when and how to use it. There are a variety of different chemical components (cannabinoids) in the marijuana plant, and research needs to be done to identify which ones might be effective for which problems. For the CP population, the two conditions for which there are anecdotes of success are seizures and muscle spasms. The American Academy of Pediatrics has stated that while cannabinoids may have potential as therapy for some medical conditions, it does not recommend its use until more research has been done.

Meningitis and Encephalitis

Meningitis is an infection of the covering over the brain (the meninges); encephalitis is an infection of the brain substance. Although these two conditions differ, the net results can be very similar. The most common cause of encephalitis is the herpes simplex virus. Meningitis can be caused by a virus (in which case it is called aseptic meningitis) or by bacteria, such as meningococcus, hemophilus influenza, and pneumococcus. Fortunately, today vaccines are given to young children for all three of these bacteria, so most young people are protected against these infections. Another bacterium, Group B streptococcus, which can be passed from the pregnant mother to her newborn infant, also can cause meningitis. There is no vaccine against this bacterium. Instead, pregnant women are tested for this infection by means of a vaginal culture; if the infection is present, it is treated with antibiotics.

Generally children with meningitis develop a fever and a stiff neck. They may also have difficulty eating, and they may vomit. Older children often complain of sensitivity to light and a headache. Infants stop feeding. A child with meningitis may fall into a coma and die. Others may survive, but with brain damage.

Care and treatment: Although the incidence of meningitis has fallen dramatically since the introduction of the *Haemophilus influenzae* type B (Hib) vaccine and, more recently, the pneumococcal vaccine, many children in the United States still contract bacterial meningitis each year. When a physician suspects meningitis, a lumbar puncture (called a spinal tap) is done, and samples of spinal fluid are sent for laboratory examination. If the infection is diagnosed and found to be bacterial, antibiotics are used to treat the infection. There is no medicine that treats most kinds of viral meningitis, and most patients with viral meningitis recover without treatment. Infection of young infants with herpes virus can be treated with a medication called acyclovir. Infections from polio, rubella (German measles), and mumps, all of which can cause encephalitis or meningitis, are preventable with immunizations.

The aftereffects of meningitis or encephalitis include brain damage or death, though most children recover without severe complications. Those with brain damage may have cerebral palsy and/or cognitive impairment. Up to 40 percent of children with bacterial meningitis (especially meningitis caused by pneumococcus) suffer hearing impairment in one or both ears.

Metabolic Disorders

There are many types of metabolic disorders, which vary considerably in their clinical and pathological aspects. However, all are due to defects caused by a single gene that result in abnormal or deficient enzymes or proteins. Thus, their pathology is typically the result of an inability to properly make or break down compounds necessary for normal body functions.

When an enzyme is not working properly, the substance it is to metabolize builds up in excess, as do other associated compounds. Disease can result from these excess metabolites, which in many cases can be toxic to the brain and other organs. In other cases, it is the absence of the compound that would have been produced by the deficient enzyme that causes disease. Many children with metabolic disease thus appear normal at birth and may not be identified with an illness until the pattern of metabolic disease becomes apparent.

Treatment for a very few metabolic disorders involves replacing the necessary enzyme. For most, however, treatment is limited and consists in dietary manipulation and the use of dietary supplements to decrease the buildup of injurious compounds and maximize the function of any enzyme available. The success of these interventions varies widely.

The number of disorders identified as metabolic has increased dramatically over the past years. Despite this, they are still relatively rare. In most states in the United States and in many other countries, newborns are screened for a number of metabolic disorders for which early identification and treatment is often successful in preventing irreversible injury. Since metabolic disorders are rare and often have very specific treatments and symptoms, an Internet search at sites like that of the National Institutes of Health is recommended, along with getting information from your child's doctor. Most reliable Internet sites now have online family forum groups, which can be an excellent source of information.

Microcephaly

Microcephaly is the condition in which a child's head circumference is more than two standard deviations below the mean measurement for children of the same age and gender. Normally the circumference of the head is measured on a regular basis, in the first few years of life during a pediatrician's routine exam and beyond that age if there is a problem. While there are genetic conditions leading to microcephaly without any brain damage, usually microcephaly reflects poor brain growth from some damage to the brain, such as an intrauterine infection (e.g., by CMV or Zika virus), severe hypoxia at birth, or meningitis during infancy. Those with the severest forms of microcephaly usually have severe intellectual impairment, and many others may have spastic cerebral palsy.

Motor Synergy
(co-contraction of muscles)

Motor synergy, or co-contraction of the muscles, means that muscles that have opposite functions contract at the same time. For example, the quadriceps muscles, on the front of the thigh, may contract at the same time as the hamstring muscles, behind the thigh. Therefore, neither muscle is able to cause the knee to bend, and the net result is a stiff knee. Although this may feel similar to spasticity, motor synergy usually occurs during specific activities, such as walking. In the case of walking, the muscle contracts at inappropriate times, so the muscle, which normally would not be contracting, actively blocks the normal joint movement.

Exaggerated muscle synergy is a significant problem for many children with cerebral palsy. Treating the underlying spasticity will not stop muscle synergy, although physical therapy to improve muscle coordination and to develop the ability to control these co-contractions is often beneficial. With appropriate treatment, a child's muscles will continue to improve until the age of 8 or 10. The contraction patterns can be identified by gait analysis, and occasionally a muscle can be moved into an area where it functions appropriately, such as with the rectus and hamstring muscles.

Movement Disorders

This term is used to describe various abnormalities of movement. They are divided into different types, based on the kind of movement that is seen.

Ballismus: Ballismus involves extremely large recurrent, rapid, flapping, involuntary violent movements of the arms, often in a circular pattern, but may occasionally involve the legs as well. These appear to be large flailing movements that may be so eruptive and strong that they throw the person off balance and cause him to fall. This movement disorder is extremely rare and can be very difficult to control. The primary treatment is a neurosurgical procedure to remove the part of the brain that controls this type of movement. In the early stages this movement disorder may look like athetoid cerebral palsy; however, unlike CP, ballismus gets progressively worse.

Chorea: Chorea is a movement disorder that primarily involves the distal joints, mostly toes and fingers. It is characterized by small, irregular, nonstereotyped jerky types of movements. These small, uncontrolled dancing movements cannot be controlled very well and usually cause significant problems with fine motor control. Unlike tics, they cannot be voluntarily suppressed. Although similar movements occur in children with cerebral palsy, CP is rarely the main cause of this movement disorder.

Dystonia: Dystonia is a movement disorder involving prolonged muscle contractions that may cause twisting and repetitive movements or abnormal posture. Usually, the arm is drawn up and may be held in the air in a flexed position, and sometimes the face or neck is affected too. Dystonia may also involve the legs. When a child first shows signs of having dystonia, contractures do not develop; over time, however, the muscle becomes contracted from remaining in the same position. Generally, the body relaxes when the person sleeps or is at rest. Dystonic movements may then occur when movement is initiated, producing "motor overflow."

The treatments for dystonia include medications and nerve injections. The drug Artane is usually used, but often it does not effectively reduce the abnormal movement. Botulinum toxin injections work well for small muscles around the neck, face, and eyelids. Surgical releases of dystonic muscles can be very unpredictable, and even without treatment, one dystonia pattern can suddenly change into another one. This pattern change may mean that suddenly the problem that had predominantly affected one arm may start affecting a foot. More commonly, however, it means that the arm or foot was twisted in a way that pulled it into flexion, and then suddenly it switches so that the arm is held in extension. When a child with dystonia is seen briefly by a physician, the posture may look like typical hemiplegic pattern cerebral palsy. Based on one short examination, a mistake can be made that could lead to very bad outcomes following surgical procedures.

Certain components of this pattern, however, should not be missed, such as the relatively small amount of muscle contracture that is usually present and the postural changes that the family may complain about. Dystonia may be present without significant changes over many years; however, some children get progressively worse over a matter of four or five years.

Despite a major effort to more clearly define these different movement patterns, physicians' definitions vary. Therefore, a parent should not become too concerned if there is disagreement between physicians.

The use of the baclofen pump has become a common treatment for severe dystonia. Another potential treatment when all else fails is deep brain stimulation. This is still considered experimental for the pediatric CP population.

Tics: Motor tics are abnormal movements that tend to be frequently repeated and usually follow the same pattern. Examples of motor tics include sniffling, swallowing, throat clearing, coughing, eye blinking, facial grimacing, or neck stretching. In fact, any part of the body may become involved. However, most individuals who experience such tics do so only for a short time, and only 10 percent of the population may experience a tic lasting one month or more. Usually the onset is during childhood or early adolescence, with the transient tic disorder lasting anywhere from one month to one year, beyond which time it is considered to be a chronic tic disorder.

In addition to motor tics, the child may have vocal tics as well, such as grunts, barks, or clearly articulated words and phrases. A disorder that involves words or phrases often is diagnosed as Gilles de la Tourette syndrome. Although tics are not a sign of cerebral palsy, tics occur more frequently in children with CP.

Neurogenic Bladder

Neurogenic bladder is a condition in which the bladder is functioning abnormally because of damage to the nerves that control bladder function. Since cerebral palsy affects the brain above the spinal cord, if there is bladder dysfunction, it is of the upper motor neuron type. The bladder will most likely be spastic and the sphincter tone abnormally increased, with uninhibited contractions. The sphincters may contract tightly but are not under normal voluntary control. This means that the bladder may frequently empty even when it is not full and at inconvenient times for the child.

Care and treatment: Treatment, under the care of a urologist, is based on urodynamic findings. Anticholinergic medications are often used to minimize uninhibited contractions, the most common being oxybutynin (Ditropan) and tolterodine (Detrol). In addition to medications, other treatments may be necessary, including clean intermittent catheterization (CIC). On rare occasions when medication and catheterization do not prevent progressive deterioration of bladder function, a surgical procedure known as vesicostomy may be necessary. In this procedure, the bladder is drained through a small opening in the skin.

Nuclear Medicine
(bone scan, renal scan, PET, SPECT)

Nuclear medicine studies include a wide range of examinations for a wide range of indications. These exams can look at function of some organs, which x-rays, MRI, CT, and ultrasound cannot do. On the other hand, nuclear medicine studies may provide less detail about organ structure. These studies all use a small amount of a radioactive material called a radiopharmaceutical for the imaging. Particles or molecules in the radiopharmaceutical contain a very, very small amount of radioactivity. The material is safe and will not hurt your child. The radioactivity is detected by the special nuclear medicine cameras, and the information about where the radioactivity is in the body is used to make pictures. Depending on the type of nuclear medicine study being done, the patient may receive the radiopharmaceutical through intravenous (IV) line; by breathing it in; by a catheter placed into the bladder; or by eating solid food or drinking liquid containing the radiopharmaceutical before the test. Once the radiopharmaceutical has been given, the pictures may be taken right away, or your child may have to wait several hours or days to allow the radioactive molecules to travel throughout the body. The scanning, or picture-taking, part of the study may take anywhere from several minutes to a few hours to complete. Longer studies may require the child to be sedated.

There are several types of nuclear medicine studies. Two of the more detailed examinations are SPECT and PET. SPECT (single photon emission computed tomography) uses a camera that rotates around the patient while gathering information. The computer can use that information to create detailed pictures of activity within the body. This technique can be used with several different types of nuclear medicine scans and is often used with bone and brain scans. PET (positron emission tomography) scans look for areas of extra energy usage in the body. These scans are particularly useful in evaluating the brain in patients who have seizures, and they can provide information not visible on MRI or CT.

Indications: There are types of nuclear medicine studies that can be used for many areas of the body, including kidney scans, gallbladder scans, liver and spleen scans, bone scans, heart muscle scans, and brain scans. There are special tests that can be used to look at the bladder and to look for reflux in the esophagus. SPECT may be used with one of these studies if more detailed infor-

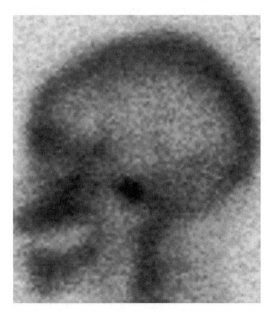

Bone scan

mation is needed. PET scans of the brain are used particularly for seizures. In special situations, PET and CT scans can be combined to look for the spread of cancer in cancer patients.

Benefits and risks: All nuclear medicine studies involve giving the child a small amount of a radioactive substance. This substance stays in the body from several hours to a few days. The amount of radiation the child gets from the radiopharmaceutical is very small; in most cases is less than the amount of radiation used for a CT scan. The radiation dose from a nuclear medicine study is believed to be safe for the child. The scanning portion of the study is not painful, but sedation may be needed if the child has to remain still for a long time. Since any sedation presents a small risk of breathing problems, the patient will need to be monitored during the sedation and afterwards until the sedatives wear off.

Nystagmus

Nystagmus is a rhythmic jerking or jumping movement of the eyes caused by spasticity. Nystagmus appears in several forms: in vertical nystagmus, the eye moves up and down; in horizontal nystagmus, it moves sideways; in rotary nystagmus, it tends to move around in a circle. Nystagmus is frequently triggered by a certain gaze, such as gazing up or to one side. Because position orientation often initiates nystagmus, many children learn to control it by avoiding looking in those directions.

Care and treatment: Children with cerebral palsy may have nystagmus, which causes significant problems for fine eye movement such as eye tracking, which is required for reading. Sometimes the nystagmus can be suppressed by immobilizing the head or preventing some head movement. Trial-and-error investigation with the individual child is required to determine what works best.

Obstructive Sleep Apnea

Obstructive apnea occurs when, despite breathing efforts, there is decreased airflow into or out of the lungs. Obstructive apnea is different from central apnea. In a central apnea event, there are no breathing efforts present. Obstructive sleep apnea occurs when there are multiple episodes of obstructive apnea, causing a person to wake up or have a drop in oxygen saturation during sleep.

Despite the impression that snoring, restless sleep, and sleep apnea are adult problems, obstructive sleep apnea is actually common in children. Snoring, the most common symptom of obstructive sleep apnea, occurs frequently in children as well. It is estimated that up to

10–12 percent of children snore regularly and that up to 1–5 percent of healthy preschool children have obstructive sleep apnea. Obstructive sleep apnea is much more common in children with abnormal muscle tone (such as those with cerebral palsy), as well as those with muscle diseases or abnormalities of the upper airway or the skull bones (craniofacial abnormalities).

Symptoms of obstructive sleep apnea include snoring and labored breathing during sleep. Family members might notice the child's chest caving in or his abdomen (belly) moving vigorously during sleep. Sometimes the child may actually gasp for air and arouse or seem to wake up during these episodes of labored breathing. Color changes to the lips and skin may occur as well, but these are rare. Some children sleep in unusual positions, with the neck extended; they may even sleep sitting up.

It is important to remember that even in children with severe symptoms at night, breathing is usually normal during the day. Some children will be congested or be chronic mouth breathers, while most will have no symptoms at all.

When breathing is labored at night and sleep is disrupted, behavioral symptoms or excessive daytime sleepiness can result. Some children with obstructive sleep apnea and severely disrupted sleep may be hyperactive, and there is growing evidence that school performance or learning can be negatively affected by poor sleep quality. Sleep disruption can occur in obstructive sleep apnea for several reasons, including the natural "arousal" response to airway obstruction and to abnormalities in the level of blood oxygen or carbon dioxide. Sleep may be disrupted many times during the night, resulting in inefficient, poor-quality sleep. Other nighttime symptoms can include bedwetting, sweating, and of course snoring and labored breathing.

In addition to behavioral and learning difficulties, obstructive sleep apnea can have other effects as well. In se-

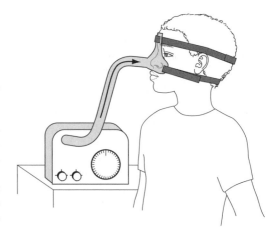

vere cases it can lead to growth failure (failure to thrive), hypertension, and even less commonly heart failure.

A careful sleep history and a sleep study to detect the presence of obstructive apnea can help diagnose obstructive sleep apnea. A sleep study is a test that is safe, painless, and highly accurate. In all cases a careful airway evaluation is indicated, since in otherwise healthy children the most common cause of obstructive sleep apnea is enlargement of the tonsils and adenoids, and removal of the tonsils and adenoids often cures the sleep apnea. In children with cerebral palsy, however, the main problem may be abnormal muscle tone, which is more difficult to overcome. Treatment may be tried with continuous or bilevel positive airway pressure (CPAP or BiPAP), supplemental oxygen, or, rarely, a tracheostomy.

Orthodontics
(malalignment of teeth)

Sometimes when a child's teeth come in, they don't meet each other in a way that best facilitates chewing and speech. Malaligned teeth can also spoil a person's appearance (this is more important to some people than to others).

Indications: Children with significant spasticity around the mouth are at risk of developing malaligned teeth. Treatment involves, first, deciding whether the malalignment presents a problem serious enough to require treatment. This determination involves considering the severity of the child's neurological defect as well as the potential effect on the child who must wear braces for several years.

For any brace to work, the child must be able to cooperate, which may be very difficult for the child with spasticity, who may bite down every time something is put into his mouth. Other considerations are the family's and the child's concern about cosmetic appearance, the availability of an experienced orthodontist, and the willingness and ability of someone to pay for the treatment. While orthodontic treatment may be desirable, it should have relatively low priority on the list of health care priorities established for an individual child. Certainly, other dental needs, such as maintaining healthy gums and preventing and treating cavities, are more important. Nevertheless, each child must be evaluated as an individual and his case considered with regard to other medical needs, family desires, and, most important, the child's desires.

Osteopenia

See Low Bone Mineral Density.

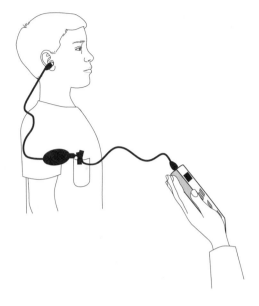

Otoacoustic Emission Testing

An otoacoustic emission test is an objective test of hearing ability. The outer hair cells of a healthy cochlea both receive and *produce* sounds. These sounds are produced spontaneously and can be elicited by a delivered sound. An audiologist can place a small probe in a child's ear canal, deliver a sound, and measure the otoacoustic emissions (OAEs). The presence of OAEs typically signifies that the cochlea is healthy and receiving sounds normally. Because the OAEs are very quiet, the child must be quiet or asleep during the test. OAEs are being used to screen hearing in newborn and young infants and children who cannot cooperate because of either age or disability, as it does not require any behavioral response on the part of the child.

If the audiologist cannot measure OAEs, this can mean that there is a hearing loss in the involved ear, but it could also mean that there is something blocking the sounds (such as earwax or fluid in the middle ear). Because of this, a child who "fails" his OAE test will often be examined by a pediatrician or an ear, nose, and throat specialist to be sure nothing is wrong with the outer or middle ear.

Palliative Care

Palliative care is an approach that focuses on improving the quality of life of patients who are facing complications associated with chronic or life-limiting disease. This care is achieved through early identification and treatment of pain and other medical or social problems.

Palliative care is often misinterpreted as hospice care. While hospice is a subset of palliative care, a child does not need to have a terminal illness to qualify for palliative care services. Many hospitals now have palliative care teams that function to support acute or chronically ill children with pain and symptom management so they can have the best quality of life possible.

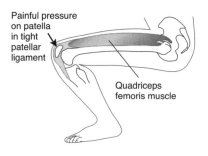

Pancreatitis

Pancreatitis is an inflammation of the pancreas that is characterized by abdominal pain, nausea, and vomiting and by an increase of the pancreatic enzymes amylase and lipase. It is usually self-limiting. Some medications that can cause pancreatitis include valproic acid and certain diuretics. Pancreatitis can also be seen after a posterior spinal fusion, a surgical procedure used for the treatment of scoliosis, which results from the pancreas being trapped in front of the spine. Treatment includes pain management and bowel rest for one to two weeks, during which food is taken intravenously. This is followed by a low-fat diet or placement of a special feeding tube beyond the stomach so that feedings are delivered into the small intestine, thus bypassing the pancreatic opening in the duodenum. The pancreatitis usually resolves between four and six weeks after the onset of the elevated enzymes.

Passive Motions

Passive motions are exercises performed upon a child without the child's assistance. Passive stretching consists in someone else stretching a child's muscles. These are common exercises that physical therapists use for children with cerebral palsy.

Patellar Pain
(chondromalacia, stress fracture of the patella, Osgood-Schlatter disease, osteochondrosis of the patella)

The patella is the kneecap. Patellar pain, or pain in the front of the knee, occurs in children with cerebral palsy, almost exclusively in those who walk with a severe crouched gait, due to hamstring tightness. Spasticity in the quadriceps muscle may also be present. Pain may be due to chondromalacia (excessive pressure behind the kneecap), stress fracture of the patella, osteochondrosis of the patella, and, uncommonly, instability (dislocation) of the patella. A child with a crouched gait stands with knees bent; the muscle in the front of the knee and kneecap is extremely tight, allowing him to stand. However, the pressure against the kneecap causes pain; if the pressure is great enough, it may cause a stress fracture through the bone and actually pull the patella apart. This

pain can become quite severe. If not treated properly, it may prevent the child from walking. This is especially true for children who develop stress fractures of the patella or significant stretching of the tendon.

Osteochondrosis of the patella occurs if the tendon that inserts into the patella pulls off. A similar situation, an inflammatory response called Osgood-Schlatter disease, occurs where the patellar tendon hooks onto the tibia. These are common problems in active, growing adolescents and even more so in children with CP and spasticity. As the child continues to grow, both of these conditions eventually resolve if the stress is not too high.

Care and treatment: The treatment of a crouched gait, osteochondrosis of the patella, and Osgood-Schlatter disease involves stretching the hamstrings in an attempt to get the child to stand up straighter and place less strain on the knees. If the knees cannot be adequately stretched out with physical therapy, surgical hamstring lengthening should be considered. Stress fractures through the bone, causing the patella to pull apart, are treated with casting until healing occurs.

Instability of the patella may be caused by a combination of hamstring and quadriceps tightness, a high-riding patella (too highly placed on the knee), and torsional problems (external tibial torsion and femoral anteversion). Therapy to stretch and strengthen muscles should be attempted first but is often unsuccessful in the child with cerebral palsy. Chronic instability causing pain should be treated surgically by correcting the causes above if they are present.

Pelvic Osteotomy
(Chiari osteotomy, Pemberton osteotomy, Dega osteotomy, acetabular shelf procedure)

The pelvic bone may be cut in a number of places, usually with the goal of redirecting or reshaping the acetabulum, which is the cup, or socket, part of the hip joint.

Indications: This procedure is performed on children with spastic hip disease because the socket is deformed from abnormal pressure and has not developed normally. The socket needs to be reshaped in order to provide better coverage if the hip is to stay in the socket.

The surgery: A variety of procedures have been developed (each named after the person who developed it), but each surgery involves making a cut in the pelvis above the hip joint socket, the acetabulum. For children with CP, if the operation has a name, it may be called Dega, San Diego, or peri-ileal osteotomy; all are essentially the same operation. This surgery reshapes the socket (acetabulum) to make it more cup shaped so as to fit the ball of the hip better. Over the last 20 years this has become almost the universal surgery to treat the deformed socket in children with CP by surgeons who are experienced in treating this condition.

After-surgery care: For the pelvic procedure a cast is not usually required, although some surgeons believe that children are more comfortable wearing a cast for several weeks. The child may return to full weight bearing immediately for walking or to full physical therapy, depending on the bone quality.

What to expect: Generally one can expect that the socket will successfully hold the ball of the hip joint permanently. A few children who are very young (under age 6) and have severe dislocations and older children with severe socket deformities develop recurrent dislocations, but this is uncommon.

Pneumonia

Pneumonia, or pneumonitis, is characterized by inflammation of the lung, primarily caused by infection. The diagnosis of pneumonia is usually a clinical one, with fever, increased respiratory rate, retractions of the chest wall muscles, and, if measured, a drop in the oxygen saturation in the blood. Often a chest x-ray is done to confirm this clinical impression. The infection is most commonly either viral or bacterial, though some cases of infectious pneumonia can be caused by fungi. In children with CP, many cases of pneumonia are caused by aspiration of material from the throat, causing either infectious or chemical pneumonitis.

Most of the pneumonias in infancy are of viral origin. Bacterial infections are treated with antibiotics, whereas

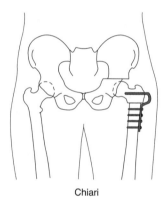

Chiari

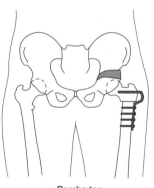

Pemberton

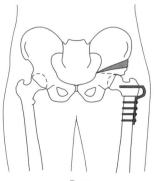

Dega

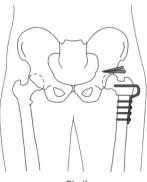

Shelf

viral infections usually are not. Aspiration pneumonia is usually treated with antibiotics to prevent either a primary infection caused by whatever was aspirated or a super-infection, a bacterial infection following injury to the lung caused by the aspiration.

Children with CP who also have problems with swallowing are much more likely to aspirate their own saliva, food that they are eating, or stomach acid and food that may be refluxing from their stomach. The resulting pneumonia can be quite severe. Sometimes however, children who are aspirating have chronic mild subclinical symptoms, such as chronic wheezing or congestion without typical symptoms of pneumonia.

If the child with pneumonia is not having severe respiratory distress, he or she can often be treated as an outpatient with oral antibiotics if there is a suspicion of bacterial infection. If the pneumonia is felt to be viral, such as that caused by influenza or respiratory syncytial virus (RSV), then antibiotics are of no help and treatment is of the symptoms alone, such as Tylenol for fever and nebulized medications for wheezing. For children with more significant respiratory symptoms, admission to the hospital and treatment with intravenous antibiotics is often necessary. Children with severe respiratory distress may end up in the intensive care unit on a ventilator. While any child can have an acute episode of pneumonia, a history of two or three such episodes in a child with CP would make one very suspicious that the child is aspirating and needs some investigation to see if there is either severe reflux or aspiration of food or secretions from the mouth.

Porencephalic Cyst

A porencephalic cyst within the brain results from damage to the brain tissue, such as that caused by a stroke or an infection, during late fetal or early infant life. Sometimes these cysts cause no problems at all and the child develops normally. Other times they can cause neurological deficits localized to one limb or side. Porencephalic cysts are quite common in children with cerebral palsy. These cysts sometimes progressively enlarge and eventually impinge on the ventricles (the fluid cavities) of the brain, causing hydrocephalus, which is the increased accumulation of cerebrospinal fluid within the ventricles. Shunt surgery may be indicated in the unusual circumstance that porencephaly is causing abnormal enlargement of the head and progressive loss of motor skills.

Prematurity

The normal gestational period is considered to be 40 weeks from the first day of the mother's last menstrual period. By definition, normal gestation can vary by two weeks; that is, it can be anywhere from 38 to 42 weeks. Prematurity is defined as birth before 38 weeks. Many children with cerebral palsy were born prematurely. Being born prematurely puts the child at risk for a variety of medical and neurological problems. However, with the improved care for premature infants that is delivered in intensive care nurseries, many of these problems are now rare except in the smallest of premature babies. Those born between 23 and 30 weeks of gestation are at the highest risk for CP, attention deficit disorder, and various learning disorders, with the most immature infants at the greatest risk.

Pressure Mapping

Children who do not have normal movement ability often develop pressure sores, also called bedsores or decubitus ulcers. This skin breakdown occurs because of too much pressure over too long a period. A tool that is used to determine where this high pressure is coming from is the pressure-mapping mat. This is a soft mat or blanket with sensors embedded in it to measure the pressure when the child sits or lies on it. The mat is attached to a computer, which shows an image of the contact area and measures the amount of pressure in any small area.

The pressure mat can be used in a wheelchair to see whether a problem with the seat back or the seat is causing the skin ulcer. It can also be placed under the child while the child is lying down to see if the pressure is caused by a specific position. Pressure mapping is an important part of the treatment of pressure sores, since the goal of treatment should be not only to heal the sore but also to determine what caused it and prevent it from happening again. See illustration on page 433.

Psychological Evaluation

Psychological evaluations typically include various testing activities, an interview with parents or guardians regarding a child's history, and direct observations. Often, teacher interviews, behavioral and social and emotional rating scales, developmental questionnaires, and a review of relevant medical and/or educational records are also completed. Testing activities can involve a variety of problem-solving tasks, including answering questions, hands-on activities, using a computer, and paper-and-pencil tasks. A comprehensive psychological evaluation could provide information regarding a child's intellectual abilities, learning and memory, attention and executive functioning (organization, planning, self-monitoring, cognitive flexibility), language, academic achievement, motor coordination, behavioral and emotional functioning, and/or general adaptive behavior.

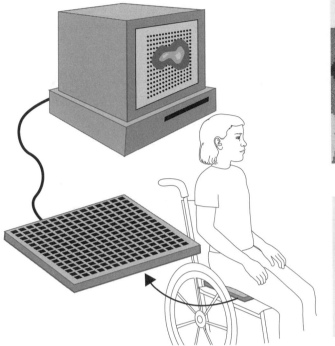

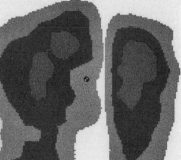

Normal pressure seating map

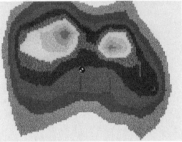

High pressure seating map

Children with cerebral palsy, however, often require unique testing. Sensory, motor, or language limitations may make it difficult to utilize common standardized measures. For example, a child with manual motor difficulties may find it difficult to efficiently complete a timed activity requiring motor skills. Children with limited language may find it challenging to produce verbal responses that reflect their knowledge or problem-solving capabilities. This makes it difficult to ascertain whether a weakness is due to a cognitive or an output deficit. Further complicating testing of children with CP is the way that tests are normed. Standardized norm-referenced assessment measures require a "standard" administration to allow comparison with appropriate age norms. While many children with cerebral palsy have adequate expressive language capabilities and motor skills, others do not and require modified testing activities. This makes some psychological findings difficult to interpret. Yet, a skilled evaluator can "adapt" many assessment measures to provide a reasonably reliable and valid indication of a child's capabilities. For example, nonverbal measures of reasoning and problem solving can be utilized when there is limited speech output. Many of these measures also allow for creative administration methods and response modes, so that the clinician has a better understanding of a child's capabilities. In addition to nonverbal assessment techniques, evaluators can choose test measures that allow pointing, multiple-choice formats, voice-

output devices, or other forms of technology. Sometimes having a child's teacher, aide, or parent participate in the evaluation provides the child the most comfortable environment in which to demonstrate his or her skills.

Quadriplegia
(pentaplegia, total body involvement, bilateral CP)

The term *quadriplegia* refers to cerebral palsy in which all four limbs are involved, with difficulty in motor control and tone imbalance. The newer term, preferred by some professionals, is *bilateral CP*. Occasionally, the term *pentaplegia* is used for those people who also have significant difficulty with motor control of the face or head. Another commonly used term is *total body involvement*, which also implies difficulty with motor control of the face, head, and neck, in addition to the four limbs. All of these terms may be used interchangeably and do not have strict independent meaning. (See Chapter 7.)

Rectus Femoris Transfer
(rectus femoris release, stiff leg walk, knee extension contracture, quadriceps contracture)

When spasticity in a child involves the quadriceps muscle (the large muscle in the front of the thigh), the rectus femoris muscle, which lies across the front of the knee,

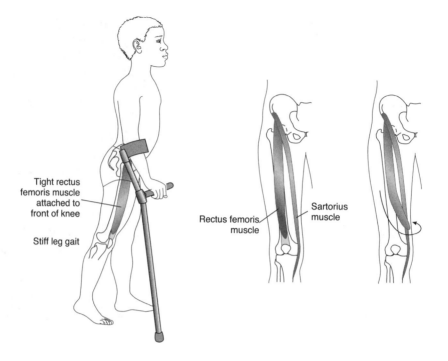

Tight rectus femoris muscle attached to front of knee

Stiff leg gait

Rectus femoris muscle

Sartorius muscle

is usually responsible. Spasticity of the rectus muscle causes stiff knee. The knee can be stiff when the child walks, specifically as he picks up his foot and attempts to bend his knee to swing the foot forward, which causes a stiff-legged gait; or the knee may be completely incapable of bending, causing difficulty sitting. If someone is unable to bend the knee in order to sit in a wheelchair, then the leg sticks out in front.

Care and treatment: Initially, treatment for spasticity of the rectus muscle should involve stretching exercises, which frequently helps the problems with seating. However, walking typically does not help stretch this muscle when it is tight. Surgical lengthening or transfer of this muscle is the most common treatment for this problem, but it is usually not an isolated procedure. Instead, it is one of a number of surgical procedures that improve the gait or the ability to sit.

The surgery: The procedure is done at the knee. It involves defining the rectus muscle and separating it from the three other muscles. It may simply be lengthened and allowed to slide; if this is done, however, the muscle usually reattaches and again becomes a problem. Instead, the operation should involve transferring the muscle to the inside of the thigh and attaching the tendon to the sartorius or semitendinous muscles. This transfer helps the hamstrings to bend the knee. Some surgeons transfer the rectus muscle to the outside of the knee to control rotational problems of the legs; the outcome of this pro-

cedure is unpredictable—though it is generally unsuccessful. This same procedure is done for those patients who have difficulty bending the knee enough to sit. In some severely involved patients, lengthening of the three muscles underlying the rectus muscle is required. This should be done if the knees do not bend.

A recently developed procedure is the rectus recession. This involves removing part of the tendon that inserts at the knee. It is a simpler procedure, with an easier recovery for the patient. The outcomes reported are relatively short term but are the same as those of the rectus transfer. Further research will be required before it can be recommended as equally effective.

Benefits and risks: The major benefit is the reduction of spasticity in the rectus muscle. The complications from this surgery are minor, and the risk of overlengthening to the point of developing the opposite deformity is minimal. Treatment after this surgery usually does not require a cast and starts with immediate ambulation and movement.

Reflexes
(normal postural reflexes, primitive reflexes, deep tendon reflexes)

The function of the central nervous system with respect to motor behavior is to coordinate the ability to move while maintaining posture and equilibrium. Every movement and change in posture produces a shift in body's relationship to the ground. Therefore, if we are

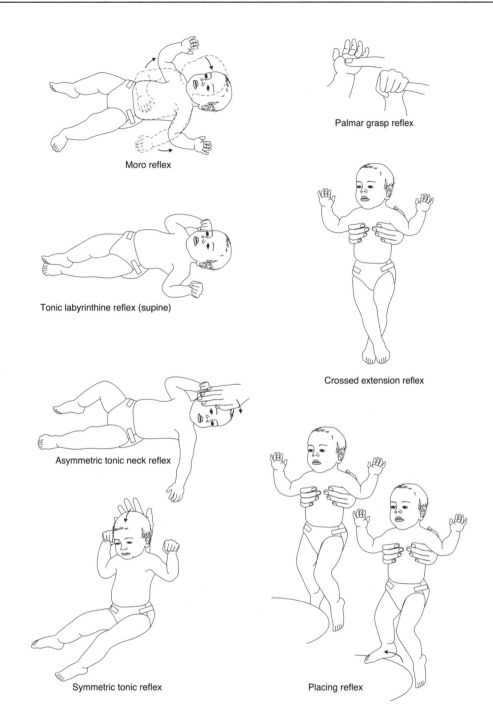

Moro reflex

Palmar grasp reflex

Tonic labyrinthine reflex (supine)

Crossed extension reflex

Asymmetric tonic neck reflex

Symmetric tonic reflex

Placing reflex

not to fall, there must be a fluctuation of tone throughout the musculature to maintain our balance while moving. These changes and patterns, known as normal postural reflexes, are brought about automatically. These reactions can be grouped as *righting reactions* and *equilibrium reactions*. Righting reactions are automatic but active responses—they maintain the normal position of the head in space and the normal alignment of the head and neck with the trunk and of the trunk with the limbs. Equilibrium reactions restore balance through complex responses to changes in posture and movement. They show themselves in slight changes of tone throughout

Table 7. Primitive Reflexes

Name	How to Elicit	Response	Appears and Disappears
Moro	Place the infant in the supine position (on the back); lift by the arm, raising the head a bit off the table, and then let go.	Extension followed by abduction of the arms with partial flexing of the elbows, wrists, and fingers.	Birth–5 months
Tonic labyrinthine	Extend the infant's head and neck 45 degrees in the midline by placing a hand between the shoulder blades.	The shoulders retract, resulting in flexion of the arms. The legs also assume a slight extensor posture. Two types of obligatory responses are always abnormal: the "decorticate" posture, in which there is primarily shoulder retraction with flexion of the arms at the elbows, and the "decerebrate" posture, where the arms assume full extension and pronation.	Birth–9 months
Asymmetric tonic neck (ATNR)	Turn the head 45 degrees to the right or left side while the infant is in the supine position.	The arm on the chin side will go out into extension, while the arm on the other side (facing the back of the head) becomes more flexed. This is known as the fencing reaction. The legs may assume a similar posture to a lesser extent.	Birth–6 months
Symmetric tonic neck (STNR)	(a) With infant held in sitting position, extend the neck backward. (b) With infant held in sitting position, flex the head.	(a) Upper extremities extend outward and legs flex. (b) The arms flex and the legs extend.	Rarely present in normal children; may be seen intermittently until 4–6 months in some normal children
Crossed extension	Apply a noxious stimulus such as a pinch or a pinprick to the sole of one foot while holding that leg in complete extension.	The other leg first flexes, followed by adduction (crosses over toward the other leg), and finally extension as if to push away the noxious stimulus.	Birth–2 months
Stepping reflex	Hold the infant in vertical position and touch the sole of one foot to the ground or tabletop. The other foot flexes, adducts, and extends.	While the second foot is flexing and adducting, the examiner immediately turns the infant so that when extension occurs that foot receives the weight, thus producing a walking or stepping response.	Birth–6 weeks
Palmar and plantar grasp	Put pressure on palm of hand or sole of foot.	Hand grasps and holds; foot flexes and grasps.	Hand: Birth–3 months (blends into voluntary activity) Foot: Birth–9 months
Upper placing	Press the back of the hand against the edge of a table.	The hand is initially lifted above the extension of the arm, thus placing the hand on the tabletop.	3 months–no stated age. These reflexes gradually merge into volitional behavior, and disappearance can't be easily assessed.

(*continued*)

Table 7. (continued)

Name	How to Elicit	Response	Appears and Disappears
Lower placing	Press the top of the foot against the edge of a table while holding the infant upright.	The leg initially flexes and then extends, "placing" the foot on the tabletop.	Birth–no stated age. These reflexes gradually merge into volitional behavior, and disappearance can't be easily assessed.
Positive support	Hold the infant in a vertical position under the arms with head in the neutral position. Bounce the child 3–5 times on the balls of the feet.	Three findings are possible: (a) absence of any response; (b) momentary extension of the legs, thus supporting the weight momentarily, followed by flexion; or (c) full extension, thus supporting the body weight.	Birth–no stated age. These reflexes gradually merge into volitional behavior, and disappearance can't be easily assessed.

the muscles and by visible countermovements to restore the disturbed balance. These reactions are needed to achieve, first, balance while sitting and, later, the ability to stand and to walk.

In the child with cerebral palsy, delay in or interference with the development of these reactions causes delay in achieving these motor abilities. The three main reasons for the delay in the appearance of the righting and equilibrium responses are the persistence of primitive reflexes past the age at which they are normally present, the presence of a primitive reflex to an abnormal degree, and the presence of hypotonia (low tone). All three are present to some degree in the child with CP. The postural reflexes do not usually appear until the latter half of the first year, between the ages of 6 and 12 months. They include the neck-righting reaction and the labyrinthine-righting reaction, among others. The parachute reaction is an equilibrium reaction that is often looked at clinically because it is delayed or asymmetrical in cerebral palsy. (The parachute reaction is what should happen when the child is thrust head first toward the examining table: she should extend both arms in front as if to break the fall.)

Primitive reflexes (see pages 436–37 [table 7]) are essentially brainstem-mediated responses that develop during fetal life and are present at birth. The majority of them disappear at between 3 and 6 months of age. At any age, if a primitive reflex is obligatory, it is always considered pathological because it signifies the presence of a motor disability, most likely cerebral palsy. A primitive reflex is described as obligatory if it is sustained for more than 30 seconds and head movements control both upper and lower extremity positioning, with the child unable to break out of the pattern, even with crying. *Absence* of reflex activity at a time when it is nor-

mally present is also an important indicator: it may reflect generalized hypotonia that could be secondary to severe central nervous system dysfunction. Asymmetry of these reflexes (that is, an abnormal reflex on one side of the body and a normal one on the other) is abnormal and may indicate developing hemiplegia. Discrepancy between upper and lower extremity activity may aid in the subclassification of cerebral palsy.

Deep tendon reflexes are stretching reflexes in which the muscles are suddenly stretched by a sudden tap with a finger or rubber hammer. In a medical examination, these reflexes are tested at the knees, ankles, elbows, and wrists. In people with cerebral palsy, the reaction is typically stronger than normal.

Rehabilitation
(continuum of care)

Rehabilitation means teaching a child to regain a function that he formerly had, such as the ability to walk or to perform activities of daily living. Teaching a new activity is technically called *habilitation*, although when speaking of the care of children, *habilitation* and *rehabilitation* are used interchangeably. Rehabilitation may take place inside or outside the hospital. Hospital stays for rehabilitation purposes generally last between two and six weeks. In the hospital, the child is handled by an integrated team that includes a physician trained in rehabilitation (usually a physiatrist), physical, occupational, and speech-language therapists, and specially trained nurses. Rehabilitation is offered in a continuum from hospital to outpatient facility, to school, and finally and most importantly, to the home. Therapies are given as close to home as is medically possible.

Indications for inpatient rehabilitation include a

recent illness or injury that acutely alters a child's capabilities to function or new medical issues that need to be sorted out. Goals might include feeding techniques, teaching parents the new care needs of their child, attention to safety in the environment, and mobility.

There are benefits from inpatient rehabilitation immediately after some surgical procedures, such as dorsal rhizotomies and some orthopedic procedures, because the child needs intense physical therapy to regain and maximize function. This may be done with the younger child, even as young as 2 or 3 years of age, though it may be very difficult emotionally for such a young child to be left by a parent for several weeks. In this age group, parents often stay with the child in the hospital.

There are also specific special needs that may be best addressed in the inpatient unit, such as the need for high-technology communication aids and mobility aids. The focus is not only on teaching the child to perform the activities himself but also on teaching the patient to direct his care.

In recent years, more and more programs have developed outpatient or day programs that provide comprehensive physician-directed rehabilitation. Length of stay for inpatient programs has decreased, and children often finish their acute rehabilitation as outpatients. Some children return for a few weeks of outpatient care each year rather than being hospitalized away from their family. Children do better sleeping in their own beds and coming in to a center for their therapies. Such centers need to have a strong multidisciplinary program that addresses the unique needs of the child living at home. The program remains in close contact with the school, and at the appropriate time the child resumes his program in his own school.

Rehabilitation involves partnership between the child, the family, and rehabilitation specialists, with the goal of maximizing the child's function in his or her own community.

Retinopathy of Prematurity
(ROP)

Children who were born prematurely and have a low birthweight are at risk for developing retinopathy of prematurity, a condition that in its severest form can cause blindness in one or both eyes. If the condition progresses to a certain stage, treatment is available that can significantly decrease the chances of severe visual impairment. Treatment most commonly consists in a laser treatment delivered to the retina inside the eye or an injection of a medication into the eye. The treatments cause the abnormal blood vessels to regress.

Rigidity

The term *rigidity* is generally synonymous with *stiffness*. Some children with cerebral palsy become very stiff, especially in the joints. This stiffness can be due to spasticity, in which the muscles become extremely tight but then suddenly relax. If the stiff muscle does not suddenly relax but slowly stretches out, with the feeling of bending a lead pipe, then the correct term is *rigidity*. For some children with CP, rigidity is a main component of their motor problem. More commonly, it becomes a mild but common feature in early adulthood of individuals with severe spasticity.

Scoliosis
(posterior spinal fusion, anterior spinal fusion, unit rod, pedicle screw and rod fixation)

Scoliosis is a side bending of the spine that occurs in many diseases. The type of scoliosis a person has is dependent on the cause. It is important to recognize that scoliosis resulting from one cause has very little relationship to scoliosis resulting from another cause. Scoliosis is a symptom or the effect of some underlying disease process. For the condition to be resolved, the treatment must be directed to the cause.

The incidence of scoliosis in children with cerebral palsy varies. It is uncommon in children with hemiplegia but slightly more common in patients with diplegia. The incidence for these two groups varies from 1 in 100 to 1 in 1,000. There may be some overlap, because having CP does not preclude one from also having idio-

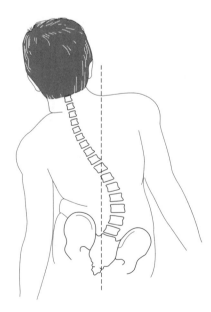

pathic scoliosis, and it may be difficult to separate the two in some patients. The highest incidence of scoliosis in children with CP is in children who are unable to walk (those classified as GMFCS IV and V). These children have a 75 to 85 percent chance of developing severe scoliosis, which requires treatment.

Scoliosis in children with cerebral palsy is caused by poor muscle control, poor coordination, or asymmetrical muscle pull. The muscles in the spine function to keep the spine straight, just as the guide wires around a radio tower function to keep the tall, slender tower standing straight. Initially, the scoliosis in young children with CP (between the ages of 2 and 8) is postural. At this age, when children sit up and do not have postural control they bend one way one time and in the opposite direction the next time. This scoliosis should be of very little concern, since it is flexible; as soon as the children lie down their spines straighten out.

During the adolescent growth spurt, which occurs between the ages of 8 and 14, the spine becomes much longer, and it is then that the side bending develops a more permanent structured curve, so that the child starts to bend only to one side. The spinal vertebrae at this time not only bend sideways but also rotate and start to stiffen into place. During this period of adolescent growth, an increasing curve combines with stiffness or resistance of the curve, and the spine no longer straightens out when the child lies down. This is termed *structural scoliosis*, which progressively worsens.

There was a time when doctors believed that applying body braces would help to prevent the progression or development of scoliosis in children with CP. The general consensus now is that braces neither delay the onset of scoliosis nor affect the curve's severity. Thus, there is no reason to prescribe spinal braces with the goal of treating the scoliosis. A brace made of a soft foamlike material can be used to help with sitting posture only in cases of a smaller, more flexible scoliosis curve. However, it should not be expected to actually keep the curve from worsening.

As the scoliosis gets worse, sitting often becomes much more difficult. Wheelchair modifications need to be made. Soon the child develops pelvic obliquity, meaning that the pelvis does not sit level to the chair seat, so that the child sits only on one side of the pelvis or hip. If the scoliosis becomes worse, the pelvis slips inside the chest cage, and the ribs start to cause irritation as they rub against the pelvis. This is usually the condition that causes pain. As the scoliosis progresses, it becomes more difficult for the abdominal muscles and the diaphragm to work, which makes breathing more difficult. Scoliosis that becomes very severe can affect the blood flow through the lungs and cause heart problems. There may be difficulty with the swallowing mechanism and with

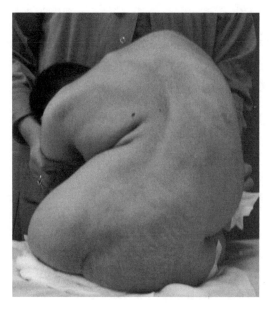

stomach function. As the scoliosis continues to progress and becomes very severe, sitting for any period of time becomes difficult. Frequently there are only one or two positions in which lying down is comfortable.

Other types of scoliosis include idiopathic scoliosis, congenital scoliosis, and the scoliosis associated with muscular dystrophy. The most common of these is idiopathic scoliosis, which occurs predominantly in preadolescent or adolescent girls. Scoliosis in children who do not have cerebral palsy is treated very differently from scoliosis in children with CP. Scoliosis screening is employed to attempt to identify the idiopathic form early in the normal child. The exact causes of idiopathic scoliosis are unknown (which is what *idiopathic* means—that we don't know what causes it). Idiopathic scoliosis is the type for which body braces and jackets are prescribed to prevent the further progression of the curve. This type of scoliosis is also treated with a spinal fusion when it becomes sufficiently severe that the risk of the curve's progression into adulthood is anticipated.

The classic instrumentation used for scoliosis in the child with CP is the unit rod. A U-shaped rod is fixed into the pelvis and then attached to the spine with wires and sometimes screws. Most surgeons not trained to treat CP are not familiar with this technique and prefer to use screws and rods, as they would for typical idiopathic scoliosis. If the fusions are from the top of the spine (T1) to the pelvis, then the outcome is often similar. The systems using screws and rods have difficulty correcting pelvic obliquity if it is severe. In this case the unit rod or the modular variation provides better correction. Correction of the pelvic obliquity is important for long-term comfortable seating.

Care and treatment: For treating scoliosis in children with cerebral palsy, the choice is between a posterior spinal fusion and no treatment at all. Without treatment, the child eventually will be unable to sit and will have increased problems breathing. Treatments such as exercises, therapy, braces, and manipulations have no impact on the outcome.

If the scoliosis is permitted to develop naturally, there is no certainty that it will become severe enough to prevent sitting, although this does occur in the majority of people. If the person is in an institutional care facility, then keeping him on his back, but with frequent changes of position so that bedsores don't develop, may be a reasonable alternative. One also needs to consider that some loss of respiratory and gastric function may occur.

For those children who can see well enough to watch television or to interact with their peers or family members, a full-time reclining position makes such activities difficult, if not impossible. It also makes feeding, as well as respiratory care and function, more difficult. In addition, when a child can no longer sit in a wheelchair, transportation and participation in activities outside the home become difficult.

Indications: The indications for a posterior spinal fusion include consideration of the child's remaining growth, as well as the severity and stiffness of the curve. For a child who still has a lot of growing ahead, the curve may be allowed to progress further, up to 90 degrees if it is not too stiff, because after the posterior spinal fusion is performed spinal growth will stop. This is usually not of major concern, since at most the procedure will remove an inch or two from the child's ultimate adult height. The posterior spinal fusion is usually performed when the child is between the ages of 10 and 15. It is best to avoid allowing the curve to become very large, and especially very stiff, because this will necessitate two operations.

If the decision is made to proceed with a spinal fusion, the goal should be to correct malalignment so the child will sit straight with a normal appearance. There is very little place today for the type of spinal fusion whose only goal is to prevent the scoliosis from progressing, since the child who sits all the time needs to be placed straight upright, with the pelvis and shoulders in a parallel position. Current technology makes it possible to perform a spinal fusion without a great deal of difficulty. Generally, a child with CP who has a spinal curve between 60 and 90 degrees is considered a candidate for fusion.

The surgery: The operation usually takes approximately four hours to complete. The patient may then need to spend time on a ventilator and in the intensive care unit.

This is a major operation that often requires transfusion of a significant amount of blood, frequently one to two times the child's blood volume. The second or third day after surgery, the child can sit up in a wheelchair. Braces or casts are not necessary with modern instrumentation systems. For young, small children, growing rods are currently a popular option in some centers. However, the children with CP who develop early scoliosis tend to have the most severe neurological disability. In addition, they usually also have seizures, weak bones, and feeding and respiratory problems and are at very high risk for complications from a procedure that may require multiple operations. Reports of use of growing rods in children with CP have shown very high significant complications. Currently we do not favor this approach except in very rare cases.

Benefits and risks: After the fusion, the child may be handled in the same way as before surgery. Frequently parents find handling their child much easier after surgery because he is straight, can sit much better, and is stiff in the midsection. Significant complications and risks associated with the spinal fusion include a very large blood transfusion, which brings with it the small risk of contracting an infection. The large amount of blood needed in debilitated patients usually means they are not able to donate their own blood. Infection of the back is also a possible complication. Injury to the spinal cord is a possibility, especially when the curve is severe. If the surgery is performed by an experienced spinal surgeon, this risk should be quite small. A fairly common complication after a posterior spinal fusion is pancreatitis. This inflammation of the pancreas can cause abdominal pain, abdominal distension, and vomiting. It can significantly delay the resumption of feeding through the stomach, making intravenous nutrition the only route for calories for days to weeks after the surgery.

Many children with CP who undergo a spinal fusion are slender, with very little body fat, and marginal nutrition can make healing large surgical wounds difficult. It is beneficial to increase feeding prior to surgery so that the child gains weight. Immediately after surgery, the child needs nutritional support. Specially placed intravenous lines or feeding tubes placed into the intestines provide ways to start extra feeding almost immediately after surgery. This is especially important in the case of severe curves that require surgery in the front of the spine. After this operation, which is a much smaller procedure, it may be a week before the posterior spinal surgery is done. If great care is not taken with nutrition, the child may go 10 to 14 days without adequate intake, a length of time that a slender child is not able to tolerate. Frequently, this type of child develops complications such as poor wound healing, infection, or pneumonia.

What to expect: Parents usually need to plan for the child to be out of school for approximately four weeks, as two weeks is the average stay in the hospital for a child undergoing a posterior spinal fusion. For those who need both front and back surgery for severe scoliosis, three weeks in the hospital and another week or two at home will be necessary. Following the surgery no special care is needed, and the child may start standing or even walking if he is able.

Seizures
(epilepsy)

The brain normally has electrical activity going on within it in a controlled manner. A seizure is a sudden burst of abnormal electrical activity in the brain that interferes with normal brain functioning. It can cause involuntary uncontrolled movements and/or behavior changes and a change in awareness. Epilepsy is a group of disorders, characterized by recurrent seizures. Epilepsy is not a disease. (See Chapter 3 for more details.)

Selective Dorsal Rhizotomy
(SDR, dorsal rhizotomy)

Selective dorsal rhizotomy (SDR) is a spinal operation to control lower limb spasticity. *Rhizotomy* is the medical term for cutting nerve rootlets. *Dorsal* refers to nerve rootlets that attach to the back side of the spinal cord. These nerve rootlets are responsible for sensation. The nerve rootlets that attach to the front, or ventral, side of the spinal cord control muscles; these rootlets are not involved in the operation. The operation is called *selective* because the rootlets most responsible for spasticity are identified for cutting by electrical recordings. Rootlets that seem to be less involved are spared.

SDR is an operation performed by a neurosurgeon, but optimal care is provided by a CP team that includes an orthopedist, a rehabilitation physician and therapists, and a developmental pediatrician. The rehabilitation program must be considered part of a coordinated, long-term plan. Most often SDR is recommended for young children with spastic diplegia who have attained independent ambulation. For such children SDR improves the mechanics and the appearance of gait. Erect posture, reduction of scissoring, and foot placement on the heel are goals that can often be achieved. Less commonly SDR may be considered for more severely affected children who need to reduce lower limb tone to facilitate care such as bathing and diapering. Pump implantation for intrathecal baclofen is the standard recommendation for such patients, but if geography or aversion to an implanted device makes this option unattractive, SDR may be considered.

SDR may be offered as part of a comprehensive, individualized care plan because on its own it does not provide everything a child with cerebral palsy needs. It does not liberate children from AFOs. It does not reliably avoid the need for later orthopedic surgery, although the tone reduction it achieves may make orthopedic surgery more successful. It does not relocate dislocated hips. It may have beneficial effects on upper limb tone, speech clarity, and even drooling, but these effects are not predictable.

The surgery takes between two and three hours, and typically a child spends four hours or a little more in the operating room. A midline incision is made over the lower spine. The length of the incision varies depending on the surgeon's preferred technique. The roof of the spinal canal is opened. The nerve rootlets float in cerebrospinal fluid (CSF) inside a sack with a thin, tough membrane called the *dura*. The dura is opened, and the rootlets are identified on the basis of anatomic landmarks and electrical stimulation. The dorsal rootlets are stimulated individually, and the reactions of the muscles of the lower limbs are recorded and observed. Rootlets that are more excitable—typically about half—are divided, and the less excitable rootlets are spared. (Some surgeons do not believe that electrical stimulation is reliable or necessary. They simply cut more or less than half the rootlets at the spinal levels that seem most involved for the individual patient.) The dura and the roof of the spinal canal are repaired, and the wound is closed. Patients remain horizontal in bed for at least 2 days after surgery to minimize the risk of CSF leakage from the wound.

What to expect: The operation is just the first step. What follows is an intensive program of therapy during which the child learns to walk without spasticity. This program is supervised by a rehabilitation physician. It begins in the inpatient unit, and it continues on an outpatient basis five days a week for at least four weeks, and often longer. This rehabilitation is a critical component of the treatment package. A child who undergoes SDR but does not receive the necessary rehabilitation will lose function. Inability to cooperate with rehabilitation or family circumstances that make compliance impossible are compelling reasons not to proceed with SDR.

Potential early complications of SDR include CSF leakage from the wound, which can interfere with wound healing and lead to infection. If the surgeon extends the operation into the second sacral level or lower, there can be disturbance of bladder function; if the operation is restricted to the first sacral level and higher, no effect on bladder function is anticipated. Tone reduction seems quite durable for as long as 10 years, but few data are available for longer periods. Exaggeration of the forward curvature of the lumbar spine (kyphosis) has been reported in long-term follow-up of children who walk independently, but this curvature has not caused symptoms or required additional surgery.

Sensorimotor Experience
(sensorimotor perception)

The ability to perceive and feel the movement of a limb when certain muscles are activated is a sensorimotor perception or experience. For example, when a child moves her arms or legs, she is able to perceive this movement by the positional senses that are present in the limbs. When she grasps an object, she can perceive its shape and the weight of the object in her hand.

The sensory feedback that is necessary for sensorimotor perception is often diminished in children with cerebral palsy. Their inability to move in space in the way a nondisabled child of the same age moves further diminishes this experience. A caregiver often discovers just how much difficulty a child with CP has when trying to teach the child to operate a motorized wheelchair. The deficit will often be more noticeable in wide-open areas outside, such as when moving along a sidewalk, than it will be within the narrow confines of a hallway or a small room. In narrow areas the child has learned to perceive movement based on her eyes alone, but this is more difficult in wide-open areas, where additional feedback is required. This deficiency can be overcome with practice and training in the use of the power chair. Gradually the child incorporates the available sensorimotor experience into a functional mechanism for perceiving the body's movement in space.

Spasticity
(spasm)

A spasm is an involuntary muscles contraction. When these contractions are persistent and cannot be voluntarily stopped, the child is said to have spasticity. When a caregiver attempts to move the child's joints, they will feel stiff; however, with gentle stretching the muscles suddenly relax. This form of stiffness caused by spasticity is substantially different from that caused by rigidity. With rigidity, the muscles do not suddenly relax and free the extremity but remain stiff regardless of any attempts to move the joints.

Spasticity is present in children with spinal cord injuries, occasionally in those with spina bifida; it may also develop with some other nerve conditions, such as multiple sclerosis. In the infant with cerebral palsy, spasticity is seldom significant in the first 6 months, but sometime between 6 months and 24 months it starts to become apparent. Initially, the child may be very floppy, but spasticity may develop with maturity. Proper positioning and postural control can decrease spasticity to some extent.

Care and treatment: Treatment of spasticity involves many different options, from nerve injections and medications by mouth to several surgical procedures. Medications used are of the benzodiazepine family—diazepam (Valium), clonazepam (Klonopin), lorazepam (Ativan), baclofen (Lioresal), tizanidine (Zanaflex), or dantrolene (Dantrium). The side effects of these medications when given by mouth, especially drowsiness, often make them unsuitable for long-term use in children with CP, though they are very useful for short-term use after surgery, for example. Some children will develop a tolerance to the sedative effects, but then there is usually less decrease in the spasticity as well. The use of an intrathecal baclofen pump, which is implanted in the abdomen and places the drug directly into the spinal fluid, where it has a direct effect on the nerves, is an effective treatment and has less sedative effect. (See Baclofen Pump.)

Treatments that are directed at the nerves involve injections with botulinum toxin. The efficacy of these treatments is limited because their effects don't last. Nerves may be surgically sectioned or crushed, but spasticity may recur in spite of this deliberate damage unless very large nerves are destroyed.

Another surgical treatment is *selective dorsal rhizotomy*, in which the nerves as they exit from the spinal cord are identified and the ones found to be most involved with the spasticity are cut (see Selective Dorsal Rhizotomy). Another option is to lengthen, release, or occasionally transfer specific muscles whose spasticity is causing problems; however, it should be confirmed that the antagonistic or opposing muscles are not also spastic, in which case the opposite deformity could then develop.

Speech-Language Therapy

Speech-language therapists diagnose and treat problems of the oral motor system, including feeding and speech issues. In the child with CP, they often evaluate the mechanical process of eating, which involves understanding how the mouth handles food, in what positions a child is best able to control the mouth muscles, how the food is moved in the mouth to the back of the throat, and how well the swallowing mechanism works.

The speech-language therapist often conducts a detailed examination using different food textures, often taking special x-rays in order to observe the swallowing mechanism on the x-ray screen. Based on this detailed examination, the speech-language therapist can decide whether oral feeding is safe for the child and make specific recommendations concerning how to place the food in the mouth, what textures of food to use, and what position the child should be in to eat safely. Speech-language therapists specialize in different areas, so it is important to be certain that the therapist who is evaluating the child for feeding problems has experience specifically in that area.

Another major effort of speech-language therapy is directed at evaluating and teaching phonation (how to breathe and to use the vocal cords to make sounds) and articulation (how to produce speech sounds in isolation, in sequences of vowels and consonants, in words, and in longer utterances that are considered "connected speech").

Indications: Speech-language therapy is recommended for a child who has difficulty with feeding, especially with swallowing, or for a child who has difficulty speaking clearly or speaking at all.

Benefits and risks: The benefits of speech-language therapy include the valuable assessment that may determine the specific cause of the child's feeding and communication problems; the instruction and education provided to the caregiver; and the techniques that may help the child to eat more easily and safely and to communicate with those around her. There are no expected risks.

Maintenance: Speech-language therapy usually requires repeated evaluation, because feeding, swallowing, and speaking tend to change as children mature. Often their abilities improve as they get older, but for some children swallowing difficulties may get worse during their adolescent growth spurt, and monitoring by a speech-language therapist is important during this period.

Spinal Fusion
(posterior spinal fusion, anterior spinal fusion, growing rods, Magec Rods)

A spinal fusion involves roughening the bone surfaces and removing the joints to allow the individual vertebrae to fuse together; a fused spine becomes in essence one long bone. The area that is fused can no longer move, and once this has healed, it lasts an entire lifetime. The most commonly performed surgery is a *posterior spinal fusion*, performed from the back of the spine, but the surgery may be performed from the front of the spine, in which case it is called an *anterior spinal fusion*.

Indications: A posterior spinal fusion is indicated if a spinal curvature is worsening and becoming functionally unmanageable or if a curvature is certain to progress at some point and become severe. A posterior spinal fu-

sion may be performed for scoliosis, kyphosis, or lordosis. For children with cerebral palsy, a posterior spinal fusion almost always involves inserting spinal rod instrumentation. Any procedure that does not involve the use of instrumentation is unlikely to provide a good result, primarily because it is extremely difficult to hold the spine straight during the healing time. If the fusion is successful, the child will be fused in a very deformed position, which obviously is not beneficial at all.

The surgery: In a posterior spinal fusion, an incision is made in the middle of the back. The bone surfaces are roughened and extra bone is applied. The extra bone may be obtained from the patient's pelvic bone—or in the case of a patient with CP, from a bone graft from the bone bank. The procedure is usually combined with the implantation of rods to hold the spine straight and in the correct position while it is healing. This surgical procedure may include the use of Harrington rods, Luque rods, unit rods, or CD rods. A newer technique that is being developed is the use of growth or growing rods, which may also be called Magec Rods. These newer systems are considered for very small and young children who still have a lot of remaining growth. The current data suggest that children with CP have very high complications rates, but these data are based on frequent sur-

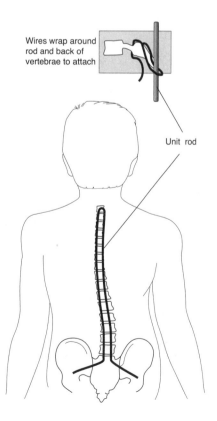

Wires wrap around rod and back of vertebrae to attach

Unit rod

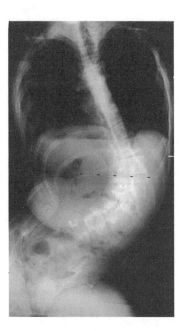

X-ray of
preoperative scoliosis

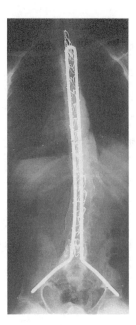

X-ray of spine
fusion scoliosis

gical lengthenings. These complications may be reduced in the future with further technological developments.

The anterior spinal fusion is performed for very severe scoliosis. It involves removing the intervertebral discs in the front of the vertebrae. This both allows much better correction and improves the ability of the vertebrae to fuse together. Usually, an anterior spinal fusion is a smaller operation than the posterior spinal fusion, takes less time, and involves less blood loss.

Benefits and risks: The benefits of fusion surgery are that it halts the progression of the curvature and straightens the spine as much as possible. Complications from a posterior spinal fusion include the possibility of infection and the need for blood transfusions. Blood loss is usually significant in spinal fusions; transfusions are frequently required. Permanent paralysis can occur but is very rare; minor nerve irritations do occasionally occur but usually resolve over several months.

Adequate nutritional intake is a problem, especially when an anterior spinal fusion is followed by a posterior spinal fusion. The nutritional requirements of the child should be very carefully monitored. Often, immediately after the surgery it is necessary to insert a feeding tube into the intestine or to insert an intravenous line to administer protein, carbohydrates, and fats.

After-surgery care: With most instrumentation systems, the child is usually sitting in a chair, taking a shower, and returning to school within four weeks. For a specific routine, consult the entry on the specific instrumentation utilized.

What to expect: Children with CP who have a spinal fusion usually remain in the intensive care unit for several days and in the hospital for approximately two weeks. They should expect to be out of school for a total of four weeks, after which they should be able to return at their normal level of function. There is seldom a need for a cast or brace after this surgery.

Splint, Elbow
(resting arm splint, extension elbow splint, spring-loaded extension splint)

Elbow splints are usually made by occupational therapists with the goal of straightening the elbow. Many children with cerebral palsy, in particular those with severe quadriplegia and moderate to severe hemiplegia, have a tendency to flex the elbow and to remain in this position. These splints are usually made of plastic and are directly applied to the arm. Sometimes these splints are made from casts that are split in half and held together with velcro straps. There is a commercially available elbow splint that has a spring, its goal being to stretch the tight elbow by means of constant pressure from the loaded spring.

Indications: The purpose of using elbow extension splints is to try to stretch out tight elbows. They should keep the elbows sufficiently loose to allow for cleaning and easy dressing of a child. For a child with cerebral palsy with hemiplegia, the goal may be to improve function, if some function already exists. Although experts disagree on which splints to use and for what length of time, chil-

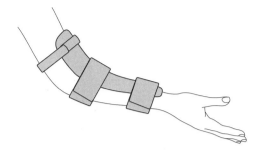

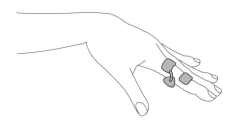

dren with spasticity and CP should use splints that are rigid and not spring-loaded. Spring-loaded splints are specifically contraindicated in children with spasticity because they further magnify the spasticity and cause the muscle to pull even harder.

Benefits and risks: The splint may improve the ability of the hand to function, but its main benefit is to prevent progressive contracture. Complications from the use of splints are primarily skin breakdown from poorly fitting splints or pain from having the elbow or wrist stretched too tightly. Generally the splints should be comfortable and fit well. Any difficulty with pain or skin breakdown needs to be addressed by the therapist who made the brace.

Maintenance and care: Most of these braces are made of low-temperature plastics. Consequently, they should be kept out of direct sunlight or areas that become very warm. They should not be washed in hot water and should only be cleaned with gentle soap. They are usually applied directly to the skin or over a sleeve and are used for several hours at a time. If the child is very comfortable, a brace may occasionally be worn all night.

Splint, Finger
(swan-neck splint)

A finger splint prevents hyperextension or the bending backward of the middle joint of the finger (PIP joint). The splint is made of metal and is applied in much the same way one puts on a finger ring. Some plastic models of this splint are also available.

Indications: This splint is used primarily for patients with athetosis who have developed some laxity (looseness), so that the fingers bend back in the wrong direction and then become stuck. This causes difficulty, because the fingers cannot bend to grasp or pick up objects. Finger splints may be used for specific activities such as typing, using a joystick, or picking up eating utensils. They usually are not worn full time.

Benefits and risks: The major benefit is to keep the finger from locking in the extended position. If there is too much pressure, the major risk is skin breakdown. If the splint causes a significant problem and cannot be modified, its use may need to be discontinued.

Maintenance and care: The splints should be kept clean and fitting well.

Splint, Hand
(wrist splint, cock-up splint, resting hand splint, functional hand splint)

Hand splints extend from below the elbow across the wrist. They are used to position the hand so as to prevent muscle contractures from developing. Made by occupational therapists, they are often custom molded out of low-temperature plastics or a nylon material. Alternatively, there are a number of off-the-shelf, ready-made models that may be used.

Indications: The indications for hand splints vary, from attempts to improve function to attempts to position the hand to prevent further contractures. The use of splints to improve function often is not very fruitful. Generally, when the splint is applied, it covers the skin, which means that the hand has less sensation. This lack of sensation usually leads to less use of the hand. There are certain circumstances in which a correctly positioned splint does place the hand in a better position and *improves* function, and the functional improvement may specifically allow the fingers to hit trip switches or to use joysticks, enabling a child to drive a chair or manipulate a computer. These uses are very child-specific and frequently require a great deal of trial and error by an experienced occupational therapist to find the right splinting position and the right material to benefit the child. If a significant attempt to try different splints does not improve the child's function, then splinting ought to be abandoned.

A second reason for the use of hand splints is to keep the hand supple as the child grows and prevent further

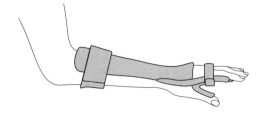

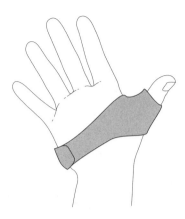

contractures, which make dressing and hygiene difficult. Resting hand splints or cock-up splints are often used. Covering the hand with these splints is not detrimental if the hand is nonfunctional. The length of time these are used varies greatly, from short periods of 30 minutes or an hour to all night long. The child should, however, spend some time out of the splint each day to keep the skin healthy and to prevent hypersensitivity. There are no recognized or generally accepted protocols for the use of this type of splinting; instead, parents needs to be guided by the philosophy and functional approach of the physician and therapists treating their child.

Benefits and risks: If a splint is used properly, it can help prevent contractures and can potentially increase function by improving hand position. Complications occur with hand splints used for functional purposes. The main problem is that they decrease rather than improve function because they decrease sensation. There may also be discomfort or skin breakdown; the skin under the splint should be checked daily to make certain that there is no irritation.

Maintenance and care: Most hand splints are made of low-temperature plastics. Consequently, they should be protected from direct sunlight and high temperatures, specifically hot water. They should be cleaned with gentle soap.

Splint, Thumb
(thumb-abduction splint)

Thumb splints are used to pull the thumb out of the palm. A fisted hand or tightly held thumb is a very common deformity in children with cerebral palsy. These braces may either be custom made by an occupational therapist or purchased commercially.

Indications: These splints have two purposes: to improve the function of the hand and to prevent a further deformity. The functional splint pulls the thumb out of the palm so that the fingers can be used for grasping large objects or manipulating joysticks or switches. The test of whether there is functional improvement is improved hand use. The second indication is to stretch the thumb

muscle to prevent it from contracting so that proper cleaning is possible.

Benefits and risks: The main benefit is preventing further contraction: children can use their fingers better when the thumb is kept out of the palm. The complications associated with these splints are related to skin breakdown from poorly fitting splints. Some of the splints can cause pain and discomfort from too much stress if a physician or therapist attempts too much correction. In these cases the splint needs to be modified.

Maintenance and care: These splints are usually made of low-temperature plastics. Consequently, they need to be kept away from hot water, direct sunlight, or other heat that might melt them. Nylon splints should not be washed, since this might damage the material.

Split Tibialis Posterior Tendon
(STPT, tibialis posterior transfer, varus foot deformity, posterior tibialis lengthening, Frost lengthening)

Below the knee, the second largest and most commonly involved muscle when there is significant spasticity is the tibialis posterior muscle. When this muscle is spastic or short, it pulls the foot in and down. This spasticity is frequently associated with spasticity of the Achilles tendon. For children who walk, the most common problem caused by this spastic muscle and its contracted tendon is that the toes drag and most of the pressure is placed on the outside edge of the sole. Also, in some children with severe involvement it may cause the foot to turn almost completely sideways, so that the child stands on the outside of the foot.

Care and treatment: In the young child, the main treatment for a spastic tibialis posterior muscle involves using a molded ankle-foot orthosis (AFO) to hold the foot flat and prevent it from rolling in. As the child gets older, however, the condition usually does not resolve; it can become so severe that the child is not able to tolerate the AFO. In that case, surgical correction is indicated.

The surgery: The most common surgical correction today is the split tibialis posterior tendon transfer, which involves taking one-half of the tendon, splitting it longitudinally, and swinging it across the back of the ankle over to the peroneal tendons on the outside of the ankle, which pulls the foot out in the opposite direction. This procedure works like a bridle, so that the spastic muscle pulls on both sides of the ankle and generally keeps the foot flat. This correction works well, remains stable, and is usually not outgrown by the child. It should seldom should be done before 8 years of age.

Lengthening of the tibialis posterior tendon, also called the Frost procedure, is a slightly less involved surgery; however, it has a higher risk of undercorrection and may be outgrown. Transfer of the entire tibialis posterior tendon is common in peroneal nerve palsy, Charcot-Marie-Tooth disease, and muscular dystrophy (all conditions that affect the nerves or muscles) but should not be utilized for children with spasticity, because it frequently causes severe deformity in the opposite direction.

Benefits and risks: The major benefit of the split tibialis posterior tendon transfer is that the foot is now kept flat, so that the child can stand and walk much more adequately than before. The complications are usually minor. The most common complication occurs when the transferred half of the tendon tears out where it is inserted, causing the deformity to recur. If this happens, the surgeon can attempt to resuture the end that tore loose. This procedure is usually successful. Overcorrection by developing a deformity in the opposite direction is unusual with this procedure. The major complications of the Frost procedure are that children often outgrow it and the

deformity recurs or overlengthening that results in the opposite type of deformity, known as severe flat foot.

After-surgery care: The usual care after the split tibialis posterior transfer is to place the child in a short leg walking cast for four weeks, although some surgeons prefer to use a long leg cast. Most surgeons allow the child to walk. An AFO may be used temporarily after the cast is removed, but frequently this is not necessary. Special physical therapy exercises are not needed after this procedure.

Stereognosis

Stereognosis is the specific sensory ability to define the shape of an object by touch. Children with cerebral palsy often lose this ability in the affected hand, often most dramatically in the hemiplegic affected hand. As a result, the child usually ignores that hand and uses the functioning hand exclusively.

Sudden Unexpected Death in Epilepsy
(SUDEP)

Sudden unexpected death in epilepsy (SUDEP) is said to occur when a person with epilepsy dies suddenly and prematurely and no other cause of death is found. A person with epilepsy has a greater risk of death than the rest of the population. Often the cause of death is known. For instance, it may be related to the cause of the epilepsy itself, or it may be related to accidents that occur because of a seizure (such as drowning, aspiration of food into the lungs, a motor vehicle accident). SUDEP is not common in children under age 16, and it is rare in children who do not have other physical or learning disabilities. This means that children with both CP and epilepsy are at risk, especially after age 16.

While sudden unexpected death occurs more often in those with epilepsy than in the general population, it is still uncommon. The death is not due to trauma or drowning. There may or may not be a sign of a seizure at the time of death. The seizure does not include status epilepticus. In addition, testing after death does not reveal an obvious cause of death.

Doctors do not know how to prevent SUDEP. The risk of SUDEP is highest in children who have uncontrolled seizures, many generalized tonic-clonic seizures, and a longer history of epilepsy. Therefore, better control of seizures is one way to decrease the risk of SUDEP. Measures you can take to try to decrease the risk include making sure your child takes the correct dose of anticonvulsant medicines at the right time every day without skipping doses, avoids known triggers for seizures, and follows through by keeping all follow-up appointments

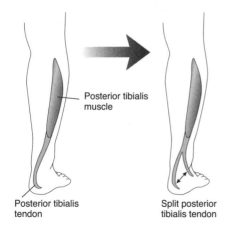

Posterior tibialis
muscle

Posterior tibialis
tendon

Split posterior
tibialis tendon

and completing all follow-up tests and blood work. Talk to your child's health care provider to determine whether other treatment options are available for your child if the anticonvulsant medicines do not control his or her seizures.

Swan-Neck Fingers
(locking fingers)

In swan-neck (locking) fingers, the end joint (DIP joint) becomes flexed and the middle joint (PIP joint) extends. The fingers lock into this position and cannot move unless another finger is used to unlock them. This problem occurs in patients with athetosis, and it can also occur in a hand in which the finger flexor sublimis tendons have been overlengthened.

Care and treatment: The primary means of treating swan-neck fingers is to identify the movements that cause the fingers to lock and to try to teach the child to avoid those movements. If the child cannot refrain from these movements, there are small figure-eight splints that may be worn. They are usually made of metal or plastic and surround the middle joint, preventing it from becoming extended. If the problem is related to certain activities, the use of splints is an excellent alternative. However, if the splints are needed all the time but cause skin irritation and discomfort, surgery should be considered.

The surgery: Surgical repair involves either suturing the sublimis tendons into part of the tendon sleeve to prevent the joints from extending or transferring the finger flexor muscles so the sublimis muscles are strengthened and do not allow the middle joint to extend. Sometimes the deformity recurs because the repair stretches out or because of a significant muscle power imbalance. Another procedure that has become popular is a minor release of the extensor tendon on the back side of the finger, which prevents too much extension; if too much of the finger extensor tendon is released, however, the finger may go into severe flexvion.

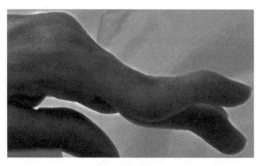
Swan neck fingers

Frequently, splints are used following the initial cast immobilization after surgery. Finger splints may be used for three to six months to protect the repair while it matures.

Syndrome

A syndrome is a constellation of physical findings that tend to occur together. Sometimes these are due to a chromosomal defect, such as with Down syndrome, which is caused by having three copies of chromosome number 21 instead of two copies. Other syndromes are associated with specific agents that can cause a birth defect. Probably the most common of these is fetal alcohol syndrome, associated with the ingestion of alcohol by a pregnant woman. Numerous other syndromes have been described and are grouped together by having similar physical findings. Many of these are known to be genetic, but many others simply describe a constellation of abnormalities that seem to occur together in more than a random fashion—and may or may not be genetic. Many syndromes are associated with cognitive impairment and seizures; others syndromes are associated with physical problems not unlike those of the child with cerebral palsy.

Therapy
(physical therapy, occupational therapy, sensory integrative therapy, neurodevelopmental therapy, NDT, conductive education, MOVE curriculum, myofascial manipulation, hippotherapy, aquatherapy, Adeli suit)

The goal of any therapy is to maximize each child's functioning. Therapy may be performed by many people, including parents, grandparents, schoolteachers, and even the child himself or herself. The professional therapists most often encountered are physical, occupational, and speech-language therapists, who are trained and licensed practitioners who direct or personally provide the therapy. (See also Speech-Language Therapy.)

Physical and occupational therapists' approaches overlap because the focus of both is to help the child develop motor skills. Areas in common include seating assessments, early intervention therapy, and developmental testing. Physical therapists, however, focus mainly on gross motor or large muscle activities involving the legs, such as walking, bracing, using crutches, and rehabilitation after surgery. Occupational therapists focus primarily on fine motor activities involving the upper extremities, including functions such as feeding, writing, and using scissors; they also splint the hand or arm as necessary. As the child grows older, occupational therapists stress activities of daily living such as dressing, bathing, and preparing food.

It is usually best to choose a physical or occupational therapist who is trained and experienced in dealing with children with developmental problems. Several of the therapeutic approaches available for a child with a physical disability are discussed below. Many have not been scientifically tested in groups of children with CP. However, since a given child may best respond to a certain type of intervention, parents can investigate these therapies. Parents need to check with their traditional medical providers to make sure that the approach they prefer has the potential to help and will do no harm.

Sensory integration therapy was developed by Jean Ayres to help children who do not understand how to execute normal movements because of decreased sensory input. The theory behind sensory integration suggests that movement disorders are caused by poor input from the sensory system, thus allowing primitive reflexes to persist and preventing children from developing normal motor movements. The treatment protocol involves a large amount of active and passive touching and muscle movement stimulation to encourage the brain to initiate better movement patterns. This technique employs swinging movements in swivel chairs as well as direct, hands-on exercises.

Neurodevelopmental therapy (NDT) was developed by Drs. Karl and Bertha Bobath. It has become one of the most commonly used intervention strategies for infants and children with developmental disabilities, including CP. As our understanding of how the brain controls movement has evolved, so has NDT therapy. NDT-trained therapists use a variety of specialized techniques that encourage active use of appropriate muscles and diminish involvement of muscles not needed for the completion of a particular task. Therapists set individual functional goals that build on one another to facilitate new motor skills or improve the efficiency of previously learned skills. In NDT the child plays an active role in treatment design. Therapists must constantly reevaluate the child's movement as they reassess and redesign the goals for the child. NDT can be used by occupational, speech, and physical therapists, as well as educators.

Conductive education was developed at the Peto Institute in Hungary and is now being provided in many countries throughout Europe, as well as the United States, Canada, Australia, and other countries. It is a system of teaching and learning for children with motor disorders. Exercises and education are broken down into basic functional movements. The exercises are performed intensively for five hours a day, five days a week, in small groups.

The *MOVE curriculum*, or Mobility Opportunities Via Education, is an activity-based curriculum designed to teach basic functional motor skills. It combines special education instruction with therapeutic methods.

The curriculum provides a framework for teaching the skills necessary for individuals with disabilities to gain greater physical independence. It combines functional body movements with an instructional process designed to help people, including those with cognitive impairment, acquire increased independence in sitting, standing, and walking. The goal is to teach especially those functional motor skills needed for adult life. The MOVE curriculum can be applied in a special school or in a regular classroom setting and provides students with increased opportunities to participate in life activities with their peers without disabilities.

Myofascial release therapy is a gentle blend of stretching and massage. It is often used to treat musculoskeletal pain such as longstanding back pain, fibromyalgia, recurring headaches, or sports injuries. However, it has also been offered to children with birth trauma, head injuries, and CP, with little evidence that it changes the course of these conditions. It is an outgrowth of chiropractic techniques. The basic therapy consists in stretching and manipulation, with the goal of stretching out the connective tissues involved in joint capsules and in the fascia overlying the muscles.

Equine therapy, also known as horseback riding therapy or hippotherapy, has become quite popular. The underlying theory is that the positioning and large movements provided by horseback riding are very helpful in establishing balance and relaxation of spastic muscles. The vertical motions of horseback riding are thought to provide sensory stimulus, which decreases muscle tone. Sitting on the horse helps stretch hip adductors and improves pelvic tilt and trunk positioning. This allows better muscle movement and range of motion for the therapist to work with after the child finishes the session. Another benefit is that many children enjoy horseback riding therapy because they have friends or siblings who ride horses too.

Aquatherapy, or *hydrotherapy*, is therapy performed in water. Being in the water gives children a feeling of weightlessness, which helps to reduce tone and allows these children better motor control. Aquatherapy is used postoperatively to allow children to start walking with reduced weight bearing. It is also a good modality for gait training, especially in an overweight child, who may be able to walk in water with relative weightlessness. In addition, swimming is an excellent recreational activity for children with CP. For many children for whom walking consumes a great deal of energy, learning to swim and swimming as a form of physical conditioning is an excellent option.

Spacesuit therapy was first investigated in Russia and later became very popular in Poland, using the Adeli suit. The suit was originally designed to help cosmonauts maintain their muscle tone in a weightless environment. It was then modified to help children with CP. It is a form-fitting suit with adjustable elastic bands designed to put the body into proper alignment. An intensive physical therapy program focuses on improving sensory stimulation and allows children to learn movement, standing posture, and balance strategies. A similar approach has been adopted in the United States, though it is not affiliated with the European program. It utilizes multiple therapeutic tools meant to promote the performance of independent and controlled movements while strengthening an isolated muscle group. The program may involve up to 20 hours per week of intensive therapy.

Indications: With such a large number of different, often conflicting types of therapy available, parents frequently have trouble deciding what is best for their child. Many therapists, parents, and other advocates for a particular therapeutic modality who embrace that method with an almost religious fervor. It is generally best to take these overenthusiastic perspectives with a grain of salt, because each therapeutic method has some bit of truth to it, and no one approach can miraculously "cure" a child, especially one who is not physically predisposed to change. Parents should choose a therapist in whom they have confidence and who seems to relate well to their child. It is better to focus on the child's progress than on the specific theory or modality.

Benefits and risks: Most pediatric physical and occupational therapy specialists who work with children with CP use a general approach, employing a combination of techniques from many therapies for the greatest benefit to the child. Most experienced therapists try working with different methods until they find the one to which the child seems to respond best. Generally speaking, if a child is responding both physically and psychologically, then the therapeutic modality is working for her.

Tibial Torsion
(internal tibial torsion, external tibial torsion, in-toeing gait, out-toeing gait)

When a child walks, his or her foot may point slightly inward (in-toeing) or slightly outward (out-toeing). There are several reasons for this, one of which is tibial torsion. Tibial torsion means that there is a twist in the tibia (the bone between the knee and the ankle) that results in a malalignment of the knee and the ankle joint. This torsion is generally due to the way a child was born or the way a child was lying in utero during the last trimester. In typically developing children under the influence of normal muscle pull and walking in early childhood, tor-

sional problems almost always completely resolve themselves. However, in children with cerebral palsy under the influence of spastic muscles that do not develop normal rotational pull, these torsional problems tend to persist and cause other problems.

Internal tibial torsion is internal rotation of the ankle with respect to the knee joint, causing the foot to point inward when the child walks. This can be present with femoral anteversion (a similar twist in the femur, or thighbone, and another common cause of in-toeing), which causes the knee to turn inward. The in-toeing may be exceedingly severe; in some cases, the heel may be in front of the toes as the child walks, causing the feet to turn backward. However, a child may have femoral anteversion with the knee pointing in and have compensatory external tibial torsion, so that the foot is pointing outward. In this situation, the foot looks like it is pointing in the right direction, but the knee appears to bend in the wrong direction when the child walks, causing the knees to knock together. There are some children who have normal alignment above the knee joint but have foot problems such that they almost roll over the inside of the foot instead of walking with the normal heel-to-toe movement.

Indications: These torsional problems tend not to improve in children who have spasticity, although as they mature

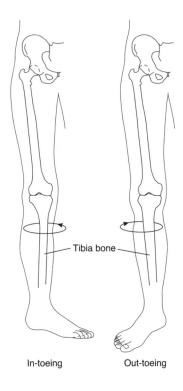

In-toeing   Out-toeing

they may gain better motor control and growth may improve their appearance. A child who is having severe difficulty learning to walk because of rotational problems of the legs ought to have surgery. There are no braces, exercises, or other devices that have a permanent impact upon these rotational problems. However, surgical correction at any age is usually permanent, with recurrence very rare.

The surgery: Tibial torsion is usually corrected just above the ankle joint. A number of holes are drilled across the tibia and the small bone (the fibula) on the lateral side. The bone is then cracked and rotated into the proper alignment. Another technique for making this correction is to make a small incision just below the knee joint and cut the bone at this level. Holding the bone in proper alignment is slightly harder in this area, and the osteotomy above the ankle joint is generally favored.

Benefits and risks: The primary benefit of this surgery is the improvement of the child's ability to walk by improving his alignment. The complications of tibial torsional osteotomies are few; however, either insufficient correction or overcorrection is possible. Further, there needs to be some way to make sure the correction is maintained during healing: if insufficient casting is applied, the proper alignment may be lost. Generally a pin is placed through the tibia just below the knee, and the foot and knee are placed in the cast to maintain the correction. This method also allows the child to start walking as soon as the pain subsides. Another technique may involve placing a plate on the bone to hold it in place until it heals.

Another complication of torsional osteotomies done to correct severe torsional problems may be the stretching of nerves. Any correction of over 40 degrees requires great caution because the procedure is like wringing a dishcloth: this "wringing-out effect" can cause both nerves and arteries to be stretched, causing difficulty with nerve function or blood flow to the foot.

After-surgery care: Postoperative management depends on the type of procedure used. If a short leg cast and pin are used, the child may start walking immediately. If a long leg cast is used with the knee bent, at four weeks it is frequently converted to a short leg cast, at which time the child may start walking. Casts must be kept dry. Physical therapy is usually prescribed to work on teaching the child a new gait pattern after the cast is removed. After the cast comes off, it usually takes three to four weeks for the foot to have normal sensation and for the child to really feel comfortable walking.

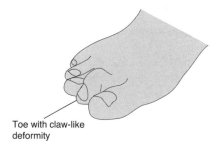

Toe with claw-like deformity

Toe Deformities
(claw toes, hammer toes)

Small toes can develop deformities from spasticity, and usually a claw or hammer toe deformity develops when toes flex severely. Inside the shoe, the end of the toe may become very sore from digging down into the sole; alternatively, one of the toe knuckles may become sore from pushing against the top of the shoe. Padding or modifying shoes may be helpful, but these conditions may cause lifelong pain that can only be improved with very simple surgical procedures.

The surgery: If the patient is relatively young and the toes are not too stiff, releasing the tendons on the underside of the toes is sufficient. If the toes have become very stiff, however, the middle toe joint often needs to be removed to fuse the joint, and a small pin is placed across the joint for approximately four weeks. In cooperative teenagers or adults, this procedure is done under local anesthesia, often in the doctor's office. General anesthesia is needed for children.

Benefits and risks: In most cases, the procedure gives a nice correction that is maintained for life. The complications from these procedures are relatively minimal, with the worst being recurrence of the deformity in the rare instance of initial undercorrection. Operations on the small toes usually do not require a cast, only soft dressing and wearing open-toe shoes for approximately four weeks.

Toe Walking
(toe dragging, idiopathic toe walking, Achilles tendon contracture)

Toe walking is a very common condition in young children as they start to walk, and it is normal for children up to 2 years of age. However, by the time a child is 2½ years old, he should be walking with his heel down and the remainder of his foot flat. Persistent toe walking can be an early sign of cerebral palsy, but there is a condition called idiopathic toe walking, in which children do not have any other signs of CP but are persistently up on their toes.

Indications: By 2½ to 3 years of age this pattern should be treated with a brace, such as an ankle-foot orthosis (AFO). If it is ignored, some children who do not have CP gradually develop a flatfooted walking pattern; others develop such tight Achilles tendons that they need surgical lengthening by age 7 or 8. The child with cerebral palsy should be treated with an ankle-foot orthosis, especially if the toe walking causes difficulty with balance and muscle coordination. Initially, an AFO that does not have a hinge is best; as the child gains more muscle control, coordination, and balance, he can use an AFO with a hinged joint, which lifts the foot up so the toe does not drag. For children with spasticity, the Achilles tendon becomes tight because the muscle does not grow adequately, and manual stretching often improves this. For some children, using the AFO may help the muscle grow.

Once the Achilles tendon contracture becomes too tight to wear an AFO, surgical lengthening of the tendon should be considered. The use of the ankle-foot orthosis is also necessary for toe dragging; however, even for adolescents with CP, if the Achilles tendon is not too tight, they should be able to pick the foot up sufficiently so the toes do not drag. Occasionally, children and young adults continue to wear AFOs because they cannot pick up their feet due to weak muscles in the front of the calf.

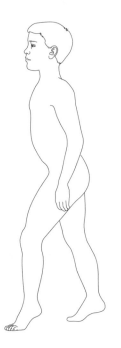

Toe dragging also is often caused by knee stiffness and is significantly improved with rectus transfer surgery at the knee.

Toe walking fosters further contractures of the Achilles tendon and also limits balance and motor coordination, since the child does not have a rigid foundation on which to stand. In the older child, toe dragging mainly causes rapid wear of shoes, can make the child look very clumsy, and causes the child to trip.

Total Parenteral Nutrition
(TPN, hyperalimentation)

TPN is an intravenous infusion of nutrients that one normally would get from the foods we eat. It contains protein as amino acids, carbohydrates as dextrose, and fat as lipids, as well as vitamins and minerals. This intravenous (IV) solution is usually given centrally, meaning through a catheter that is placed into a large vein in the chest and ends in the heart. It can be given peripherally, through a regular IV in the arm or leg, but only for a few days and with much lower concentrations of nutrients. Some children require TPN if their gastrointestinal (GI) tract is not working properly or if they are not able to eat by mouth. While there are many different reasons why a child might need TPN, it would typically be used in a child with CP following surgery for scoliosis, after abdominal surgery, or if the child develops pancreatitis, which would result in vomiting and intolerance to feedings. Rarely, children (including those with CP) develop severe dysmotility of their gastrointestinal system, meaning that their system no longer works well, and they cannot tolerate feedings through their stomach or even small intestine. Such children might need TPN for a long time or even chronically if their system does not resume normal function.

Tracheostomy
(laryngotracheal separation, tracheal diversion)

A tracheostomy is an operation that creates an opening from the neck into the trachea (windpipe). One reason to perform a tracheostomy is to bypass a tracheal obstruction and provide an airway. It is occasionally performed on children with cerebral palsy, since they may aspirate (inhale) food or liquids into the windpipe. This condition leads to frequent bouts of pneumonia, a chronic cough or bronchitis, and sometimes asthma. Over time, it may cause permanent damage to the lungs and be life threatening.

Indications: If recurrent pneumonia due to aspiration or airway obstruction is persistent and not improving, the growing child may require a tracheostomy. An opening

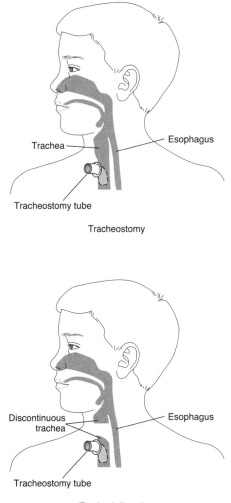

Trachea — Esophagus

Tracheostomy tube

Tracheostomy

Discontinuous — Esophagus
trachea

Tracheostomy tube

Tracheal diversion

is made in the neck and a tube is then placed through this opening so that air can directly enter into the lungs. If the aspiration is severe, then a laryngotracheal separation or diversion may be needed. This is a procedure in which the trachea is divided, permanently separating the lower windpipe from the mouth. This prevents saliva from entering the lower airway. Because this procedure results in the loss of the ability to speak or even make sounds (because air is no longer passing the vocal cords), a laryngotracheal separation or diversion is generally considered for children who previously were not speaking.

The surgery: The operation usually takes less than 30 minutes. It involves opening the trachea and inserting a plastic tube.

After-surgery care: A tracheostomy may seem intimidating to a parent. Caring for a child with a tracheostomy, however, need not be complicated. It is generally easy for parents and school personnel to learn to manage a tracheal tube, including cleaning and changing it when necessary. Usually, however, the first change of the tracheostomy tube should be done by the surgeon. The tracheostomy makes suctioning to help the child deal with secretions easy. A laryngotracheal separation prevents aspiration of secretions. A tracheostomy, however, makes finding respite care and care in some facilities more difficult because the person needs to stay with someone trained in caring for the tracheostomy. Although it is not difficult, training is mandatory. Caregivers must learn to recognize the signs of an obstructed tracheostomy tube (due to thick secretions) so they can quickly suction the tube or remove it and replace it with a new tube if suctioning is not successful. For this reason, the child must always keep a spare tracheostomy tube with him.

What to expect: Increased care is usually necessary for the child who has a tracheostomy or laryngotracheal separation. The air now bypasses the mouth and is not moisturized, so some source of moisture is often necessary. A parent or other caregiver must also be trained to suction and change the tube.

Transition of Medical Services

There are two major transitional milestones that must be achieved by the adolescents or young adults, whether or not they have a disability. These are the transition from the pediatric health care system to the adult health care system and the transition from school to whatever comes next, whether it be further education, a job, or a change in living situation.

As adolescents become adults, they need to assume responsibility for their own health care. For the adolescent with special health care needs, such as cerebral palsy, this may be difficult. It is often hard to find an adult care provider who is trained in caring for a pediatric condition such as CP or willing to assume primary responsibility for that care. Many pediatricians and pediatric hospitals will transition patients from their care at age 18 or age 21, sometimes even 25. However, at some age this transition needs to happen, and it can be emotionally difficult for the physician, the family, and the child.

A summary of the child's health history is often a good place to begin. If possible, this summary form of the child's health and medical history should be filled out by the teen himself, with help from the parents if necessary. It should include a description of the child's special needs, the medications he or she is currently taking and why, any allergies or adverse reactions to medications or foods, past hospitalizations or surgeries, and any past serious illnesses. This helps the teen learn more about his or her general health and specific health care needs and how to articulate knowledge of his or her own condition when meeting with new doctors. It also shows the parents what the teen still needs to learn before transitioning to adult health care and more independence. For the child with CP who may not be able to assume this kind of responsibility, for instance, because of cognitive limitations, the parents themselves will need to complete such a form.

One of the first priorities of the child transitioning care will be to try to find a primary care provider who can provide a "medical home" for the young adult. This may be a family doctor who has monitored the child since infancy, or it may be the parents' own doctor, who has cared for them but not for the child and may now be willing to assume that responsibility as well. Or it may be someone entirely new to the child and family. This primary care doctor would then help identify which specialists will be needed and who they might be. Alternatively, the pediatric subspecialists who have cared for the child until now may be able to identify colleagues of theirs who treat adults.

Healthy People 2010, a plan generated by the US Department of Health and Human Services in 2000, established a goal that all young people with special health care needs would receive the services needed to make necessary transitions to all aspects of adult life, including health care, work, and independent living. There continue to be significant barriers to reaching this goal, which can be divided into three major components that promote or impede the movement from child-centered to adult systems: service needs, structural issues, and personal preferences. *Service needs* refers to the availability or absence of treatment services and the degree to which these services will satisfy the young adult and his or her family. Such services must be developmentally appropriate and address the changing and maturing needs of young adults; they should include services that address young adults' reproductive issues and concerns. *Structural issues* include insurance coverage, institutional policies, and medical practices that either promote or impede the transition. Lack of adequate health insurance is one major barrier. Young adults can now be covered by their parents' health insurance until 26 years of age, after which they may not have a job that provides health insurance. Many health insurance safety-net programs that are available to children are not available to young adults. The third component comprises personal preferences and interpersonal dynamics. On the one hand, young adults often want to make the transition because they no longer want to be treated as a child. Barriers include the fact that the adult health providers may not recognize the family and young adult herself as being knowledgeable members of the treatment team in the way that the pediatric team did. In addition, many families and pediatricians have built up a very close personal relationship through the years and will have a hard time separating as this phase approaches.

Although not all these problems can be addressed, the following suggestions might make the transition a bit easier. The family, the young adult, and the provider must be aware that the child will likely live into adulthood (which is certainly true for most children with CP) and the transition process should be started early, during adolescence. This includes planning for insurance coverage, providers, and equipment. Family members and health care providers need to foster as much personal and medical independence as the child is capable of. The pediatric health care workers and families need to learn to "say goodbye" and to celebrate transitions as they occur. As part of this process, they should develop a written transition plan that anticipates future needs and use the plan as a means to document what has been completed and what still needs to be done. (See Chapter 8 for more on this topic.)

Triplegia

Triplegia is a term that may be confusing. There is not a typical pattern of involvement, although the term is best used to describe children who have significant involvement in three limbs and have one limb that is much more functional. Usually it describes involvement of both legs and one arm. There is tremendous variation in this pattern—it is usually a combination of hemiplegia overlaying diplegia. However, some children have quadriplegia, with much less involvement in one arm.

Ultrasonography
(ultrasound)

Ultrasonography is an imaging technique employing high-frequency sound waves (above the level that we can hear) that bounce off body tissues. When sound waves are sent through body tissue, some bounce back and can be used to make a picture, similar to radar being used to see storms and predict the weather, which can then be viewed on a video screen. The echo pictures that show solid and fluid structures in the body are interpreted by a radiologist who has been specially trained to recognize them. The ultrasound apparatus consists of a console with one or more video monitors. Only the transducer actually comes in contact with the patient. This device emits and receives the sound waves and is connected by a cable to the console. The technologist doing the scan puts a clear gel over the area to be scanned, which helps form a better connection between the transducer and the patient. The technician then slides the transducer around until the appropriate images have been seen and recorded on the video monitor. An ultrasound exam involves no pain or discomfort.

Indications: Ultrasound is used extensively for imaging the fetus during pregnancy, and it is used to evaluate the brain in newborn infants when the skull is not completely closed. It is also used to evaluate hip dislocation in infants and to view the liver, spleen, and kidneys.

Benefits and risks: The major benefit of ultrasound examination is that it involves no radiation and is performed quickly without sedation. The major risk is that the images obtained are often difficult to interpret; the outcome may depend on the skill of the technician or physician doing the examination. For this reason, ultrasound is most helpful when it is used by technicians and physicians with special training.

Undescended Testicles
(testicles, testicular torsion, orchidopexy)

When a male fetus is growing in his mother's womb, his testicles form high up in his abdomen. Gradually, in the last trimester of pregnancy, they move down from the abdomen into the scrotum, where they normally are located at the time of birth. If the testicles do not move down into the scrotum, they are considered undescended. Premature infants are more likely to have undescended testicles than full-term infants. Both testicles should be descended into the scrotum by the first birthday.

Some boys have testicles that are called "retractile." Retractile testicles are not in the scrotum most of the time but can be felt high at the top of the scrotum at the edge of the groin, but when they are pulled, they come down into the scrotum without any discomfort or much tension. Generally, retractile testicles do not become undescended but with growth relax and come down into the scrotum. These should be monitored by the pediatrician, however, because occasionally they can become stuck in the high position, which is technically a form of undescended testicles.

Boys with spasticity due to cerebral palsy have a high incidence of undescended testicles, which may be due in part to the frequency of prematurity at birth but is probably also due to the spasticity, which is present in the muscles and pulls the testicles back into the abdomen.

The surgery: The operation to bring the testicles down into the scrotum is called an orchidopexy. It is usually rec-ommended for boys whose testicles have not descended into the scrotum by age 1. The surgical descending of the testicles is performed to keep the testicles from becoming entrapped or twisted, thereby cutting off their blood supply and causing them to die, which requires an emergency operation. There is also an increased risk of developing testicular cancer later in life if testicles are not descended into the scrotum. Bringing the testicles down into the scrotum, however, does not necessarily reduce the risk of cancer, but it does make the testicles much easier to examine for the presence of any lumps or masses. Also, boys who are active are much more likely to injure the testicles if they are partially descended, as they often sits right in front of the pubic bone, so any pressure in that area can damage them. Another reason for surgically bringing the testicles down into the scrotum is to enhance the boy's self-esteem, especially when he grows older.

The surgery is usually performed on an outpatient basis. The child comes to the hospital, has general anesthesia, and then leaves the same day. An incision is made in the groin, the testicle is identified and brought down into the groin, and a suture is placed, holding it down to the bottom of the scrotum. Afterwards, boys are often limited in their activities, partially because of the discomfort and partially because the procedure needs time to heal.

Benefits and risks: The procedure has a very high success rate, and complications are rare. Usually recovery is very quick, with the boy resuming full activity without any problems within two weeks. Parents should follow up with a physical examination every year until puberty to make certain that the testicles continue to grow normally. When complications occur, infection is the most common and can easily be treated with antibiotics. Symptoms of infection include fever, lack of appetite, and an inflamed incision. Occasionally, the blood supply to the testicle is insufficient, and the testicle has

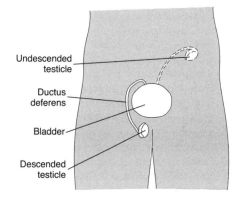

Undescended testicle

Ductus deferens

Bladder

Descended testicle

to be removed. If this occurs, a simple procedure, called *placement of a testicular prosthesis*, is recommended at puberty. Rarely, the testicle may remain undescended even after the surgical procedure, and a repeat operation is sometimes necessary.

Children with one undescended testicle have a slightly lower fertility rate than the general population. When both testicles are undescended, infertility is very common.

Urinary Tract Infections

Urinary tract infections include a range of infections by microorganisms in the urinary tract. Fever may be the only symptom of a urinary tract infection, especially in young children. Boys are affected far more often than girls during the newborn period, and it has been found that uncircumcised boys are affected far more frequently than those who have been circumcised. This has led to a change in thinking regarding circumcision, which until recently was felt to be an unnecessary procedure that was done for cultural but not medical reasons.

After the newborn period, urinary tract infections are far more common in girls, but for both boys and girls, there needs to be further evaluation of the urinary tract system if an infection occurs. A major contributor to infections may be vesicoureteral reflux. In vesicoureteral reflux, when the bladder attempts to empty, some urine goes back up into the ureters toward the kidney rather than out of the body. Other predisposing factors are incomplete drainage and/or stasis in the urinary system, which means that the bladder does not empty completely and some urine remains in the bladder, allowing bacteria to multiply. In addition, if infected urine comes back up from the bladder into the kidney because of vesicoureteral reflux, it can cause kidney damage. This is the situation in some patients with cerebral palsy, whose neurological condition can cause poor bladder functioning.

Patients with urinary tract infections should undergo radiological studies to evaluate the anatomy of the kidney and the bladder and to determine whether there is vesicoureteral reflux. Ultrasound examination of the kidney, the ureters, and the bladder shows the anatomy of this system. The evaluation for reflux is done by a procedure called a voiding cystourethrogram (VCUG), which consists in placing dye into the bladder and watching to see whether it is all emptied out or whether some is pushed up toward the kidney.

The degree of reflux is graded on a scale from 1 to 5, with 1 being the mildest and 5 the most severe. Mild forms of reflux are usually managed with prophylactic antibiotics (a lower dose of an antibiotic to prevent a urinary tract infection), whereas more severe reflux may

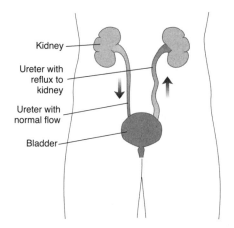

need to be treated with surgery by a urologist. If both the ultrasound and the VCUG are normal, then no further evaluation is necessary. If the VCUG shows reflux or if the ultrasound of the kidney is abnormal, then a renal scan is performed. This is the most sensitive means of detecting scarring of the kidney.

Urodynamic Testing

For people who have cerebral palsy and who are not able to be toilet trained, the incontinence may be due to delayed toilet training or an abnormal function of the bladder. Urodynamic testing may be necessary to assess the bladder function. This test consists in measuring the pressure and volume of the bladder as well as the sphincter muscles, which should relax and contract at various times during urination. If these various processes are not working normally, testing will aid in assessing the problem and may indicate a medication that will help relieve these symptoms.

Indications: Children who are 5 years of age or older and have the mental capacity to understand the concept of going to the bathroom but are unable to control their bladder should have urologic evaluation including uroflometry and urodynamic testing. Children who have periodic incontinence that they seem unable to control should also undergo urologic evaluation. The child who has to urinate very frequently may have a very small bladder volume, and this too can be measured and detected with urodynamic testing. A comprehensive urodynamic evaluation includes noninvasive assessment of urination (uroflometry and post-void residual measurements) and invasive testing (a catheter in the bladder measures bladder pressure).

Benefits and risks: The benefit of urodynamic testing is that it can measure the bladder's capacity and the functioning of the sphincter muscles, so that the cause of incontinence can be determined. The major risk is that it requires inserting a catheter, which has a very small chance of causing an infection in the bladder.

Maintenance and care: If the child develops burning upon urination or a fever after urodynamic testing, it may indicate an infection. In this case, the child may need antibiotics for several days. No other aftercare is required.

Vagus Nerve Stimulator

In 1997 the US Food and Drug Administration approved the vagus nerve stimulator (VNS) for use in the treatment of uncontrolled seizures. The precise mechanism of action is unknown. However, it has been shown to effectively control seizures in some patients and significantly reduce seizure frequency and/or duration in many others. The device also gives the patient, family member, or other caregiver an active part in the reduction of seizures.

The child or adolescent has an evaluation with a neurologist and health care team that is trained in the use of the VNS. Tests such as video electroencephalograms (EEGs) and medical imaging studies may be conducted. Once it is determined that the child is a candidate for surgery, a surgical evaluation is done by either a neurosurgeon or a cardiovascular surgeon, either of whom can perform this procedure. Once these evaluations are complete, the child or adolescent is scheduled for surgery. The device is placed under the skin, usually in the left chest area. It has wires that are threaded up under the skin and wrapped around the left vagus nerve in the neck. The vagus nerve has a link to the brain. The device is programmed by a special computer to stimulate the left vagus nerve throughout the day, which ultimately stimulates the base of the brain. This stimulus helps to control seizures in some individuals. The VNS also comes with a special, very strong magnet. This magnet can be moved over the device in the chest by the patient, family member, or other caregiver to cause an additional stimulus to try to prevent or stop a seizure.

The VNS can be effective for all seizure types. It is available to all patients who have failed or are unable to tolerate other modalities, such as antiepileptic drugs or the ketogenic diet, and are not candidates for epilepsy surgery. Side effects are few. In regard to the surgical procedure, there are the risks that accompany any procedure, such as infections and bleeding, as well as anesthesia risks. There is also the rare possibility that the body will reject the device. In addition, some individuals experience hoarseness, coughing, gagging, and/or tingling when the device is activated.

Once the individual has the device implanted, he or

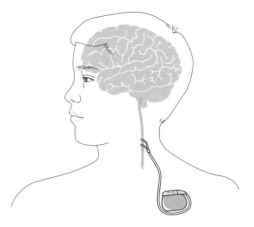

she must keep routine appointments with a health care provider, usually a neurologist, who is knowledgeable about the VNS device. The health care provider will continue to manage the individual's response to the device and its effectiveness. In some situations, antiepileptic medications may be either reduced or discontinued completely.

Valgus
(valgus foot, valgus hip, valgus knee)

Valgus is an anatomical term that refers to the bending away from the midline by a part of the body. The term *valgus* is generally applied to the legs. When applied to the hip, it means an increased angle of the femoral head and neck with the shaft of the femur (thighbone). When applied to the knee, it means that the lower leg is bending away from the midline; in other words, the child is knock-kneed. When applied to the foot and ankle, the term refers to the foot's turning away from the midline and is approximately synonymous with the term *eversion*, which means that the sole points away from the midline of the body.

Varus
(varus hip, varus knee, varus foot)

Varus is an anatomical term meaning that a part of the body is bending toward the midline. When the term is applied to the hip, it means that the angle between the femoral head, the neck, and the femoral shaft is decreasing. When the term is applied to the knee, it means that the leg below the knee is bending toward the midline (also known as bowlegs). When it is applied to the foot, it means that the sole is pointing toward the midline of the body; *varus foot* is synonymous with *inversion of the foot*.

Visual Impairment
(low vision, legal blindness, cortical visual impairment)

The term *blindness* has been replaced with *mild* (20/40–20/60), *moderate* (20/70—better than 20/200) and *severe* (20/200 or worse) *visual impairment*. The visual acuity defining the level of impairment is based on corrected vision and is determined by the ophthalmologist.

Legal blindness is defined as a visual acuity of 20/200 or less in the better eye after the best possible correction, or a visual field of 20 degrees or less. This definition is used by the federal government and other agencies to determine eligibility for federal programs such as Supplemental Security Income (SSI).

The educational system defines a child with a visual impairment as one whose visual limitations interfere with his or her ability to learn. There is no specific level of visual impairment a child must have in order to qualify for services. Determination of eligibility for services will depend upon the state or the agency providing services.

Up to 70 percent of children with cerebral palsy may have cortical visual impairment (CVI). CVI is defined as deficient visual function caused by damage to the parts of the brain responsible for vision. Children with significant CVI typically display characteristic behaviors such as poor visual response, difficulty with complexity and novelty, and improved visual function with movement.

Vocational Rehabilitation
(job training)

Vocational rehabilitation is a set of services used to assess people with physical and/or cognitive disabilities and to assist people with those disabilities in overcoming barriers to obtaining further education and employment. Every state has a federally funded agency for vocational rehabilitation (VR). The services generally include educational support, job services, supported employment, and independent (and sometimes assisted) living services. VR is often thought of as an adult resource, but most programs will start working with individuals and families during high school, with some integrating into the school-based IEP planning and setting up postsecondary programs.

Interested individuals apply through their local VR program and are assigned a counselor, who will meet with them to discuss goals and formulate a plan. In order to succeed, rehabilitation must take into account the whole person, including her or his specific interests; visual, cognitive, and physical abilities; and psychological and behavioral stability. The goal is to develop a realistic plan that will match the individual with an educational program or job that is appropriate for his or her abilities and interests and to then provide the necessary support for a successful transition into the job or educational program. Vocational programs offer many services, including vocational counseling, academic or literacy and vocational training, job search and placement assistance, transportation and technology assistance, and more. Five services in particular—on-the-job training, job placement assistance, on-the-job support, maintenance services, and rehabilitation technology—have been shown to have positive correlation with good employment outcomes.

✌ RESOURCES

PART ONE

Chapter 1
CPdailyliving.com

Chapter 3
Epilepsy Foundation of America: 800-332-1000; www
.efa.org.

MyHealth Passport: https://www.sickkids.ca/my
healthpassport/. This is a useful tool for organizing a
child's medical information.

National Vaccine Injury Compensation Program:
800-338-2382; www.hrsa.gov/vaccinecompensation/.
This program compensates parents of children who
may have been injured by certain vaccines.

Traveler's health information: wwwnc.cdc.gov/travel.

Vaccine Adverse Events Reporting System (VAERS):
800-822-7967; http://www.cdc.gov/vaccinesafety
/ensuringsafety/monitoring/vaers/. VAERS is a
national vaccine safety monitoring program that
collects reports about illnesses or adverse reactions
that occur after a vaccine is given.

Vaccine Information Statements (VISs): www.cdc.gov
/vaccines/hcp/vis/index.html. VISs explain the
benefits and risks of each vaccine.

Vaccine schedules: www.cdc.gov/vaccines/schedules
/easy-to-read/index.html.

Chapter 9
Sign up for medical insurance through the Federal
Insurance Exchange at www.healthcare.gov.

Chapter 10
Developmental Disabilities Council: There is a separate
web address for each state. For instance, in Delaware
it's ddc.delaware.gov.

Easter Seals: www.easterseals.com. Easter Seals offers
a variety of services to help people with disabilities
address life's challenges and achieve personal
goals.

Family Voices: www.familyvoices.org. This is a grass-
roots organization run by parents who have children
with special health care needs. Contact Family
Voices for information on state programs and eligibility, insurance questions, advocacy support, and
general information.

National Association of Councils on Developmental
Disabilities: www.nacdd.org. The website has links
to individual state councils.

Office of Intellectual/Developmental Disabilities: These
state-specific offices are under the Department of
Health and Human Services in each state. They
often list their providers for residential, vocational,
respite care, and family support.

Parent Training and Information (PTI) Center: There
is a center in each state. The Center for Parent
Information and Resources (CPIR) website, www
.parentcenterhub.org, has links to the state centers.
The centers specialize in education law, IEPs, 504
plans, accommodations, and parent support.

United Cerebral Palsy (UCP): www.ucp.org. Each
region has a local chapter.

Chapter 11
Branch Military Parent Technical Assistance Center:
https://branchta.org/.

Center for Parent Information and Resources (CPIR):
www.parentcenterhub.org. The CPIR serves as
central source of information and products for the
community of Parent Training Information (PTI)
Centers and Community Parent Resource Centers
(CPRCs), allowing them to focus their efforts on
serving families of children with disabilities.

Native American Parent Technical Assistance Center:
www.naptac.org.

Parent Technical Assistance Center (PTAC): The six
regional PTACs help the Parent Training and Information (PTI) Centers in their regions build capacity
to provide information and training to families of
children with disabilities and to manage the administrative challenges of running a PTI Center.

Parent Training and Information (PTI) Center: There
is a center in each state. The Center for Parent
Information and Resources (CPIR) website, www
.parentcenterhub.org, has links to the state centers.
The centers specialize in education law, IEPs, 504
plans, accommodations, and parent support.

Chapter 12

National Association of Councils on Developmental Disabilities: www.nacdd.org. The website has links to councils in all 50 states.

National Disability Rights Network (NDRN): www.ndrn.org. The NDRN website has background information and links to all state protection and advocacy agencies (P&As). Every state has a P&A agency. These agencies provide advocacy and legal services to persons with disabilities, usually for free.

Parent Training and Information (PTI) Center: There is a center in each state. The Center for Parent Information and Resources (CPIR) website, www.parentcenterhub.org, has links to the state centers. The centers specialize in education law, IEPs, 504 plans, accommodations, and parent support.

Partners in Policymaking online courses: www.partnersonlinecourses.com. The goal of Partners in Policymaking is to educate participants to be active partners with those who make policy. Some states offer a "junior" Partners in Policymaking program to teach teens and young adults self-advocacy.

Wrightslaw.com. The website is a valuable and highly respected source of parental information on special education.

Other: A useful overview of the impact of the Affordable Care Act on individuals with developmental disabilities is published at http://autisticadvocacy.org/policy-advocacy/reports-and-brief-materials/the-affordable-care-act-and-the-idd-community-an-overview-of-the-law-and-advocacy-priorities-going-forward/.

PART TWO

Home Modifications

There are agencies that help plan for and carry out changes to accommodate the needs of individuals with disabilities. There are four with a national focus:

1. ABLEDATA, a database of products, devices, and equipment for people with disabilities (800-227-0216; www.abledata.com)
2. The National Rehabilitation Information Center (800-246-2742; www.naric.com)
3. The National Council of Independent Living (703-525-3406; www.ncil.org)
4. Americans with Disabilities Act Information Hotline (202-514-0301; www.ada.gov)

Purchasing a Wheelchair

United Cerebral Palsy (www. ucp.org). There are local chapters throughout the United States.

Variety Club (www.usvariety.org) . There are local chapters throughout the United States.

Service Dogs

US Dog Registry (usdogregistry.org)

Hospitalization

KidsHealth.org

Nemours Get Well Network

OTHER RESOURCES

Safety and Emergency Planning

For information about preparing for emergencies and disasters, see the following:
- www.ready.gov/individuals-access-functional-needs
- www.redcross.org/prepare/location/home-family/disabilities
- www.allreadyde.org

For help in developing an emergency preparedness plan, contact the Center for Disabilities Studies at the University of Delaware (302-831-7464; www.udel.edu/cds/health-wellness.html).

Complex Child

a monthly online magazine written by parents

Nemours YouTube videos

regarding estate planning and transitions, particularly for teens with health needs transitioning to adulthood. www.nemours.org/about/mediaroom/press/dv/transition-videos.html

Professional Organizations

American Academy of Cerebral Palsy and Developmental Medicine (AACPDM)
www.aacpdm.org
This organization is a multidisciplinary scientific society devoted to studying cerebral palsy and other childhood-onset disabilities; promoting professional education for the treatment and management of these disabilities; and improving the quality of life for people with these disabilities.

American Academy of Pediatrics (AAP)
www.aap.org
The AAP is a professional membership organization of 64,000 primary care pediatricians, pediatric medical subspecialists, and pediatric surgical specialists dedicated to the health, safety, and well-being of infants, children, adolescents, and young adults.

American Academy of Physical Medicine & Rehabilitation (AAPMR) .
www.aapmr.org

The AAPMR is a national medical society representing more than 6,000 physicians who are specialists in the field of physical medicine and rehabilitation. The society provides continuing education opportunities, increases awareness of the specialty, and advocates public policies.

American Congress of Rehabilitation Medicine (ACRM)
www.acrm.org
The mission of the ACRM is to promote the art, science, and practice of rehabilitation care for people with disabilities.

American Occupational Therapy Association (AOTA)
www.aota.org/

American Physical Therapy Association (APTA)
www.apta.org

Association of Rehabilitation Nurses (ARN)
www.rehabnurse.org
ARN's mission is to promote and advance professional rehabilitation nursing practice through education, advocacy, collaboration, and research to enhance the quality of life for those affected by disability and chronic illness.

National Association for Home Care (NAHC)
www.nahc.org/
NAHC is a trade association that represents the interests of more than 6,000 home care agencies, hospices, and home care aide organizations. Its members are primarily corporations or other organizational entities, as well as state home care associations, medical equipment suppliers, and schools.

National Institute of Neurological Disorders and Stroke (NINDS)
NIH Neurological Institute
Bethesda, MD 20824
www.ninds.nih.gov

National Organization for Rare Disorders (NORD)
www.rarediseases.org
NORD is an organization with a database on over 1,000 rare diseases, with educational materials for parents and health professionals. It also has links to parent support groups and hundreds of organizations that can help families deal with these rare conditions.

Pediatric Orthopaedic Society of North America (POSNA)
https://posna.org

Rehabilitation Engineering and Assistive Technology Society of North America (RESNA)
www.resna.org
RESNA is as an interdisciplinary society that promotes the transfer of science, engineering, and technology to meet the needs of individuals with disabilities.

♦ INDEX

Page numbers in *italics* refer to illustrations; those in **boldface** refer to primary Encyclopedia descriptions; those followed by "t" refer to tables.

role of, 51–52; sending specialists' reports to, 241; what they do, 242

primitive reflexes, 30, 35, **434–35**, 436t, **437**

privacy: of children and adolescents, 216; legal right to, 335, 338

professional organizations, 460–61

profundus muscle, 385, 386

prognosis, 14–16, 142, 188, 360

prokinetic medications, 92

pronation, 154, 387, 436t

pronator teres transfer, 156, **386–87**

prone stander, 191–92, 318–20, 421; photo, *319*

proprioception, 84, 416

protection and advocacy (P&A) agencies, 274, 460

Protection and Advocacy for Assistive Technology (PAAT), 274

Protection and Advocacy for Beneficiaries of Social Security (PABSS), 274

Protection and Advocacy for Developmental Disabilities (PADD), 274

protective equipment, 73–74

protein, in diet, 63–64, 343, 344

proton pump inhibitors (PPI), 92–93

Proventil (albuterol), 99

proximal femoral excision, 211

pseudobulbar palsy, 85

psychiatrists, 181, 232

psychological evaluation, 67, 221, 417, **432–33**

psychologists, 15, 25, 117, 232, 264; and adolescents, 48, 181; assessments by, 74, 134, 268; and caregivers, 138, 228

puberty, 106–10; in boys, 106; delayed, 49, 95, 423; in girls, 106–8; precocious, 48–49

public guardians, 280–81

quadcanes, **391**

quadriplegia, 185–219; from birth to one year, 186–87; at ages one to three, 188–94; at ages four to six, 194–201; at ages seven to twelve, 201–7; at ages thirteen to eighteen, 207–19; adults with, 224–25; ankle-foot orthosis for, 194, 200, 206; arm problems with, 207; bone and joint problems with, 193–94; and bone fractures, 205–6; caregivers for, 217–18; communication problems with, 195; defined and described, 185, **433**; diagnosis of, 186; drooling with, 204; foot problems with, 200–201, 206, 212–13; hip problems with, 199, 206–7, 210–12; knee problems with, 200, 206, 212; and kyphosis, 193–94, 199, 207, 210; scoliosis with, 193–94, 199, 207, 208–10, 212; sitting difficulties with, 185, 190, 191, 196, 206, 209, 210, 212; spinal problems with, 194, 199, 207, 208–10; surgery for, 193, 198–99, 200–10, 211–12, 219; therapy for, 187, 188–89, 195, 201–4; toe problems with, 201, 213–14; types of, 185–86; vision and hearing screening for,

195; walkers and standers for, 190–92, 194, 197, 198–99; wheelchairs for, 192, 196–98, 205

radial head dislocation, **394**

radiologists, 88–90, 91, 92, 93, 97, 347, 454

range of motion, 342; and diplegia, 163, 171; and quadriplegia, 188; therapy exercises to maintain, 385, 387, 394, 423, 449

ranitidine (Zantac), 92

rape, 107

reactive airway disease, **361–62**. *See also* asthma

reading: by children, 99, 126, 132, 303, 363; to children, 169

"reasonable accommodation," 287–88

recommended dietary intake (RDI), 205

rectal medications or suppositories, 353–55

rectus femoris transfer, **433–34**

reflex epilepsy, 61

reflexes, **434–37**

refractive errors, 76, 77

Reglan (metoclopramide), 491

regression, term, 14

rehabilitation, **437–38**; facilities for, 216; vocational, 225, 229, 329, **458**

Rehabilitation Act of 1973: Section 503 of, 287; Section 504 of, 266, 286–87

Rehabilitation Engineering and Assistive Technology Society of North America (RESNA), 461

Reimer's migration index, **394–96**

renal scan, **427–28**, 456

representational thought, 124–25

respiratory distress syndrome, 377, 379, 432

respiratory syncytial virus (RSV), 55, 377, 432

respite care, 218, 258, 282, 418, 453, 459

restraints, 190, 314

retinopathy of prematurity (ROP), 75, **438**

retractile testicles, 105, 455

Rett syndrome, 142, 360

revocable trusts, 295

Rifton Activity Chair, 311

righting reactions, *435*, 437

rigidity, 6–7, **438**, 442

Ritalin (methylphenidate), 70

Robinul (glycopyrrolate), 97, 398

Ronald McDonald Houses, 303

round back, **420–21**. *See also* kyphosis

rubella (German measles), 4, 10, 54, 68, **384–85**

safety: car seats and, 313; helmets for, 60, 66, 177, 190; individual's sense of, 171, 309, 416; monitoring of vaccines for, 56, 459; and self-injurious behavior, 72, 73–74, 189–90, 367; and walkers, 144, 165, 191, 199; and wheelchairs, 197, 313, 315, 328

salivagram, 89, 98